Medical Nutrition and Disease

A Case-Based Approach

Editor-In-Chief

Lisa Hark PhD, RD

Consultant, Department of Medicine
Jefferson Medical College
Thomas Jefferson University
Philadelphia, PA, USA

Senior Editor

Gail Morrison, MD

Vice Dean of Education, Professor of Medicine
University of Pennsylvania School of Medicine
Philadelphia, PA, USA

FOURTH EDITION

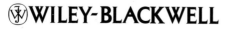
WILEY-BLACKWELL

A John Wiley & Sons, Ltd., Publication

This edition first published 2009, © 1995, 1999, 2003, 2009 by Blackwell Publishing Ltd

Blackwell Publishing was acquired by John Wiley & Sons in February 2007. Blackwell's publishing program has been merged with Wiley's global Scientific, Technical and Medical business to form Wiley-Blackwell.

Registered office: John Wiley & Sons Ltd, The Atrium, Southern Gate, Chichester, West Sussex, PO19 8SQ, UK

Editorial offices: 9600 Garsington Road, Oxford, OX4 2DQ, UK

The Atrium, Southern Gate, Chichester, West Sussex, PO19 8SQ, UK

111 River Street, Hoboken, NJ 07030-5774, USA

For details of our global editorial offices, for customer services, and for information about how to apply for permission to reuse the copyright material in this book please see our website at www.wiley.com/wiley-blackwell

The right of the author to be identified as the author of this work has been asserted in accordance with the Copyright, Designs and Patents Act 1988.

Wiley also publishes its books in a variety of electronic formats. Some content that appears in print may not be available in electronic books.

Designations used by companies to distinguish their products are often claimed as trademarks. All brand names and product names used in this book are trade names, service marks, trademarks or registered trademarks of their respective owners. The publisher is not associated with any product or vendor mentioned in this book. This publication is designed to provide accurate and authoritative information in regard to the subject matter covered. It is sold on the understanding that the publisher is not engaged in rendering professional services. If professional advice or other expert assistance is required, the services of a competent professional should be sought.

Library of Congress Cataloging-in-Publication Data

Medical nutrition and disease : a case-based approach / [edited by] Lisa Hark, Gail Morrison. – 4th ed.

p. ; cm.

Includes bibliographical references and index.

ISBN 978-1-4051-8615-5

1. Dietetics.   2. Diet therapy.   3. Nutrition.   I. Hark, Lisa.   II. Morrison, Gail.

[DNLM: 1. Nutrition Physiology–Case Reports.   2. Diet Therapy–Case Reports.   3. Nutritional Support–Case Reports.   WB 400 M4896 2009]

RM216.M456 2009

613.2–dc22   2008045733

A catalogue record for this book is available from the British Library.

Set in 9.5/12 pt Minion by Aptara® Inc., New Delhi, India

Printed in Singapore by Ho Printing Singapore Pte Ltd

1   2009

Contents

Contributors

Editors-in-Chief

Lisa Hark, PhD, RD
Former Director
Nutrition Education Program
University of Pennsylvania School of Medicine
Philadelphia, PA

Gail Morrison, MD
Vice Dean for Education
University of Pennsylvania School of Medicine
Philadelphia, PA

Associate Editors/Contributors

Tamara Bockow, BS
Medical Student
University of Pennsylvania
Philadelphia, PA

Jeremy Brauer, MD
Resident
Ronald O. Perelman Department of
   Dermatology
New York University
Langone Medical Center
New York, NY

Darwin Deen, MD,MS
Medical Professor
Department of Family and Community
   Medicine
Sophie Davis School of Biomedical
   Education
City College of New York
New York, NY

John B. Swaney, PhD
Professor of Biochemistry and Molecular
   Biology
Drexel University College of Medicine
Philadelphia, PA

Managing Editor/Contributor

Diana Fischmann, MsEd
Editorial Research Assistant
University of Pennsylvania School of Medicine
Philadelphia, PA

Contributors

Diane Barsky, MD
Assistant Professor of Pediatrics
The Children's Hospital of Philadelphia
Philadelphia, PA

Vicki Bovee, MS, RD
Clinical Dietitian
Western Bariatric Institute
Reno, NV

Frances Burke, MS, RD
Senior Clinical Dietitian
Department of Cardiovascular Medicine
University of Pennsylvania School of Medicine
Philadelphia, PA

Jo Ann S. Carson, PhD, RD
Professor, Department of Clinical Nutrition
UT Southwestern Medical Center
Dallas, TX

Robert DeChicco, MS, RD, CNSD
Nutrition Education Coordinator
Cleveland Clinic
Cleveland, OH

Horace M. Delisser, MD
Associate Professor of Pulmonary, Allergy, and
   Critical Care Medicine
Assistant Dean, Cultural Competency and
   Spirituality
University of Pennsylvania School of Medicine
Philadelphia, PA

Ara DerMarderosian, PhD
Professor of Pharmacognosy
Research Professor of Medicinal
　Chemistry
University of the Sciences in Philadelphia
Philadelphia, PA

Jessica Dine, MD
Pulmonary and Critical Care Fellow
Division of Pulmonary, Allergy, and Critical
　Care Medicine
Hospital of the University of Pennsylvania
Philadelphia, PA

Sharon Drozdowsky, MES
Industrial Hygienist
Division of Occupational Safety & Health
Washington State Department of Labor and
　Industries
Tumwater, WA

Cade Fields-Gardner, MS, RD
Director of Services
The Cutting Edge
Cary, IL

Judith Fish, MS, RD
Nutrition Consultant
Private Practice
Asheville, NC

Marion J. Franz, MS, RD
Nutrition and Health Consultant
Nutrition Concepts by Franz, Inc.
Minneapolis, MN

M. Patricia Fuhrman, MS, RD, LD, FADA, CNSD
National Director
Nutrition Services DCRX Infusion
Ballwin, MO

Katherine Galluzzi, DO
Professor and Chair, Department of Geriatrics
Philadelphia College of Osteopathic Medicine
Philadelphia, PA

Emily Gelsomin, RD, LDN
Clinical Nutrition Specialist
Ambulatory Nutrition Services
Massachusetts General Hospital
Boston, MA

Henry Ginsberg, MD
Director
Irving Institute for Clinical and Translational
　Research
Columbia University
New York, NY

Samuel N. Grief, MD
Associate Professor in Clinical Family Medicine
Department of Family Medicine
University of Illinois at Chicago
Chicago, IL

Scott M. Grundy, MD
Director, Center for Human Nutrition
Professor, Department of Internal Medicine
University of Texas Southwestern Medical
　Center
Dallas, TX

Indira Gurubhagavatula, MD, MPH
Assistant Professor of Medicine
Division of Sleep and Pulmonary, Allergy, and
　Critical Care Medicine
Director, Sleep Disorders Clinic
Pulmonary, Critical Care and Sleep Section
Philadelphia VA Medical Center
Philadelphia, PA

Jo Ann T. Hattner, MPH, RD, CSP
Instructor, Web-Based Nutrition Course
Stanford University School of Medicine
Palo Alto, CA

Ann Honebrink, MD, FACOG
Associate Professor
Obstetrics and Gynecology
University of Pennsylvania School of Medicine
Medical Director Penn Health for Women at
　Radnor
University of Pennsylvania Health System
Radnor, PA

Barbara Hopkins, MS, RD
Assistant Professor, Clinical Director
Dietetic Internship Program
Division of Nutrition
Georgia State University
Atlanta, GA

Elizabeth Horvitz, BA
Medical Student
University of California at Irvine
Irvine, CA

Satya S. Jonnalagadda, PhD, RD, LD
Principal Scientist
General Mills Bell Institute of Health and
 Nutrition
Minneapolis, MN

**Wahida Karmally, DrPH, RD,
CDE, CLS**
Associate Research Scientist
Lecturer in Dentistry
Director of Nutrition
Irving Institute for Clinical and Translational
 Research
Columbia University
New York, NY

John A. Kerner, MD
Director of Nutrition
Director of Pediatric Gastroenterology
 Fellowship
Pediatric GI, Hepatology and Nutrition
Stanford University Medical Center
Medical Director
Children's Home Pharmacy
Lucile Packard Children's Hospital/Stanford
 University
Palo Alto, CA

Doina Kulick, MD, MS, FACP
Assistant Professor of Medicine
University of Nevada School of Medicine
Reno, NV

Ruth Lawrence, MD, FAAP, FABM
Professor of Pediatrics and Obstetrics/
 Gynecology
Director, Breastfeeding and Human Lactation
 Study Center
University of Rochester School of Medicine and
 Dentistry
Rochester, NY

Ronald H. Lands, MD
Associate Professor
Director, Geriatric Fellowship
Department of Family Medicine
Graduate School of Medicine
University of Tennessee
Knoxville, TN

Gary R. Lichtenstein, MD
Professor of Medicine
University of Pennsylvania School of
 Medicine
Director
Center for Inflammatory Bowel Diseases
Gastroenterology Division
University of Pennsylvania Health System
Philadelphia, PA

Maria R. Mascarenhas, MD
Associate Professor of Pediatrics
University of Pennsylvania School of
 Medicine
Director, Nutrition Support Service
Section Chief, Nutrition
Division of Gastroenterology, Hepatology, and
 Nutrition
Children's Hospital of Philadelphia
Philadelphia, PA

**Laura Matarese, PhD, RD, LDN,
FADA, CNSD**
Assistant Professor of Surgery
University of Pittsburgh School of
 Medicine
Director of Nutrition
Intestinal Rehabilitation and Transplantation
 Center
Thomas E. Starzl Transplantation Institute
Pittsburgh, PA

Andrea J. Nepa, MS, RD, CSP, LDN
Clinical Dietitian
The Children's Hospital of Philadelphia
Philadelphia, PA

Xavier Pi-Sunyer, MD
Professor of Medicine, Columbia University
Chief, Division of Endocrinology, Metabolism,
 and Nutrition
Director, Obesity Research Center
St. Luke's Roosevelt Hospital
New York, NY

Alix Pruzansky
Student School of Arts and Sciences
University of Pennsylvania
Philadelphia, PA

Elizabeth B. Rappaport, MD
Associate Professor
Department of Family and Community
 Medicine
Jefferson Medical College
Thomas Jefferson University
Philadelphia, PA

José Antonio Ruy-Díaz, MD
Professor of Surgery
Head of the Department of Postgraduate
 Studies and Research
Chairman of the Department of Medical
 Sciences
Anahuac University School of Medicine
Mexico City, Mexico

Douglas Seidner, MD, FACG
Associate Professor of Medicine
Division of Gastroenterology, Hepatology, and
 Nutrition
Director, Vanderbilt Center for Human
 Nutrition
Vanderbilt University Medical Center
Nashville, TN

Ezra Steiger, MD
Professor of Surgery, Cleveland Clinic
Consultant in General Surgery and
 Gastroenterology
Departments of General Surgery and
 Gastroenterology
Codirector, Nutrition Support
Cleveland Clinic Lerner College of Medicine
 of Case Western Reserve University
Cleveland, OH

Jean Stover, RD, LDN
Renal Dietitian, DaVita Dialysis
Philadephia, PA

Catherine Sullivan, PhD, RD
North Carolina Breastfeeding Coordinator
Nutrition Services Branch
Raleigh, NC

Andrew M. Tershakovec, MD
Senior Director, Clinical Research
Merck Research Laboratories
North Wales, PA

Jennifer Thorpe, MBA, RD, CSP, LDN
Clinical Dietitian, Home Care
The Children's Hospital of Philadelphia
Philadelphia, PA

Brian W. Tobin, PhD
Associate Dean for Medical Education
Professor and Founding Chair
The Department of Medical Education
Texas Tech University Health Sciences Center
Paul L. Foster School of Medicine
El Paso, TX

Lisa D. Unger, MD, FACP
Assistant Professor of Clinical Surgery
Attending Physician, Nutrition Support Service
University of Pennsylvania School of Medicine
Philadelphia, PA

Julie Vanderpool, MPH, RD, CNSC
Clinical Dietitian
Brigham and Women's Hospital
Boston, MA

Jane White, PhD, RD
Professor, Department of Family Medicine
Graduate School of Medicine
University of Tennessee
Knoxville, TN

Jennifer Williams, MS, RD, CNSD
Advanced Clinical Dietitian Specialist
University of Pennsylvania Health System
Philadelphia, PA

Judith Wylie-Rosett, EdD, RD
Professor and Head
Division of Behavioral and Nutritional
 Research
Department of Epidemiology and Population
 Health
Albert Einstein College of Medicine
Bronx, NY

Susan Zogheib, RD
Graduate Student, Ryerson University
Toronto, ON

Preface

We are extremely proud to introduce the fourth edition of *Medical Nutrition and Disease: A Case-Based Approach*. The new edition of this best-selling text has been updated by nationally recognized nutritionists and physicians to include the most current evidenced-based medical nutrition therapy. Two new chapters have been added: Vitamins, Minerals, and Dietary Supplements and Cancer Prevention and Treatment. Four new cases have also been developed: Bariatric Surgery, Hypertension, Metabolic Syndrome and Lpa Genetic Defect, and Sleep Apnea.

The scientific evidence supporting medical nutrition therapy in health promotion and disease prevention continues to be strong. With this growth in knowledge, skills and attitudes, major changes have occurred in curriculum development and national nutrition guidelines have been amended. These include the National Heart, Lung, and Blood Institute, National Cholesterol Education Program, American Cancer Society, American Heart Association, American Diabetes Association, *Healthy People 2010*, and the Joint National Committee on the Prevention, Detection, Evaluation, and Treatment of High Blood Pressure.

Medical Nutrition and Disease: A Case-Based Approach is written for medical, nursing, and physician assistant students, residents, dietetic interns, and health professionals in practice. Registered dietitians can also earn **45 pre-approved continuing education credits** from the American Dietetic Association by successfully completing the multiple choice questions included in the book. There are no additional fees. For more information on how to successfully incorporate nutrition into your curriculum or clinical practice, contact:

Lisa Hark, PhD, RD
Consultant, Department of Medicine
Jefferson Medical College, Thomas Jefferson University
840 Walnut Street, Suite 1430
Philadelphia, PA. 19107-5109
215-928-3045
hark@LisaHark.com
www.LisaHark.com

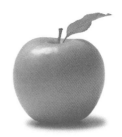

Part I
Fundamentals of Nutrition Assessment

1 Overview of Nutrition Assessment in Clinical Care

Lisa Hark[1], Darwin Deen[2], and Alix Pruzansky[3]

[1] Jefferson Medical College, Philadelphia, PA
[2] City College of New York, New York, NY
[3] University of Pennsylvania, Philadelphia, PA

OBJECTIVES*

- Recognize the value of nutrition assessment in the comprehensive care of ambulatory and hospitalized patients.

- Take an appropriate patient history, including medical, family, social, nutrition/dietary, physical activity, and weight histories; use of prescription medicines, over-the-counter medicines, dietary and herbal supplements; and consumption of alcohol and other recreational drugs.

- Demonstrate how to conduct an appropriate physical examination, calculate body mass index, measure waist circumference, and evaluate growth and development and signs of nutritional deficiency or excess.

- Describe the diagnosis, prevalence, health consequences, and etiology of obesity and undernutrition.

- Identify the most common physical findings associated with obesity, undernutrition, and vitamin/mineral deficiencies or excesses.

- List the laboratory measurements commonly used to assess the nutritional status of patients.

*Source: Objectives for chapter and cases adapted from the *NIH Nutrition Curriculum Guide for Training Physicians*. (www.nhlbi.nih.gov/funding/training/naa)

Nutrition Assessment in Clinical Care

Nutrition assessment is the evaluation of an individual's nutritional status based on the interpretation of clinical information. Nutrition assessment is an important tool in clinical medicine because malnutrition (both obesity and undernutrition) is a common clinical finding. Many patients can benefit from medical nutrition therapy (MNT) using established evidence-based protocols. The purpose of nutrition assessment is to:

- accurately evaluate an individual's dietary intake and nutritional status;
- determine if medical nutrition therapy and/or counseling is needed;
- monitor changes in nutritional status; and
- evaluate the effectiveness of nutritional interventions.

Medical Nutrition and Disease: A Case-Based Approach, 4th edition. Edited by Lisa Hark.
© 2009 Wiley-Blackwell Publishing, ISBN: 978-1-4051-8615-5.

Integrating Nutrition into the Medical History and Physical Examination

The following illustrates how to integrate nutrition into all components of the clinical evaluation and nursing assessment, including the medical history, diet history, review of systems, physical examination, laboratory data, and treatment plan.

Medical History

Past Medical History

Standard past medical history such as immunizations, hospitalizations, surgeries, major injuries, chronic illnesses, and significant acute illnesses can have nutritional implications. Detailed information should be obtained about current or recent prescription medications and use of vitamins, minerals, laxatives, topical medications, over-the-counter medications, and products such as nutritional or herbal supplements that patients frequently do not recognize as medications. Nutritional supplements include any products that a patient uses to increase his or her caloric, vitamin, or protein intake. Whether the patient has any known food allergies or suffers from milk (lactose) intolerance is also important.

Family History

In assessing risk for future diseases, patients are asked to identify their parents, siblings, children, and partner, give their respective ages and health status, and indicate the cause of death of any deceased family members. Familial occurrences of disease are also recorded here. Family history of food intolerance reflects nutritional risk as does family history of diabetes, heart disease, obesity, hypertension, osteoporosis, food allergies, eating disorders, or alcoholism.

Social History

Pertinent non-medical information recorded in the social history includes the patient's occupation, daily exercise pattern, and marital and family status. Information is also solicited regarding the patient's education, economic status, residence, emotional response and adjustment to illness, and any other information that might influence the patient's understanding of his or her illness and adherence to a nutritional program. Details concerning the duration and frequency of the patient's use of substances such as alcohol, tobacco, illicit drugs, and caffeine are also documented. These data can be extremely useful when formulating the treatment plan. Economic limitations that influence access to an adequate diet, difficulties shopping for or preparing food, participation in feeding programs (e.g. Women, Infants, and Children (WIC), Meals on Wheels) are relevant to nutritional assessment. The social history is typically where the patient's diet history is explored.

The Importance of Taking a Diet History

The purpose of obtaining dietary information from patients is to assess their nutritional status and, if necessary, formulate a treatment plan. Infants, children, adolescents, pregnant women, older adults, and patients with a family history of or who have diabetes, hypertension, heart disease, hyperlipidemia, obesity, eating disorders, alcoholism, osteoporosis, gastrointestinal or renal disease, cancer, or weight loss or gain should always be asked about their eating habits, even during routine visits. Dietary information may be collected using any of the methods described in this section. In addition, the patients' past and/or current food intake patterns, such as vegetarian or kosher diet practices, cultural background, and social situations should be considered during the interview. Family members who purchase and prepare the food should be involved in the interview process whenever possible. Diet-related questions should ideally take only a few minutes by physicians, if properly directed (See Table 1-1). Registered dietitians typically spend more time taking a diet history and report these results to the physician, nurse practitioner or physician assistant. This detailed history may include information on food preferences, portion sizes, frequency of eating out, and emotional responses to eating. Dietary intake information is used to determine total calories, fat, protein, sodium, fiber, and adequacy of vitamin and mineral intake and serves as a basis for counseling. Numerous brief

Table 1-1 Key Diet History Questions for Brief Intervention

Questions for All Patients
- How many meals and snacks do you eat every day?
- Do you feel that you eat a healthy balanced diet? Why or why not?
- What do you like to drink during the day, including alcohol? How many glasses?
- How often do you eat fruits and vegetables?
- How often do you eat dairy products? Low-fat or regular type?
- How often do you eat out? What kinds of restaurants?
- Do you usually finish what is on your plate or leave food?
- How often do you exercise, including walking?

In addition to the questions above
Questions for Patients with Hyperlipidemia (Chapter 6)
- How often do you eat fatty meats? (hot dogs, bacon, sausage, salami, pastrami, corned beef)
- How often do you eat fish? How is it prepared?
- What types of fats do you use in cooking and baking?
- What do you spread on your bread?
- What type of snacks and desserts do you eat?

Questions for Patients with Hypertension (Chapter 6)
- Do you use a salt shaker at the table or in cooking?
- Do you read food labels for sodium content? (<400 mg/serving permitted)
- How often do you eat canned, smoked, frozen, or processed foods?

Questions for Patients with Diabetes (Chapter 8)
- What times do you take your diabetes medication (including insulin)?
- What times do you eat your meals and snacks?
- Do you ever skip meals during the day?
- How many servings of starchy foods such as breads, cereals, rice, pastas, corn, peas, or beans do you eat during a typical day?

Source: Lisa A. Hark, PhD, RD. Used with permission.

24-Hour Recall

Purpose This informal, qualitative, questioning method elicits all foods and beverages the patient has consumed in the preceding 24 hours. This method is recommended for patients with diabetes because of the ability to assess the timing of meals, snacks, and insulin injections.

Questions "Please describe everything that you ate and drank within the past 24 hours (meals and snacks), including quantities, and how you prepared these foods." Begin with the last meal eaten and work backwards or ask for a description of everything that the patient ate the day before. Family members are usually consulted if the patient is a child or unable to convey adequate detail. Patients can be asked to write down what they ate the day before while they are waiting to be seen. Hospitalized patients can be monitored through calorie counts reported by the nursing or dietary staff, who record the daily amounts of food and drink the patient consumes. Keep in mind that the 24-hour recall method, when used alone, may underestimate or overestimate a person's usual caloric intake since the patient's recollection may not reflect long-term dietary habits.

Usual Intake/Diet History

Purpose Similar to the 24-hour recall, a usual intake/diet history is a retrospective method to obtain dietary information by asking the patient to recall his or her normal daily intake pattern, including amounts of foods consumed. This method is suggested for older adults who frequently skip meals, and for those interviewing pediatric patients whose diets may not be varied. This approach provides more information about usual intake patterns than others and tends to reflect long-term dietary habits with greater accuracy.

Questions "What do you usually eat and drink during the day for meals and snacks?" As a busy clinician, this question may be all that you will have time to ask, but it can serve as a screening mechanism to identify patients who need further counseling with a registered dietitian. When using this approach it is important to be flexible. Begin by asking patients to describe their usual intake and if they cannot recall their usual diet, ask what they ate and drank the day before (a switch to the 24-hour recall method). You can then ask if these 24 hours are typical. Also bear in mind that some patients tend to report having eaten only those foods that they know are healthy.

Food Frequency Questionnaire

Purpose The food frequency questionnaire is another retrospective approach used to determine trends in a patient's usual frequency of consumption of specific foods.

Questions The patient is usually asked several key questions regarding the frequency of intake of particular foods. Frequencies can be listed to identify daily, weekly, or monthly consumption patterns. Patients can be asked these questions during the history, or these items can be added to the written form for new patients while they are in the waiting room or mailed prior to their visit. For the clinician, the questions can be geared toward the patient's existing medical conditions, which is why this method is best for patients with diabetes, heart disease, hypertension, or osteoporosis and can be used for evaluating current intake of fruits, vegetables, dairy products, or processed foods.

Numerous questionnaires have been developed for brief diet assessment and counseling. These include "Rapid Eating Assessment for Patients" (REAP), "Quick Weight, Activity, Variety, and Excess Screener (WAVE) for Adults and Adolescents," and "Rate Your Plate" (see references).

Review of Systems

This subjective reexamination of the patient's history is organized by body systems. It differs from the past medical history by concentrating on symptoms, not diagnoses, and by emphasizing current more than past information. All positive and negative findings are listed. Nutrition questions vary according to the patient's age. One goal of this part of the history is to determine whether any dietary changes have occurred in the patient's life, either voluntarily or as a consequence of illness, medication use, or psychological problems. Examples within the review of systems that may have nutritional implications (and their potential significance) include weakness and fatigue (anemia), clothes tighter or looser (weight gain or weight loss), vomiting, nausea, diarrhea (poor nutritional intake, lactose intolerance), dehydration, constipation (low fiber or fluid intake), amenorrhea (anorexia nervosa), or changes in appetite.

Physical Examination

The physical examination begins with the patient's vital signs (blood pressure, heart rate, respiration rate, temperature), height, weight, body mass index (BMI), and general appearance. For example, "On examination, she is a well-developed, thin woman." When terms such as obese, overweight, undernourished, thin, well-nourished, well-developed, or cachectic (profound, marked state of ill health and undernutrition) are used, they should be supported by findings in the physical examination and noted in the problem list.

Body Mass Index (BMI)

To calculate BMI using the metric system:

$$BMI = \frac{weight\ (kg)}{height\ (m^2)}$$

To calculate BMI using English units:

$$BMI = \frac{weight\ (lbs) \times 703}{height\ (in^2)}$$

Table 1-2 Classifications of BMI

Underweight	<18.5 kg/m^2
Normal weight	18.5–24.9 kg/m^2
Overweight	25–29.9 kg/m^2
Obesity (Class 1)	30–34.9 kg/m^2
Obesity (Class 2)	35–39.9 kg/m^2
Extreme obesity (Class 3)	≥40 kg/m^2

Source: National Heart, Lung, and Blood Institute, NIH. *Clinical Guidelines on the Identification, Evaluation, and Treatment of Overweight and Obesity in Adults.* 1998. Used with permission.

Body mass index provides a more accurate measure of total body fat than body weight alone. The BMI value is also more accurate than the older height–weight tables, which were based on a homogeneous population, primarily Caucasian, with higher than average socioeconomic status. BMI has also been shown to more accurately estimate obesity than bioelectrical impedance tests. BMI associated with the lowest mortality increases slightly as people age. However, there are some limitations: BMI may overestimate body fat in very muscular people and underestimate body fat in some underweight people who have lost lean tissue, such as the elderly. BMI values can be determined based on height and weight measurements as shown in Figure 1-1. Classifications of underweight, normal weight, overweight, and obesity are shown in Table 1-2. Health professionals should routinely assess height, weight, and BMI, and evaluate growth and development in infants, children, and adolescents.

Waist Circumference

Waist circumference is an independent measure of risk in normal weight, as well as overweight and obese individuals. Excess fat located in the abdominal area (termed visceral adipose tissue) is reflected by waist circumference measurement. Waist circumference is a predictor of morbidity, and is considered an independent risk factor for diabetes, dyslipidemia, hypertension, and cardiovascular disease even when BMI is not markedly increased. In patients with a BMI greater than 35 kg/m^2, there is little additional risk from elevated waist circumference, as severe risk is already present. Therefore, measuring waist circumference is recommended in patients with a BMI less than 35 kg/m^2. The waist circumference measurement is particularly important for patients with a family history of diabetes and those who may be borderline overweight.

In order to obtain an accurate waist circumference measurement, patients should be standing in only their underwear. A horizontal mark should be drawn just above the uppermost lateral border of the right iliac crest, which should then be crossed with a vertical mark in the midaxillary line. The measuring tape is placed in a horizontal plane around the abdomen at the level of this mark on the right side of the trunk. The plane of the tape should be parallel to the floor and the tape should be snug but not tight. Patients should be advised to breathe normally when the measurement is taken. Waist circumference values greater than 102 cm (40 inches)

Body Mass Index Chart

in/cm	lbs/kg 100/45	105/48	110/50	115/52	120/55	125/56	130/59	135/61	140/64	145/66	150/68	155/70	160/73	165/75	170/77	175/79	180/82	185/84	190/86	195/89	200/91	205/93	210/95	215/98	220/100	225/102	230/104	235/107	240/109	245/111	250/114
5'0"/153	20	21	21	22	23	24	25	26	27	28	29	30	31	32	33	34	35	36	37	38	39	40	41	42	43	44	45	46	47	48	49
5'1"/155	19	20	21	22	23	24	25	26	26	27	28	29	30	31	32	33	34	35	36	37	38	39	40	41	42	43	43	44	45	46	47
5'2"/158	18	19	20	21	22	23	24	25	26	27	27	28	29	30	31	32	33	34	35	36	37	37	38	39	40	41	42	43	44	45	46
5'3"/160	18	19	19	20	21	22	23	24	25	26	27	27	28	29	30	31	32	33	34	35	35	36	37	38	39	40	41	42	43	43	44
5'4"/163	17	18	19	20	21	21	22	23	24	25	26	27	27	28	29	30	31	32	33	33	34	35	36	37	38	39	39	40	41	42	43
5'5"/165	17	17	18	19	20	21	22	22	23	24	25	26	27	27	28	29	30	31	32	32	33	34	35	36	37	37	38	39	40	41	42
5'6"/168	16	17	18	19	19	20	21	22	23	23	24	25	26	27	27	28	29	30	31	31	32	33	34	35	36	36	37	38	39	40	40
5'7"/171	16	16	17	18	19	20	20	21	22	23	23	24	25	26	27	27	28	29	30	31	31	32	33	34	34	35	36	37	38	38	39
5'8"/173	15	16	17	17	18	19	20	21	21	22	23	24	24	25	26	27	27	28	29	30	30	31	32	33	33	34	35	36	36	37	38
5'9"/176	15	16	16	17	18	18	19	20	21	21	22	23	24	24	25	26	27	27	28	29	30	30	31	32	32	33	34	35	35	36	37
5'10"/178	14	15	16	17	17	18	19	19	20	21	22	22	23	24	24	25	26	27	27	28	29	29	30	31	32	32	33	34	34	35	36
5'11"/181	14	15	15	16	17	17	18	19	20	20	21	22	22	23	24	24	25	26	27	27	28	29	29	30	31	31	32	33	33	34	35
6'0"/183	14	14	15	16	16	17	18	18	19	20	20	21	22	22	23	24	24	25	26	26	27	28	28	29	30	31	31	32	33	33	34
6'1"/186	13	14	15	15	16	16	17	18	18	19	20	20	21	22	22	23	24	24	25	26	26	27	28	28	29	30	30	31	32	32	33
6'2"/188	13	13	14	15	15	16	17	17	18	19	19	20	21	21	22	22	23	24	24	25	26	26	27	28	28	29	30	30	31	31	32
6'3"/191	12	13	14	14	15	16	16	17	17	18	19	19	20	21	21	22	22	23	24	24	25	26	26	27	27	28	29	29	30	31	31
6'4"/193	12	13	13	14	15	15	16	16	17	18	18	19	19	20	21	21	22	23	23	24	24	25	26	26	27	27	28	29	29	30	30

Underweight	Normal	Overweight	Obese
<18.5	19–24.9	25–29.9	>30

Figure 1-1 BMI Values Based on Height and Weight

in men and greater than 88 cm (35 inches) in women are considered indicators of increased risk, although this may differ among ethnic groups . These values also represent one of the diagnostic criteria of metabolic syndrome (Chapter 1: Case 1). In patients trying to lose weight by exercising, waist circumference may decrease without significant weight loss.

Percent Weight Change

Weight loss is very common in hospitalized and nursing home patients. Weight loss is also frequently seen in older adults or those with significant appetite changes due to chronic illnesses such as cancer, gastrointestinal problems, or secondary to surgery, chemotherapy, or radiation therapy. If weight loss is identified in the medical history or review of systems, it is essential to take a diet and weight history and determine the percent weight change over that period of time using the patient's current body weight and usual weight. Severity of weight loss is defined by percent change in a defined period of time (Table 1-3).

$$\textbf{Percent weight change} = \frac{\text{Usual Weight} - \text{Current Weight}}{\text{Usual Weight}} \times 100$$

Table 1-3 Interpretation of Percent Weight Change

Time	Significant Weight Loss	Severe Weight Loss
1 week	1–2%	>2%
1 month	5%	>5%
3 months	7.5%	>7.5%
6 months	10%	>10%
1 year	20%	>20%

Physical Examination Findings

Nutrition-oriented aspects of the physical examination focus on the skin, head, hair, eyes, mouth, nails, extremities, abdomen, skeletal muscle, and fat stores. Areas to examine closely for muscle wasting include the temporal muscles and the interosseous muscles on the hands. The skeletal muscles of the extremities also serve as an indicator of undernutrition. Subcutaneous fat stores should be examined for losses due to a sudden decrease in weight or for excess accumulation that commonly occurs in obesity. Isolated vitamin deficiencies such as scurvy and pellagra are rarely seen in modern clinical practice. At the present time, the most commonly encountered nutritional problem seen in clinical practices in the United States and many developed countries is obesity and its associated complications. Specific clinical signs that are attributable to nutrient deficiencies and significance on physical examination appear in Table 1-4.

Table 1-4 Physical Examination Findings with Nutritional Implications

Vital Signs:	temperature, blood pressure, pulse, respiratory rate, height, weight, BMI, waist circumference, percent weight change.
General:	wasted, cachectic, overweight, obese, muscle weakness, anorexic
Skin:	acanthosis nigricans (obesity, metabolic syndrome, insulin resistance, diabetes)
	ecchymosis (vitamin K, C deficiency)
	dermatitis (marasmus, niacin, riboflavin, zinc, biotin, EFA deficiency)
	follicular hyperkeratosis (vitamin A deficiency)
	petechiae (vitamin A, C, K deficiency)
	pigmentation changes (niacin deficiency, marasmus)
	pressure ulcers/delayed wound healing (kwashiorkor, diabetes, vitamin C, zinc deficiency)
	psoriasiform rash, eczematous scaling (zinc deficiency)
	purpura (vitamin C, K deficiency)
	scrotal dermatosis (riboflavin deficiency)
	pallor (iron, folic acid, vitamin B_{12}, copper, vitamin E deficiency)
	thickening and dryness of skin (linoleic acid deficiency)
Hair:	dyspigmentation, easy pluckability (protein), alopecia (zinc, biotin deficiency)
Head:	temporal muscle wasting (marasmus and cachexia)
	delayed closure of fontanelle (pediatric undernutrition or growth retardation)
Eyes:	night blindness, xerosis, Bitot spots, keratomalacia (vitamin A deficiency)
	photophobia, blurring, conjunctival inflammation, corneal vascularization (riboflavin deficiency)
Mouth:	angular stomatitis (riboflavin, iron deficiency)
	bleeding gums (vitamin C, K, riboflavin deficiency)
	cheilosis (riboflavin, niacin, vitamin B_6 deficiency)
	dental caries (fluoride deficiency)
	hypogeusia (zinc, vitamin A deficiency)
	glossitis (riboflavin, niacin, folic acid, vitamin B_{12}, vitamin B_6 deficiency)
	nasolabial seborrhea (vitamin B_6 deficiency)
	papillary atrophy or smooth tongue (riboflavin, niacin, iron deficiency)
	Fissuring, scarlet or raw tongue (niacin, folate, B_{12}, B_6 deficiency)
Neck:	goiter (iodine deficiency)
	parotid enlargement (marasmus)
Thorax:	thoracic and rachitic rosary (vitamin D deficiency)
Abdomen:	abdominal obesity (metabolic syndrome, diabetes, heart disease)
	diarrhea (niacin, folate, vitamin B_{12} deficiency) (marasmus)
	hepatomegaly/ascites (kwashiorkor, alcoholism)
Cardiac:	heart failure (thiamin, selenium deficiency, anemia)
Genital/urinary:	delayed puberty (marasmus, eating disorder)
	hypogonadism (zinc deficiency)
Extremities:	ataxia (vitamin B_{12} deficiency, vitamin B_6 toxicity)
	bone ache, joint pain (vitamin C deficiency)
	bone tenderness, kyphosis
	edema (thiamin and protein deficiency)
	growth retardation, failure to thrive (energy deficiency)
	hyporeflexia (thiamin deficiency)
	kyphosis (calcium, vitamin D deficiency)
	muscle wasting and weakness (vitamin D, magnesium deficiency, marasmus)

Table 1-4 (*Continued*)

	tenderness at end of long bones (vitamin D deficiency)
	squaring of shoulders—loss of deltoid muscles (kwashiorkor)
Nails:	spooning (koilonychias) (iron deficiency)
	transverse lines (kwashiorkor)
Neurological:	dementia, delirium, disorientation (niacin, thiamin, vitamin E deficiency)
	loss of reflexes, wrist drop, foot drop (thiamin deficiency)
	ophthalmoplegia (vitamin E, thiamin deficiency)
	peripheral neuropathy (thiamin, vitamin E, vitamin B_{12} deficiency)
	tetany (vitamin D, calcium, magnesium deficiency)

Source: Lisa A. Hark, PhD, RD. Used with permission.

Laboratory Data to Diagnose Nutritional and Medical Problems

No single blood test or group of tests accurately measures nutritional status. Therefore clinical judgment is important in deciding what tests to order based on the individual's history and physical findings. The following tests are grouped according to medical condition.

Alcoholism: Aspartate aminotransferase (AST), alanine aminotransferase (ALT), gamma-glutamyl transferane (GGT), thiamin, folate, and vitamin B_{12}.

Anemia: Complete blood count (CBC), serum iron and ferritin, total iron binding capacity (TIBC), transferrin saturation, mean corpuscular volume (MCV), reticulocyte count, red blood cell folate, and serum vitamin B_{12}.

Diabetes: Fasting serum glucose, hemoglobin A1c, insulin levels, C-reactive protein (CRP), serum and urinary ketone bodies.

Eating Disorders: Potassium, albumin, serum amylase, thyroid studies, beta carotene aspartate amino transferase (AST), alanine aminotransferase (ALT), and anemia.

Fluid, Electrolyte, and Renal Function: Sodium, potassium, chloride, calcium, phosphorus, magnesium, blood urea nitrogen (BUN), creatinine, urine urea nitrogen, urinary and serum, oxalic acid, and uric acid.

Hyperlipidemia: Cholesterol, triglyceride, low density lipoprotein-cholesterol (LDL-C), high density lipoprotein-cholesterol (HDL-C), homocysteine, and thyroid stimulating hormone (TSH) (secondary cause).

Musculoskeletal pain, weakness: 25(OH) vitamin D, phosphate, PTH.

Malabsorption: 24-hour fecal fat, barium studies, electrolytes, albumin, serum triglycerides, and hydrogen breath test.

Metabolic Syndrome: Fasting serum glucose, lipid panel, and uric acid.

Refeeding Syndrome: Albumin, calcium, phosphorous, magnesium, and potassium

Undernutrition: Protein Status

Clinically, visceral protein status may be depleted by increased protein losses in the stool and urine, as a result of wounds involving severe blood loss, or by poor dietary protein intake. The following serum protein levels may prove useful in conjunction with other nutrition assessment parameters. Once again, however, each of these tests has limitations because serum protein levels are affected not only by nutrition and hydration status, but by disease states, surgery, and liver dysfunction.

The half-life ($t_{1/2}$) of each protein is given because knowing its duration allows the clinician to use these tests to monitor changes in protein nutrition:

- **Serum Albumin** Serum albumin has a half-life of 18 to 20 days and reflects nutritional status over the previous 1 to 2 months. Levels may decrease with acute stress, overhydration, trauma, surgery, liver disease, and renal disease. False increases often occur with dehydration. This test is not a good indicator of recent dietary status or acute changes in nutritional status (less than 3 weeks) given its long half-life. Significantly reduced levels of serum albumin are associated with increased morbidity and mortality (<3.5 mg/dL).
- **Serum Transferrin** Serum transferrin has a half-life of 8 to 9 days. Changes in serum transferrin levels are influenced by iron status, as well as by protein and calorie intake. Results of this test reflect intake over the preceding several weeks.
- **Serum Prealbumin** With a half-life of 2 to 3 days, serum prealbumin reflects nutritional status as well as protein and calorie intake over the previous week. Prealbumin levels may be falsely elevated with renal disease. However, as with albumin, the level is reduced with severe liver disease.

Assessment and Problem List: Medical Nutrition Therapy

The health care professional clinically assesses the individual patient based on his/her history, review of systems, physical examination, and laboratory data.

Active problems are listed in order of their importance. Inactive problems are also recorded. Evidence of a nutrition disorder should be considered primary if it occurs in an individual with no other etiology that explains signs and symptoms of undernutrition. A primary nutrition problem is usually the result of imbalances, inadequacies, or excesses in the patient's nutrient intake. Manifestations may include obesity, weight loss, undernutrition, or poor intake of vitamins or minerals such as iron, calcium, folate, vitamin D, or vitamin B_{12}.

Patients having normal weight and no other risk factors should be encouraged to maintain their weight. Overweight patients with co-morbidities, such as diabetes, hypertension, or heart disease, should be advised to lose weight by increasing their physical activity level and reducing their total calorie and saturated fat intake, as well as portion sizes.

Secondary nutrition problems occur when a primary pathologic process results in inadequate food intake, impaired absorption and utilization of nutrients, increased loss or excretion of nutrients, or increased nutrient requirements. Common causes of secondary nutritional disorders include anorexia nervosa, malabsorption, diabetes, trauma, acute medical illness, and surgery. Undernutrition may occur as a result of a chronic condition or an acute episode complicating an underlying disease. After assessing each problem, medical nutrition therapy should be recommended

Table 1-5 Key Dietary Issues by Age and Disease

Infants	Fluoride, iron, calories, protein, fat for growth and development
Children	Fluoride, iron, calcium, calories, protein, fat for growth and development
Teenagers	Iron, calcium, calories, protein for pubertal development (screen for eating disorders)
Pregnancy	Folate, iron, calcium, protein, appropriate weight gain
Alcoholism	Folate, thiamin, vitamin B_{12}, calories
Anemia	Iron, vitamin B_{12}, folate
Ascites	Sodium, protein
Beriberi	Thiamin
Cancer	Adequate protein, calories, and fiber
COPD, Asthma	Vitamin D, calcium, weight loss, calories
Diabetes	Carbohydrates, saturated fat, cholesterol, calories, fiber
Heart Disease	Saturated fat, monounsaturated fat, cholesterol, fiber
Hyperlipidemia	Saturated fat, monounsaturated fat, cholesterol, fiber
Heart Failure	Sodium
Hypertension	Sodium, calcium, potassium, alcohol, total calories
Kidney Stones	Calcium, oxalate, uric acid, protein, sodium, fluid
Liver Disease	Protein, sodium, fluid
Malabsorption	Vitamins A, D, E and K
Obesity	Total calories, portion sizes, saturated fat
Osteoporosis	Vitamin D and calcium
Pellegra	Niacin
Renal Failure	Protein, sodium, potassium, phosphorous, fluid
Rickets	Vitamin D and calcium
Scurvy	Vitamin C
Vegetarian diet	Protein, vitamin B_{12}, iron, calcium

Source: Lisa A. Hark, PhD, RD. Used with permission.

that includes both a diagnostic component and a treatment plan. Patient education is an essential part of medical nutrition therapy. Key dietary issues by age and disease are summarized in Table 1-5.

Estimating Energy Requirements

Resting Energy Expenditure (REE)

The amount of energy required to maintain vital organ function in a resting state over 24 hours is referred to as the resting energy expenditure (REE). The basal metabolic rate (BMR) is the minimum caloric requirement at a neutral environmental temperature and fasting. BMR is generally impractical to measure. REE is approximately 10 percent above the BMR. Thus, the REE is used in clinical medicine for estimation of BMR. REE accounts for approximately 65 percent of total daily energy expenditure and varies considerably among individuals with different height, weight, age, body composition, and gender. REE significantly correlates with lean body mass. Regular physical activity, especially weight-bearing exercises, can increase lean muscle mass, and thus increase REE. Since REE decreases as people age

Table 1-6 Definition of Energy/Calorie

Energy is expressed in kilocalories (kcal) and is produced by the oxidation of dietary protein, fat, carbohydrate, and alcohol.
- One gram of **protein** yields approximately 4 kcal.
- One gram of **carbohydrate** yields approximately 4 kcal.
- One gram of **fat** yields approximately 9 kcal.
- One gram of **alcohol** yields approximately 7 kcal.

A calorie is the amount of heat required to raise the temperature of 1 gram of water by 1 degree Celsius. A kilocalorie is the amount of heat required to raise the temperature of one kilogram of water by 1 degree Celsius.

---

due to the loss of lean body mass over time, regular exercise can play a significant role in maintaining REE, especially in older adults. The energy produced by the oxidation of dietary macronutrients is shown in Table 1-6. Equations to estimate energy requirements have been developed as part of the Dietary Reference Intake recommendations and are shown in Table 1-7. Physical activity coefficients to use when estimating energy requirements are shown in Table 1-8.

Energy and Protein Needs of Hospitalized or Critically Ill Patients

Activity factors are added to the REE as necessary to calculate total daily caloric needs, which vary for active and inactive patients. Total energy expenditure (TEE) is equal to the REE times the appropriate physical activity factor. The physical activity factor for hospitalized patients or those confined to bed is 1.2; for non-hospitalized, sedentary patients, use 1.3. Many hospitals still use the Harris–Benedict equations to estimate calorie requirements, which are shown in Table 1-9.

Table 1-7 Dietary Reference Intakes: Equations to Estimate Energy Requirement

---

Adults 19 years and older
Estimated Energy Requirement (kcal/day) = Total Energy Expenditure

---

Men	EER = 662 − (9.53 × age [y]) + PA × {(15.91 × weight [kg]) + (539.6 × height [m])}
Women	EER = 354 - (6.91 × age [y]) + PA × {(9.36 × weight [kg]) + (726 × height [m])}

Source: Food and Nutrition Board, Institute of Medicine. *Dietary Reference Intakes for Energy, Carbohydrates, Fiber, Fat, Fatty Acids, Cholesterol, Protein, and Amino Acids*. Washington, DC: National Academies Press, 2002.

Table 1-8 Physical Activity Coefficients (PA values) for Use in EER Equations

	Sedentary (PAL 1.0–1.39)	Low Active (PAL 1.4–1.59)	Active (PAL 1.6–1.89)	Very Active (PAL 1.9–2.5)
	Typical daily living activities (e.g household tasks, walking to the bus)	Typical daily living activities PLUS 30–60 minutes of daily moderate activity (ex. walking at 5–7 km/h)	Typical daily living activities PLUS at least 60 minutes of daily moderate activity	Typical daily living activities PLUS at least 60 minutes of daily moderate activity PLUS an additional 60 minutes of vigorous activity or 120 minutes of moderate activity
Men 19 y +	1.00	1.11	1.25	1.48
Women 19 y +	1.00	1.12	1.27	1.45

Source: Food and Nutrition Board, Institute of Medicine. *Dietary Reference Intakes for Energy, Carbohydrates, Fiber, Fat, Fatty Acids, Cholesterol, Protein, and Amino Acids*. Washington, DC: National Academies Press, 2002.

Table 1-9 Harris–Benedict Equations to Estimate Calorie Requirements

The Harris–Benedict equations estimate the basal (resting) energy expenditure in adults, which varies with both body size and gender.

REE equation for males:
$$66 + [13.7 \times \text{weight (kg)}] + [5.0 \times \text{height (cm)}] - [6.8 \times \text{(age)}] = \text{kcal/day}$$

REE equation for females:
$$655 + [9.7 \times \text{weight (kg)}] + [1.85 \times \text{height (cm)}] - [4.7 \times \text{(age)}] = \text{kcal/day}$$

Total Energy Expenditure (TEE):

Multiply the REE by an activity factor to estimate the TEE: Use 1.2 for those confined to bed, 1.3 for those with a sedentary lifestyle and low physical activity. For healthy, active individuals use a factor of 1.5 to estimate caloric needs for weight maintenance.

The Harris–Benedict equation should be modified by using an adjusted body weight for patients who are obese because adipose tissue is not as metabolically active as lean body mass. The REE would be overestimated if this factor were not taken into account. The equation for calculating adjusted body weight is:

$$[(\text{Current body weight} - \text{goal weight}) \times 25\%] + \text{goal weight}$$

Protein requirements in a critically ill patient depend on the degree of catabolic stress the patient is experiencing. Protein calories should be calculated separately. Some guidelines are as follows:

- In unstressed well-nourished individuals, protein needs range from 0.8 to 1.0 gram per kilogram body weight per day.
- In post-surgical patients protein needs range from 1.5 to 2.0 grams per kilogram body weight per day.
- In highly catabolic patients (burns, infection, fever), protein needs can be over 2 grams per kilogram body weight per day.

Undernutrition
Health Consequences of Undernutrition

According to the World Health Organization (WHO), undernutrition affects all age groups across the entire lifespan, from conception to older adults. Health consequences of underweight range from intrauterine brain damage and growth failure to reduced physical and mental capacity in childhood to an increased risk of developing diet-related chronic diseases later in life.

Insufficient food intake results in loss of fat, muscle, and ultimately visceral tissue. This reduction in tissue mass is reflected in weight loss. The smaller tissue mass has reduced nutritional requirements, likely reflecting more efficient utilization of ingested food and reduction in work capacity at the cellular level. The combination of decreased tissue mass and reduction in work capacity impedes homeostatic responses, including responses to illness or surgery. The stress of critical illness inhibits the body's natural conservation response to undernutrition. In addition, undernourished individuals experience nutrient deficiencies and imbalances that exacerbate the natural reduction in cellular work capacity. They also experience a decrease in the inflammatory response and immune function. These alterations result in increased morbidity and mortality among undernourished patients. Adequate nutrition is essential for reversing these physiological effects. Aggressive nutritional support, instituted early in critical illness, may reduce the adverse effects of the critically ill patient's undernutrition.

Etiology/Causes of Undernutrition

Decreased Oral Intake Poverty, poor dentition, gastrointestinal obstruction, abdominal pain, anorexia, dysphagia, depression, social isolation, and chronic pain are some of the many possible causes of decreased oral intake.

Increased Nutrient Loss Glycosuria, gastrointestinal bleeding, diarrhea, malabsorption, nephrosis, a draining fistula, or protein-losing enteropathy can result in nutrient losses.

Increased Nutrient Requirements Hypermetabolic state or excessive catabolic processes can result in increased nutrient requirements. Common examples of situations that can dramatically affect nutrient requirements include surgery, trauma, fever, burns, hyperthyroidism, severe infection, malabsorption syndromes, cancer, COPD, cardiac cachexia, critical illness, and HIV/AIDS. Pregnant women and children are also at risk due to increased nutritional requirements during growth and development.

Diagnosis of Undernutrition

Undernutrition is defined as a suboptimal or deficient supply of nutrients that interferes with an individual's growth, development, general health, or recovery from illness. A BMI of less than $18.5 kg/m^2$ defines adults who are consistently underweight and at risk for undernutrition. Infants and children who fall below the 5th percentile for weight-for-age or BMI-for-age on the pediatric growth charts should be evaluated further. In acute undernutrition, a child's weight-for-age percentile on the growth chart falls first, followed by a decline in height growth. In extreme cases of undernutrition or starvation, a child's head circumference growth may also plateau. The importance of plotting pediatric growth parameters over time is paramount, as poor weight gain and/or weight loss are key to diagnosing undernutrition, failure to thrive, and other medical conditions associated with poor weight gain in the pediatric population, such as cystic fibrosis.

Marasmus results when the body's requirements for calories and protein are not met by dietary intake. Marasmus is characterized by severe tissue wasting, excessive loss of lean body mass, and subcutaneous fat stores, dehydration, and weight loss. Decreased protein intake is usually associated with decreased calorie intake, but can occur independently.

Kwashiorkor describes a predominant protein deficiency. Kwashiorkor is characterized by lethargy, apathy, irritability, retarded growth, changes in skin (dermatitis) and hair pigmentation, edema, and low serum albumin. Both marasmus and kwashiorkor are associated with weakness, weight loss, decline in functional status (increased difficulties with activities of daily living), impaired immune function with increased susceptibility to infection, and increased risk of morbidity and mortality.

Prevalence of Undernutrition

Children, older adults, and hospitalized and nursing home patients are particularly prone to undernutrition. According to the *Healthy People 2010* objectives, 6 percent of low-income children under the age of five years were growth retarded due to undernutrition in 2006. According to WHO, 50 percent of deaths among children less than five years of age in developing countries are associated with undernutrition. One in three people are affected by vitamin and mineral deficiencies and one out of four pre-school children suffers from undernutrition. One in six infants born in developing countries is of low birth weight.

Some degree of undernutrition occurs during most hospitalizations regardless of the type of injury or illness. The prevalence of undernutrition in the outpatient population has not been clearly determined. Risk factors for undernutrition include chronic diseases, use of multiple prescription medications, poverty, inadequate nutritional knowledge, homebound and/or non-ambulatory status, poor social support structure, major psychiatric diagnosis, and alcoholism. Undernutrition in nursing home patients has been reported in up to 50 percent of residents depending on the facility.

Food insecurity is defined by the US Department of Agriculture (USDA) as lack of access to enough food to fully meet basic needs at all times due to lack of financial resources. Households that are insecure, even when hunger is not present, have such limited resources that they may run out of food and cannot afford balanced meals. Hungry households have been defined as those that lack adequate financial resources to the point where family members, especially children, are hungry on a regular basis and adults' food intake is severely reduced.

According to the Census Bureau, 13 million US households (11.1 percent) experienced food insecurity for at least some time during 2007. This represented 36.2 million people, including 12.4 million children. Nationally, food insecurity is more prevalent in households with children under 6 years (15.8 percent) and food insecurity is lower for those without children (8.7 percent). Food insecurity increases generally among low-income households with children (41.5 percent). Households with WIC-eligible incomes experience food insecurity more than those with higher income levels. Studies have shown that the federally funded Women, Infants, and Children program (WIC) is an effective means of decreasing rates of food insecurity while positively influencing nutrient intakes.

Unfortunately, with the shift from welfare to work, many low-income working families who are eligible for Food Stamps do not participate in the program, leaving children more vulnerable to food insecurity than ever before. Bills have been introduced in Congress to improve the Food Stamp Program, to better target low-income working families and those making the transition from public assistance. Currently, there are approximately 38 million individuals eligible to participate in the Food Stamp Program.

Food insecurity and poor diet quality exist at unsettling levels throughout the United States despite attempts to create a food and nutrition safety net. Studies show that specific populations, including rural, low-income women with children, are at increased risk for experiencing food insecurity. Providing nutrition education to all food assistance program participants, including the benefits associated with the recommended intake of fruits and vegetables as well as the availability and affordability of fresh produce, should be a priority.

Overweight and Obesity

Health Consequences of Overweight and Obesity

Obesity is a complex, multi-factorial disease that is becoming increasingly common among adults and children worldwide. Once considered a problem only in developed countries, overweight and obesity are now dramatically on the rise in developing countries as well, particularly in urban settings. This is of particular concern for health professionals because according to a recent NIH study, obese individuals have 50 to 100 percent increased risk of premature death from all causes

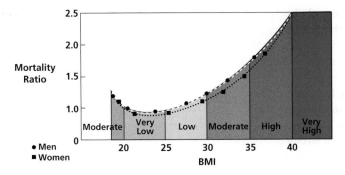

Figure 1-2 Obesity and Mortality Risk
Source: Bray GA. *Med Clin North Am.* 1989; 73(1):161–84.

compared to normal weight individuals. The National Heart, Lung, and Blood Institute (NHLBI) *Clinical Guidelines on the Identification, Evaluation, and Treatment of Overweight and Obesity in Adults* states, "next to smoking, obesity is the second leading cause of preventable death in the US today." Obese individuals have an increased risk of diabetes, coronary heart disease, hyperlipidemia, hypertension, stroke, gallbladder disease, sleep apnea, osteoarthritis, respiratory problems, and certain types of cancers (endometrial, breast, prostate, and colon), all of which increase their risk of mortality as shown in (Figure 1-2).

The life expectancy of a moderately obese person could be shortened by 2 to 5 years while the life expectancy of a morbidly obese man with a BMI greater than 40 kg/m² is likely to be reduced by almost thirteen years. The WHO predicts that deaths from diabetes complications will increase 50 percent worldwide in the next ten years. Cardiovascular diseases, mainly heart disease and stroke, are already the world's number one cause of death, killing over 17 million people each year. Obesity accounts for 5 to 7 percent of national health expenditures in the United States. A report from the non-profit business group Conference Board suggests obesity is costing United States businesses $45 billion annually in medical expenses and lost productivity. The NIH estimates total costs for obesity treatment to be approximately $117 billion.

There is strong evidence that a modest weight loss of 10 percent of body weight will result in a reduction of blood pressure, fasting glucose, and lipid levels. Treatment should be aggressive for obese individuals who have three or more of the following risk factors: cigarette smoking, hypertension, high LDL-cholesterol levels, low HDL-cholesterol levels, elevated fasting glucose levels, and/or family history of coronary heart disease and age over 45 and 55 years for men and women, respectively.

Etiology of Overweight and Obesity

The etiology of obesity can be explained by a combination of biological and environmental factors. Biological factors that have been identified include an individual's genetic predisposition, the size and number of adipose cells, and resting energy expenditure. Environmental factors that have been identified as contributory to overweight and obesity include excessive caloric intake and inadequate physical activity. These are the most likely environmental factors associated with the significant increase in overweight and obesity seen in the United States and developed countries over the past several decades.

Genetics In humans, 426 variants of 127 different genes have been associated with obesity. According to the latest update of the Human Obesity Gene Map, single mutations in 11 genes were strongly implicated in 176 cases of obesity worldwide. Additionally, 50 chromosomal locations have been mapped that contain genes that may be related to obesity. According to the CDC, "recently, several independent population-based studies reported that a gene of unknown function, referred to as fat mass and obesity-associated gene (FTO), may be responsible for up to 22 percent of all cases of obesity. Interestingly, the FTO gene also shows a strong association with diabetes. The mechanism by which FTO operates is currently under investigation."

Family history reflects genetic susceptibility and environmental exposures shared by close relatives. Genetic studies over the past several decades investigating adopted twins and their biological and adoptive parents show that adoptees' weight correlates most strongly with their biological parents' weight. Additional research has shown that children of one overweight parent have a 40 percent chance of becoming overweight as adults. This risk increases to 80 percent if both parents are overweight. Regardless of the strong evidence for genetic influences on human obesity, genetics accounts for no more than one-third of the variance in body weight. Experts agree that since there has been no change in the gene pool over the past three decades, the dramatic increase in the prevalence of obesity in both children and adults in the United States, likely reflects environmental influences.

Adipose Cell Size and Number The size and number of fat cells have been studied for many years and vary between normal, overweight, and obese individuals. During infancy, adolescence, and pregnancy, fat cells normally increase in number. With modest weight gain, fat cells increase in size, and with significant weight gain, fat cells increase in both size and number. With weight loss, fat cells decrease in size but not in number. The lack of reduction in fat cell number may help explain why it is difficult for obese individuals to maintain weight loss for an extended period of time after a significant weight loss.

Excess Caloric or Energy Intake Humans require energy (calories) to support normal metabolic functions, physical activity, and growth and repair of tissues. According to the latest National Health and Nutrition Examination Survey III (NHANES), Americans are eating 220 more calories per day compared to twenty years ago. This increase in calories can be partially attributed to a combination of increased portion sizes or "super-size" servings and the increased frequency of eating outside the home, especially at fast food restaurants. This calorie increase may also be secondary to increased body weight, which increases energy requirements.

Decreased Physical Activity The dramatic increase in sedentary activities and labor-saving devices (sitting at the computer, watching television, using the remote

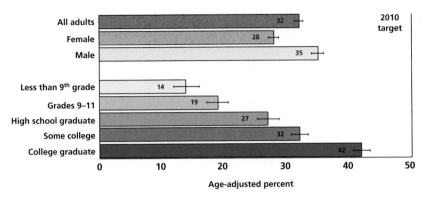

Figure 1-3 Adults Engaging in Physical Activity, by Gender and Education, 2000
Source: National Health Interview Survey, CDC, NCHS.

control, taking escalators, elevators, or moving sidewalks, using drive-through windows to pick up food, and using garage door openers as examples) have reduced the amount of energy we expend as a society. According to the Centers for Disease Control and Prevention (CDC), in 2006, 62 percent of adults never engaged in any periods of vigorous leisure-time physical activity (lasting 10 minutes or more per week) while only 24 percent engaged in such activity three or more times per week. Gender differences indicate that 57 percent of men do not meet this activity standard compared with 66 percent of women. Ethnic differences also exist. Fifty-eight percent of non-Hispanic white adults did not meet the standard compared with 67 percent of non-Hispanic black adults and 72 percent of Hispanic adults. In addition, the Behavioral Risk Factor Surveillance System indicates that participation in physical activity declines as people age.

Because regular physical activity modestly contributes to caloric expenditure, reduced abdominal fat, and increased cardio-respiratory fitness, it should be strongly encouraged, along with a reduced calorie diet, to improve the health of overweight and obese individuals. Recent studies from the National Weight Control Registry have indicated that regular physical activity is the single best predictor of long-term weight control in overweight and obese individuals who have lost weight.

Diagnosis and Assessment of Overweight and Obesity
Body Mass Index (BMI)
According to the NHLBI's *Clinical Guidelines*, BMI provides a more accurate measure of total body fat than body weight alone. The NHLBI *Clinical Guidelines* classify BMI as shown in Table 1-2. Since many people with a BMI of 25 kg/m^2 or greater begin to experience complications, such as elevated low-density lipoprotein cholesterol (LDL-C) and total cholesterol levels, high blood pressure, and glucose intolerance, as shown in Figure 1-2, the guidelines define overweight individuals as those with a BMI of 25 to 29.9 kg/m^2 and obese individuals as those with a BMI of 30 kg/m^2 and above.

Prevalence of Overweight and Obesity

According to the CDC, more than one-third of US adults or 72 million Americans were obese in 2005 to 2006. Although obesity prevalence has not measurably increased in the past few years, levels are still high at 34 percent of US adults aged 20 and over. Adults aged 40 to 59 have the highest obesity prevalence compared with other age groups. From an international perspective, the WHO stated in 2005 that more than 1.6 billion adults (ages 15 years and older) across the globe were overweight, and at least 400 million were obese. The CDC's Behavioral Risk Factor Surveillance System (BRFSS) shown in Figures 1-4 and 1-5 illustrates that during the past 20 years there has been a dramatic increase in US obesity rates. These two US maps from 1985 and 2007 demonstrate this trend by mapping the increased prevalence of obesity across each of the states. In 1985, there were thirteen states that had 10 percent or less prevalence of obesity; in 2007 no states had less than 10 percent prevalence of obesity. In 1985 no states had more than a 14 percent increase in prevalence of obesity. In 2007, only one state had a prevalence of obesity less than 20 percent. Also in 2007, twenty-three states had prevalence equal to or greater than 25 percent; two of these states, Mississippi, Tennessee and West Virginia, had a prevalence of obesity equal to or greater than 30 percent.

According to data based on NHANES 2001–2004, 133.6 million (66 percent) adults age 20 and older are overweight or obese (BMI > 25 kg/m^2), while 63.6 million (31.4 percent) of United States adults age 20 and older are obese (BMI > 30 kg/m^2). The prevalence has steadily increased over the years among both genders, all ages, all racial and ethnic groups, all educational levels, and all smoking levels.

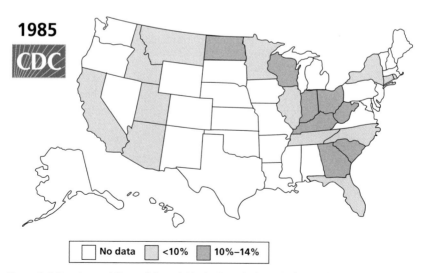

Figure 1-4 Prevalence of Overweight and Obesity Rates in the United States by State (1985). Source: Centers for Disease Control. National Center for Health Statistics. Prevalence of Overweight and Obesity Among Adults: US, 2003-2004. Available from http://www.cdc.gov.

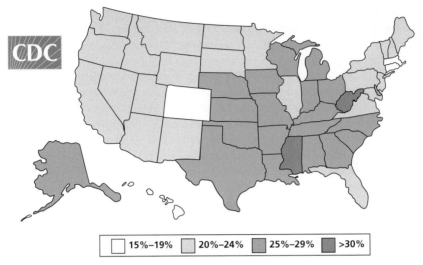

| 15%–19% | 20%–24% | 25%–29% | >30% |

Figure 1-5 Prevalence of Overweight and Obesity Rates in the United States by State (2007) Source: Centers for Disease Control. National Center for Health Statistics. Prevalence of Overweight and Obesity Among Adults: US. Available from http://www.cdc.gov.

Among women, the age-adjusted prevalence of overweight or obesity in racial and ethnic minorities is higher among non-Hispanic black and Mexican–American women than among non-Hispanic white women. Among men, the difference is less pronounced, as shown in Figure 1-6. For children and adolescents as well, overweight is defined as BMI above the 85th percentile and obesity is greater than the 95th percentile-for-age. Approximately 13.9 percent of children age 2 to 5, 18.8 percent of children age 6 to 11, and 17.4 percent of adolescents age 12 to 19 were obese in 2003–4, as shown in Figure 1-7.

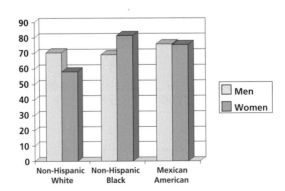

Figure 1-6 Prevalence of Obesity in Adults by Race/Ethnicity: Sources: Ogden CL, et al. *JAMA* 2006; 295:1549–1555.

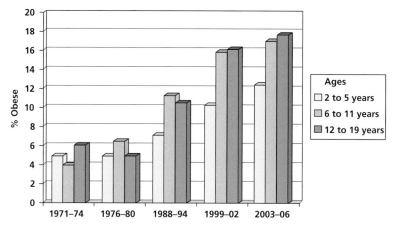

Figure 1-7 Prevalence Data of Obese Children and Adolescents By Age
Sources: Ogden CL. *JAMA* 2006;295(13):1549–55. Ogden CL, Carroll MD, Flegal KM.
JAMA. 2008;299(20):2401–2405.

Effective Counseling for Lifestyle and Behavior Change

Lifestyle and behavior changes often require many attempts, large and small, over many years. The first principle of behavior change is to understand the long-term nature of lifestyle changes, to encourage a person who has not met goals or has relapsed, and for health care providers who also can become discouraged with apparent lack of immediate success.

In making a change, people move through a series of steps: Precontemplation, Contemplation, Preparation, Action, Maintenance, and Relapse (Prochaska Stage of Change Model). This model is often used to clarify for people and their providers their readiness for change. Health care providers can provide information and motivational counseling to help patients move from one stage to another. Providers can help the patients by considering behavioral beliefs, such as personal perceived risk of negative outcome from the behavior, normative beliefs (similar behavior by family members and individuals important to them), and efficacy beliefs (they believe they can make the change). People often need skills (label reading and menu planning) to help turn their intention to action. Providers who model or perform a specific behavior are more likely to help patients perform this behavior. Reviewing barriers to a change, the circumstances of previous behavior change and relapse, and motivations to change can also provide useful insights to patients.

Important questions that could be asked of all patients seen for follow-up to assess their level of change include:

- How have you changed your diet or exercise since the last visit?
- What problems did you encounter in making these changes?
- Do you feel confident that you can maintain the changes you have made?
- What changes would you still like to make in your diet or exercise pattern to improve your health?
- How can I help you with these changes?

- What one behavior could you change that would result in the most significant change in your health?
- What one or two behaviors would you be unlikely to change now?

In conclusion, the value of nutrition assessment in the clinical care of both ambulatory and hospitalized patients cannot be overemphasized. Considering nutrition during the medical history and physical examination to evaluate growth and development in children and signs of nutrient excess or deficiencies in children and adults should be routine parts of clinical care. Development of a realistic treatment plan that includes lifestyle counseling can help patients change their behaviors and lead healthier lives.

Case 1 **Obesity and Metabolic Syndrome**

Xavier Pi-Sunyer

St. Luke's Roosevelt Hospital, New York, NY

OBJECTIVES

- Identify methods to appropriately diagnose obesity and the metabolic syndrome.
- Describe the metabolic and health consequences associated with being overweight or obese.
- Given the anthropometric and laboratory data, and usual diet of a patient, assess the patient's risk for metabolic complications associated with excess weight gain.
- Describe the components of a successful weight management program, including specific nutrition, physical activity, and behavioral recommendations.
- Describe the efficacy of medications (over-the-counter and prescription) and surgical approaches to the treatment of obesity.

RS is a 44-year-old African–American woman who works as a management consultant. She presents to her family physician with elevated blood pressure and obesity. She has a history of dieting but has been unable to maintain a healthy weight. This is approximately the twelfth time in the past 15 years she has tried a weight loss diet. RS states her weight problems began when she had her first child 18 years ago. Although she understands the medical consequences associated with being overweight, she is primarily motivated to lose weight for cosmetic reasons.

Past Medical History

RS has no past medical history of cardiovascular or gallbladder disease. (She has not had an EKG for the past 5 years). She takes no medications, vitamins, or herbal supplements although she states that she should be taking calcium. When asked about sleep disturbances, she admits to snoring at night, but denies waking up in the middle of the night or falling asleep during daytime activities.

Family History

The family history is positive for overweight and obesity. RS's one brother and a sister are overweight. Her father and another sister are normal weight. Her mother is obese, hypertensive, and had a myocardial infarction at the age of 67. RS states that her mother does not have diabetes although her blood glucose was elevated in a recent blood test.

Medical Nutrition and Disease: A Case-Based Approach, 4th edition. Edited by Lisa Hark.
© 2009 Wiley-Blackwell Publishing, ISBN: 978-1-4051-8615-5.

Social History

RS does not smoke. She averages two to three 4 ounce glasses of wine per week. She eats three meals per day and admits to nibbling whenever food is available at work or when she is bored. She states she has no time to exercise due to her work and family schedule. RS is currently at her highest adult weight.

Obstetrical history

RS delivered three healthy, full-term children, who are now 18, 13, and 10 years old. She gained 35 to 40 pounds (16 to 18 kg) with each pregnancy and lost about 20 pounds (9 kg) after each birth. RS has never been able to reach her pre-pregnancy weight.

Review of Systems

Skin: No history of rashes or unusual skin pigmentation
HEENT: No visual complaints
Neurologic: No headaches, tremors, seizures, or depression
Endocrine: Normal menstrual cycle; denies abnormal heat or cold intolerances
Cardiovascular: Normal rate and rhythm. No orthopnea, or dyspnea
Joints: No swelling, heat, or redness

Physical Examination
Vital signs

Temperature: 98.4 °F (36.9 °C)
Heart rate: 88 BPM
Blood pressure: 135/88 mm Hg
Height: 5′3″ (160 cm)
Current weight: 208 lbs (94.5 kg)
BMI: 36.8 kg/m^2
Waist circumference: 38 inches (96.5 cm)
Weight history: Her highest adult weight is her current weight while her lowest adult weight of 150 pounds (68 kg) was before she had children at age 25. Her weight has averaged 175 pounds (79.4 kg).

Exam

General: Obese woman in no acute distress; no cushingoid features, negative for hirsutism, no dorsal, cervical, or supraclavicular fat
Skin: No striae, no acanthosis nigricans
HEENT: Unremarkable
Neck: Nonpalpable thyroid
Chest: Clear
Heart: S$_1$ and S$_2$ normal rate and rhythm
Abdominal: Obese, no organomegaly
Extremities: No edema

Laboratory Data

Patient's Fasting Values	Normal Values
Glucose: 116 mg/dL	70–99 mg/dL
Potassium: 3.8 mEq/L	3.5–5.0 mEq/L
Cholesterol: 216 mg/dL	desirable <200 mg/dL
Triglycerides: 175 mg/dL	desirable <150 mg/dL
HDL-C: 42 mg/dL	desirable for female ≥50 mg/dL
Calculated LDL-C: 139 mg/dL	desirable <130 mg/dL

RS provides vague information on serving sizes particularly when she feels guilty about them. The following represents her usual diet:

Breakfast (home)

Coffee	8 ounces (240 mL)
Half and half cream	1 ounce (30 mL)
Bagel	1 large
Cream cheese	2 Tbsp.
Orange juice	8 ounces (240 mL)

Lunch (office)

Chef salad	2 cups
(Turkey, ham, cheese, boiled egg)	
French dressing	3 Tbsp.
Bread sticks	2 small
Iced tea (presweetened)	12 ounces (360 mL)

Snack (office)

Pretzels	1.5 ounce bag
Diet soda	12 ounces (360 mL)

Dinner (home)

Spaghetti	2 cups
Tomato sauce	½ cup
Beef meatballs	3 ounces (85 g)
Garlic bread	1 piece
Red wine	5 ounces (150 mL)

Snack (home)

Vanilla wafers	10 small
Lemonade	12 ounces (360 mL)

Total Calories: 2691 kcal
Protein: 94 g (14% of calories)
Fat: 90 g (30% of calories)
Saturated fat: 33 g (11% of calories)
Monounsaturated fat: 21 g (7% of calories)
Cholesterol: 334 mg
Carbohydrate: 355 g (53% of calories)
Dietary fiber: 13 g
Sodium: 4800 mg
Calcium: 601 mg

Case Questions

1. How are overweight and obesity clinically assessed in this patient?
2. What are the medical risks associated with obesity in this patient?
3. Does RS meet the criteria to diagnose metabolic syndrome?
4. What are the appropriate treatment goals for RS?
5. RS is interested in trying a high-protein, low-carbohydrate diet. Describe the biochemical and metabolic effects of high protein, low carbohydrate diets.
6. Is this popular diet appropriate for RS based on her medical history?
7. What dietary and exercise guidelines would you recommend for RS considering her diagnosis of metabolic syndrome and her current diet?
8. On a subsequent visit, RS is interested in medication for weight loss. Discuss the current criteria and options for pharmacologic therapy.

Answers to Questions: Case 1
Part 1: Assessment and Diagnosis

1. How are overweight and obesity clinically assessed in this patient?

Body mass index (BMI) is a useful clinical calculation for documenting obesity because it assesses the relative risk of excess weight. BMI is defined as weight/height^2 (kg/m^2).

The amount of intra-abdominal adipose tissue, independent of BMI, correlates strongly with increased risk of cardiovascular disease, stroke, dyslipidemia, hypertension, and type 2 diabetes in both men and women. Abdominal obesity can be assessed by measuring the patient's waist circumference, in the horizontal plane around the abdomen at the level of the iliac crest.

RS is clinically assessed as having Class 2 obesity since she has a BMI of 36.8 kg/m^2. In addition, she has excess adipose tissue located in her abdomen, as indicated by her waist circumference of 38 inches (96.5 cm), increasing her risk for heart disease and diabetes.

2. What are the medical risks associated with obesity in this patient?

Obesity increases a person's risk of developing cardiovascular disease, dyslipidemia, hypertension, type 2 diabetes, osteoarthritis, gallstones, respiratory disease, cholecystitis, and certain types of cancer. Obesity also increases a patient's risk during surgical procedures because increased subcutaneous fat can make surgery technically more difficult and prolongs the procedure. Post-operative complications are more common in obese patients.

Evidence exists to indicate that RS is experiencing some signs of physical stress related to obesity which include the following:

1. RS complains of snoring, which combined with obesity, places her at risk for sleep apnea in the future.
2. Borderline high LDL-C according to the Adult Treatment Panel (ATP III) (2001) Guidelines from the National Cholesterol Education Program (NCEP) (Chapter 6).
3. Elevated fasting glucose level, indicating impaired fasting glucose and suggesting impaired glucose tolerance and insulin resistance, although not frank diabetes. RS is at risk for type 2 diabetes due to the constellation of risk factors: obesity, abdominal fat distribution, sedentary lifestyle, and impaired glucose tolerance.
4. Elevated blood pressure adding to her risk of disease according to the Joint National Committee on Prevention, Detection, Evaluation, and Treatment of High Blood Pressure (JNC-VII).
5. Elevated triglyceride level and a low HDL-C level for a woman.

3. Does RS meet the criteria to diagnose metabolic syndrome?

Recent attention regarding risk for coronary heart disease has focused on a cluster of metabolic abnormalities that arise primarily out of obesity. According to the National Cholesterol Education Program (NCEP) Adult Treatment Panel III (ATP III) Guidelines, patients can be diagnosed with metabolic syndrome if they exhibit any three of the following five conditions (Table 1-10). (Note differences in low normal ranges for HDL-C cholesterol for men and women.) RS has all five of the criteria for metabolic syndrome.

Table 1-10 Diagnosing Metabolic Syndrome: 3 or More of the following 5 Criteria

Abdominal obesity	Waist circumference Men >40 inches Women >35 inches
Pre-Hypertension	BP >130/>85 mm Hg
Glucose intolerance	FBG >110 mg/dL
High triglycerides Low HDL-C	>150 mg/dL Men <40 mg/dL Women <50 mg/dL

Source: Adult Treatment Panel (ATP) III Guidelines. NCEP 2001 Report.

Part 2: Medical Nutrition Therapy

4. What are the appropriate treatment goals for RS?

The first line of treatment for patients with obesity and the metabolic syndrome is weight reduction and increased physical activity. However, one does not need to lose a lot of weight to be successful.

Weight Reduction: Clinical research has demonstrated that obese individuals who achieve and maintain a 10 percent reduction in body weight, regardless of initial BMI, are likely to lower their blood pressure, serum glucose, and LDL-cholesterol and triglyceride levels, thereby reducing their risk of developing diabetes and cardiovascular disease. The Diabetes Prevention Program (DPP), a national study comparing lifestyle changes to medication, found that type 2 diabetes can be prevented or delayed with just a 5 to 7 percent weight loss due to lifestyle changes. For a more complete review of the Diabetes Prevention Program (DPP), see Chapter 8; Case 2.

Lifestyle modifications may also prevent the onset of hypertension as well as reduce elevated blood pressure. RS has a blood pressure of 135/88 mm Hg. According to JNC VII, patients with a blood pressure in the high normal range of 130/85 to 139/89 mm Hg should begin an aggressive lifestyle modification program to lower blood pressure to less than 130/85 mm Hg to reduce their risk of cardiovascular disease.

A linear association has been demonstrated between excess body weight (BMI greater than 27 kg/m^2) and severity of hypertension. A mean weight loss of 20 pounds (9.2 kg) is associated with a 6.3 mm Hg reduction in systolic BP and a 3.1 mm Hg reduction in diastolic BP. In addition, weight loss enhances the blood pressure lowering effect of anti-hypertension medications.

The incidence of other health problems associated with obesity, such as sleep apnea and osteoarthritis, also decrease with moderate weight loss.

Thus, if RS were to lose 20 pounds (9.2 kg) or about 10 percent of her weight, it is likely that the clinical abnormalities associated with the metabolic syndrome will improve.

Increased Physical Activity: Exercise has been shown to be the single best predictor of long-term weight maintenance and therefore should always be encouraged for weight loss. Patients who participate in regular exercise have lower blood pressure levels as well as a reduced risk of cardiovascular disease and osteoporosis compared to those who do not exercise. The Centers for Disease Control and Prevention (CDC) recommend a minimum of 30 minutes a day of physical activity, five days a week for adults. The Institute of Medicine (IOM) currently recommends adults to reach one hour a day of exercise, which is consistent with the CDC'S recommendations for physical activity for children and teenagers. Current research indicates that this level of physical activity can be accumulated throughout the day. Both observational and interventional studies suggest that even brisk walking 3 hours per week can reduce the risk of cardiovascular disease and type 2 diabetes by at least 30 percent.

An active lifestyle has also been shown to prevent or delay the development of type 2 diabetes, since both moderate and vigorous exercise decrease the risk of impaired glucose tolerance and type 2 diabetes.

It is likely that the beneficial effects of exercise on the prevention of cardiovascular disease are associated with improvements in the metabolic syndrome. In hypertensive patients with hyperinsulinemia, regular exercise has consistently demonstrated a reduction in blood pressure levels. Regular exercise has also been shown to reduce levels of triglyceride-rich VLDL particles, and raise HDL-C levels.

5. RS is interested in trying a high-protein, low-carbohydrate diet. Describe the biochemical and metabolic effects of high-protein, low-carbohydrate diets.

High-protein, low-carbohydrate diets remain popular today: the most controversial being those that exclude almost all carbohydrate (less than 5 percent of total calories). These extremely low-carbohydrate diets, such as the Atkins diet, may consist of greater than 150 grams of protein, 100 grams of total fat (much of which is saturated fat), 500 mg cholesterol, and less than 28 grams of carbohydrate per day during the induction phase of the diet.

These diets cause the body to go into ketosis. Ketosis can be defined as an increased level of ketone bodies in the blood. Ketones are acetoacetic acid and beta-hydroxybutyric acid, which form from the breakdown of free fatty acids. Ketosis also occurs during starvation, but due to lack of calories and protein, significant lean body mass is lost. In the weight loss diets that try to promote ketosis, the dietary protein is excessive and therefore, lean body mass seems to be preserved (although research is sparse).

When ketone bodies build up in excess amounts in the blood (ketonemia), they spill into the urine (ketonuria) and are excreted as sodium or potassium salts, resulting in a net loss of these two minerals. In addition, excess dietary animal protein may also lead to hyperuricemia (increased uric acid in the blood) and hyperuricosuria (increased excretion of uric acid in the urine). This increases the patient's risk of developing gout, uric acid kidney stones, and possibly bone loss. It is therefore critical to drink at least 64 ounces (1920 mL) of water per day on such a high-protein diet, and maintain an adequate electrolyte intake.

The question then is why do people lose weight on high-protein, low-carbohydrate diets? Most experts agree that when patients adhere to any weight loss program, plan their meals, and focus on what and how much they are eating, they lose weight. In addition, when entire food groups, such as carbohydrates, are avoided, caloric intake is significantly reduced.

The rationale for this low-carbohydrate, high-protein diet is the theory that high-carbohydrate diets promote insulin resistance and cause obesity. Insulin resistance occurs as a result of increased body weight, lack of exercise, or medical conditions such as type 2 diabetes. Protein also stimulates insulin secretion. Consuming more calories than your body requires from any food source potentially leads to weight gain if not balanced with increased exercise.

6. Is this popular diet appropriate for RS based on her medical history?

Given the cardiovascular concerns and the lack of data from well-controlled studies, a ketogenic weight loss diet may not be appropriate for RS. If she feels that she is eating too many carbohydrates from starches and simple sugars, suggest that she become more aware of serving sizes, eat more vegetables and fruit and ingest her carbohydrates from predominantly whole grains.

On a ketogenic diet, when carbohydrates are reduced to 28 grams per day, fat and protein intake are significantly increased. Depending on the choice of protein-containing foods, a high saturated fat diet may result. It is well established from epidemiological data and clinical trials that a high saturated fat intake increases serum LDL-C levels and therefore the risk of cardiovascular disease. The current ATP III Therapeutic Lifestyle Changes Diet advocates less than 7 percent of the total calories coming from saturated fat, less than 200 milligrams of cholesterol and up to 20 percent of calories from monounsaturated fat per day (Chapter 6).

In addition, in order to keep carbohydrates low enough so that ketosis occurs, fruits, fruit juices, grains and dairy products are severely limited or avoided. Therefore these diets may be lacking in vitamins (A, B, C, D) and minerals (calcium). Patients are advised in these ketogenic diet books to take many vitamin and mineral supplements.

The Dietary Approaches to Stop Hypertension (DASH) diet, an excellent diet evaluated in a multi-center randomized, controlled trial that assessed the effects of dietary patterns on blood pressure, supports eating plenty of fruits, vegetables, and dairy foods for patients with high blood pressure. This trial enrolled 459 adults with mean base-line blood pressure levels of 131.3/84.7 mm Hg. Subjects were randomized to the control diet rich in fruits and vegetables with an average fat content or a combination diet with low-fat dairy and reduced total and saturated fat. Results showed a 5.5 mm Hg greater decrease in systolic pressure and 3.0 mm Hg greater decrease in diastolic pressure with the intervention diet as compared to the control diet. The average sodium intake was 3000 mg/day. Reduction in blood pressure began within two weeks and was maintained for the duration of the study. Further blood pressure reductions were achieved with sodium restriction.

7. What dietary and exercise guidelines would you recommend for RS considering her diagnosis of metabolic syndrome and her current diet?

Considering the fact that RS has tried unsuccessfully to diet twelve times over the past fifteen years, it is important to assess what RS feels is her biggest vulnerability and also what lifestyle changes she is willing to incorporate. RS needs to focus on decreasing her total caloric intake and increasing her level of physical activity to lose weight and improve her metabolic syndrome.

Dietary Goals: Specifically, RS would benefit from decreasing her consumption of saturated fat, simple carbohydrates, sodium and low fiber foods intake. The current IOM report recommends 45 to 65 percent of total calories coming from carbohydrates and 20 to 35 percent from fat. Because of the beneficial effects of increasing monounsaturated fat (MUFA) on triglyceride and HDL-C levels, RS could replace saturated fat with MUFA by using olive oil on her salad instead of French dressing and substituting low-fat cream cheese for the full-fat varieties. Snacking on hummus and raw carrots rather than pretzels, crackers, or cookies should also be suggested. She could also choose carbohydrate-containing, high fiber foods such as fresh fruits, vegetables, and whole grain breads instead of bagels and pasta. RS needs to be counseled on reducing her serving size of pasta. She can add cooked frozen vegetables to her spaghetti to fill her up at dinner. Water and other non-caloric drinks should be substituted for sugar-sweetened drinks or fruit juice, as these drinks are contributing a significant number of empty calorie carbohydrates to her diet.

As shown in the revised menu, we recommend that RS substitute a small amount of peanut butter, a good source of MUFA and protein, rather than butter or cream cheese at breakfast. We also suggest she skip the cheese and egg yolk on the Chef's salad at lunch. Turkey, boiled ham, and egg whites are good sources of lean, low fat protein. If RS skips the garlic bread with dinner and limits her pasta to one cup cooked, she will be successful in decreasing calories, carbohydrate, saturated fat, and cholesterol. By adding vegetables RS will improve the nutritional value of her diet while keeping total calories low. Finally, RS should be advised to take a calcium supplement (500 mg per day) since her calcium intake is far below her daily requirement of 1200 mg per day.

Physical Activity Goals

RS states that she does not have time to exercise due to her work and children's schedule. She currently works as a management consultant and travels several times a month. Therefore, in order to realistically encourage RS to increase her activity, it would be helpful to address these time barriers and to help her identify strategies to achieve increased physical activity. When she is traveling and does not have child care responsibilities, she could walk if she brings her exercise clothes and sneakers. When she is at home, she might be able to take a walk at night after dinner, or she could walk during her lunch break at work. In RS's case, she can benefit from using a pedometer that measures the number of steps taken each day. Metabolic fitness goals could be set at five thousand steps (or 30 minutes) per day, which can be gradually achieved over time. Keeping a record of her exercise may help RS stick with her commitment.

Realistic Weight Goals

The healthcare provider should discuss the appropriate rate of weight loss. A safe rate of weight loss is 1 to 2 pounds or 1 percent of body weight per week. RS's current weight is 208 pounds (94.3 kg), and she is 63 inches (160 cm) tall. If RS is able to adhere to these dietary recommendations and increase her physical activity, she should be able to reduce her weight by 10 to 20 pounds (4.5 to 9.0 kg) over a period of 6 months. Studies have shown that weight loss slows or stops after about the 24th week of most diets. This "plateau" occurs because the calories consumed and energy expended are now sufficient to maintain, rather than allow for additional weight loss.

After attaining this goal, a new weight goal can be negotiated. Since RS would like to lose more, it is helpful to reiterate how much healthier she will be when she meets her first goal, and the fact that she is very successful if she maintains that weight loss. A potential next goal of 175 pounds (79.4 kg) can be set.

Recommended revised diet for weight loss:
Breakfast (Home)
Coffee	8 ounces (240 mL)
Whole grain bread	1 slice
Peanut butter	1 Tbsp.
Low fat milk (1%)	4 ounces (120 mL)
Banana	1 small

Lunch (office)
Chef salad (no cheese)	2 cups
(Turkey, ham, egg whites,	
tomato, raw broccoli)	
Olive oil	2 Tbsp.
Balsamic vinegar	2 Tbsp.
Diet soda or water	12 ounces (360 mL)

Snack (office)
Hummus	4 Tbsp.
Raw carrots	2 ounces (57 g)
Water	8 ounces (240 mL)

Dinner (home)
Spaghetti	1 cup
Mixed vegetables	10 ounces (283 g)
Lean beef meatballs	3 ounces (85 g)
Water	8 ounces (240 mL)

Snack (home)
Fat-free yogurt	8 ounces (240 mL)

Total Calories: 1506 kcal
Protein: 78 g (20% of calories)
Fat: 59 g (34% of calories)
Saturated fat: 11 g (7% of calories)
Monounsaturated fat: 29 g (17% of calories)
Carbohydrate: 178 g (46% of calories)
Dietary fiber: 34 g
Sodium: 1934 mg
Calcium: 785 mg

Part 3: Pharmacotherapy Options

8. On a subsequent visit, RS is interested in medication for weight loss. Discuss the current criteria and options for pharmacologic therapy.

Pharmacological interventions to facilitate weight loss include enhancing satiety, decreasing fat absorption, and decreasing appetite. Two medications for weight loss are currently approved by the FDA for long-term use: Meridia (sibutramine) and Xenical (orlistat). It is important to note that although most people consider stopping the drug after weight loss has resulted, this may precipitate regaining weight. Similarly, it would be inappropriate to stop a cholesterol lowering medication after blood cholesterol has been reduced or to discontinue a hypertension medication because blood pressure has normalized.

It is also important to note that both sibutramine and orlistat have very low abuse potential and both have good safety records. However, weight reduction with either of these medications is modest (7 to 11 pounds or 3 to 5 kg) over a one-year period. Orlistat can now be obtained over-the-counter under the name Alli, in a 60-mg dose. Other over-the-counter weight loss dietary supplements are available but their safety and efficacy are not assured by clinical trials.

Sibutramine (Meridia): Sibutramine is a serotonin and norepinephrine re-uptake inhibitor (SNRI). Research shows that this drug reduces body weight by decreasing food intake. Research findings in humans indicate that patients receiving 10 to 15 mg/day of sibutramine had a 6 to 8 percent weight loss compared to a 2 percent weight loss with placebo. This drug is indicated for patients with a BMI greater than 30 kg/m^2 or greater than 27 kg/m^2 in the presence of risk factors. Sibutramine is prescribed in the following dosages: 5, 10, or 15 mg once per day. It may be taken in the morning to reduce any effect of insomnia; however, the medication is best prescribed based on the patient's high risk eating time as the medication seems to peak at about seven hours in the fed state.

Since sibutramine is a serotonergic medication, it should be monitored in patients who are also taking Selective Serotonin-Reuptake Inihibitors (SSRIs) (e.g. Paxil, Zoloft, fluoxetine). Sibutramine is contraindicated in patients who take Monoamine Oxidase (MAO) Inhibitors or those patients with poorly controlled hypertension, history of coronary artery disease, congestive heart failure, arrhythmia, or stroke. Regular BP and heart rate monitoring is required since norepinephrine effects can increase heart rate (four beats per minute in clinical studies) and cause small increases in systolic and diastolic pressure (2 to 4 mm Hg). The long-term effects of these changes are unknown. Other common side effects include dry mouth and constipation. In one double-blind, two-year study, weight loss was better maintained at one year and HDL-cholesterol was raised significantly in those subjects prescribed sibutramine compared with those taking placebo.

Orlistat (Xenical): Orlistat's activity occurs in the small intestine and promotes weight loss by inhibiting gastric and pancreatic lipases, thus partially blocking the hydrolysis of triglycerides. Thirty percent of ingested fat is unabsorbed and excreted in the stool. Patients are required to follow a low-fat diet ($\leq$30 percent) in order to minimize side effects, specifically steatorrhea, associated with fat malabsorption. Orlistat is prescribed at a dose of 120 mg TID with meals containing fat. Because fat-soluble vitamins may also be malabsorbed, a multivitamin should be prescribed once per day to be taken at least two hours before or after the medication. Xenical is contraindicated for pregnant and lactating women and those with chronic malabsorption syndromes and cholestasis. In a two-year study, patients given Xenical lost more weight, maintained more weight loss and reduced serum cholesterol, LDL-cholesterol, and blood pressures compared with those subjects taking a placebo.

It is incumbent upon the physician to bring the patient back for a follow-up visit within a month in order to assess the effectiveness of the medication as well as any side effects. One criterion of success for either medication is a 4 pound (1.8 kg) weight loss in the first month. If this has not occurred it is important for the physician and patient to re-evaluate the effectiveness of the medication for improvement in behavior, adherence, etc.

Case 2 **Obesity and Bariatric Surgery**

Doina Kulick[1] and Vicki Bovee[2]

[1] University of Nevada School of Medicine, Reno, NV
[2] Western Bariatric Institute, Reno, NV

OBJECTIVES

- Describe the indications for bariatric surgery. Enumerate the commonly used bariatric operations, and provide an overview of the mechanisms by which these surgeries produce weight loss.
- Describe the components of a successful surgical weight management program, and review the efficacy of surgical approach to the treatment of obesity and its co-morbidities.
- Describe the nutritional and clinical management of bariatric patient.

CG is a 54-year-old Caucasian woman with past medical history significant for extreme obesity, diabetes mellitus, obstructive sleep apnea (OSA), hypertension, and dyslipidemia who presents to her primary care physician to ask if bariatric surgery could be an option for her. CG feels that her health is deteriorating continuously, and she believes that the current medical treatments are not controlling her health problems. CG was told at the previous visit, 3 months ago, that she needs to start insulin therapy to better manage her diabetes, but the patient was very reluctant to start it. She also rejoined a low-calorie diet program at the University Weight Management Clinic. In spite of CG's motivation she was only able to lose four pounds during these three months, and her blood glucose levels have not improved. She was also given an appetite suppressant, but was forced to stop 2 weeks later because it gave her palpitations, and her systolic blood pressure went up 8 mmHg.

CG also complains of increase daytime sleepiness and fatigue, worsening shortness of breath, and edema of both lower extremities. She was diagnosed with obstructive sleep apnea (OSA) eight years ago and was placed on Continuous Positive Airway Pressure (CPAP). The pressure of her CPAP machine has been gradually titrated up. Two weeks ago she saw a pulmonologist who increased the CPAP pressure to 20 cm H_2O.

Past Medical History and Medications

- Obesity; CG has been "heavy" all her life and had enrolled in numerous weight loss programs (commercial and medically supervised) with only minor and transitory success.

Medical Nutrition and Disease: A Case-Based Approach, 4th edition. Edited by Lisa Hark.
© 2009 Wiley-Blackwell Publishing, ISBN: 978-1-4051-8615-5.

- Type 2 diabetes for 22 years. She is treated with Metformin 2000 mg/day, glipizide 40 mg/day, and pioglitazone (Actos) 30 mg/day which was added one year ago. Her last HgbA1c, three months ago, was 8.6 percent.
- Sleep apnea for 8 years. She is treated with CPAP 20 cm H_2O.
- Hypertension for 18 years. She is treated with lisinopril 80 mg/day, labetalol 900 mg twice/day, amlodipine 10 mg once a day, and hydrochlorothiazide 25 mg/day.
- Dyslipidemia for 20 years. She is treated with simvastatin 80 mg/day.
- Gastro esophageal reflux disease (GERD) diagnosed 14 years ago, treated with omeprazole 40 mg/day.
- Severe degenerative joint disease affecting both knees for the last 6 years. She is currently treated with acetaminophen/hydrocodone, with only minimal pain relief.
- Laparoscopic cholecystectomy for symptomatic gallstones, 10 years ago.

Family History

CG's family history is positive for overweight and obesity, hypertension, diabetes mellitus, stroke, and coronary artery disease. CG's one brother and mother are both obese; her father and a sister are overweight. Her mother has diabetes and hypertension, and had a myocardial infarction at the age of 69. Her father is hypertensive and had a stroke at the age of 68. Her brother has diabetes.

Social History

CG never smoked. She drinks two to three 12 ounce bottles of beer per month. She uses no illegal drugs. It was recommended that she follow a diabetic diet, but she feels she is not doing a very good job at this. She states she has no time to exercise due to her work schedule and cannot do much because of the pain in her knees. She works at a loan office; she is happily remarried and has two children from her first marriage.

Diet History

Breakfast - She eats this meal 3 to 4 times per week at work and skips breakfast the other days. When she does eat breakfast, it typically consists of a breakfast burrito with bacon or one 5 ounce bagel with 2 Tbsp. regular cream cheese; coffee, (24 Fluid ounces), with flavored creamer
Snack - Granola bar or cereal bar
Lunch - Fast food on workdays (1/4 lb. hamburger or crispy chicken sandwich, medium French fries, 32 ounces ice tea with Splenda)
Snack - Candy bar, 100 calorie cookie snack packs;12 fluid ounce diet soda
Dinner - Home cooked meals 3 to 4 times/week, take-out or restaurant meals for the rest of the days: chicken breast or other kind of meat, baked or broiled, 4 to 6 ounces; 1 to 1 1/2 cups pasta from a box mix; 1 cup vegetables with butter, usually corn or green beans; water; dessert 2 times per week, usually 1 cup regular ice cream, no toppings

Snack - 2 to 3 medium commercial cookies or 1 to 2 cups wheat crackers
Bedtime Snack -1.5 cups Cheerios with 2 percent milk (6 fluid ounces)
No nocturnal eating

Daily caloric and macronutrient extrapolation from food history:
Total Calories: 2700 kcal
Protein: 100 g (15% of calories)
Fat: 110 g (35% of calories)
Saturated fat: 35 g (12% of calories)
Monounsaturated fat: 32 g (11% of calories)
Carbohydrate: 345 g (50% of calories)
Dietary fiber: 23 g

Review of Systems
General: Fatigue
Skin: Venous stasis dermatitis involving both ankles
HEENT: No visual complaints; last diabetic eye examination done 10 months ago showed mild non-proliferative diabetic retinopathy.
Neurologic: Occasional headaches responding to Tylenol, no tremors, seizures, or depression
Endocrine: Irregular menstrual cycles, last mensus was 10 months ago, denies abnormal heat or cold intolerances.
Gastrointestinal: Heartburns, normal bowel movements
Cardiovascular: No palpitations, no orthopnea, no chest pain; the patient had a stress echocardiogram 6 months ago when she presented to ER with chest pain (CP); the test showed no ischemia and a normal left ventricular ejection fraction, and the CP was determined to be due to GERD.
Joints: Pain both knees; patient had an intra-articular steroid injection in her right knee 2 months ago.

Physical Examination
Vital signs
Temperature: 98.4 °F (36.9 °C)
Heart rate: 80 BPM
Blood pressure: 145/98 mm Hg
Height: 5'8" (173 cm)
Current weight: 294 lbs (134 kg)
BMI: 44.7 kg/m^2

General: Obese woman in no acute distress; Pickwickian body habitus, no Cushingoid features
HEENT: No palpable thyroid; no acanthosis nigricans
Respiratory: Lungs clear to auscultation bilaterally
CV: Distant heart sounds, regular rhythm, no murmur heard
Abdominal: Abdomen soft, normal bowel sounds, difficult deep palpation due to subcutaneous adipose tissue, but no hepatomegaly or mass appreciated

Extremities: 2+ pitting edema involving both ankles
Skin: Brownish pigmented skin of both ankles

Laboratory Data

Patient's Fasting Values	**Normal Values**
Glucose: 156 mg/dL	70–99 mg/dL
Potassium: 3.8 mEq/L	3.5–5.0 mEq/L
Cholesterol: 216 mg/dL	Desirable <200 mg/dL
Triglycerides: 308 mg/dL	Desirable <150 mg/dL
HDL-C: 42 mg/dL	Desirable ≥50 mg/dL
Calculated LDL-C: 112 mg/dL	Desirable <100 mg/dL
Hemoglobin A1C 8.3%	<7.0%
Thyroid-stimulating hormone (TSH): 3.4	0.5–5.0 μU/mL
Free thyroxin (T4): 1.8 ng/dL	0.9–2.4 ng/dL

A stress echocardiogram two weeks ago shows no left ventricular wall motion abnormalities; left ventricular ejection fraction of 60 percent; right atrial and ventricular enlargement, diagnosed as pulmonary hypertension.

Case Questions

1. Does CG meet the criteria for bariatric surgery?
2. CG wants to know what are the commonly performed types of bariatric surgery.
3. What could we tell CG about the expected benefits and risks of bariatric surgery?
4. There are several bariatric surgeons in the area where CG lives. She is asking her primary care physician to help her choose "the best." What should be the advice regarding this issue?
5. Describe the pre-surgical nutritional evaluation of CG.
6. Should CG lose weight before the surgery?
7. What is the nutritional impact of bariatric surgery?
8. CG undergoes laparoscopic RYGB. No surgical and peri-operative complications occur. Outline the nutritional and medical management of this patient for the first three months following the surgery.
9. CG comes to the Bariatric Center for her six-month follow-up visit. She complains of nausea, shaking, diaphoresis, and diarrhea after eating. What is the most likely cause of these symptoms and how should she be treated?
10. Outline the long-term nutritional and medical management of this patient.

Answers to Questions: Case 2
Part 1: Screening and Procedure Options

1. Does CG meet the criteria for bariatric surgery?

The indications for the surgical management of obesity are outlined in NHLBI's *The Clinical Guidelines on the Identification, Evaluation, and Treatment of Overweight and Obesity in Adults: The Evidence Report*. Adults with a BMI 40 or 35 kg/m² with co-morbid conditions (diabetes, sleep apnea, obesity-related cardiomyopathy, or severe joint disease) may be candidates for bariatric surgery. In addition, they must have acceptable risk for surgery and have failed previous non-surgical weight loss interventions. It is also very important that potential bariatric patients understand the role of bariatric surgery in treating obesity, and display commitment to enduring lifestyle changes. Contraindications to bariatric surgery include patients with untreated major depression or psychosis, binge eating disorders, ongoing drug and alcohol abuse, severe cardiovascular diseases with prohibitive operative risks, severe coagulopathy, or inability to comply with nutritional requirements including life-long vitamin replacement. Age alone should not preclude surgical treatment for obesity in adult men and women. Review of the literature shows that bariatric surgery in adolescents (age 12–18) is safe and is associated with significant weight loss, correction of obesity comorbidities, and improved self-image and socialization.

CG has a BMI of 44.7 kg/m², which alone would qualify her for bariatric surgery. In addition, she has significant comorbidities: diabetes mellitus (poorly controlled on oral medication), uncontrolled hypertension, sleep apnea (severe symptoms and pulmonary hypertension in spite of recent titration of the pressure on her CPAP to the upper limit), and debilitating degenerative joint disease. Possible secondary causes for obesity (hypothyroidism and Cushing syndrome) have been excluded by clinical evaluation and blood work. She has diligently undergone multiple lifestyle and pharmaceutical interventions, with modest and transitory success. She has no history or current use of illicit drugs or alcohol, and she appears to have a good family support system. In addition, the psychological evaluation also showed that CG has no signs of depression or eating disorders, and that she is very motivated to proceed with the surgery. Her operative risk assessment indicates she is an acceptable candidate for bariatric surgery.

2. CG wants to know the commonly used types of bariatric surgery.

Bariatric surgery encompasses several operative techniques that could be classified based on the main mechanism of weight loss in primarily restrictive or malabsorptive procedures (Table 1-xx). The restrictive procedures limit caloric intake by decreasing the stomach's capacity. Currently, the most commonly used restrictive procedure in the United States is the laparoscopic adjustable gastric band (as shown in Figure 1-8). Used in Europe and Australia for almost two decades, this procedure was approved by the FDA in June 2001. Gastric banding has rapidly gained popularity among patients and surgeons, primarily because of its simplicity and lower complication rates when compared to more involved procedures such as Roux-en-Y gastric bypass (RYGB). The band consists of a hollow silicone ring, and is placed just

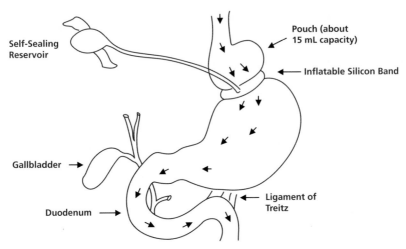

Figure 1.8 Laparoscopic Adjustable Gastric Banding (LAP-BAND). An Inflatable Silicone Band is Placed Around the Gastric Cardia to Achieve a 15-mL Gastric Pouch with an Adjustable Outlet that is Determined by the Volume of Fluid Inserted into the Band Reservoir. The Reservoir is Placed in the Subcutaneous Tissue of the Upper Abdomen, and can be Easily Accessed with a Syringe, Under Local Anesthesia (the Small Arrows Show the Path of the Ingested Food)
Source: Doina Kulick, MD, FACP. Used with Permission.

a few centimeters below the cardia of the stomach, creating a 15 mL gastric pouch. The band is connected to an infusion port placed in the subcutaneous tissue of the upper abdominal wall. The port may be accessed with relative ease by a syringe and needle, under topical anesthesia. Injection of saline into the port leads to reduction in the band diameter, which results in an increased degree of gastric restriction.

Other procedures have both restrictive and malabsorptive components. RYGB is a classic example: even though it is primarily a restrictive operation in which a small gastric pouch limits food intake, the small bowel reconfiguration produces mild malabsorption. There are possibly some neuronal and gut hormonal changes as well, all of which provide additional mechanisms to facilitating weight loss. RYGB is still the most common bariatric surgery performed in the United States, and is considered the "gold standard" (see Figure 1-9).

The malabsorptive techniques produce primarily a decrease in the efficiency of nutrient absorption by shortening the length of the functional small intestine. Even though these procedures promote significant weight loss, the nutritional and metabolic complications, such as protein-caloric malnutrition and various micronutrient deficiencies, often offset the benefits of weight loss. All the above mentioned procedures can be performed by minimally invasive techniques. The laparoscopic approach offers the advantages of decreased post-operative pain, shorter hospital stay, and decreased rates of wound infection and hernia formation. Currently there are no guidelines or algorithms for choosing the most appropriate type of surgical procedure for the patient. The choice is based on clinical judgment, patient and surgeon preferences, patient's surgical risk, and reimbursement issues. After discussing it with her physician, nutrition specialist, and the bariatric surgeon, CG chooses to undergo RYGB (Table 1-11).

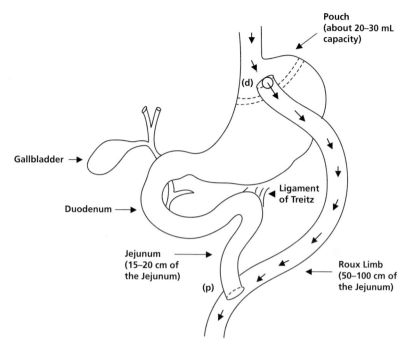

Figure 1.9 Roux-en-Y Gastric Bypass: The Stomach is Stapled Just Beneath the Gastroesophageal Junction. The Small Bowel (jejunum) is Divided Approximately 30 cm Distal to Ligament of Treitz. The Distal Cut End of the Small Bowel (d) is Anastomosed to the Proximal Gastric Pouch. The Proximal Cut End of the Small Bowel (p) is Anastomosed to the Limb 40 cm Distal to the Gastrojejunostomy (the Small Arrows Show the Path of the Ingested Food).
Source: Doina Kulick, MD, FACP. Used with Permission.

Table 1-11 Types of bariatric procedures

Restrictive
– Laparoscopic adjustable gastric band
– Vertical banded gastroplasty
– Intragastric balloon

Primary Restrictive with a malabsorptive component
– Roux-en-Y gastric bypass

Malabsorptive
– Biliopancreatic diversion with duodenal switch
– Jejunoileal bypass
– Biliopancreatic diversion

Source: Doina Kulick MD, FACP and Vicki Bovee, MD. Used with permission.

3. What could we tell CG about the expected benefits and risks of bariatric surgery?

Bariatric surgery is not a cure for obesity, but is the most effective modality currently available for weight management, and was proven in prospective studies to reduce morbidity and mortality in obese patients. A meta-analysis published in 2004 showed that the average percentage of weight loss was 61.2 percent (95 percent Confidence Interval (CI) of 58.1–64.4 percent) for all patients; 47.5 percent (95 percent CI of 40.7–54.2 percent) for patients who underwent gastric banding; 61.6 percent (95 percent CI of 56.7–66.5 percent) for gastric bypass; and 70.1 percent (66.3–73.9 percent) for biliopancreatic diversion or duodenal switch.

In general, after RYGB, patients lose an average of 1/2 to 1 pound (0.22–0.45 kg) daily for the first 3 months, 1/4 to 1/2 pound (0.11–0.22 kg) daily from 3 to 9 months, and 1/4 pound (0.11 kg) daily thereafter for up to 12 to18 months. This analysis also shows that type 2 diabetes mellitus was completely resolved in almost 80 percent of patients, and hyperlipidemia improved in 70 percent of patients. About 61 percent of patients can be taken off or have discontinued their blood pressure medication and obstructive sleep apnea resolves in 86 percent of patients.

You could inform CG that she could expect to lose approximately 90 to 100 pounds (or one-third of her pre-operative weight) within 12 to 18 months after undergoing the RYGB procedure. This weight loss would bring her body weight to 196 pounds (BMI <30 kg/m^2), which is a change in classification from extreme obesity to overweight. Her diabetes mellitus, hyperlipidemia, hypertension, and obstructive sleep apnea would likely improve significantly following bariatric surgery.

Regarding mortality data after bariatric surgery, a recent meta-analysis shows that the early (less than 30 days) and late (more than 30 days and up to 2 years) mortality rates after bariatric surgery are low. Mortality in the first 30 days post-operative was 0.07 percent (95 percent CI, 0.02–0.12) for the laparoscopic restrictive procedures; 0.16 percent (95 percent CI, 0.09–0.23) for laparoscopic restrictive/malabsorptive (gastric bypass); and 1.11 percent (95 percent CI, 0.00–2.70) for laparoscopic malabsorptive.

4. There are several bariatric surgeons in the area where CG lives. She is asking her primary care physician to help her choose "the best." What should be the advice regarding this issue?

A successful long-term outcome of bariatric surgery is dependent on the patient's understanding of the role of bariatric surgery in weight management and his/her commitment to a lifetime of dietary and lifestyle changes. Bariatric surgery is only a point in the continuum of care for obesity and the patient will need adequate support. Thus CG should be advised to seek a bariatric surgeon who operates as part of an experienced and knowledgeable multidisciplinary team of health-care providers. This team will provide the pre-operative and post-operative education and health care. Usually the team consists of the following health professionals:

Obesity specialist: An internist, endocrinologist, or a physician nutrition specialist who has a special interest and training in obesity. This physician, in close collaboration with the other health professionals team members, coordinates the peri-operative care in order to optimize the patient's co-morbidities and reduce the surgical risk and adjust medical treatments in accordance with the rapidly changing metabolic status following surgery (especially for the procedures containing a malabsorptive component). This physician may also follow-up with patients annually, often in close collaboration with the patient's primary care physician.

Bariatric Surgeon: A bariatric surgeon is a surgeon with special training in bariatric surgery, who has substantial experience with the procedure, but also with the pre- and post-operative management of severely obese patients. Bariatric surgery is considered one of the most challenging procedures performed by general surgeons. Recent studies that look at outcomes after bariatric surgical procedures found that the surgeon's experience inversely correlated with the incidence of post-operative complications.

Registered Dietitian: A very important member of the bariatric team. As mentioned, bariatric surgery does not cure obesity, but significantly facilitates the patient's adherence to long-lasting lifestyle changes. Thus the decision to operate must include an assessment of the patients' dietary habits, and his/her ability to comply with the post-operative dietary regimen. A dietitian performs a pre-op dietary assessment and provides instructions to help patients initiate dietary changes consistent with surgery. In anticipation of surgery, the dietitian helps patients prepare their kitchens with the needed appliances (e.g., food processor, blender, and standardized measuring cups and spoons) and appropriate foods for a transition diet upon discharge from the hospital. He/she also provides counseling for patients as they advance their diet during the early (3 months) post-operative period, and periodically thereafter, especially when the patient has difficulties in meeting his/her nutritional goals.

Psychologist: Psychological testing is a recommended part of the pre-operative assessment. Almost half of the patients referred for bariatric surgery may present with one of the following diagnoses: somatization, social phobia, obsessive–compulsive disorder, substance abuse/dependence, binge-eating disorder, night eating syndrome, post-traumatic stress disorder, generalized anxiety disorder, and depression. The psychologist may use various psychological tests and tools (the Beck Depression Inventory or the Minnesota Multiphasic Personality Inventory, the Boston interview for gastric bypass, or the structured clinical interview with the Weight and Lifestyle Inventory from the University of Pennsylvania) to reveal potential problems, and help patients adopt new lifestyle behavior changes needed for a successful long-term surgical outcome.

Primary care physician (PCP): The PCP needs to become an active member of the team in the peri-operative stage, and most importantly facilitate the long-term care of the bariatric patient. Many times it is the PCP who will see the patient annually for his/her post-op evaluation, and will refer the patient to the nutrition specialist and dietitian whenever he /she considers appropriate follow-up is indicated.

Part 2: Pre-Surgery Nutrition Assessment

5. Describe the pre-surgical nutritional evaluation of CG.

Ideally, the medical assessment of patients considering bariatric surgery should be done, as mentioned before, by a multidisciplinary team of health care professionals from the fields of nutrition, medicine, psychiatry, and surgery, who have special interest and expertise in bariatric surgery. This detailed assessment helps determine if the patient meets the recommended criteria for bariatric surgery. Furthermore, it aids in assessment of the patient's dietary risk factors that may diminish long-term successful weight loss or influence the long-term complications.

CG was evaluated and approved for surgery and her operative risk was assessed as being low to moderate. A comprehensive nutritional evaluation of CG shows the following: CG has been "heavy" all her life, and is now at the highest weight of her adult life. Her lowest adult body weight was 150 pounds at the age of 20, just before she got married (when she underwent a 16-week low-calorie diet program). She has gained weight progressively since that time, with spurts related to pregnancies and family/social stressor events. CG has enrolled in numerous commercial and medically supervised weight loss programs (more than a dozen times over last 34 years) with only minor and transitory success. She has also used prescription weight loss drugs four times in the last 34 years, most recently when she enrolled in a university medically supervised weight loss program. The pharmacotherapy was always of brief duration (2 to 4 weeks) because of side effects (palpitations, anxiety, GI side effects).

A food record is used to estimate food intake over a period of days and appears to be more reflective of eating patterns than a 24-hour recall. The food record reveals that because of her work schedule, she frequently eats out or skips meals. For greater compliance to dietary recommendations after surgery, it is critical to have an understanding of meal patterns, eating habits, and typical foods consumed. With this information, plus an estimation of nutrient intake, the dietitian can work with the patient to develop pre-operative goals that will set a foundation for post-operative eating. Information about current physical activity and/or exercise habits, and perceived obstacles to successful weight management, are also very important.

CG's diet is deficient in dairy foods, vegetables, and fruits. She appears to consume adequate protein and grains, however she eats sweets in excess. She has roughly 2 to 3 bottles of beer per month and her other drinks are usually calorie free. CG does not drink sufficient amounts of water. She takes no vitamin and/or mineral supplements. She is not participating in any intentional physical activity at this time due to knee pain. In addition to the lack of physical activity, she states that her biggest challenges in managing her weight are her sweet tooth, eating when bored, and not enough time for meal planning and preparation.

When asked about her support system for surgery, CG states that her children are very supportive of her decision but her husband is reluctant because of his expectations that her shopping habits and foods available in the home will change post-operatively. CG has two coworkers who have previously had weight loss surgery and she states that her friends at work have been answering her questions and are helping her prepare for surgery.

The patient displays the following behaviors associated with increased risk of surgery failure: high intake of high-fat foods, high intake of sweets, grazing, evening eating, emotional eating, and time or schedule constraints for meal planning and preparation.

The dietitian's recommendation is that the patient is a good candidate for gastric surgery but adherence to post-operative dietary changes may be difficult. Together, the dietitian and the patient have developed a pre-operative nutrition plan until a surgery date has been scheduled when further guidelines will be provided:

1. Reduce intake of high-fat foods.
   a Use of meal replacement shake for breakfast
   b Pack lunch or choose lower fat, fast food options at lunch
2. Reduce intake of sweets
   a Afternoon snack of fresh fruit or protein-based food
   b Replace evening snack with a meal replacement shake
3. Take prescribed dietary supplements as directed

6. Should CG lose weight before the surgery?

Regarding the recommendation for pre-operative weight loss, most experts agree that patients should be advised and provided with instructions to lose 5 to 10 percent of excess body weight (EBW). Clinical studies concerning the effect of pre-operative weight loss on surgical outcome indicate that a 5 to 10 percent EBW loss may be beneficial to improving surgical risk by ameliorating the patients' co-morbidities (OSA, blood pressure, blood sugar control); decreasing the operative time and complications; reducing the intra-operative need of conversion to open surgical technique; and possibly improving long-term weight loss success. The choice for the pre-op weight loss regimen (low-calorie diets (LCD), very low-calorie diets (VLCD), or pharmacotherapy) should be based on clinical judgment and the patient's history of previous weight loss interventions.

The patient had recently undergone a low-calorie diet program plus pharmacotherapy with unsatisfactory weight loss. It is possible that the recently added medication to her diabetic treatment, Actos (which is known to produce water retention), could have tempered her weight loss. Four weeks of a VLCD (800 calories) would be a reasonable pre-op weight loss treatment for CG.

The physician nutrition specialist prescribed a liquid meal replacement diet consisting of 800 calories per day. Attention was given to the macronutrient composition, and she was provided with an adequate amount of daily proteins and essential fatty acids. She was also recommended to take a daily multivitamin and two tablets of fiber supplements. The Actos and glipizide were discontinued at the beginning of the VLCD. She remained on metformin, and supplemental short-acting insulin was added as need (PRN). She was instructed to monitor her blood glucose three times a day. The patient lost 23 pounds by the end of the fourth week.

Part 3: Post- Surgical Assessment and Medical Nutrition Therapy

7. What is the nutritional impact of bariatric surgery?

The nutritional goals following bariatric surgery are to produce a significant caloric deficit, while maintaining an adequate intake of essential macro and micronutrients. Usually the more significant the component of malabsorption, the greater the success of weight loss; however, nutritional deficiencies follow the same trend.

Proteins are absorbed mainly in the jejunum and mid ileum, sites commonly bypassed by many bariatric procedures that have a malabsorptive component. Nonetheless, restrictive procedures could also lead to protein malnutrition due to significantly reduced food intake. The clinical signs of protein malnutrition are edema, alopecia, and low serum albumin level (less than 3.5 g/dL). Testing patient's serum albumin concentration is considered to be an effective and convenient method of monitoring protein nutritional status. The incidence of protein malnutrition in purely restrictive procedures is very low (0 percent to 2 percent), and has been found in 13 percent of patients after RYGB.

Iron deficiency is among the most common nutritional problem following bariatric surgery. Decreased ability to convert the dietary Fe^{3+} into the more absorbable Fe^{2+} form (due to low gastric acid production) and the bypassing of the duodenum and proximal jejunum (which are the main sites of iron absorption) are the main mechanisms leading to iron deficiency. Up to 50 percent of the RYGB patients have iron deficiency at 4 years, and it is two times more common in females compared to males. The prevalence of iron deficiency is even higher in jejuno–ileal bypass and duodenal switch. Measurement of serum ferritin is the single best diagnostic test for iron deficiency and is the first test to show abnormal results. Occurrence of microcytic anemia is usually a late finding and denotes severe iron deficiency.

Calcium and Vitamin D deficiencies are also commonly encountered in the bariatric patient. Calcium absorbs primarily in the duodenum and proximal jejunum, and absorption is facilitated by the presence of gastric acid secretion and vitamin D. Calcium status can be monitored by serum total calcium concentration, but calcium levels may be artificially low in the setting of hypoalbuminemia. Vitamin D is primarily absorbed in the jejunum and ileum. Being liposoluble, the absorption of vitamin D requires adequate mixing and action of pancreatic and billiary secretions. Even before surgery, up to 25 percent of obese patients have subclinical calcium deficiency (elevated PTH, with normal calcium), and 50 percent are vitamin D deficient. After surgery, the procedures with malabsorptive component cause significantly more calcium and vitamin D deficiency compared to the restrictive procedures. The best marker for vitamin D deficiency is the measurement of 25-hydroxy vitamin D. Low vitamin D and calcium levels trigger secondary hyperparathyroidism, which can be suspected by the increased levels of intact parathyroid hormone. All these nutritional and metabolic changes accelerate the bone loss after bariatric surgery.

Vitamin B$_{12}$ and Folic Acid. Vitamin B$_{12}$ is almost entirely absorbed in the terminal ileum in the presence of the intrinsic factor which is secreted from the antrum of the stomach. Adequate gastric and pancreatic enzyme secretion and mixing are also required in order to release vitamin B$_{12}$ from food and then from binding protein, so that vitamin B$_{12}$ is made available to bind to the intrinsic factor for absorption in the ileum. The human body stores substantial amounts of vitamin B$_{12}$ (about 2000 micrograms), but at 3 years, deficiency occurs in approximately one-third of patients who have had gastric bypass.

Folic acid deficiency is less common, because it is absorbed throughout the small intestine and deficiency is largely due to severely reduced dietary intake. Purely restrictive procedures are generally not associated with vitamin B$_{12}$ or folic acid deficiencies. Serum levels of vitamin B$_{12}$ and folic acid are used to monitor nutritional status of these vitamins. The use of methylmalonic acid to detect vitamin B$_{12}$ deficiency is not routinely recommended.

Thiamin is absorbed primarily in the duodenum, mostly in the more acidic environment of its proximal portion. The pathogenesis of thiamin deficiency is believed to be due to decrease in acid production (resulting from a decreased gastric capacity) and restriction of food intake, in the context of profuse and protracted vomiting. Symptomatic thiamin deficiency in bariatric patients is rare, but can occur even in the case of a restrictive procedure. The clinical presentation of thiamin deficiency most often consists of Wernicke's encephalopathy: altered mental status, ataxic gait, double vision, nystagmus, and acute polyneuropathy with paralysis. Clinical recognition of this syndrome may be lifesaving, since the symptoms respond very well to prompt intravenous administration of thiamin. Deficiency of thiamin can be confirmed by measuring the serum thiamin levels, or the erythrocyte thiamine transketolase (ETKA) (which is the most reliable method, but not often used in practice).

Other Vitamins and Minerals Low serum levels of vitamin A, K, and E were noticed after bariatric surgery, but clinical manifestation of such deficiencies has not yet been described. No clinical complications due to lack of vitamin C, magnesium, and selenium have been reported. Cases of zinc deficiency were found to occur following malabsorptive procedures, and usually manifest as alopecia. It is important to emphasize to patients that nutritional deficiencies following bariatric surgery can be avoided or corrected by routine monitoring, adequate nutrition, and supplementation.

8. CG undergoes laparoscopic RYGB. No surgical and peri-operative complications occur. Outline the nutritional and medical management of this patient for the first three months following the surgery.
Prior to surgery CG attended a nutrition class where she received written and oral instructions, including recommendations of foods to include and avoid for dietary progression upon discharge from the hospital. She was advised to follow a full-liquid diet for the remainder of the first week while at home. She was instructed

to keep the volume small, no more than $1/4$ cup per meal, and to try to eat five to six times per day. Week two post-operatively, CG was instructed to begin adding pureed foods with an emphasis on including higher protein foods. Meal volume remained small and she was advised to slowly increase the volume of food. She was advised to begin adding semi-solid/soft foods into her diet as tolerated, usually about 10 to 14 days after surgery, and reminded to chew each small bite thoroughly. Previously the patient was provided with food lists and the clinician reviewed foods to avoid. Foods not well tolerated during the first few months after surgery are red meat, chicken and turkey, white flour products, foods high in sugar and fat, and most raw fruits and vegetables.

The guidelines for continued weight loss were reviewed: keep portions small, no beverages 30 minutes before eating and 30 to 60 minutes after eating, a minimum intake of 60 grams protein per day, eat at scheduled times and avoid grazing, and include physical activity most days of the week. The patient was fairly adherent to her diet progression regime and slowly added new foods. At her three-month postoperative visit, she was eating approximately $1/2$ to 1 cup of food per meal, averaging 50 to 60 grams of protein every day and 48 ounces of water. She had not yet tried to eat red meat or raw vegetables. She stated even though she was not hungry, she still felt the desire to eat more food than she could tolerate.

9. CG comes to the Bariatric Center for her six-month follow-up visit. She states that for the last four weeks she has experinced nausea, shaking, diaphoresis, and diarrhea after eating. What is the most likely cause of these symptoms and how should she be treated?

The symptoms described at this visit are suggestive of dumping syndrome. Dumping syndrome occurs innitially in 70 to 76 percent of patients with RYGB. The clinical manifestations of dumping include GI and vasomotor symptoms. Dumping syndrome can be divided into early and late phases depending on the relation of symptoms to the time elapsed from meal intake. Symptoms of early dumping occur within 10 to 30 minutes after eating. They result from accelerated gastric emptying of hyperosmolar content into the small bowel, followed by fluid shifts from the intravascular compartment into the intestinal lumen. These events are believed to be responsible for GI symptoms such as nausea, bloating, abdominal cramps, and explosive diarrhea. The majority of patients have early dumping. Late dumping occurs 1 to 3 hours after eating, and it is characterized predominantly by systemic vascular symptoms including flushing, dizziness, palpitations, and light-headedness. Physical examination of these patients may reveal profound orthostatic changes. Late dumping occurs in approximately one-quarter of patients with dumping syndrome. Late dumping is considered to be the consequence of hypoglycemia from an exaggerated release of insulin.

An important element of the history that needs to be obtained from any patient presenting with these symptoms is a detailed food history, with particular attention to the intake of foods with a high content of sugar and /or fat. Our patient admitted that she had been snacking on her favorite cookies for the past month. Dumping syndrome usually responds to dietary interventions: reduction of carbohydrate intake, with preference for complex, rather than simple carbohydrates, avoidance of liquids for at least 30 minutes after a solid meal, and small portion size. In very rare cases drug therapy may be required (octreotide). CG responded well to dietary interventions.

10. Outline the long-term nutritional and medical management of this patient.

For her long-term diet, CG should continue to spend at least 30 minutes at each meal, taking her time to eat. She should slowly sip her fluids between meals (8 FO of fluids over 30–40 minutes), but not 30 minutes before or 30 to 60 minutes after eating. Food and liquids should continue to be low in fat and sugar. She was advised to eat at least 60 grams of protein daily. Protein-rich foods include lean meat, low-fat milk and dairy products, beans, peas, lentils, eggs, and protein supplements if needed. Vitamins and minerals should be taken regularly.

During the first year following bariatric surgery CG was seen at 1, 3, 6, and 12-month visits. She should be monitored on an annual basis by an obesity specialist or her primary care physician. Visits with a dietitian or behavioral therapist should be recommended anytime patients have difficulty maintaining their dietary goals or regain weight. One year after her surgery CG lost 101 pounds, which was what was initially predicted. Her BMI is 27.8 kg/m^2. Her annual visits focus on building long-term healthy dietary behavior, continuing physical activity, and monitoring and correcting potential nutritional deficiencies.

Routine blood tests for her annual post-operative visits include a CBC, chemistry panel including liver enzymes, lipid panel, HbA1c, ferritin, iron, TIBC, TIBC saturation, vitamin B_{12}, 25(OH) vitamin D, and intact PTH. A DEXA scan and other lab tests should be done based on clinical judgment. Our patient, who was perimenopausal before surgery, has not had a period for the last 16 months, and is considered post-menopausal. This status, along with rapid weight loss, increases her risk of osteoporosis, and most clinicians would agree that she should have a DEXA scan.

Evaluation of her co-morbidities and adjustment of medical management should be done as part of the continuum of care. Her medications were drastically reduceds she is only taking Metformin, 1000 mg once daily, and her HbA1c is 6.9 percent. She no longer requires hydrochlothiazide or labetalol to control her blood pressure, and her amlodipine was reduced to 5 mg once daily. She only needs half of the pre-operative dose of Zocor to keep her lipid panel at the ideal level. Her CPAP machine was adjusted two weeks ago to 10 cm H_2O, which represents a significant improvement from the pre-operative status; she no longer has lower extremity edema or shortness of breath. She has been able to discontinue her GERD medication without return of symptoms. She hopes that by losing more weight, she will be able to discontinue using her CPAP device. CG should remain for the rest of her life on the following daily nutritional supplements:

- Prenatal multivitamins/ minerals one tablet (prenatal vitamins usually have the adequate amount of 1 mg folic acid/day and higher iron content).
- Oral vitamin B_{12}, 500 to 1000 micrograms/day or 500 micrograms/week intranasally (alternative, 1000 micrograms IM once a month).
- Calcium citrate 1200 mg to 1500 mg/day (depending on dietary calcium intake).
- Vitamin D_3, 800 to 1000 IU/day.
- Iron (65 mg/day elemental iron, preferably in the reduced ferrous form; may add vitamin C to increase absorption).
- Thiamin, 10 mg/day.

It is important to mention that these recommendations are based mainly on expert opinion, and more clinical studies in this area are needed.

Chapter and Case References

Alami RS, Hsu G, Safadi BY, et al. The impact of preoperative weight loss in patients undergoing laparoscopic Roux-en-Y gastric bypass. *Obes Surg* 2005;15(9):1282–1286.

Appel LJ, Moore TJ, Obarzanek E, et al. for the DASH Collaborative Research Group. A clinical trial for the effects of dietary patterns on blood pressure. *N Engl J Med* 1997;336:1117–1124.

Barner CW, Wylie-Rosett J, Gans KM. WAVE: A pocket guide for a brief nutrition dialogue in primary care. *Diabetes Educator* 2001;27(3):352–362.

Bish CL, Blanck HM, Sedula MK, et al. Diet and physical activity behaviors among Americans trying to lose weight: 2000 Behavioral Risk Factor Surveillance System. *Obes Res* 2005;13(3):596–607.

Bray GA. Medical therapy for obesity – current status and future hopes. *Med Clin North Amer* 2007;91:1225–1254.

Bray GA. Classification and evaluation of the obesities. *Med Clin North Am.* 1989; 73(1):161–84.

Buchwald H, Avidor Y, Braunwald E, et al. Bariatric surgery: a systematic review and meta-analysis. *JAMA* 2004;292(14):1724–1237.

Buchwald H, Estok R, Fahrbach K, et al. Trends in mortality in bariatric surgery: a systematic review and meta-analysis. *Surgery* 2007;142(4):621–632; discussion 632–635.

Centers for Disease Control and Prevention. National Center for Health Statistics. Prevalence of overweight and obesity among adults: US, 2003–2004. Available from http://www.cdc.gov/nchs/products/pubs/pubd/hestats/overweight/overwght_adult_03.htm.

Centers for Disease Control and Prevention. Vital and Health Statistics. Summary health statistics for US adults: National Health Interview Survey 2006. Available from http://www.cdc.gov/nchs/data/serioes/sr_10/sr10_235.pdf.

Centers for Disease Control and Prevention. Behavioral risk factor surveillance system. US Obesity Trends 1985–2006. Available from http://www.cdc.gov/nccdphp/dnpa/obesity/trend/maps/index.htm.

Centers for Disease Control and Prevention. National Office of Public Health Genomics. Obesity and Genetics. Available from http://www.cdc.gov/genomics/training/perspecitves/files/obesedit.htm.

Centers for Disease Control and Prevention. New CDC study finds no increase in obesity among adults; but levels still high. Available from http://www.cdc.gov/nchs/pressroom/07newsreleases/obesity.htm.

Christakis NA, Fowler JH. The spread of obesity in a large social network in the last 32 years. *N Engl J Med* 2007;357(4):370–379.

Daniels SR, Arnett DK, Eckel RH, et al. Overweight in children and adolescents: pathophysiology, consequences, prevention, and treatment. *Circulation* 2005;111:1999–2010.

Davidson MH, Hauptman J, DiGirolamo M, et al. Weight control and risk factor reduction in obese subjects treated for 2 years with orlistat: a randomized controlled trial. *JAMA* 1999;281(3):235–242.

Department of Health and Human Services. Healthy People 2010 Midcourse Review. Executive Summary. Available from http://www.healthypeople.gov/data/midcourse/html/execsummary/introduction.htm.

Davies DJ, Baxter JM, Baxter JN. Nutritional deficiencies after bariatric surgery. *Obes Surg* 2007;17:1150–1158.

Dorsey KB, Wells C, Krumholz HM, et al. Diagnosis, evaluation, and treatment of childhood obesity in pediatric practice. *Arch Pediatr Adolesc Med* 2005;159:632–638.

Eckstein KC, Mikhail LM, Ariza AJ, et al. Parents' perception of their child's weight and health. *Pediatrics* 2006;117(3):681–690.

Erickson SJ, Gerstle M, Feldstein SW. Brief interventions and motivational interviewing with children, adolescents, and their parents in pediatric health care settings. *Arch Pediatr Adolesc Med* 2005;159:1173–1180.

Ferreira I, Twisk JWR, Mechelen WV, et al. Development of fatness, fitness, and lifestyle from adolescence to the age of 36 years: determinants of the metabolic syndrome in adults: The Amsterdam Growth and Health Longitudinal Study. *Arch Intern Med* 2005;165:42–48.

Flegal KM, Graubard BI, Williamson DF, et al. Excess deaths associated with underweight, overweight, and obesity. *JAMA* 2005;293:1861–1867.

Food and Nutrition Board, Institute of Medicine, *Dietary Reference Intakes for Energy, Carbohydrates, Fiber, Fat, Fatty Acids, Cholesterol, Protein, and Amino Acids*. National Academi Press, Washington, DC: 2002.

Fujioka K. Follow up of nutritional and metabolic problems after bariatric surgery. *Diabetes Care* 2005;28:481–484.

Gans KM, Ross E, Barner CW, et al. REAP and WAVE: new tools to rapidly assess/discuss nutrition with patients. *J Nutrition* 2003;133(2):556S–62S.

Gans KM, Risica PM, Wylie-Rosett J, et al. Development and evaluation of the nutrition component of the Rapid Eating and Activity Assessment for Patients (REAP): a new tool for primary care providers. *J Nutr Educ Beh* 2006;38(5):286–92.

Gans KM, Hixson ML, Eaton CE, et al. Rate Your Plate: An eating pattern assessment and educational tool for blood cholesterol control. *Nutr Clin Care* 2000;3(3):163–169, 177–178.

Grundy SM, Hansen B, Smith SC Jr., et al. Clinical management of metabolic syndrome: a report of the American Heart Association/National Heart, Lung, and Blood Institute/American Diabetes Association conference on scientific issues related to management. *Circulation* 2004;109(4):551–556.

Grundy SM, Cleeman JI, Daniels SR, et al. Diagnosis and management of the metabolic syndrome: an American Heart Association/National Heart, Lung, and Blood Institute Scientific Statement. *Circulation* 2005;112(17):2735–2752.

Hedley AA, Ogden CL, Johnson CL, et al. Prevalence of overweight and obesity among US children, adolescents, and adults, 1999–2002. *JAMA* 2004;291:2847–2850.

International Diabetes Federation. IDF task force on epidemiology and prevention of diabetes. *Diabetes Voice* 2007;52(4):29–32.

Katzmaryzyk PT, Janssen I, Ross R, et al. The importance of waist circumference in the definition of metabolic syndrome. *Diabetes Care* 2006;29(2):404–409.

Kini S, Herron DM, Yanagisawa RT. Bariatric surgery for morbid obesity: a cure for metabolic syndrome? *Med Clin North Amer* 2007;91:1255–1271.

Lobstein T, Jackson-Leach R. Child overweight and obesity in the USA: prevalence rates according to IOTF definitions. *Int J Pediatr Obes* 2007;2(1):62–64.

Maggard MA, Shugarman LR, Suttorp M, et al. Meta-analysis: surgical treatment of obesity. *Ann Intern Med* 2005;142(7):547–559.

Muennig P, Lubetkin E, Jia H, Franks P. Gender and the burden of disease attributable to obesity. *Am J of Pub Heal* 2006;96(9):1662–1668.

National Center for Health Statistics. *Chartbook on Trends in the Health of Americans. Health, United States, 2006.* Hyattsville, MD: Public Health Service. 2006.

National Cholesterol Education Program, *Third Report of the NCEP Expert Panel on Detection, Evaluation, and Treatment of High Blood Cholesterol in Adults.* National Institutes of Health Publication No. 02-5215; September 2002. Available from www.nhlbi.nih.gov/guidelines/cholesterol/atp3_rpt.htm.

National Institutes of Health, National Heart, Lung, and Blood Institute. *Clinical guidelines on the identification, evaluation, and treatment of overweight and obesity in adults: the evidence report. Obes Res* 1998;6S2:51S–210S.

National Institute of Health. Weight-control Information Network. Statistics Related to Overweight and Obesity. Available from http://win.niddk.nih.gov/statisics/index.htm#preval.

Narayan KMV, Boyle JP, Thompson TJ, et al. Effect of BMI on lifetime risk for diabetes in the US. *Diabetes Care* 2007;30(6);1562–1566.

Nguyen NT, Silver M, Robinson M, Needleman B, et al. Result of a national audit of bariatric surgery performed at academic centers: a 2004 University Health System Consortium Benchmarking Project. *Arch Surg* 2006;141:445–449.

Ogden CL, Carrol MD, Curtin LR, et al. Prevalence of overweight and obesity in the US, 1999–2004. *JAMA* 2006;295:1549–1555.

Ogden CL, Carrol MD, McDowell MA, et al. Obesity among adults in the US – no statistical change since 2003–2004. *CDC* 2007;1:1–6.

Ogden CL, Carroll MD, Flegal KM. High body mass index for age among US children and adolescents, 2003–2006. *JAMA.* 2008;299(20):2401–2405.

Otten JJ, Pitzi Hellwig J, Meyers LD. *Dietary reference intakes: essential guide to nutrient requirements.* Institute of Medicine. National Academies Press: Washington DC, 2006.

Pi-Sunyer FX, Aronne LJ, Heshmati HM, et al. Effect of rimonabant, a cannabinoid-1 receptor blocker, on weight and cardiometabolic risk factors in overweight or obese patients: RIO-North America: a randomized controlled trial. *JAMA* 2006;295(7):761–775.

Powers KA, Rehrig ST, Jones DB. Financial Impact of Obesity and Bariatric Surgery. *Med Clinics N Am.* 2007; 91(3):321–38.

Price GM, Uauy R, Breeze E, et al. Weight, shape, and mortality risk in older persons – elevated waist-hip ration, not high body mass index, is associated with a greater risk of death. *Am J Clin Nutr* 2006;84(2):449–460.

Rubenstein AH. Obesity: a modern epidemic. *Trans Am Clin Climatol Assoc* 2005;116:103–113.

Sjöström L, Lindroos AK, Peltonen M, et al. Lifestyle, diabetes, and cardiovascular risk factors 10 years after bariatric surgery. *N Engl J Med* 2004;351(26):2683–2693.

Sjostrom L, Narbro K, Sjostrom CD, et al. Effects of bariatric surgery on mortality in Swedish obese subjects. *N Engl J Med* 2007;357(8):741–752.

Snow V, Barry P, Fitterman N, et al. Pharmacologic and surgical management of obesity in primary care: a clinical practice guideline from the American College of Physicians. *Ann Intern Med* 2005;142(7):525–531.

Soroudi N, Wylie-Rosett J, Mogul D. Quick WAVE Screener: a tool to address weight, activity, variety, and excess. *Diabetes Educ.* 2004;30(4):616, 618–22, 626–8.

Still CD, Benotti P, Wood GC, et al. Outcomes of preoperative weight loss in high-risk patients undergoing gastric bypass surgery. *Arch Surg* 2007;142(10):994–998.

Sugerman HJ, Sugerman EL, DeMaria EJ, et al. Bariatric surgery for severely obese adolescents. *J Gastrointest Surg* 2003;7(1):102–107

USDA. Economics research service. *Household food security in the US,* 2007.

US Department of Health and Human Services. Healthy people 2020: the road ahead. Available from http://www.healthypeople.gov/hp2020/.

US Department of Health and Human Services and US Department of Agriculture. *Dietary Guidelines for Americans, 2005.* 6th ed., Washington, DC: US Government Printing Office, January 2005.

Walley AJ, Blakemore AIF, Froguel P. Genetics of obesity and the prediction of risk for health. *Hum Mol Genet* 2006;15(2):R120–R130.

Wirth A, Krause J. Long-term weight loss with sibutramine: a randomized controlled trial. *JAMA* 2001;286(11):1331–1339.

World Health Organization. Nutrition: global programming note 2005–2006. Available from http://www.who.int/nmh/donorinfo/nutrion/en/index.html.

World Health Organization. Obesity and overweight. Fact sheet no. 311. 2006. Geneva: World Health Organization.

Xanthakos SA, Inge TH. Nutritional consequences of bariatric surgery. *Curr Opin Clin Nutr Metab Care* 2006;9:489–496.

2 Vitamins, Minerals, and Dietary Supplements

Jeremy Brauer[1], Elizabeth Horvitz[2], and John Swaney[3]

[1] New York University Langone Medical Center, New York, NY
[2] University of California, School of Medicine, Irvine, CA
[3] Drexel University College of Medicine, Philadelphia, PA

OBJECTIVES *

- Know the major roles played by the various vitamins and the pathological consequences of deficiency or toxic excess.
- Be aware of the physiological functions of the major minerals and their role in any disease processes.
- Understand how laboratory measurements can be used for the diagnosis of pathologies involving vitamins or minerals.
- Appreciate the various circumstances that might warrant the use of supplements

*Source: Objectives for chapter and cases adapted from the *NIH Nutrition Curriculum Guide for Training Physicians*. (www.nhlbi.nih.gov/funding/training/naa)

The Need for Vitamins

Vitamins are organic chemical substances required for normal growth, development, and metabolism throughout all stages of life. While humans mostly rely on exogenous sources of vitamins and minerals, certain intestinal microorganisms produce vitamin K and biotin, while vitamin D and niacin are synthesized from their chemical precursors, cholesterol and tryptophan, respectively.

As the importance of adequate vitamin balance for health and disease prevention has been increasingly discussed in the lay press, the annual expenditure for over-the-counter dietary supplements in the United States has grown to over $16 billion. Therefore, it is essential for clinicians to assume a stronger patient education role regarding supplements while simultaneously emphasizing the importance of a varied diet as a source of most vitamins and minerals.

It is also important to be aware of those individuals who have increased vitamin and mineral requirements. These populations include, but are not limited to, pregnant and lactating women; those who have suffered severe trauma including burns, fractures, or major surgery; those who have or are at high risk for infections, such as HIV and malabsorption syndromes; alcohol, cigarette, and illicit substance abusers; and those taking medications that may interfere with the absorption and/or metabolism of nutrients.

Medical Nutrition and Disease: A Case-Based Approach, 4th edition. Edited by Lisa Hark.
© 2009 Wiley-Blackwell Publishing, ISBN: 978-1-4051-8615-5.

Vitamin Intake Standards

The requirements of each vitamin and mineral change throughout various stages of life. The Food and Nutrition Board of the National Research Council established a Recommended Daily Allowance (RDA) for most nutrients based on a review of published scientific data. A considerable body of knowledge exists for certain vitamins and minerals, and RDAs for various gender and age categories have been established. These levels are set at two standard deviations above the mean requirement to cover the needs of practically all healthy persons.

It is important to note two caveats with regard to these recommendations. The first is that suggested levels were established by the Food and Nutrition Board for groups of healthy people. Thus, the requirements of individuals with special nutritional needs or medical conditions were not specifically addressed. Second, the RDAs were developed with prevention of classic nutrient deficiencies in mind, rather than the enhancement of overall health and well-being. Vitamin requirements for patients with acute or chronic disease and the potential for supplements to improve health are active areas of research.

To address the changing needs for information, the Institute of Medicine of the National Academy of Sciences established the first Dietary Reference Intakes (DRIs) in 1997. The new DRIs move beyond the traditional RDAs to focus on the prevention of chronic disease. See Tables 2-1, 2-2, and 2-3 on pages 60–67. Dietary Reference Intake is a collective term that refers to three nutrient-based dietary reference values for every stage of life and both genders in addition to the conventional RDA: Estimated Average Requirement (EAR), Adequate Intake (AI), and the Tolerable Upper Intake Level (TUL).

Estimated Average Requirement (EAR)

The EAR is the most useful DRI for assessing the nutrient intake of a population. This is the daily intake expected to meet the requirement of 50 percent of the individuals in a particular life-stage and gender category. Individuals are advised to take in the EAR plus 2 standard deviations (the RDA) to ensure that their intake is adequate. A population whose mean intake is below the EAR is, on average, getting insufficient amounts of that nutrient.

Adequate Intake (AI)

The AI is an approximation of the average nutrient intake by a population or subgroup that appears to be healthy and not at increased risk of a particular chronic disease. The AI is a rough equivalent of the RDA, but is based upon estimation where adequate data for determining an EAR are unavailable.

Tolerable Upper Intake Level (TUL)

The TUL is the level of daily nutrient intake that is unlikely to pose risks of adverse health effects to almost all (97 to 98 percent) of the individuals in a specified life-stage and gender group. These levels, taken together, allow one to estimate a range of safe levels for supplementation.

Table 2-1 Dietary Reference Intakes (DRIs): Recommended Intakes for Individuals, Vitamins Food and Nutrition Board, Institute of Medicine, National Academies

Life Stage Group	Vitamin A (μg/d)[a]	Vitamin C (mg/d)	Vitamin D (μg/d)[b,c]	Vitamin E (mg/d)[d]	Vitamin K (μg/d)	Thiamin (mg/d)	Riboflavin (mg/d)	Niacin (mg/d)[e]	VitaminB_6 (mg/d)	Folate (μg/d)[f]	VitaminB_{12} (μg/d)	Pantothenic Acid (mg/d)	Biotin (μg/d)	Choline[g] (mg/d)
Infants														
0–6 mo	400*	40*	5*	4*	2.0*	0.2*	0.3*	2*	0.1*	65*	0.4*	1.7*	5*	125*
7–12 mo	500*	50*	5*	5*	2.5*	0.3*	0.4*	4*	0.3*	80*	0.5*	1.8*	6*	150*
Children														
1–3 y	300	15	5*	6	30*	0.5	0.5	6	0.5	150	0.9	2*	8*	200*
4–8 y	400	25	5*	7	55*	0.6	0.6	8	0.6	200	1.2	3*	12*	250*
Males														
9–13 y	600	45	5*	11	60*	0.9	0.9	12	1.0	300	1.8	4*	20*	375*
14–18 y	900	75	5*	15	75*	1.2	1.3	16	1.3	400	2.4	5*	25*	550*
19–30 y	900	90	5*	15	120*	1.2	1.3	16	1.3	400	2.4	5*	30*	550*
31–50 y	900	90	5*	15	120*	1.2	1.3	16	1.3	400	2.4	5*	30*	550*
51–70 y	900	90	10*	15	120*	1.2	1.3	16	1.7	400	2.4[h]	5*	30*	550*
>70 y	900	90	15*	15	120*	1.2	1.3	16	1.7	400	2.4[h]	5*	30*	550*
Females														
9–13 y	600	45	5*	11	60*	0.9	0.9	12	1.0	300	1.8	4*	20*	375*
14–18 y	700	65	5*	15	75*	1.0	1.0	14	1.2	400[i]	2.4	5*	25*	400*
19–30 y	700	75	5*	15	90*	1.1	1.1	14	1.3	400[i]	2.4	5*	30*	425*
31–50 y	700	75	5*	15	90*	1.1	1.1	14	1.3	400[i]	2.4	5*	30*	425*
51–70 y	700	75	10*	15	90*	1.1	1.1	14	1.5	400	2.4[h]	5*	30*	425*
>70 y	700	75	15*	15	90*	1.1	1.1	14	1.5	400	2.4[h]	5*	30*	425*
Pregnancy														
≤18 y	750	80	5*	15	75*	1.4	1.4	18	1.9	600[j]	2.6	6*	30*	450*
19–30 y	770	85	5*	15	90*	1.4	1.4	18	1.9	600[j]	2.6	6*	30*	450*
31–50 y	770	85	5*	15	90*	1.4	1.4	18	1.9	600[j]	2.6	6*	30*	450*

Lactation													
≤18 y	**1,200**	**115**	5*	75*	**19**	**1.4**	**1.6**	**17**	**2.0**	**500**	2.8	7*	35*	550*
19–30 y	**1,300**	**120**	5*	90*	**19**	**1.4**	**1.6**	**17**	**2.0**	**500**	2.8	7*	35*	550*
31–50 y	**1,300**	**120**	5*	90*	**19**	**1.4**	**1.6**	**17**	**2.0**	**500**	2.8	7*	35*	550*

NOTE: This table (taken from the DRI reports, see www.nap.edu) presents Recommended Dietary Allowances (RDAs) in **bold type** and Adequate Intakes (AIs) in ordinary type followed by an asterisk (*). RDAs and AIs may both be used as goals for individual intake. RDAs are set to meet the needs of almost all (97 to 98 percent) individuals in a group. For healthy breastfed infants, the AI is the mean intake. The AI for other life stage and gender groups is believed to cover needs of all individuals in the group, but lack of data or uncertainty in the data prevent being able to specify with confidence the percentage of individuals covered by this intake.

[a] As retinol activity equivalents (RAEs). 1 RAE = 1 μg retinol, 12 μg β-carotene, 24 μg α-carotene, or 24 μg β-cryptoxanthin. The RAE for dietary provitamin A carotenoids is two-fold greater than retinol equivalents (RE), whereas the RAE for preformed vitamin A is the same as RE.

[b] cholecalciferol. 1 μg cholecalciferol = 40 IU vitamin D.

[c] In the absence of adequate exposure to sunlight.

[d] As α-tocopherol. α-Tocopherol includes RRR-α-tocopherol, the only form of α-tocopherol that occurs naturally in foods, and the 2R-stereoisomeric forms of α-tocopherol (RRR-, RSR-, RRS-, and RSS-α-tocopherol) that occur in fortified foods and supplements. It does not include the 2S-stereoisomeric forms of α-tocopherol (SRR-, SSR-, SRS-, and SSS-α-tocopherol), also found in fortified foods and supplements.

[e] As niacin equivalents (NE). 1 mg of niacin = 60 mg of tryptophan; 0–6 months = preformed niacin (not NE).

[f] As dietary folate equivalents (DFE). 1 DFE = 1 μg food folate = 0.6 μg of folic acid from fortified food or as a supplement consumed with food = 0.5 μg of a supplement taken on an empty stomach.

[g] Although AIs have been set for choline, there are few data to assess whether a dietary supply of choline is needed at all stages of the life cycle, and it may be that the choline requirement can be met by endogenous synthesis at some of these stages.

[h] Because 10 to 30 percent of older people may malabsorb food-bound B_{12}, it is advisable for those older than 50 years to meet their RDA mainly by consuming foods fortified with B_{12} or a supplement containing B_{12}.

[i] In view of evidence linking folate intake with neural tube defects in the fetus, it is recommended that all women capable of becoming pregnant consume 400 μg from supplements or fortified foods in addition to intake of food folate from a varied diet.

[j] It is assumed that women will continue consuming 400 μg from supplements or fortified food until their pregnancy is confirmed and they enter prenatal care, which ordinarily occurs after the end of the periconceptional period—the critical time for formation of the neural tube.

Table 2-2 Dietary Reference Intakes (DRIs): Recommended Intakes for Individuals, Elements Food and Nutrition Board, Institute of Medicine, National Academies

Life Stage Group	Calcium (mg/d)	Chromium (µg/d)	Copper (µg/d)	Fluoride (mg/d)	Iodine (µg/d)	Iron (mg/d)	Magnesium (mg/d)	Manganese (mg/d)	Molybdenum (µg/d)	Phosphorus (mg/d)	Selenium (µg/d)	Zinc (mg/d)
Infants												
0–6 mo	210*	0.2*	200*	0.01*	110*	0.27*	30*	0.003*	2*	100*	15*	2*
7–12 mo	270*	5.5*	220*	0.5*	130*	11*	75*	0.6*	3*	275*	20*	3
Children												
1–3 y	500*	11*	340	0.7*	90	7	80	1.2*	17	460	20	3
4–8 y	800*	15*	440	1*	90	10	130	1.5*	22	500	30	5
Males												
9–13 y	1,300*	25*	700	2*	120	8	240	1.9*	34	1,250	40	8
14–18 y	1,300*	35*	890	3*	150	11	410	2.2*	43	1,250	55	11
19–30 y	1,000*	35*	900	4*	150	8	400	2.3*	45	700	55	11
31–50 y	1,000*	35*	900	4*	150	8	420	2.3*	45	700	55	11
51–70 y	1,200*	30*	900	4*	150	8	420	2.3*	45	700	55	11
>70 y	1,200*	30*	900	4*	150	8	420	2.3*	45	700	55	11
Females												
9–13 y	1,300*	21*	700	2*	120	8	240	1.6*	34	1,250	40	8
14–18 y	1,300*	24*	890	3*	150	15	360	1.6*	43	1,250	55	9
19–30 y	1,000*	25*	900	3*	150	18	310	1.8*	45	700	55	8
31–50 y	1,000*	25*	900	3*	150	18	320	1.8*	45	700	55	8
51–70 y	1,200*	20*	900	3*	150	8	320	1.8*	45	700	55	8
>70 y	1,200*	20*	900	3*	150	8	320	1.8*	45	700	55	8
Pregnancy												
≤18 y	1,300*	29*	1,000	3*	220	27	400	2.0*	50	1,250	60	13
19–30 y	1,000*	30*	1,000	3*	220	27	350	2.0*	50	700	60	11
31–50 y	1,000*	30*	1,000	3*	220	27	360	2.0*	50	700	60	11

Lactation												
≤18 y	1,300*	44*	1,300	3*	290	10	360	2.6*	50	1,250	70	14
19–30 y	1,000*	45*	1,300	3*	290	9	310	2.6*	50	700	70	12
31–50 y	1,000*	45*	1,300	3*	290	9	320	2.6*	50	700	70	12

NOTE: This table presents Recommended Dietary Allowances (RDAs) in **bold type** and Adequate Intakes (AIs) in ordinary type followed by an asterisk (*). RDAs and AIs may both be used as goals for individual intake. RDAs are set to meet the needs of almost all (97 to 98 percent) individuals in a group. For healthy breastfed infants, the AI is the mean intake. The AI for other life stage and gender groups is believed to cover needs of all individuals in the group, but lack of data or uncertainty in the data prevent being able to specify with confidence the percentage of individuals covered by this intake.

SOURCES: *Dietary Reference Intakes for Calcium, Phosphorous, Magnesium, Vitamin D, and Fluoride* (1997); *Dietary Reference Intakes for Thiamin, Riboflavin, Niacin, Vitamin B_6, Folate, Vitamin B_{12}, Pantothenic Acid, Biotin, and Choline* (1998); *Dietary Reference Intakes for Vitamin C, Vitamine E, Selenium, and Carotenoids* (2000); and *Dietary Reference Intakes for Vitamin A, Vitamin K, Arsenic, Boron, Chromium, Copper, Iodine, Iron, Manganese, Molybdenum, Nickel, Silicon, Vanadium, and Zinc* (2001). These reports may be accessed via www.nap.edu.

Table 2-3 Dietary Reference Intakes (DRIs): Tolerable Upper Intake Levels (UL^a), Vitamins Food and Nutrition Board, Institute of Medicine, National Academies

Life Stage Group	Vitamin A (μg/d)^b	Vitamin C (mg/d)	Vitamin D (μg/d)	Vitamin E (mg/d)^c,d	Vitamin K	Thiamin	Riboflavin	Niacin (mg/d)^d	Vitamin B$_6$ (mg/d)	Folate (μg/d)^d	Vitamin B$_{12}$	Pantothenic Acid	Biotin	Choline (g/d)	Carotenoids^e
Infants														
0–6 mo	600	ND^f	25	ND	ND	ND	ND	ND	ND	ND	ND	ND	ND	ND	ND
7–12 mo	600	ND	25	ND	ND	ND	ND	ND	ND	ND	ND	ND	ND	ND	ND
Children														
1–3 y	600	400	50	200	ND	ND	ND	10	30	300	ND	ND	ND	1.0	ND
4–8 y	900	650	50	300	ND	ND	ND	15	40	400	ND	ND	ND	1.0	ND
Males, Females														
9–13 y	1,700	1,200	50	600	ND	ND	ND	20	60	600	ND	ND	ND	2.0	ND
14–18 y	2,800	1,800	50	800	ND	ND	ND	30	80	800	ND	ND	ND	3.0	ND
19–70 y	3,000	2,000	50	1,000	ND	ND	ND	35	100	1,000	ND	ND	ND	3.5	ND
>70 y	3,000	2,000	50	1,000	ND	ND	ND	35	100	1,000	ND	ND	ND	3.5	ND

Pregnancy															
≤18 y	2,800	1,800	50	800	ND	ND	ND	30	80	800	ND	ND	ND	3.0	ND
19–50 y	3,000	2,000	50	1,000	ND	ND	ND	35	100	1,000	ND	ND	ND	3.5	ND
Lactation															
≤18 y	2,800	1,800	50	800	ND	ND	ND	30	80	800	ND	ND	ND	3.0	ND
19–50 y	3,000	2,000	50	1,000	ND	ND	ND	35	100	1,000	ND	ND	ND	3.5	ND

[a] UL = The maximum level of daily nutrient intake that is likely to pose no risk of adverse effects. Unless otherwise specified, the UL represents total intake from food, water, and supplements. Due to lack of suitable data, ULs could not be established for vitamin K, thiamin, riboflavin, vitamin B$_{12}$, pantothenic acid, biotin, or carotenoids. In the absence of ULs, extra caution may be warranted in consuming levels above recommended intakes.

[b] As preformed vitamin A only.

[c] As α-tocopherol; applies to any form of supplemental α-tocopherol.

[d] The ULs for vitamin E, niacin, and folate apply to synthetic forms obtained from supplements, fortified foods, or a combination of the two.

[e] β-Carotene supplements are advised only to serve as a provitamin A source for individuals at risk of vitamin A deficiency.

[f] ND = Not determinable due to lack of data of adverse effects in this age group and concern with regard to lack of ability to handle excess amounts. Source of intake should be from food only to prevent high levels of intake.

Table 2-3 (*continued*) Dietary Reference Intakes (DRIs): Tolerable Upper Intake Levels (UL[a]), Elements Food and Nutrition Board, Institute of Medicine, National Academies

Life Stage Group	Arsenic[b]	Boron[b] (mg/d)	Calcium (g/d)	Chromium	Copper (μg/d)	Fluoride (mg/d)	Iodine (μg/d)	Iron (mg/d)	Magnesium (mg/d)[c]	Manganese (mg/d)	Molybdenum (μg/d)	Nickel (mg/d)	Phosphorus (g/d)	Selenium (μg/d)	Silicon[d]	Vanadium (mg/d)[e]	Zinc (mg/d)
Infants
0–6 mo	ND[f]	ND	ND	ND	ND	0.7	ND	40	ND	ND	ND	ND	ND	45	ND	ND	4
7–12 mo	ND	ND	ND	ND	ND	0.9	ND	40	ND	ND	ND	ND	ND	60	ND	ND	5
Children
1–3 y	ND	3	2.5	ND	1,000	1.3	200	40	65	2	300	0.2	3	90	ND	ND	7
4–8 y	ND	6	2.5	ND	3,000	2.2	300	40	110	3	600	0.3	3	150	ND	ND	12
Males, Females
9–13 y	ND	11	2.5	ND	5,000	10	600	40	350	6	1,100	0.6	4	280	ND	ND	23
14–18 y	ND	17	2.5	ND	8,000	10	900	45	350	9	1,700	1.0	4	400	ND	ND	34
19–70 y	ND	20	2.5	ND	10,000	10	1,100	45	350	11	2,000	1.0	4	400	ND	1.8	40
>70 y	ND	20	2.5	ND	10,000	10	1,100	45	350	11	2,000	1.0	3	400	ND	1.8	40
Pregnancy
≤18 y	ND	17	2.5	ND	8,000	10	900	45	350	9	1,700	1.0	3.5	400	ND	ND	34
19–50 y	ND	20	2.5	ND	10,000	10	1,100	45	350	11	2,000	1.0	3.5	400	ND	ND	40

Lactation																
≤18 y	ND	17	2.5	ND	8,000	10	900	45	350	9	1,700	1.0	4	400	ND	ND	34
19–50 y	ND	20	2.5	ND	10,000	10	1,100	45	350	11	2,000	1.0	4	400	ND	ND	40

[a] UL = The maximum level of daily nutrient intake that is likely to pose no risk of adverse effects. Unless otherwise specified, the UL represents total intake from food, water, and supplements. Due to lack of suitable data, ULs could not be established for arsenic, chromium, and silicon. In the absence of ULs, extra caution may be warranted in consuming levels above recommended intakes.

[b] Although the UL was not determined for arsenic, there is no justification for adding arsenic to food or supplements.

[c] The ULs for magnesium represent intake from a pharmacological agent only and do not include intake from food and water.

[d] Although silicon has not been shown to cause adverse effects in humans, there is no justification for adding silicon to supplements.

[e] Although vanadium in food has not been shown to cause adverse effects in humans, there is no justification for adding vanadium to food and vanadium supplements should be used with caution. The UL is based on adverse effects in laboratory animals and this data could be used to set a UL for adults but not children and adolescents.

[f] ND = Not determinable due to lack of data of adverse effects in this age group and concern with regard to lack of ability to handle excess amounts. Source of intake should be from food only to prevent high levels of intake.

Sources: *Dietary Reference Intakes for Calcium, Phosphorous, Magnesium, Vitamin D, and Fluoride* (1997); *Dietary Reference Intakes for Thiamin, Riboflavin, Niacin, Vitamin B₆, Folate, Vitamin B₁₂, Pantothenic Acid, Biotin, and Choline* (1998); *Dietary Reference Intakes for Vitamin C, Vitamine E, Selenium, and Carotenoids* (2000); and *Dietary Reference Intakes for Vitamin A, Vitamin K, Arsenic, Boron, Chromium, Copper, Iodine, Iron, Manganese, Molybdenum, Nickel, Silicon, Vanadium, and Zinc* (2001). These reports may be accessed via www.nap.edu.

THE VITAMINS

Vitamin A

Vitamin A is a group of fat-soluble compounds that includes retinoic acid, retinol, and carotenoids. Retinol, also known as pre-formed vitamin A, is the most active form and is mostly found in foods of animal origin. Beta-carotene, also known as provitamin A, is the most common of the plant carotenoids, and is converted in the body to retinol.

Forms and Absorption Following ingestion of beta-carotene (or other carotenoids), the body enzymatically cleaves some of these compounds to retinol, which is esterified in the intestinal cell to retinyl esters that, along with the remaining carotenoids, are incorporated into chylomicrons in the enterocytes for transport into the lymph and eventually the blood. Dietary retinyl esters follow a similar path and are likewise incorporated into chylomicrons, eventually delivering the retinyl esters and carotenoid pigments to the liver for storage. When a particular part of the body, such as the eyes, requires vitamin A, the liver releases the retinol, bound to RBP (retinol binding protein).

Function Vitamin A plays an essential regulatory role in the following physiological functions:
1) In the eye, vitamin A is involved in the development or maintenance of the mucus membranes, cornea, and conjunctiva.
2) In a process known as phototransduction, all-*trans* retinal is linked to a protein to form rhodopsin in the rod cells, and iodopsin in the cone cells, of the retina. These cells are required for night vision and the perception of color in bright light.
3) Normal integrity and growth of skin and tissue cells, including the mucus membranes of the mouth, intestinal, respiratory, genitals, and urinary tracts.
4) Production of keratin, which is a component of skin and epithelia.
5) In the form of all-trans retinoic acid, vitamin A plays a role in the functioning of testicles and ovaries and aids in the development of the embryo.
6) Many carotenoids function as antioxidants.

Retinol Equivalents Vitamin A is ingested either as preformed vitamin A (retinol or retinyl ester), or a beta-carotene that can be split into retinol in the intestine. Beta-carotene is the most abundant carotenoid present in green, yellow, and orange fruits and vegetables. Due to inefficient conversion, 12 μg of beta-carotene in food yields only about 1 μg retinol, and therefore a serving of food that contains 12 μg of beta-carotene is said to contain 1 μg RAE (retinol activity equivalent; the older literature uses a similar concept with the abbreviation RE, for retinol equivalent). Because other carotenoids are even less efficiently converted to retinol, 1 μg RAE equates to 24 μg of these other carotenoid species.

International units (IU) are also used to express the amount of vitamin A in supplements and occasionally in foods. 100 IU of retinol in supplements translates to 30 μg RAE, while 100 IU of beta-carotene equates to 5 μg RAE.

Deficiency Vitamin A deficiency is one of the most common forms of malnutrition in the world, with infants and young children most affected. Primary deficiency is due to inadequate intake of vitamin A and its precursors, whereas secondary deficiency occurs from poor absorption of fat-soluble vitamins, which may occur in patients with cystic fibrosis, Crohn's disease, tropical sprue, or liver disease, or in those who abuse alcohol.

Clinical problems associated with vitamin A deficiency include perifollicular hyperkeratosis, night blindness, xerophthalmia (which can progress from conjunctival thickening to corneal ulceration and eventual irreversible blindness), and impairment of both the humoral and cell-mediated immune systems; this latter effect is known to increase mortality from certain infectious diseases, such as measles, in developing countries.

Toxicity Chronic excesses in vitamin intake of 30 mg/day (100,000 IU/day) or acute doses of 150 mg (500,000 IU) can cause a variety of symptoms ranging from bone and skin changes and liver abnormalities (hepatomegaly) to headache, nausea, vertigo, blurred vision, and lack of muscle coordination. Recently, attention has been directed at elucidating whether chronic vitamin intakes only modestly higher than recommended levels might have an adverse effect on bone health and the risk of osteoporosis. The results have been mixed and complicated by inadequate measures of vitamin A status. However, vitamin A intake tends to be adequate or more than adequate in the United States, and supplementation with preformed vitamin A resulting in total intake which exceeds the RDA should be discouraged.

Consuming too much vitamin A, especially retinoic acid, during the first trimester of pregnancy can cause birth defects to the developing embryo. Therefore, women who are using vitamin A for the treatment of acne, or for other purposes, should cease using these products.

Because only limited amounts of beta-carotene are converted to vitamin A, excessive intake of beta-carotene has not been shown to produce toxic effects. People who consume large doses of beta-carotene, either through dietary sources or supplements, may however develop a yellow tinge to the skin. This carotenosis, commonly seen in babies whose caretakers give them squash and sweet potatoes as early solid food, has no harmful effects. While many in vivo and in vitro studies have supported a link between vitamin A and the treatment of epithelial cancers, intervention trials have been disappointing.

Supplemental Issues Certain forms of vitamin A, specifically the all-*trans* form of retinoic acid, have proven useful for the treatment of dermatological disease such as acne and psoriasis, presumably because of its effects on gene expression and cell differentiation. Retinoic acid has also been found to be effective in the treatment of acute promyelocytic leukemia. However, studies attempting to establish a role for retinoic acid for treatment of other cancers have generally been disappointing.

Similarly, randomized trials of beta-carotene have shown no benefit for the prevention of coronary heart disease (CHD). Recent studies suggest that vitamin A and beta-carotene, used alone or in combination with other anti-oxidant supplements, may in fact increase overall mortality.

Vitamin A Food Sources See Appendix A.

Vitamin D

Vitamin D is a fat-soluble vitamin, naturally occurring in two forms, vitamin D_2(ergocalciferol) and vitamin D_3(cholecalciferol). Vitamin D_2 is a plant or yeast steroid that is commonly used to fortify milk, while vitamin D_3 is from animal sources or produced in the skin upon exposure to adequate amounts of sunlight. Five to 30 minutes of sun exposure between 10 am and 3 pm at least twice a week without sunscreen has been suggested to provide sufficient vitamin D synthesis in temperate zones.

Forms and Absorption Since vitamin D is a fat-soluble vitamin, some fat is required in the diet for its absorption, and fat malabsorption conditions adversely affect vitamin D absorption. Once absorbed and transported to the liver as a component of chylomicrons or bound to a serum carrier protein, vitamin D binding protein (DBP), vitamin D undergoes hydroxylation to 25-hydroxy vitamin D [25(OH)D or calcidiol] with further conversion to its physiologically active form, 1,25-dihydroxy-vitamin D [1,25(OH)$_2$D or calcitriol], in various tissues. The synthesis and metabolism of vitamin D are closely coupled to calcium homeostasis; therefore when calcium levels in the blood are low, the body releases parathyroid hormone (PTH), which stimulates the kidney to convert 25(OH)D to 1,25(OH)$_2$D. Elevations in 1,25(OH)$_2$D stimulate the gastrointestinal tract to increase calcium absorption from about 10 to 30 percent and phosphorous absorption from about 60 to 80 percent. Serum 25(OH)D is the best indicator of vitamin D status. It reflects vitamin D produced cutaneously and that obtained from food and supplements, and has a half-life of 15 days.

Units The most common unit reported for vitamin D is International Units (IU). Vitamin D may also be listed in micrograms. Use the following conversion: 1 microgram $=$ 40 IU.

Functions Vitamin D plays an essential regulatory role in the following bodily functions:
1) Intestinal absorption of calcium and phosphorus.
2) Regulation of calcium and phosphorous deposition in the bones, teeth, and cartilage in children and adults.
3) Maintenance of blood calcium and phosphorus levels.

4) Vitamin D is associated with a variety of physiological functions, including immunity, neuromuscular functions, blood pressure regulation, insulin production, reduction of inflammation, and apoptosis.

Deficiency Vitamin D deficiency can be due to impaired availability of vitamin D (inadequate dietary intake or fat malabsorptive disorders, coupled with a lack of sun exposure) or impaired metabolism (at the level of the liver, kidney, or end organs). Serum levels less than 20 ng/mL are indicative of low serum vitamin D. Groups with increased risk for low vitamin D levels are breastfed infants, older adults, obese individuals (BMI > 30 kg/m^2), people with dark skin, and those with limited sun exposure. Strict vegetarians, and those who have a milk allergy or lactose intolerance, are also at risk. Older adults and seniors are at increased risk for vitamin D deficiency, especially those who are bed-ridden or who live in nursing homes and may not have adequate exposure to sunlight coupled with inadequate dietary intake. In fact, recent studies in healthy college and medical students in Boston have documented deficient serum levels at the end of winter.

Vitamin D deficiency results in rickets in infants and children and osteomalacia (softening of the bones) in adults. Rickets causes retarded growth, swelling and tenderness at the ends of the bones, and malformation of the joints. Rickets in infants also leads to a delay in the closure of the skull bones, possibly leading to a larger skull ("frontal bossing"), as well as bowed legs, pigeon breast, and beaded ribs ("rachitic rosary") seen in older children. Osteomalacia may lead to pain in the legs, ribs, hips, and muscles, and easily breakable bones. Osteomalacia may occur when long-term anticonvulsant medications such as phenobarbital or phenytoin are taken because they increase the liver's breakdown of vitamin D. Individuals with chronic kidney disease often develop osteodystrophy, secondary to the kidney's inability to convert vitamin D to its active form.

Toxicity Chronically elevated doses of vitamin D may lead to kidney stones, nausea, headaches, weakness, anorexia, frequent urination, weight loss, irregular heartbeat, and weak bones and muscles. Excess levels may also lead to an elevation in serum calcium, which can cause calcification of soft tissues such as organs and blood vessels, possibly resulting in irreversible damage. In infants and children, too much vitamin D can lead to retarded growth, rounding of the skull, mental retardation, and death. However, excessive levels of vitamin D are believed to occur only through the use of supplements rather than from food or too much sun exposure. The tolerable upper limit for vitamin D has been established at 50 μg /day (2000 IU/day) but recently, vitamin D researchers have questioned whether this level is set too low.

Supplement Issues There are two forms of supplements, D$_2$ and D$_3$. Vitamin D$_3$ has been shown to be more effective at raising and maintaining serum 25(OH)D levels. A meta-analysis of randomized controlled trials indicated that vitamin D$_3$ supplementation led to a decreased risk of all-cause mortality with a relative risk of 0.93. The mean daily dose was 528 IU (with a range of 300 to 2000 IU). Although the basis for this is unclear, studies have suggested that the risk for certain cancers, notably colorectal and breast, may be significantly reduced in individuals with higher than normal serum levels of vitamin D, corresponding to intakes of 1000 to 4000 IU/day. Studies with supplement dosages at the current RDA levels (400 IU/day) showed no benefit, but arguments have been made that the RDA is too low and that the upper limit of 2000 IU/day is too restrictive and could be raised by a factor of five. Compounding the problem is that the vitamin D content of most foods is quite low, and even 8 ounces of milk provides only 100 IU. Five to 30 minutes of sun exposure several times a week yields blood levels of vitamin D much higher than is achievable orally, and is argued to represent the "natural" level for this vitamin.

Studies of the effect of vitamin D on fractures showed no benefit at the standard dosage of 400 IU/day, but recent meta-analyses of studies using higher vitamin D dosages (800 IU/day or greater), when accompanied by significant calcium supplementation, showed significant reduction in hip fractures (18 percent to 24 percent reduction). (See Chapter 4 for current vitamin D recommendations in infants and children).

Vitamin D Food Sources: See Appendix B.

Vitamin E

Vitamin E is another fat-soluble vitamin group made up of alcohol compounds called tocopherols and tocotrienols. Each series comes in alpha, beta, gamma, and delta forms for a total of 8 compounds with vitamin E activity. Of the various tocopherols, alpha-tocopherol has the highest biological activity.

Forms and Absorption Vitamin E is absorbed passively in the ileum, requiring the presence of bile salts. Vitamin E absorption requires dietary fat, as absorption of all of the fat-soluble vitamins depends upon bile-acid mediated fat digestion and absorption processes, with incorporation of these vitamins into chylomicrons for delivery to the liver and adipose tissues.

Functions Vitamin E plays an essential regulatory role in the following bodily functions:
1) Acts as an antioxidant, protecting polyunsaturated fatty acids within cell membranes from peroxidation.
2) Inhibits cell proliferation, platelet aggregation, and monocyte adhesion.
3) Plays an important role in the maintenance of fertility.

Deficiency Vitamin E deficiency is rare, except in people who cannot absorb fat, such as patients with pancreatic insufficiency. Clinical signs include neurologic dysfunction, loss of deep tendon reflexes, and diminished vibratory or position sense. Infants who are treated with oxygen may develop retrolental fibroplasias, leading to vision impairment and possibly blindness. This may be prevented by vitamin E supplements.

Toxicity Vitamin E is considered non-toxic except at very high doses. Reports indicate that very large doses of vitamin E can interfere with the vitamin K formation of functional clotting factors, resulting in hemorrhage. For this reason, large doses of vitamin E should be avoided 2 weeks before and after surgery as well as when taking anticoagulation medications, such as Coumadin. It has also been reported that premature infants may be especially sensitive to excess vitamin E, resulting in hemorrhage and sepsis. The tolerable upper intake level for vitamin E has been established at 1000 mg/day.

Relationship to Disease Prevention Vitamin E is considered to be nature's most effective lipid-soluble antioxidant, protecting cell membranes from oxidative damage. In spite of its popularity as a supplement to prevent heart disease, recent studies have failed to demonstrate any benefit from vitamin E in reducing the risk of heart attacks or deaths from heart disease. Interestingly, additional studies have suggested that individuals with type 2 diabetes might reduce their risk of cardiovascular disease by taking E supplements.

Vitamin E Food Sources See Appendix C.

Vitamin K

Vitamin K is a fat-soluble vitamin that is obtained from dietary sources and also produced by intestinal bacteria. Phylloquinone is the predominant form of vitamin K from dietary sources and menaquinone is produced by gut micro-flora.

Forms and Absorption Absorption of vitamin K occurs primarily in the proximal small bowel and requires bile salts. Following intestinal absorption, vitamin K is transported by chylomicrons for storage mostly in the liver.

Function Vitamin K is a required cofactor for enzymes involved in forming calcium-binding gamma-carboxyglutamate (gla) residues required for activity in coagulation factors VII, IX, X, and prothrombin. Additionally, anticoagulant proteins S and C require vitamin K for their activity. Vitamin K is also necessary for bone mineralization, because it is required for the formation of gla-residues in osteocalcin and gla matrix protein.

Deficiency Deficiency of vitamin K in an otherwise healthy individual is rare, although deficiency may occur in people with fat malabsorption or those on prolonged antibiotic therapy, which destroys the intestinal microorganisms that produce vitamin K. Symptoms of vitamin K deficiency include signs of impaired coagulation such as easy bruisability, mucosal bleeding, melena, and hematuria.

A recent observational study suggested that a low plasma level of vitamin K might be associated with a higher prevalence of osteoarthritis of the hands and knees. Also, a meta-analysis of randomized controlled trials suggested that vitamin K supplementation reduced bone loss, with a positive effect on fractures.

Infants are given a vitamin K injection at birth, as a precaution to prevent hemorrhagic disease of the newborn. Infants' intestinal tracts lack the necessary bacteria to adequately synthesize vitamin K until approximately one week after birth and the newborn liver is therefore unable to produce adequate levels of coagulation factors.

Toxicity Toxicity is virtually unknown to phylloquinone or menaquinone, although allergic reactions to mega doses of vitamin K have been reported. Severe jaundice may occur in infants treated with doses of menadione. There is no tolerable upper level for vitamin K. Patients taking warfarin (Coumadin) as an anticoagulant are cautioned to avoid marked changes in their intake of vitamin K-rich foods or supplements since the dose of Coumadin is titrated to maintain a narrow range of anticoagulation, which may be reversed by increased intake of vitamin K.

Vitamin K Food Sources See Appendix D.

Ascorbic Acid (Vitamin C)

Ascorbic acid is a water-soluble vitamin commonly known as vitamin C. It is the least stable of all the vitamins, and is easily destroyed during cooking and processing.

Form and Absorption The jejunum and ileum efficiently absorb vitamin C. The amount of vitamin C in the blood is modulated by renal excretion, with levels exceeding the reabsorption threshold being excreted in the urine.

Functions Vitamin C plays an essential role in the following:
1) Formation of collagen, which is responsible for strengthening bones and blood vessels, anchoring teeth into the gums, as well as forming the substances necessary for body growth, tissue repair, and wound healing.
2) Synthesis of neurotransmitters such as norepinephrine.
3) Antioxidant activity.

Deficiency Individuals who do not have access to fresh citrus fruits and juices, such as urban or poor older adults, may have insufficient vitamin C intake. Individuals with severe burns, fractures, pneumonia, rheumatic fever, and tuberculosis, as well as those who have recently undergone surgery, have increased requirements for vitamin C. Alcohol decreases absorption and cigarette smoking depletes tissue levels. Thus, alcoholics and smokers should increase their dietary intake or take supplemental vitamin C.

Vitamin C deficiency is characterized by the development of scurvy, in which impaired collagen synthesis results in muscle weakness, joint pain, impaired wound healing, loose teeth, bleeding and swollen gums, bruised skin, fatigue, and depression.

Toxicity Since vitamin C is a water-soluble vitamin, the body excretes the excess when intake exceeds the body's requirements. However, because vitamin C is metabolized to oxalic acid, consuming too much may cause increased excretion of oxalate, which suggests that patients with a history of forming oxalate kidney stones should avoid high doses of this vitamin. Doses in excess of the UL (2000 mg/day) can have other side effects including nausea, diarrhea, and abdominal cramps.

Relationship to Disease Prevention Vitamin C is a powerful antioxidant that provides the first line of defense against free radicals in aqueous compartments of the body. However, to date, studies have been unable to demonstrate a clear protective role for vitamin C in cancer prevention or in the development of atherosclerosis. The role of vitamin C in the prevention and treatment of the common cold remains controversial.

Vitamin C Food Sources See Appendix E.

Thiamin (Vitamin B$_1$)

Form and Absorption Thiamin is a water-soluble vitamin. It is primarily absorbed in the jejunum via active transport when intake levels are low and passive transport when intake levels are high. Absorption is significantly reduced in the presence of alcohol, as well as in individuals with folate deficiency. Once absorbed, thiamin is primarily found in the skeletal muscles, liver, heart, kidneys, and brain; however, it is not stored in the body to any great extent, so daily intake is required.

Functions Thiamin is an essential prosthetic group in a number of enzymes that play key roles in the production of energy from carbohydrate and protein.

Deficiency Primary thiamin deficiency (beriberi), which is due to poor intake of thiamin-containing foods, is rare in the United States because the majority of grain products are fortified with thiamin. However, thiamin deficiency does typically occur in individuals who abuse alcohol because excessive alcohol intake significantly decreases thiamin absorption and interferes with its metabolism. Early thiamin deficiency is characterized by poor appetite, irritability, apathy, confusion, and weight loss. Advanced stages of beriberi affect the nervous and cardiovascular system, causing abnormal heart rhythms and heart failure. Wet beriberi refers to a form characterized primarily by cardiomyopathy and edema.

Causes and Effects of Toxicity Thiamin toxicity has not been described.

Relationship to Disease Prevention While thiamin is not generally associated with disease prevention, prompt administration of thiamin is indicated for the alcoholic patient who shows signs of Wernicke disease, which is usually a consequence of thiamin deficiency due to reduced absorption.

Riboflavin (Vitamin B$_2$)

Riboflavin is water soluble. It functions as a precursor to the flavin category of enzyme prosthetic groups (FAD, FMN) that participate in oxidation/reduction reactions, many of which are involved with energy production.

Form and Absorption   Free riboflavin is released from foods by digestive enzymes and is actively absorbed by an ATP-requiring process in the jejunum. Some of the riboflavin circulating in the blood is loosely associated with albumin, although significant amounts complex with other proteins. Once riboflavin is delivered to a variety of cells, it is converted into flavin mononucleotide (FMN) and flavin-adenine dinucleotide (FAD).

Functions   Riboflavin plays an essential role in the following bodily functions:
1) Aids in normal growth and development.
2) Helps glucose breakdown to yield energy for all cells.
3) Facilitates glycogen production and digestion of fats.
4) Helps change the amino acid tryptophan into niacin.
5) Serves to maintain normal mucous membranes and protects the nervous system, skin, and eyes.

Deficiency   Riboflavin deficiency can result from inadequate intake, poor absorption, lack of utilization, or increased excretion. Riboflavin deficiency symptoms include inflammation of the mucosa of the mouth or tongue, cheilitis, stomatitis, glossitis, seborrheic dermatitis, and normocytic-normochromic anemia. The eyes may also become bloodshot, itchy, watery, and sensitive to bright light. Riboflavin deficiency typically develops in conjunction with deficiencies of other water-soluble vitamins, as the B vitamins, which are commonly found in the same foods.

Toxicity   No adverse effects from high intake of riboflavin have been reported and hence there is no tolerable upper limit established for this vitamin.

Relationship to Disease Prevention   None known.

Niacin (Vitamin B$_3$)

Niacin is a water-soluble vitamin, found in two common forms: nicotinic acid and nicotinamide. Niacin is the precursor to the coenzymes nicotinamide adenine dinucleotide (NAD) and NAD phosphate (NADP), which are electron carriers used in both synthetic reactions and for ATP production. Some but not all of our niacin requirement can also be met by conversion from the amino acid tryptophan.

Form and Absorption   Niacin and nicotin amide are absorbed through the intestine by simple diffusion. Niacin and nicotinamide are metabolized via different pathways.

Functions Niacin plays an essential role in the following bodily functions:

1) Normal enzyme production in at least 200 reactions in the body involved in energy production. Most enzymes require niacin to accept electrons or donate hydrogen molecules.
2) Normal production and breakdown of glucose, fats, and amino acids, thereby helping the body to metabolize these substances.
3) Required for normal development, maintenance, and function of the skin, gastrointestinal tract, and nervous system.
4) Aids the body in synthesizing DNA.

Deficiency Niacin is found primarily in protein-rich foods, and a deficiency is rare in the United States. Historically, the deficiency developed in those whose diet mainly consisted of corn, which is low in niacin and lacks tryptophan (a precursor to niacin). A vitamin B_6 deficiency can also contribute to a niacin deficiency, as the synthesis of niacin from tryptophan requires a vitamin B_6-dependent enzyme. Individuals who abuse alcohol also are at increased risk of niacin deficiency because alcohol significantly reduces niacin absorption.

The initial signs of niacin deficiency include fatigue, loss of appetite, weakness, mild gastrointestinal disturbance, anxiety, irritability, and depression. A severe deficiency causes a disease state known as pellagra ("rough skin") commonly showing symptoms of diarrhea, dermatitis (pigmented skin rash, especially to sun-exposed skin), dementia, and if left untreated, death ("4 Ds"). Additional symptoms include inflammation of the mucous membranes of the mouth (magenta tongue), apathy, fatigue, and loss of memory.

Toxicity Niacin toxicity from food sources has not been documented to the best of our knowledge. Pharmacologic doses of niacin have been used to treat hypercholesterolemia, which commonly causes minor adverse effects, including flushing and dizziness. Based upon estimated minimum levels that produce these symptoms, a tolerable upper limit for niacin has been established at 35 mg/day. Niacin at pharmacological doses (greater than 2000 mg/day) over a long period has been associated with elevated liver enzymes and elevated blood sugar levels in some individuals.

Recently, it has been reported that individuals seeking to "beat" urine drug screening have presented at Emergency Departments with symptoms of niacin toxicity, sometimes life-threatening. This misguided use of niacin can result in intake exceeding even normal pharmacologic doses and have resulted in symptoms ranging from nausea and vomiting to metabolic acidosis and electrocardiogram abnormalities.

Relationship to Disease Prevention Although excessive amounts of niacin may have adverse effects in some individuals, pharmacological doses of nicotinic acid (between 1 and 3 grams/day) have been used to successfully treat individuals with high blood cholesterol levels. Niacin has also been used to treat dizziness and tinnitus, as well as prevent premenstrual headaches. Side effects of mega doses of niacin include flushing, itching, and burning of the skin, particularly in the face, which may be minimized by administering an aspirin prior to ingesting each dose of niacin or by using a sustained release preparation.

Pantothenic Acid

Pantothenic acid is a B-complex vitamin. It is a precursor of two components necessary for the metabolism of fats, carbohydrates, and proteins called coenzyme A (CoA) and the acyl-carrier protein (ACP) moiety of the enzyme fatty acid synthase. CoA derived from food is hydrolyzed in the small intestine to form pantothenic acid, which is then absorbed in the jejunum.

Functions Pantothenic acid, as a component of Coenzyme A, is essential for the following bodily functions:
1) Synthesis of fatty acids, triglycerides, cholesterol, and acetylcholine.
2) Metabolism of protein and amino acids, fat, and carbohydrates.
3) Synthesis of cell membranes.

Deficiency Lack of pantothenic acid in the body is very unlikely and there is no evidence that a deficiency of this vitamin can occur naturally. However, by inducing a deficiency in test subjects, the following symptoms occur: indigestion, abdominal pain, burning sensation in the feet, arm and leg cramps, insomnia, and nerve inflammation (neuritis). Damage to the adrenal cortex, nervous system, skin, and hair has also been observed. It is thought that alcoholics may exhibit neuritis due to a lack of pantothenic acid; however, further evidence is needed for confirmation.

Toxicity: Unknown.

Biotin

Biotin is a member of the water-soluble B-complex of vitamins.

Forms and Absorption Biotin is absorbed in the proximal small intestine. Intestinal bacteria also synthesize biotin as a by-product, which contributes to body stores.

Functions: Biotin is an important prosthetic group in the class of enzymes called carboxylases, which use bicarbonate to attach a CO_2 group onto various metabolic substrates; as such, biotin plays a key role in glucose synthesis.

Deficiency Biotin deficiency in humans is rare. Experimentally, biotin deficiency has been induced in humans who consume large quantities of raw egg whites. These contain the protein avidin, which binds to biotin in the intestine preventing biotin absorption. Symptoms of biotin deficiency include inflammation of the skin, hair loss, muscle pain, abnormally increased sensitivity of the skin, loss of appetite, nausea, mental problems, high cholesterol, and decreased hemoglobin levels. Low levels of biotin have been found in some pregnant women, dialysis patients, and people who lack sufficient amounts of an enzyme needed for biotin absorption called biotinidase, although the symptoms of biotin deficiency and biotinidase deficiency are not identical.

Toxicity There is no evidence of biotin toxicity.

Pyridoxine (Vitamin B$_6$)

Vitamin B$_6$ is a water-soluble vitamin that is one of a group of compounds that includes pyridoxine and pyridoxamine, mainly found in plants, and pyridoxal, derived from animal products. All of these compounds are easily converted to pyridoxal phosphate, a coenzyme involved in the metabolism of amino acids.

Forms and Absorption Vitamin B$_6$ and its related compounds are absorbed in the jejunum. Once absorbed, vitamin B$_6$ is widely distributed in the body, primarily found in muscle tissue.

Functions Vitamin B$_6$-dependent enzymes perform a number of biochemical functions, such as:
1) Varied reactions involving amino acids, including transamination.
2) Synthesis of a variety of biogenic amines, including serotonin, dopamine, norepinephrine, and histamine.
3) Heme synthesis.
4) Conversion of the amino acid tryptophan to niacin; breakdown of glycogen to glucose phosphate; and the conversion of homocysteine to cysteine.

Deficiency Vitamin B$_6$ deficiency, while relatively rare, can occur as a consequence of an adverse interaction with the antitubercular drug, isoniazid, or penicillamine. This deficiency is characterized by cheilosis, glossitis, a pellagra-like dermatitis, depression, confusion, and EEG abnormalities.

Certain medical conditions have been associated with a decrease in the blood levels of pyridoxal phosphate: asthma, renal disease, Hodgkin's disease, sickle cell anemia, and diabetes.

Toxicity The tolerable upper intake level for vitamin B$_6$ has been established at 100 mg/day. Reports of toxicity have been noted in individuals taking 100 to 300 mg/day. Megadoses of 500 mg/day or higher of vitamin B$_6$ for two months or more can cause a polyneuropathy characterized by failure of muscular coordination and severe sensory damage, as well as photosensitivity.

Relationship to Disease Prevention Vitamin B$_6$, in the form of pyridoxine hydrochloride, has been utilized to treat Down's syndrome, autism, high oxalate levels in the urine, diabetes during pregnancy, carpal tunnel syndrome, asthma, depression, and diabetic neuropathy.

Vitamin B_{12}

Vitamin B_{12} is a water-soluble vitamin also known as cyanocobalamin (a synthetic form used in supplements); the term cobalamins refers to several forms of the vitamin of which cyanocobalamin and methylcobalamin are the most important. Cobalamins are produced by bacterial fermentation (e.g., in the rumen of cattle); therefore animal products provide the only dietary sources.

Form and Absorption Adequate absorption of Vitamin B_{12} depends on the presence of stomach acid and pepsin, pancreatic proteases, intrinsic factor (IF), and IF receptors on the terminal ileum. Because there is a low (~1 percent) rate of absorption even in the total absence of IF, individuals with B_{12} malabsorption may be maintained with large oral doses of vitamin B_{12} (250 to 1000 μg/day) after initial parenteral loading.

Functions Vitamin B_{12} is a prosthetic group required for two enzymatic reactions and is essential for cell replication and neurological function.

Deficiency Those at greatest risk of a vitamin B_{12} deficiency include strict vegetarians (vegans) who avoid all animal products, including meat, chicken, fish, eggs, and dairy products. Individuals with pernicious anemia lack intrinsic factor, and thus develop a B_{12} deficiency due to the inability to absorb the vitamin. Some people develop pernicious anemia as a consequence of autoimmune inactivation of IF. Others at risk include patients who have had their terminal ileum surgically removed as therapy for inflammatory bowel disease, cancer, or trauma. Patients taking proton pump inhibitors on a long-term basis may develop B_{12} deficiency secondary to malabsorption. Many older people develop achlorhydria and lose their ability to release B_{12} from protein, so they absorb less vitamin B_{12}. Alcohol abuse is also a risk factor for dietary B_{12} deficiency.

Symptoms of vitamin B_{12} deficiency include megaloblastic anemia, nerve damage (tingling in the hands and feet), and a swollen, painful, red tongue. Long-term vitamin B_{12} deficiency, if not treated, can cause severe, irreversible nerve damage and dementia.

Toxicity No toxic or adverse effects have been associated with large intakes of vitamin B_{12}. When high doses of vitamin B_{12} are given orally, only a small percentage is absorbed, which may explain its low toxicity. There is no tolerable upper intake level.

Vitamin B_{12} is a product of bacterial fermentation. The only dietary sources of vitamin B_{12} are foods of animal origin such as meat, chicken, fish, eggs, and dairy products. Fortified foods, such as brewers yeast and soy milk, may also contain added vitamin B_{12}. Seaweed, algae, spirulina, and fermented plant foods, such as tempeh and miso, are touted as vegetarian sources of vitamin B_{12} but contain only trace amounts.

Folate (Folic Acid)

Folate is a water-soluble B vitamin also known as folacin or folic acid. Folate is found in both plant and animal food sources. Dietary folate in the form of the polyglutamates is digested to the monoglutamate form and actively absorbed in the jejunum.

Functions Folate plays an essential role in transferring single carbon units to acceptor molecules and thus is important for the following:

1) Synthesis of DNA and RNA, cell division, and growth and development.
2) Synthesis of heme for the formation of blood cells.
3) Serving as a methyl donor for the enzyme involved in the conversion of homocysteine to methionine.

Deficiency Folate deficiency in humans is attributed to sub-optimal dietary intake of folate, inadequate absorption (e.g., as a consequence of gluten enteropathy), inadequate utilization (e.g., from drug antagonists like methotrexate or enzyme deficiencies), increased demands (e.g., pregnancy), or increased losses (e.g., liver disease or dialysis). Although folate deficiency is rare in the United States, it occurs in alcoholics, as well as individuals who are unable to absorb folate from their intestinal tract, such as those with Crohn's disease, ulcerative colitis, or short bowel syndrome.

Folate deficiency in the elderly may be the result of a poor diet or the use of drugs that impede the absorption of folate. Antacids hinder the absorption of folate by raising the pH levels of the upper intestine. Cimetidine, sulfasalazine, and phenytoin also impede the absorption of folate. Folate supplementation can reverse the macrocytic anemia in pernicious anemia; however, it will not reverse the neurologic damage caused by pernicious anemia (see vitamin B_{12}).

A lack of folate results in abnormalities in red blood cell formation in the bone marrow, affecting cell division. Symptoms of folate deficiency commence with macrocytosis and progress to macrocytic anemia. As the oxygen-carrying capacity of the blood gradually diminishes symptoms such as weakness, fatigue, irritability, headache, palpitations, and shortness of breath may appear. Folate deficiency also results in elevated blood homocysteine levels. It is estimated that two-thirds of individuals with high homocysteine levels have poor folate intake.

Toxicity The upper intake limit for folate has been set at 1 mg/day. Although folate appears to have little or no toxicity *per se*, the UL was established because excessive consumption of folic acid may mask vitamin B_{12} deficiency, allowing neurologic sequelae to progress even though the anemia associated with this deficiency resolves.

Relationship to Disease Prevention Since folate is involved in the synthesis of DNA and proteins, adequate levels are particularly important at times of rapid cell growth, such as in fetal development. It is thought that neural tube defects occur for a combination of two reasons: dietary deficiency of folate and a genetic defect in the production of enzymes involved in folate metabolism. Folate administration in the very early stages of pregnancy has been convincingly demonstrated as important in preventing neural tube defects. Fortification of certain foods with folate has been credited with substantially reducing the incidence of neural tube defects and perhaps some other birth defects. (Chapter 5: Case 2)

People with high blood levels of the amino acid homocysteine (HCys) have been shown to have an increased risk of developing heart disease. The "salvage" of homocysteine (a product of methylation reactions) by conversion to methionine requires methyl tetrahydrofolate; thus, a block in this reaction from inadequate folate or inadequate B_{12}, a required coenzyme for this conversion, results in elevations of HCys in the body. As vitamin B_6 is required for the lone alternative pathway for HCys utilization, a lack of any of these B vitamins causes especially high levels of HCys. Therefore, researchers have suggested that increasing folate, either through the diet or supplements, will reduce homocysteine levels in the blood and cut the risk of heart disease as well. However, recent findings report no beneficial vascular effects in high-risk populations, suggesting that elevated homocysteine may be a marker for increased risk of cardiovascular disease rather than a causative agent.

Folate Food Sources See Appendix F.

Minerals

Mineral elements are inorganic substances that occur as salts, such as sodium chloride (NaCl), or as a component of organic compounds, such as the iron in the tetrapyrrole ring of heme (e.g., hemoglobin) or the sulfur found in certain amino acids. Minerals are classified as macrominerals or microminerals, based on their percentages of total body weight.

Macrominerals constitute more than 0.005 percent of the body's weight, or 50 parts per million (ppm). Examples include calcium, chloride, phosphorus, potassium, magnesium, sodium, and sulfur.

Microminerals fall into two categories:
- Minerals with identified roles in health maintenance, including chromium, cobalt, copper, fluoride, iodide, iron, manganese, molybdenum, selenium, and zinc.
- Minerals with currently unestablished roles in health maintenance, such as arsenic, boron, cadmium, nickel, silicon, tin, and vanadium.

In foods, minerals commonly occur as salts, such as sodium chloride or as enzyme cofactors. Because salts are usually water soluble, some loss occurs during cooking, such as when vegetables are boiled. The body is capable of storing some minerals (e.g., iron in ferritin, calcium in bone) so that deficiencies may require a prolonged period of poor intake before symptoms develop.

Calcium

Calcium is abundant in the body, with 99 percent present in the bones and teeth. The remaining 1 percent is used for a variety of functions such as enzyme activation, blood clotting, and muscle contraction. Most calcium absorption occurs in the duodenum, but the jejunum and ileum contribute substantially to overall calcium absorption, as well. Vitamin D levels in the body regulate calcium absorption. The parathyroid gland responds to low serum calcium levels by releasing parathyroid hormone (PTH), which stimulates many tissues to convert vitamin D to its active form (calcitriol). Activated vitamin D, in turn, increases absorption of calcium from the intestine and regulates calcium excretion.

When calcium levels in the blood are elevated, the hormone calcitonin, released from the parafollicular cells (or "C cells") in the thyroid gland, prevents the bone from releasing calcium and promotes calcium excretion in the kidney. Individuals who have poor vitamin D intake and low sun exposure have poor calcium absorption. Lactose, the sugar in dairy products, improves calcium absorption in infants, whereas oxalate (which is present in spinach and rhubarb) and, to a lesser extent phytate, can inhibit calcium absorption. Calcium excretion is related to dietary protein intake – high protein diets increase urinary excretion of calcium; however protein intake accompanied by adequate calcium intake promotes bone growth. Adults with a history of calcium oxalate kidney stones should be advised to limit their protein intake to the RDA level of 0.8 (g/kg bodyweight)/day, avoid oxalate-rich foods, and limit salt intake.

Function Calcium plays an essential role in the following bodily functions:
1) Bone mineralization. Calcium levels are maintained in equilibrium by the movement of 250 to 1000 mg of calcium in and out of bone tissue every day.
2) Maintenance of cell membrane permeability.
3) Muscle contraction.
4) Blood clotting.
5) Nerve impulse conduction.

Calcium Deficiency Calcium deficiency usually remains undiagnosed for years because the bones serve as a reservoir and continue to release calcium into the blood. Symptoms of calcium deficiency (hypocalcemia) include irritability, "pins and needles" in hands and feet (paresthesia), muscle cramps and twitching (tetany), and possible seizures (convulsions). Eventually, low calcium can manifest as osteoporosis, with accompanying bone fractures and loss of height. Calcium deficiency in children is characterized by paresthesia of the mouth or extremities, stunted growth, tetany, and seizures.

Problems related to poor calcium intake include the following:
1) Rickets is caused most commonly by vitamin D deficiency, but lack of calcium and phosphorus can also be a basis for this disease. Rickets is characterized by abnormal bone formation, bending and distortion of the bones, nodular enlargements of the boney epiphyses, delayed closure of the fontanels, and bone pain.
2) Osteoporosis is defined as a reduction in bone density, rendering bones brittle and susceptible to fractures. Symptoms of osteoporosis may include altered posture caused by deformity of the spine, postural slumping due to acute pain,

waddling gait, loss of height, muscle weakness, and kyphosis. The bones most commonly affected include the hip, spine, wrist, and upper arm. A low calcium diet and lack of adequate physical activity are primary factors believed to contribute to the development of osteoporosis. Excessive alcohol intake, family history of osteoporosis, race, early menopause, short stature, and cigarette smoking are major contributors as well.

Calcium Toxicity Hypercalcemia may be seen in people with a hyperactive parathyroid gland, excessive intake of vitamin D, or certain cancers, including breast and lung cancer. Hypercalcemia may result in dehydration, lethargy, nausea, vomiting, anorexia, and possibly death. The tolerable upper limit for calcium intake has been established at 2500 mg/day.

Supplement Issues With the lifetime risk for osteoporotic fractures in women estimated as high as 50 percent, and costs associated with hip fracture alone estimated at $13 to $18 billion/year in the United States, combined with exponential increases expected for the future, prevention is key. While osteoporosis is a multifactorial disorder, calcium intake during adolescence and throughout life is critical to achieving optimal peak bone mass and also may play a significant role in preventing degenerative bone diseases in later years. Adolescents need to be educated about the importance of calcium for health, recommended intake (no s), and good food sources of calcium, particularly lower-fat dairy products. Calcium supplements are recommended for the following populations:
1) Post-menopausal women.
2) Amenorrheic women.
3) Patients who avoid dairy foods, or those who do not ingest 3 servings of dairy per day, including strict vegetarians, vegans, and lactose-intolerant persons.

Calcium supplementation to pregnant women with low calcium intakes reduced the severity of preeclampsia, maternal morbidity, and neonatal mortality. However, meta-analysis of cohort studies and clinical trials failed to show any reduction in fractures with increased calcium intake. More focus on the contribution of vitamin D and phosphate in combination with calcium supplementation is required.

Calcium Food Sources (including fortified sources) See Appendices G, H.

Magnesium
Forms and Absorption Magnesium is absorbed primarily in the distal jejunum and ileum and when intake is low, magnesium is more efficiently absorbed. Magnesium competes with calcium for absorption, and its absorption is also slightly enhanced by vitamin D. Magnesium is found in bone, muscle, cells, and extracellular fluid. The kidney is the principal modulator of magnesium homeostasis through filtration and reabsorption.

Functions Magnesium plays a role in the following physiological functions:

1) As a necessary chelator for the highly negatively-charged ATP and ADP molecules, it is involved in hundreds of ATP-requiring reactions in metabolism and active transport.
2) In conjunction with calcium, sodium, and potassium, magnesium is involved in transmitting neural impulses and thereby eliciting muscle contractions.
3) It is found as a component of bones and teeth.
4) Protein synthesis and cell replication are very sensitive to magnesium depletion.
5) Parathyroid hormone secretion; magnesium suppresses PTH secretion as does calcium, but is only about one-half as effective as Calcium.

Magnesium Deficiency While magnesium deficiency is rare due to its presence in a wide variety of foods, deficiency can occur in individuals who have absorption or excretion problems. These conditions include intestinal malabsorption, surgical removal of the lower part of the intestine, diuretic medications, severe vomiting, and kidney disease. Individuals with protein-calorie malnutrition, chronic alcohol abuse, hyperparathyroidism, and liver cirrhosis may have low levels of magnesium in their blood. Since magnesium is required for normal parathyroid functioning, low magnesium levels may alter calcium and phosphorous homeostasis.

Indications of magnesium deficiency include low levels of calcium and potassium in the blood, as well as changes in the gastrointestinal, neuromuscular, and cardiovascular systems. Individuals may also have fatigue, lethargy, weakness, poor appetite, impaired speech, anemia, irregular heartbeat, tremors, and failure to thrive. Clinical signs of advanced magnesium deficiency include rapid heart rate, cardiac fibrillation, and convulsions.

Magnesium Toxicity Elevated blood magnesium levels may be seen in people with renal failure or those receiving high doses of magnesium. High blood levels may result in changes in mental status, muscle weakness, nausea, extremely low blood pressure, difficulty breathing, and an irregular heartbeat. The tolerable upper limit for magnesium has been established at 350 mg/day for adults and adolescents.

Supplement Issues Low magnesium intake has been correlated with diabetes and heart disease risk in several studies of older Americans. Recent research has demonstrated that low magnesium intake is associated with increased risk of developing metabolic syndrome and type 2 diabetes. Additionally, low magnesium levels have been observed in obese children with insulin resistance, although a cause-and-effect relationship has not yet been established.

Magnesium supplementation may benefit the following patients:

1) Patients with asthma.
2) Patients taking antidiuretics or certain medications for the treatment of cancer.
3) Patients with malabsorptive diseases, such as gluten enteropathy.
4) Persons with chronically low levels of potassium and calcium.
5) Patients with diabetes or pre-diabetes.
6) Older adults.

For patients with renal disease, serious accumulation of magnesium can occur. High doses (1000 to 5000 mg) may cause toxicity symptoms.

Magnesium Food Sources (including enriched sources): See Appendix K.

Phosphorus

Phosphorus is second in abundance to calcium and is an essential mineral present in bones and teeth, as well as phospholipids, proteins, carbohydrates, enzymes, DNA, and ATP.

Form and Absorption Phosphorous is absorbed in the form of phosphate primarily in the small intestine. Absorption rates are generally high (about 2/3 is absorbed), and this is fairly constant; however, while vitamin D may promote uptake by active transport, the observed constancy of phosphate fractional absorption suggests that most uptake occurs by a passive, concentration-dependent process. Aluminum-containing antacids can reduce phosphate absorption, however.

Function Phosphorous plays an essential role in the following bodily functions:
1) Normal construction of bones and teeth.
2) DNA and RNA synthesis.
3) Energy synthesis (ATP, ADP).
4) Aids in protein, fat, and carbohydrate metabolism.
5) Phosphate helps to maintain the body's normal pH levels.
6) Normal cell membrane structure.

Phosphorus Deficiency Phosphorous deficiency is generally regarded as rare, but occurs most commonly in chronic alcoholics during withdrawal or in persons who have experienced diabetic ketoacidosis. It may be observed in individuals who consume excessive and prolonged amounts of aluminum hydroxide-containing antacids; the aluminum binds dietary phosphorous preventing its absorption. Symptoms of phosphorous deficiency are primarily a consequence of decreased levels of ATP and include weakness, anorexia, and bone pain; proximal myopathy is observed in some instances. Prolonged deficiency can result in rickets or osteomalacia, due to the need for phosphate for hydroxyapatite formation in bone.

Phosphate Toxicity Abnormal elevated blood phosphorus levels appear in individuals with renal failure and can give rise to the precipitation of calcium phosphate in tissues (metastatic calcification), further compromising kidney function. High dietary intake of phosphate in persons with normal kidney function does not seem to cause this toxicity. Recent data have suggested that elevated phosphorus levels are a risk factor for cardiovascular disease. The tolerable upper limit for phosphorus has been established at 4000 mg/day.

Supplement Issues None.

Phosphorous Food Sources See Table 10-4.

Iron

Iron is an essential element in all cells of the body. As a component of hemoglobin, myoglobin, and cytochrome enzymes, iron plays a key role in oxygen transport and normal cellular respiration.

Forms and Absorption Iron is absorbed in the duodenum via iron-binding proteins that transfer it across the intestinal mucosa. Non-heme iron absorption requires an acidic gastric pH to convert it from ferric (Fe^{+++}) to ferrous (Fe^{++}) forms. The absorption of iron from plants (non-heme iron) is enhanced by the concurrent ingestion of vitamin C (which aids in reducing the valence of ferric iron) and is increased in iron-deficient individuals through upregulation of the divalent metal transporter in mucosal cells. Heme iron is absorbed considerably more efficiently than non-heme iron.

Function Iron plays an essential role in the following physiological functions:
1) Hemoglobin and myoglobin synthesis. About 70 to 75 percent of the body's iron is bound to hemoglobin and myoglobin while the other 25 to 30 percent is stored as ferritin and hemosiderin in the liver, bone marrow, and spleen. Iron is transported in the serum bound to transferrin, which represents about 1 percent of the body's iron stores.
2) Cytochrome protein synthesis. Many cytochrome proteins contain iron bound to heme; these enzymes function in a variety of roles, including many metabolic reactions, electron transport, and drug detoxification.

Iron Deficiency Iron deficiency is one of the most prevalent nutritional problems in the world, with pregnant women, infants and children, and menstruating females at greatest risk. Iron deficiency is most frequently caused by inadequate dietary intake, or a diet with low bioavailable iron, as seen with vegetarians or infants who are not given iron-fortified formula or cereal after the age of six months. In the United States, the iron intake of most boys and men exceeds the RDA, while intake of most girls and women (up to the age of 50) is less than the RDA. Iron deficiency is characterized by weakness, fatigue, poor work performance, adverse pregnancy outcomes, developmental delays, and cognitive impairment. Symptoms of iron deficiency include poor capillary bed refill, pale mucosa, fatigue, feelings of faintness, cold or abnormal sensations of the extremities, shortness of breath, greater susceptibility to infections, and concave shaped or brittle nails. Infants and young children with iron deficiency may have low IQ levels and learning and/or behavioral problems.

Iron Toxicity Excessive iron ingestion may cause deposition of iron in the tissues. Prolonged iron overload (e.g., hemochromatosis) may cause bronzed pigmentation to the skin and damaged liver and pancreas tissue and may possibly cause diabetes. The hemochromatosis gene is present in 1 in 200 non-Hispanic white Americans, although even among homozygote individuals, only 1 percent develop signs of iron overload. The tolerable upper limit (UL) for iron has been established at 45 mg/day for normal adults based upon gastrointestinal side effects.

Supplementation Issues Iron deficiency anemia is an important cause of morbidity in several populations (i.e. infants, pregnant women, women with heavy menstruation losses). Iron supplementation for infants is indicated for pre-term or low birth weight infants, children whose diet does not include foods fortified with iron, or those with frank anemia. However, iron can be toxic at doses not much higher than the therapeutic range, and a meta-analysis of data currently available indicates that giving iron supplementation to children who are already iron replete can cause adverse effects on weight gain and possibly increased susceptibility to infection. Similarly, while iron deficiency is a common cause of anemia in pregnancy and benefits from supplementation, recent data suggest that iron supplementation in non-anemic pregnant women can cause increases in hypertension and small-for-gestational age births.

Although it is commonly believed that older adults are at high risk for iron deficiency, results are mixed and data from the Framingham Heart Study showed that elevated iron stores (evidenced by high serum ferritin) are 4 to 5 times more common than iron deficiency among white Americans aged 67 to 96 years; similar results have been obtained in other countries. Because of known risks for heart disease and cancer attributable to excessive iron, the older population should be advised against taking iron supplements unless iron deficiency is documented by laboratory results.

Iron Food Sources (including fortified sources) See Appendix L.

Zinc

Forms and Absorption Zinc status is determined through a balance of absorption in the intestine (principally the jejunum) and secretion of endogenous reserves; zinc depletion increases the efficiency of its absorption. Zinc absorption is reduced in the presence of copper, iron, oxalate, calcium, phytate, and fiber. Once absorbed, zinc is widely distributed throughout the body, with highest levels found in the prostate, skin, brain, liver, pancreas, bone, and blood.

Function Zinc plays an essential role in the following bodily functions:
1) Acts as a cofactor for over 100 enzymes, playing an important role in carbohydrate, fat, and protein metabolism.
2) Normal cell division, growth, and repair at all stages of life, especially during fetal growth.
3) Synthesis of DNA and RNA and gene regulation.
4) Normal immune function including wound healing and skin integrity.
5) Sexual maturation, fertility, and reproduction.
6) Maintenance of normal sense of taste and smell.

Zinc Deficiency Zinc deficiency, which can occur due to poor intake or with malabsorption syndromes, can be manifested as symptoms of poor appetite, changes in perception of taste and smell, hair loss, skin problems, poor wound healing, impaired cell mediated immunity, and growth retardation in infants, children and adolescents. If affected, the cornea, which has a very high zinc concentration, may develop edema and opacification.

Zinc Toxicity Zinc toxicity is rare, but high intakes can cause diarrhea, nausea, and vomiting. Chronic toxicity can impair copper status, and may depress immune function. High doses of zinc have also been associated with urinary tract infections and other negative effects on the urinary tract. The tolerable upper limit for zinc has been established at 40 mg/day.

Zinc Requirements Individuals with intestinal resection or surgical removal of all or part of their intestines may require zinc supplementation, as both transit time and surface area influence zinc absorption.

Supplementation Issues Individuals who may benefit from zinc supplementation include
1) Those with malabsorption or chronic diarrhea.
2) Vegetarians, due to lower efficiency of zinc absorption from plant material.
3) Alcoholics, as alcohol inhibits zinc absorption and promotes excretion.
4) Children who exhibit growth failure accompanied by zinc deficiency.
5) Lactating women, as there is a greater need for zinc during this period.

Zinc supplements should not be taken simultaneously with either calcium or iron supplements as these interfere with zinc absorption. Long-term high doses can cause copper deficiency, which produces brittle nails, weaken immune function, and cause urinary complications. Doses exceeding 40 mg per day may interfere with white blood cell function. Zinc supplementation has been shown to significantly reduce the frequency and severity of childhood diarrhea and respiratory illnesses.

Copper
Form and Absorption Copper absorption occurs in the small intestine. Absorption is enhanced in an acidic medium and decreased by the presence of calcium, phytates, fiber, or zinc. About 30 to 50 percent of the copper in the diet is absorbed.

Functions Copper plays an essential role in the following bodily functions:
1) Production of skin, hair, and eye pigment (melanin).
2) Synthesis of connective tissue (copper functions in the development of healthy bones, teeth, and vascular structures).
3) Protection of cells from oxygen damage (as a component of antioxidant enzymes).
4) Maintenance of the myelin sheath surrounding nerve fibers.

5) Metabolism of catecholamines required in the functioning of the nervous system.
6) Essential for iron metabolism (anemia is a consequence of copper deficiency).

Copper Deficiency Copper deficiency is rare though it can occur in malnourished infants, and poor copper absorption can occur in certain disease states (e.g., Menkes syndrome). Copper deficiency results in anemia and connective tissue damage, which can cause lung damage or excessive bleeding. Low levels of copper in the blood are seen in nutritional disorders such as kwashiorkor, anemia, tropical sprue, and celiac disease.

Copper Toxicity Excessive copper intake or poisoning may occur with consumption of acidic beverages stored in containers made with copper. Symptoms of copper toxicity include nausea, diarrhea, vomiting, anemia, anuria, and, in extreme cases, death.

The genetic syndrome Wilson's disease results in decreased blood copper levels, but with increased copper deposits in certain organs such as the brain, kidney, cornea, and liver. Untreated, it can result in nervous system and liver damage. The tolerable upper limit for copper has been established at 10,000 µg/day.

Supplement Issues None.

Sodium

Functions Sodium functions together with chloride to regulate hydration and cell membrane potentials. Sodium is the predominant extracellular cation.

Sodium Deficiency Sodium deficiency is uncommon. Most Americans consume 3000 to 4000 mg of sodium daily (about 9 g of table salt), while the recommended upper limit for daily intake is 2300 mg. Fluid retention or sodium loss can cause low serum sodium levels (hyponatremia) which may represent relative deficiency of sodium. Prolonged vomiting, diarrhea, excessive or persistent sweating (such as marathon runners, or those who participate in triathlons), and certain forms of kidney disease also cause sodium deficiency. A "salt-wasting" crisis can also occur as a consequence of insufficient aldosterone production, as seen in congenital adrenal hyperplasia. Symptoms of hyponatremia include headache, nausea, vomiting, muscle cramps, fainting, fatigue, and death.

Sodium Toxicity Excess serum sodium (hypernatremia) is generally caused by inadequate hydration rather than excess sodium intake. Symptoms of hypernatremia include vomiting, diarrhea, excess sweating, mental status changes due to cerebral edema, seizures, and death.

Relationship to Disease Prevention
Hypertension Hypertension affects about one in four adults or about 50 million Americans. It is a leading cause of stroke and can contribute to a heart attack, heart

failure, and kidney failure. It is well-known that diets high in sodium are associated with a higher risk of developing hypertension in salt-sensitive populations. Studies, including the DASH Trials, have shown that restricting sodium intake to below 1.2 g/day (<3 g of salt, sodium chloride) is effective in lowering systolic blood pressure by 6–9 mm Hg and can improve the action of certain medications, such as diuretics, in lowering blood pressure. However, other studies have reported that for the US population mean intake, increases in sodium actually correlated with a decreased risk of cardiovascular disease and all-cause mortality, although a few studies of populations with high sodium intakes (4.4 to 5.4 g/day) showed reductions in cardiovascular disease with salt restriction. Thus, health benefits from salt restriction may be limited to persons with excessive intake or other conditions that alter risk.

Osteoporosis Along with decreasing the risk of hypertension, lowering an individual's sodium intake may decrease the risk of osteoporosis because high salt intake has been shown to increase the amount of calcium excreted in the urine. By decreasing salt intake, more calcium remains in the body thereby decreasing the risk for bone loss.

Sodium Food Sources See Appendix I.

Potassium
The predominant intracellular cation; even small changes in the concentration of extracellular potassium greatly affect the extracellular:intracellular potassium ratio and thereby affect neural transmission, muscle contraction, and vascular tone.

Function Potassium is an extremely important electrolyte that functions in the maintenance of the following:
1) Water balance and distribution.
2) Acid-base balance.
3) Muscle and nerve cell function.
4) Heart function.
5) Kidney and adrenal function.
6) Potassium is needed for glycogen storage, perhaps because low potassium suppresses insulin secretion.

Potassium Deficiency Low levels of potassium in the blood, referred to as hypokalemia, is most commonly a result of excess potassium losses. These losses can occur from vomiting, diarrhea, kidney disease, or metabolic disturbances, as well as sweat-producing exercise where potassium and electrolytes are not replenished. Diuretics (prescribed for patients with hypotension or congestive heart failure) or excessive use of laxatives can also cause hypokalemia (defined as a serum potassium level below 3.5 mmol/L). Because potassium is found mainly in fruits and non-grain vegetables, a diet lacking in these foods can lead to potassium deficiency. In potassium deficiency there may not be sufficient glycogen reserves, and muscle weakness progressing to respiratory failure can occur. Other symptoms include fatigue, constipation, impaired renal function resulting in excessive urination (polyuria), and adverse cardiac effects on persons taking digitalis. Severely low levels can lead to cardiac arrhythmias.

Potassium Toxicity Potassium toxicity is unlikely, except in patients with poor renal function or excessive supplementation. Hyperkalemia can be seen in trauma or severe burns that lead to significant tissue damage resulting in release of potassium into the blood. Symptoms of hyperkalemia include tingling in the hands and feet, muscle weakness, and temporary paralysis. Severe hyperkalemia, if left untreated, can cause EKG changes characterized by ventricular asystole and fibrillation and eventually cardiac arrest.

Supplementation Issues Potassium can help to maintain proper function of both the heart and nervous system. Regular consumption of high-potassium foods or potassium supplements may help to lower and control blood pressure. People with heart failure or high blood pressure must receive adequate amounts of this mineral. An elevated potassium intake has also been linked to decreasing the risk of stroke, osteoporosis, and calcium-containing kidney stones.

Potassium Food Sources See Appendix J.

Selenium

Selenium is an essential trace mineral in the body that contributes to antioxidant defense mechanisms.

Form and Absorption Selenium absorption is efficient and is not regulated. Selenium enters in the body from the diet in the form of selenocysteine and selenomethionine. It is absorbed in the gastrointestinal tract in the range of 50 to 100 percent. Selenium leaves the body via urine, feces, skin, and as an exhaled metabolite that is exhaled.

Functions:
1) Selenium is an essential component of the enzyme glutathione peroxidase, which protects cells from the damaging effects of free radicals. For example, LDL oxidation is reduced by selenium.
2) Selenium is essential for normal functioning of the immune system and thyroid gland.
3) Epidemiological and animal studies have shown that selenium may have anti-cancer properties, possibly from its antioxidant function.

Selenium Deficiency Selenium deficiency is not common in the United States and seldom causes frank illness when it occurs in isolation. However, selenium deficiency has been seen in people maintained on total parenteral nutrition (TPN) as their only source of nutrition. People with gastrointestinal problems can have impairment of selenium absorption. Low selenium intake has been seen in children with kwashiorkor because selenium is found only in protein.

Signs of selenium deficiency are seen in countries where the selenium content in the soil is very low and therefore selenium intake is poor. These areas include China, New Zealand, and Venezuela. Furthermore people living in areas of China, New Zealand, and Venezuela may develop an enlarged heart with poor cardiac function as a result of selenium deficiency.

Selenium Toxicity Selenium toxicity is rare in the United States and the few reported cases have been associated with industrial accidents and a manufacturing error that led to an excessively high dose of selenium in a supplement. High blood levels of selenium called selenosis lead to symptoms including gastrointestinal upset, hair loss, and fatigue. Acute toxicity can lead to respiratory distress syndrome, myocardial infarction, and renal failure. The tolerable upper limit established for selenium is 400 µg per day.

Supplement Issues Most cases of selenium deficiency occur as a consequence of a gastroenterological disturbance, such as Crohn's disease. Preliminary studies have shown a correlation between low plasma selenium levels and cancer risk. Currently, a large clinical trial is underway to study the use of selenium supplements for the prevention of prostate cancer. The Selenium and Vitamin E Cancer Prevention Trial (SELECT) is a phase III randomized, placebo-controlled trial of selenium (200 µg/day) and/or vitamin E (400 IU/day) supplementation for a minimum of 7 years (maximum of 12 years) in American men 50 years of age and older. The Nutritional Prevention of Cancer study has also reported that selenium supplementation is associated with reduced risk of colorectal cancer and adenomas in subjects with a low baseline selenium level. However, this same trial recently reported that selenium supplementation on top of adequate dietary selenium may increase the risk for type 2 diabetes.

Fluoride

Fluoride is found at varying concentrations in drinking water and soil. It is not an essential nutrient in the customary sense, but helps protect the teeth against dental caries. Although found in bone, fluoride has not convincingly been shown to prevent fractures or osteoporosis. About 99 percent of the fluoride in the body is in the bone and teeth. When fluoride is consumed in optimal amounts from water and food, or used topically in toothpastes, mouth rinses, and professionally applied office treatments it functions to

1) Increase tooth mineralization and bone density.
2) Reduce the risk and prevalence of dental caries.
3) Promote enamel re-mineralization throughout life for individuals of all ages.

Fluoride Deficiency As there is no known metabolic function for fluoride, a deficiency state cannot be defined.

Water Fluoridation Fluoridation of public water supplies has been endorsed by over 90 professional health organizations as the most effective dental public health measure in existence. Still, about half of the US population fails to receive the maximum benefits possible from community water fluoridation and the use of fluoride products. Although fluoride treatment has long been recognized as being of benefit to children, a recent meta-analysis indicated that fluoride also causes significant reduction in dental caries in adults of all ages.

Fluoride Toxicity: Fluoride can be toxic when consumed in excessive amounts, so concentrated fluoride products should be used with caution. To prevent the possibility of acute fluoride poisoning, fluoride products should be kept out of reach of small children. Fluorosis results from excessive fluoride ingestion prior to tooth eruption and results in a disruption of tooth enamel formation. Fluorosis can range from mild to severe. In cases of mild fluorosis, teeth are highly resistant to dental caries but may have chalky white spots or patches. Severe fluorosis can result in teeth with brown discoloration and is most often seen in areas of the country that have excessive concentrations of natural fluoride in water supplies, such as wells.

Swallowing of fluoride toothpaste in early years, misuse of dietary fluoride supplements, or long-term use of infant formula (particularly powder concentrates reconstituted with fluoridated water) can lead to fluorosis. To minimize the risk of excessive exposure the American Dental Association requires toothpaste manufacturers to include the phrase "use only a pea-sized amount (of toothpaste) for children under six" on labels.

Supplement Issues Fluoride supplementation may benefit children and patients who do not have fluoride added to their public drinking water.

Fluoride Sources The primary dietary source of fluoride is fluoridated water. The average child under age 6 consumes less than a half liter of water a day and would consume less than 0.5 mg/day of fluoride from drinking optimally fluoridated water. The TUL for infants 0 to 6 months is 0.7 mg/day and 1.3 mg/day for children ages 1–3 years.

Iodine

Iodine is essential for humans as a component of thyroid hormones (thyroxine). Approximately 40 percent of the body's iodine is stored in the thyroid gland.

Forms and Absorption Iodine is absorbed in the gastrointestinal tract in the ionized form (I^-). Extra iodine in the body is excreted via the urine.

Iodine Deficiency If there is not enough iodine in the body, there is a decrease in the production of the thyroid hormones (T_3 and T_4). To compensate for this lack of production of the thyroid hormones, the thyroid gland hypertrophies (goiter). Symptoms of iodine deficiency include lethargy, dry skin, thick lips, enlarged tongue, reduced muscle and skeletal growth, and mental retardation (cretinism).

Iodine Toxicity Excessive dietary intake of iodine results in inhibition of thyroid hormone synthesis. Generally, the body will adapt to the higher intake, but a few individuals will develop goiters due to reduced iodine absorption when iodine blood levels are too high. The tolerable upper limit for iodine has been established at 1100 µg/day.

Supplement Issues Iodine deficiency affects 1.9 billion people worldwide, and is a common worldwide cause of endemic goiter and cretinism in children who do not have access to iodized salt or live in mountainous places where iodine is not found. Congenital hypothyroidism has been reported to occur at a rate of about one out of every 4000 children and early treatment with iodine is necessary to avoid mental retardation. Many people are interested in potassium iodide supplements to prevent radioactive iodine uptake in the event of a nuclear accident or after exposure to medical radiation. Supplementation with iodine has been shown to be effective in reducing the risk of an iodine-deficient child developing thyroid cancer after exposure to radiation from a radiation accident or from medical procedures.

Chromium

Chromium is proposed to potentiate the action of insulin and has been identified as a "glucose tolerance factor."

Form and Absorption Chromium exists in various inorganic forms; most chromium found in food is in the trivalent chromium (III) form. Chromium absorption depends upon the form and physiochemical reactions in the intestinal lumen, but generally the efficiency of absorption is low (<3 percent). Fiber and phytates reduce absorption and a deficient diet results in higher fractional absorption rates.

Functions Chromium is hypothesized to potentiate the action of insulin via an oligopeptide that as been named "chromodulin," which binds to the insulin receptor stimulating its tyrosine kinase activity.

Chromium Deficiency A diet high in simple sugars promotes chromium excretion and may lead to long-term deficits. Since it is not possible to determine chromium status, it is difficult to determine the impact of low chromium intake.

Chromium Toxicity As no adverse effects have been observed from excess chromium intake from food no TUL has been established. The predominant form of chromium in food and supplements is the trivalent form (Cr^{+++}), which is not believed to have any toxic effects. However, in the light of reports that hexavalent chromium at high levels in drinking water in a Chinese province is believed to be responsible for increased mortality from stomach cancer, concerns about overuse of chromium supplements remains. However, meta-analysis of reports indicated that hexavalent chromium was only weakly linked to lung cancer and not to any other cancers.

Supplement Issues In diabetic subjects chromium supplementation, usually with chromium picolinate or chloride, has been shown to improve insulin sensitivity and reduce serum lipids in some studies, although conflicting results continue to be reported. A recent review of 41 separate studies concluded that while chromium supplementation in patients with type 2 diabetes had a modest beneficial effect on glycemia and dyslipidemia, the overall poor quality of the studies limited the strength of the conclusion. The Office of Dietary Supplements of the National Institutes of Health has concluded that "the value of chromium supplements for diabetics is inconclusive and controversial." Newer forms of chromium bound to niacin or biotin are available and may have improved efficacy.

Case 1 **Iron Deficiency Anemia in Women**

Lisa Hark

University of Pennsylvania School of Medicine, Philadelphia, PA

OBJECTIVES

- Describe the prevalence of and risk factors for iron deficiency in US women.
- Recognize signs and symptoms of iron deficiency.
- Evaluate and interpret laboratory values used to diagnose iron deficiency.
- Become familiar with methods for prevention and treatment of iron deficiency.

AP, a 36-year-old Chinese–American woman, presents to her family physician complaining of fatigue lasting over the past year and of "always being cold." One year ago, she gave birth to a full-term healthy baby. She initially assumed her symptoms were due to the demands of caring for her infant, but reports that her fatigue is much greater in severity than that experienced after delivering her first child seven years ago. She was an avid runner throughout her adult years, but has been unable to run even a mile over the last few months due to the overwhelming fatigue. She feels a lack of energy throughout the day, and has difficulty focusing while at work.

AP has a history of heavy menses; she typically uses more than five sanitary pads on each of the first two days of her period, which lasts seven days. She resumed menstruating four months after giving birth. She occasionally has small amounts of blood in her stool from hemorrhoids, but has not had any frank gastrointestinal bleeding and denies other sources of blood loss.

Past Medical History

AP has a recent history of iron deficiency anemia. At six months gestation, routine hemoglobin screening revealed a normal value of 12.5 g/dL. One month after giving birth, AP's hemoglobin was tested by her gynecologist, revealing a significantly reduced level of 7.4 g/dL. Iron deficiency anemia was suspected. Her laboratory results confirmed the diagnosis and AP's gynecologist prescribed ferrous sulfate (325 mg, three times per day) for six months. Unfortunately, AP found that the iron supplements caused constipation and abdominal pain. She discontinued them and began taking a multivitamin containing iron.

Diet History

AP avoids red meat due to its saturated fat content, and eats chicken and fish each about once a week each. In an effort to increase the calcium in her diet, she reports

---

Medical Nutrition and Disease: A Case-Based Approach, 4th edition. Edited by Lisa Hark.
© 2009 Wiley-Blackwell Publishing, ISBN: 978-1-4051-8615-5.

that she generally tries to eat a dairy food at each meal: milk with cereal for breakfast, yogurt and fruit at lunch, and cheese with pasta or in a casserole for dinner. She obtains most of her vegetable intake from salads containing lettuce, cucumbers, and tomatoes. She does not each much fruit.

Physical Examination
Vital Signs
Temperature: 98.6 °F (37 °C)
Heart rate: 80 BPM
Respiration: 26 BPM
Blood pressure: 110/60 mm Hg
Height: 5′8″ (173 cm)
Current weight: 145 lbs (65.8 kg)
BMI: 24 kg/m^2

Exam
General: Well-developed, well-nourished female in no acute distress.
Skin: Pallor
Eyes: Conjunctiva pale conjunctiva?
Nails: No spoon nails

Laboratory Data

Current Labs:	Normal Values
Hemoglobin: 9.5 mg/dL	12–16 g/dL
Hemotocrit: 35%	37–48%
MCV: 82 fL	86–98 fL
Ferritin (serum): 7 ng/mL	Females: 12–150 ng/mL
Iron (serum): 40 µg/dL	50–150 µg/dL
TIBC: 425 µg/dL	250–370 µg/dL

Case Questions
1. What are the prevalence of and risk factors for iron deficiency anemia in pre-menopausal women in the United States?
2. Which signs and symptoms of iron deficiency did this patient exhibit?
3. How was the diagnosis of iron deficiency anemia confirmed in this patient?
4. What diet history questions should be asked of patients suspected of iron deficiency? How would you counsel this patient to improve her dietary iron intake and absorption?
5. How should iron deficiency be treated?

Answers to Questions: Case 1
Part 1: Prevalence and Diagnosis

1. What are the prevalence of, and risk factors for, iron deficiency anemia in pre-menopausal women in the United States?
Iron deficiency is a fairly prevalent problem in pre-menopausal women. According to the NHANES III data (1994–1998), five percent of women aged 20 to 49 have

iron deficiency anemia, and 11 percent have iron deficiency without anemia. The prevalence of iron deficiency was similar in NHANES III and NHANES 1999–2000 in most age and sex groups, with the exception of males aged 12–69 years and women aged 50–69 years. In these groups, the prevalence was substantially higher in NHANES 1999–2000 than in NHANES III as determined by a t-test.

Risk for iron deficiency is a function of levels of iron loss, iron intake, iron absorption, and physiologic demands. Populations most at risk include pregnant women, women of child-bearing age, and women with heavy menses. Other populations at risk include strict vegetarians and vegans, infants, toddlers, and adolescents. Low iron intake and decreased iron absorption are the most common etiologies.

Women in their child-bearing years have greater iron needs than men due to menstrual blood losses, iron demands of the developing fetus during pregnancy, and blood loss during childbirth. Uterine fibroids (common, benign tumors often found in women of child-bearing age) may cause heavy and prolonged menses, resulting in increased blood loss. In order to avoid the development of iron deficiency during this time, dietary iron intake must keep pace with increased demands. Those not consuming adequate quantities of iron-rich foods may be at risk for iron deficiency.

Iron deficiency in women (and in men) may also be caused by other sources of blood loss including frequent blood donation, gastrointestinal bleeding, neoplasms, inflammatory bowel disease, parasitic infections (more common in third world populations than developed countries), and hemorrhoids. Chronic blood loss may occur from the urinary tract as well.

In this case, AP's heavy menstrual periods and aspects of her dietary intake increase her risk for iron deficiency. Occasional bleeding from hemorrhoids is most likely not a contributing factor.

2. What are the clinical signs and symptoms of iron deficiency?

Clinical signs of anemia include pallor, mouth changes such as glossitis (atrophy of the lingual papillae), and angular stomatitis, as well as tachycardia. Symptoms are generally non-specific and may include fatigue, palpitations, or dyspnea. Fatigue is a common presentation of iron deficiency with or without anemia. Iron is necessary for hemoglobin synthesis in red blood cells, which functions in oxygen transport and delivery from the lungs to the tissues. Iron deficiency can lead to fatigue as oxygen is needed for energy (ATP) production. In addition, iron serves as a cofactor for many physiologically important enzymes, including those involved in oxidative metabolism, dopamine, DNA synthesis, and free radical formation in neutrophils.

Presumably due to a lack of oxygen needed for energy and heat production, iron deficiency may cause a sensation of feeling cold, affect work capacity and exercise tolerance, affect neurotransmitter function, and diminish immunologic and inflammatory defenses. Other symptoms of iron deficiency include cold intolerance, pica (compulsive eating of non-food items), and pagophagia (compulsive eating of ice). Patients having any of these signs and symptoms should receive a laboratory evaluation for iron deficiency.

3. How was the diagnosis of iron deficiency anemia confirmed in this patient?

Laboratory evaluation along with physical signs and symptoms can confirm a diagnosis of iron deficiency. Serum ferritin, iron, and TIBC were outside the normal reference range. A complete blood count revealed a microcytic anemia with a low mean corpuscular volume (MCV) of 82 fL. In this patient, serum ferritin was low at 7 ng/mL. Serum iron was low at 40 μg/dL, and total iron binding capacity (TIBC) was high at 425 μg/dL (the TIBC, or transferrin, concentration increases to compensate for low iron availability), confirming the diagnosis of iron deficiency. The patient's hemoglobin, hematocrit, and MCV were low, indicating a microcytic anemia, and reticulocyte count was low, indicating decreased red blood cell production.

Serum ferritin is the single best non-invasive, sensitive marker of iron status. Serum ferritin concentrations reflect body iron stores (one microgram/liter of serum ferritin concentration is equivalent to approximately 10 mg of stored iron). Compared to the gold standard of a bone marrow biopsy, serum ferritin is a sensitive and specific indicator of iron depletion. Levels below 15 mg/mL are 75 percent sensitive and 98 percent specific for iron deficiency. However, because serum ferritin is an acute phase reactant, chronic infection, inflammation, or diseases causing tissue and organ damage can raise its concentration independent of iron status masking depleted tissue stores of iron.

Transferrin saturation (which is equivalent to serum iron concentration divided by the total-iron binding capacity (TIBC) × 100) reflects the extent to which iron binding sites are vacant on transferrin. It is another commonly used measure to assess iron deficiency. Normal saturation falls between 30 and 35 percent, whereas levels less than 15 percent indicate decreased iron availability for erythropoiesis in the bone marrow.

Overall, this measure does not perform as well as ferritin among non-pregnant women of childbearing age. As with ferritin measurements, factors other than iron status can affect results of this test. Serum iron varies diurnally (higher in the a.m., lower in the p.m.), increases after meals, and is decreased by infection and inflammation. Inflammation, chronic infection, malignancies, liver disease, nephrotic syndrome, and malnutrition can reduce TIBC and oral contraceptive use and pregnancy can increase it.

Erythrocyte protoporphyrin concentration can also be used to assess whether adequate iron is available for red blood cell synthesis. Protoporphyrin levels remain elevated when there is inadequate iron available to be integrated into hemoglobin. Normal protoporphyrin levels vary from 16 to 65 μg/dL in adults. Anemia produces levels over 100 μg/dL.

Iron deficiency often exists without anemia, but deficiency without anemia will progress to anemia if the causes of deficiency are not corrected. Red blood cells are small, or microcytic, due to insufficient hemoglobin production, and numbers of new red blood cells, or reticulocyte counts, are low indicating decreased bone marrow production of red blood cells.

In the presence of an inflammatory or infectious state, when iron deficiency risk factors or symptoms of iron deficiency are present but ferritin is in the normal range, a complete blood count (CBC) and a reticulocyte count may be quite helpful. If iron deficiency is indeed present, erythrocyte indices (e.g., MCV) should improve with iron administration, and a therapeutic trial of supplementation will help to confirm or rule out iron deficiency.

Part 2: Medical Nutrition Therapy and Treatment

4. What diet history questions should be asked of patients suspected of iron deficiency? How would you counsel this patient to improve her dietary iron intake and absorption?

Sources of dietary iron include red meat, poultry, fish and shellfish, nuts and seeds, legumes and bean products, green leafy vegetable, raisins, whole grains, and fortified cereals. In evaluating a patient for iron deficiency, the clinician should inquire about dietary intake of iron-rich foods, as well as dietary factors that may influence the absorption of iron (e.g., low vitamin C intake). Ascorbic acid can reduce ferric iron to its more soluble ferrous form, thus decreasing the formation of insoluble complexes. Thus, ascorbic acid can enhance iron absorption by forming soluble complexes with iron at low pH that remains soluble in the more alkaline environment of the duodenum.

Iron absorption is not directly correlated to iron intake. As physiologic iron levels decrease, the efficiency of gastrointestinal absorption of iron increases. The bioavailability of iron, or the percentage of dietary iron absorbed and ultimately physiologically available, varies depending on the dietary source of the iron and other foods consumed at the same time as the iron-containing foods. Heme (dietary iron attached to heme-containing proteins, such as myoglobin or hemoglobin) and non-heme iron are absorbed by different receptors on the intestinal mucosa. Iron bound to heme is highly absorbable and represents 40 percent of iron from animal sources. The absorption of non-heme iron can be increased or decreased by various factors. Phytates, or inositol phosphate salts that store minerals in plant matter, bind to iron in the lumen of the intestine and decrease its absorption. Polyphenols in tea, coffee, cocoa, spinach, and oregano inhibit iron absorption as well.

Iron is best absorbed in its ferrous form, and thus ascorbic acid in fruits, vegetables, and fortified cereals, increases iron absorption. Calcium inhibits the absorption of both heme and non-heme iron by an unknown mechanism, and epidemiologic studies show a correlation between intake of milk and the prevalence of iron deficiency. Thus, it is important for patients to also be asked about their intake of dairy foods. Those eating dairy foods or taking a calcium supplement or calcium-containing antacids at each meal may have lower iron absorption.

One of the easiest ways for this patient to increase her dietary iron would be to add red meat to her diet at least on a weekly basis, and to increase her consumption of chicken. She could also be counseled to eat iron-rich grains and vegetables at two meals a day with fruits, and she may be advised to eat iron fortified foods such as oatmeal or breakfast cereal.

5. How should iron deficiency be treated?

A ferritin level of less than 12 ng/mL in women is indicative of sub-optimal iron stores, and patients with levels in this range should receive a course of replacement therapy. Iron is best absorbed in its ferrous form, and ferrous salts of iron are generally used for oral supplementation. Ferrous sulfate, succinate, lactate, fumarate, glycine sulfate, glutamate, and gluconate are all about equally well-absorbed and tolerated. Standard doses are 50 to 60 mg of oral elemental iron twice daily. Vitamin C taken concurrently with the iron will increase absorption. Constipation and gastrointestinal distress are common side effects of oral iron supplementation. In the event these symptoms occur, the dose should be reduced by one-half but continued. Enteric-coated or delayed-release preparations should not be used; with these preparations iron is released distally in the small intestine or in the colon where it is not well-absorbed.

Parenteral iron therapy, which is administered via intramuscular or intravenous routes, may be required in patients with severe malabsorption, ongoing blood loss, those requiring chronic hemodialysis, and those who are unable to tolerate oral iron. Iron dextran is the most widely available parenteral form and contains 50 mg/mL of elemental iron. However, there are multiple serious side effects associated with parenteral iron including muscle necrosis, phlebitis, and in rare cases, anaphylaxis. The most serious side effect of parenteral iron is anaphylaxis. For this reason, small test doses (25 mg of iron dextran) should be administered and the patient should be observed in a controlled setting for one hour before full doses are administered for the first time.

With iron dextran, a delayed reaction can be seen 24 to 48 hours after administration and can include symptoms such as arthralgias, backache, chills, dizziness, fevers, headache, malaise, myalgia, nausea, and vomiting. Symptoms generally subside within a week. This syndrome is most common in settings where a total replacement dose is administered during a single infusion and is less likely if smaller doses are administered on separate occasions. Intramuscular administration of iron dextran may cause local skin site reactions and potentially carry a risk of carcinogenesis at the injection site and are not recommended by this author. Other intravenous preparations such as iron sucrose, iron saccharate, and sodium ferric gluconate are becoming more widely used and may be better tolerated than iron dextran.

A 3 month course of oral therapy is recommended for the treatment of iron deficiency. In the presence of anemia, reticulocyte counts will begin to rise after a few days of supplementation and will peak in approximately seven days. Hemoglobin will begin to rise after 10 to 14 days, and will generally normalize in two months. Some hematologists recommend continuing supplementation for six to twelve months. However, as iron status improves, a lower proportion of the supplement dose is absorbed and the benefits of supplementation are thus reduced as the course of therapy is lengthened. During therapy, patients should be monitored carefully for adherence since side effects are common.

During the course of supplementation, patients should be advised concerning diets higher in iron containing foods and given advice to optimize absorption. Patients with sources of ongoing physiologic blood loss, such as heavy menses, may require continuous low dose supplementation, such as an iron-containing multivitamin, after a full course of supplementation is complete.

Any correctable causes of blood loss should be addressed while replacement therapy is administered. In situations such as this case, when heavy menses are the most likely cause of iron deficiency, low dose oral contraceptives may also be helpful to reduce menstrual flow.

If the anemia does not correct with iron supplementation, several causes must be considered, including:

- Impaired absorption (may be seen with celiac disease, malabsorptive disease, or concomitant use of binders).
- Poor adherence due to side effects.
- Excess iron loss or increased need.
- Thalassemia.

Case 2 **Drug–Herb Interaction with St. John's Wort**

Ara DerMarderosian

University of the Sciences in Philadelphia, Philadelphia, PA

OBJECTIVES

- Describe the hypothesized mechanism of action and metabolism of St. John's Wort.
- Evaluate the safety and efficacy of St. John's Wort for the treatment of depression.
- Provide effective dietary counseling for patients on Warfarin therapy.
- Recognize the importance of quality control when recommending over-the-counter dietary and herbal supplements.
- Recognize the potential for toxicity and drug–herb interaction of St. John's Wort and other commonly used botanicals.

LB is a 54 year-old Caucasian woman who was in good health until 2 weeks ago when she developed acute shortness of breath and palpitations while driving to work. On arrival in the emergency room she was found to have atrial fibrillation with a rapid ventricular response. She was admitted to the cardiac intensive care unit and treated medically with beta-blockers to slow down her heart rate. She was treated with intravenous and then oral anticoagulants to reduce her risk of stroke. She was discharged on the fourth hospital day and now comes to see her physician for management of her warfarin anticoagulation one week later, post-hospital discharge. LB has been stable on a warfarin dose of 3 mg/day with an International Normalized Ratio (INR) in the appropriate therapeutic range of 2.0 to 3.0. At today's visit, it is noted that her INR is sub-therapeutic at 1.2. She denied any changes in medication compliance or diet, and denied starting any recent antibiotics.

Upon further questioning, LB admits to taking some over-the-counter dietary supplements. She currently takes vitamin E 400 IU once daily as a "cardioprotective antioxidant," calcium carbonate 500 mg B.I.D. (twice per day) for bone health, and St. John's Wort 300 mg B.I.D. which she buys from her local health food store. She states that she started St. John's Wort three weeks ago because a friend told her it might help her "lift her spirits."

She has no known food or drug allergies.

Medical Nutrition and Disease: A Case-Based Approach, 4th edition. Edited by Lisa Hark.
© 2009 Wiley-Blackwell Publishing, ISBN: 978-1-4051-8615-5.

Past Medical History
LB has a history of mild hypertension that has been primarily managed with a sodium-restricted diet. She also has a history of mild depression, which she attributes to being perimenopausal. She has never had an episode of major depression or psychiatric hospitalization and has never been treated with prescription antidepressants. She denies any thoughts of suicide.

Medications
Warfarin (Coumadin): 3 mg at bedtime
Atenolol: 50 mg daily in the morning

Social History
LB lives with her husband and their two cats. Her children are grown and in college. She explains that she has not been feeling like her usual self since the hospitalization. She often awakens during the night and has a difficult time going back to sleep. She still enjoys playing bridge and gardening but describes herself as frequently distracted and occasionally "blue." She avoids alcohol and tobacco and drinks one cup of coffee daily.

Review of Systems
General: She reports losing about 5 pounds since her admission
GI: Poor appetite

Physical Examination
Vital Signs
Temperature: 98.6 °F (37 °C)
Heart rate: 72 BPM
Respiration: 16 BPM
Blood pressure: 138/84 mmHg
Height: 5′4″ (152.4 cm)
Current weight: 150 lbs (68.04 kg)
Usual weight: 155 lbs (70.31 kg)
BMI: 25.7 kg/m^2

Exam:
General: Well-developed, well-nourished woman in no apparent distress.
Skin: Warm and dry
HEENT: Within normal limits
Cardiac: Irregularly irregular radial pulse. Normal S1 & S2 without S3 or S4.
Abdomen: Soft, non-tender, non-distended
Extremities: No clubbing, cyanosis, or edema
Neurologic mental status exam: Alert and oriented to person, place, and time with slightly depressed affect. Sensory and motor exams are grossly intact.

Laboratory Data:

Patient's Lab Values	Normal Values
Prothrombin time = 13.4 seconds	<13 seconds
International normalized ratio (INR) = 1.2	*
Thyroid stimulating hormone (TSH) = 3.1	0.5–5.0 µU/mL

*Target therapeutic range for patients being anticoagulated for stroke prevention in fibrillation with warfarin therapy = 2–3

Case Questions

1. What is known about the mechanism of action and metabolism of St. John's Wort?
2. What safety issues are of concern for patients taking St John's Wort alone or in combination with other drugs?
3. Is St. John's Wort effective in the treatment of depression?
4. What are the issues related to the product quality are important to consider when assessing over-the-counter dietary supplements?
5. Based on LB's medical history, what treatment recommendations for depression would be appropriate at this time?
6. What dietary advice should be provided to all patients on warfarin (anticoagulant) therapy?

Answers to Questions: Case 2
Part 1: Mechanisms of Action and Safety

1. What is known about the mechanism of action and metabolism of St. John's Wort?

St. John's Wort (SJW), also known as *Hypericum perforatum*, is one of the most commonly used herbal remedies in the Western world. Extracts of this popular botanical have been used since the early nineteenth century to treat mood disorders. The exact mechanism of action of SJW remains largely unknown, but like many herbs it likely involves multiple pathways due to its several constituents. A number of early studies suggested that *Hypericum* inhibits monoamineoxidase (MAO), an enzyme involved with the breakdown of some neurotransmitters that influence mood. Other postulated mechanisms from animal studies include the inhibition of serotonin reuptake, the down regulation of serotonin receptors, and inhibition of GABA pathways.

St. John's Wort's major active constituents are thought to be hypericin and hyperforin. Hypericin has anti-viral properties while hyperforin appears to be the major active anti-depressant. It has been shown to inhibit the uptake of 5-HT, dopamine, noradrenaline, GABA, and glutamate. However, even hyperforin-free extract of SJW has anti-depressant effects, hence other ingredients are likely involved.

Metabolism of SJW constituents is especially relevant when one considers the potential for toxicity and drug–herb interaction. In a study of the action of *Hypericum* on human cytochrome P450 activity, it was found that long-term administration in humans resulted in a significant and selective induction of CYP3A4 and CYP2C9 activity in the intestinal wall. CYP3A4 is one subtype of the many cytochrome P450 enzymes that help to detoxify and metabolize drugs. If an herbal supplement induces one of these enzymes, then other drugs may be metabolized faster. If an herbal supplement inhibits this enzyme, then the functional level of other drugs may rise and cause toxicity. In this case, blood levels of drugs metabolized by this enzyme, such as cyclosporine, digoxin, warfarin, theophylline, and protease inhibitors (antiretrovirals) can be expected to fall during chronic administration of SJW.

2. What safety issues are of concern for patients taking St. John's Wort alone or in combination with other drugs?

When used in monotherapy at doses up to 900 mg/day, SJW has been shown to be safe with a better side-effect profile than prescription anti-depressant agents. One study found that 3 percent of SJW treated patients dropped out secondary to side effects (gastrointestinal irritation, dizziness, confusion, tiredness, and restlessness) compared to a 16 percent drop out rate in the imipramine group. In the most recently published multicenter trial involving 340 subjects, 900 mg of SJW caused more anorgasmia and frequent urination compared to placebo, but SJW caused fewer side effects compared to 50 to 100 mg of sertraline. Importantly, a systematic review of SJW clinical trials concluded that this herb can decrease the bioavailability of several conventional drugs if taken at the same time.

Relevant to this case, SJW can reduce the efficacy of warfarin and thus lead to under anti-coagulation. This might increase the risk of thromboembolic complications in patients with atrial fibrillation. Thus, while LB was previously therapeutically anticoagulated on her 3 mg dose of warfarin, her recent daily use of SJW has likely caused her INR to be sub-therapeutic, thereby possibly increasing her risk of stroke.

When used in combination with other drugs, SJW can cause clinically significant toxicities related to the upregulation of CYP3A4. As a result, there are several reports of transplanted organ rejection related to concomitant use of SJW and cyclosporine. Additionally, SJW can reduce the levels of the antiarrythmic digoxin used to treat patients with heart failure or atrial fibrillation. These are just some of the examples of possible drug–herb interactions. Table 2-4 below lists other drug–herb interactions for commonly used botanicals.

Part 2: Treatment and Recommendations

3. Is St. John's Wort effective in the treatment of depression?

There are well over 20 randomized, placebo-controlled studies evaluating the safety and efficacy of SJW in treating mild to moderate depression. St. John's Wort has also been compared with tricyclic antidepressants (amitryptilline, imipramine) and more recently with two selective serotonin reuptake inhibitors (SSRIs) fluoxetine and sertraline. The majority of placebo-controlled studies have shown that standardized extracts of SJW in the dose range of 300 mg to 900 mg daily are moderately

Table 2-4 Selected Drug-Herb Interactions

Botanical	Common Usage	Drug/drug class	Potential Interaction
Green tea extract	Antioxidant	Warfarin	Decreased drug activity
Kava	Anxiety	Benzodiazepines	Additive sedative effect. Kava has recently (2004) been related to possible hepatotoxicity.
Valerian	Insomnia	Barbituates	Additive sedative effect
St. John's Wort	Depression	Cyclosporine digoxin, warfarin, indanavir, oral contraceptives, amitryptiline, theophylline	Decreased drug activity
St. John's Wort	Depression	SSRIs	Increased drug activity
St. John's Wort	Depression	Oral contraceptives	Intermenstrual bleeding
Echinacea	Immune stimulant	Immunomodulatory drugs (prednisone, Methotrexate, Cyclosporine)	Decreased drug activity
Garlic	Hypercholesterolemia	Warfarin	Decreased drug activity
Gingko	Memory enhancement	Warfarin, aspirin	Increased risk of bleeding
Panax Ginseng	Increase well-being	Warfarin	Decreased drug activity
Panax Ginseng	Increase well-being	Hypoglycemic drugs	Enhanced drug activity
Yohimbine	Increase libido	TCA	Hypertension
Ephedra	Weight loss/energy	Antihypertensives	Decreased drug activity
Cranberry Juice	Reduce urinary tract infection	Warfarin	Possibly potentates anticoagulant action of Warfarin

Source: Adapted from *Guide to Natural Products. 2nd edition.* (DerMarderosian A, editor) Facts & Comparisons, St. Louis MO. 2001. (Reprinted with permission).

effective in the treatment of mild-to-moderate depressive symptoms. Some studies have shown equivalence of 900 mg of SJW to low dose imipramine and low dose fluoxetine. A recent study of patients with major depression failed to show improvement over both placebo and standard doses of sertraline. Differences in study design (lack of active control and placebo), study populations (major vs. mild/moderate depression), and dosing of SJW or comparator agents is likely responsible for some variance in results.

4. What issues related to the product quality are important to consider when assessing over-the-counter dietary supplements?

The Dietary Supplement and Health Education Act (DSHEA) of 1994 created a new class of compounds called "dietary supplements" that do not need to meet the same regulatory scrutiny as prescription pharmacologic agents. As a result of DSHEA, herbal remedies marketed as dietary supplements cannot make claims that their products can be used to "diagnose, prevent, mitigate, treat, or cure a specific disease." DSHEA thus led to a marked increase in the availability and popularity of dietary supplements in the United States. While DSHEA required that botanicals be labeled with the parts of the plant used and the strength of its ingredients, many herbal products have been found to contain less or none of the proposed active compounds. This stems in part from the complexity of herbal preparations, which can contain several potentially bioactive constituents. The strength and potency of an herbal extract can depend, among other things, on the time of year the plant was cultivated, the quality of the soil, the parts of the plant that are used, and variations in processing of the herb.

The problems of quality control can be illustrated with the case of SJW. The most common analytical "marker" compound used in standardizing SJW extracts is hypericin, even though it is not the only active principle. SJW also contains among other substances pseudohypericin, protohypericin as well as flavonoids and volatile oils. The majority of the American products are standardized to contain at least 0.3 percent hypericin. Some more recent products are standardized to what is believed to be the major anti-depressive agent, hyperforin, at a level range of 3 to 5 percent. Some products are sold as capsules while others are alcoholic liquid extracts. Finally, many products contain SJW as one of several possibly active compounds. Of note, the majority of the European clinical studies used a specific extract called LI-160 delivering 900 mg/day of the aerial parts (leaves and flowers) of the dried herb. Even when products are standardized, batch to batch variability can also lead to inconsistent therapeutic effects. Thus, the quality of a dietary supplement is difficult to ascertain for consumers who must rely on independent testing of products (www.consumerlabs.com) or use products specifically tested in clinical trials. A recent study of 16 SJW products found that most did not pass quality tests. Some had lower amounts of hypericin and hyperforin, and some had not labeled the plant part used. Aerial parts are required.

5. Based on LB's medical history, what treatment recommendations for depression would be appropriate for LB at this time?

By taking a thorough medication and supplement history, the astute clinician will recognize that the recent addition of SJW may have reduced the effectiveness of warfarin. LB was counseled to stop the SJW and increase the dose of warfarin for 3 days before returning to her stable dose of 3 mg. A more in-depth psychosocial history did not reveal evidence for major depression. LB was diagnosed with adjustment disorder and will follow-up in one week's time for a re-evaluation of her INR.

6. What dietary advice should be provided to all patients on Warfarin therapy?

It is widely believed that vitamin K intake will inversely influence the efficacy of warfarin-based anticoagulant therapy. Therefore, the most important dietary advice to give patients is to keep their intake of vitamin K-containing foods and dietary supplements fairly constant from day to day. Phylloquinone is the predominant dietary form of vitamin K. An understanding of the dietary vitamin K–Warfarin interaction and knowledge of high, medium, and low dietary sources of vitamin K is necessary for successful anticoagulation.

Higher concentrations of vitamin K are found in dark green leafy vegetables such as spinach, kale, and collard greens, and in the outer peels of certain fruits, such as apples and grapes. Other significant dietary sources of vitamin K are certain oils including soybean, canola, cottonseed, and olive although values fluctuate since these oils are highly susceptible to both daylight and fluorescent light (See Appendix D for foods high in vitamin K).

Chapter and Case References

Aggarwal R, Sentz, J, Miller, MA. Role of zinc administration in prevention of childhood diarrhea and respiratory illnesses: A meta-analysis. *Pediatrics* 2007;119:1120–1130.

Araujo AB, Travison TG, Harris SS, et al. Race/ethnic differences in bone mineral density in men. *Osteoporos Int* 2007;18:943–953.

Autier P, Gandini S. Vitamin D supplementation and total mortality: a meta-analysis of randomized controlled trials. *Arch Intern Med* 2007;167(16):1730–1737.

Balk EM, Tatsioni A, Lichtenstein AH, et al. Effect of chromium supplementation on glucose metabolism and lipids: a systematic review of randomized controlled trials. *Diabetes Care* 2007;30(8):2154–2163.

Barbagallo M, Dominguez L. Magnesium metabolism in type 2 diabetes mellitus, metabolic syndrome and insulin resistance. *Arch Biochem Biophys* 2007;458(1):40–47.

Baribeault SR, Rosenberg CL. Safe administration of iron sucrose in a patient with a previous hypersensitivity reaction to ferric gluconate. *Pharmacotherapy* 2007;27(4):613–5.

Belin RJ, He K. Magnesium physiology and pathogenic mechanisms that contribute to the development of the metabolic syndrome. *Magnes Res* 2007;20(2):107–129.

Bischoff-Ferrari H, Dawson-Hughes B, Baron JA, et al. Calcium intake and hip fracture risk in men and women: a meta-analysis of prospective cohort studies and randomized controlled trials. *Am J Clin Nutr* 2007;86:1780 –1790.

Bjelakovic G, Nikolova D, Gluud LL, et al. Mortality in randomized trials of antioxidant supplements for primary and secondary prevention: systematic review and meta-analysis. *JAMA* 2007;297(8):842–57.

Bleie O, Semb AG, Grundt H, et al. Homocysteine-lowering therapy does not affect inflammatory markers of atherosclerosis in patients with stable coronary artery disease. *J Int Med* 2007;262:244–253.

Bleys J, Miller ER 3rd, Pastor-Barriuso R. Vitamin-mineral supplementation and the progression of atherosclerosis: a meta-analysis of randomized controlled trials. *Am J Clin Nutr* 2006;84(4):880–887.

Boonen S, Lips P, Bouillon R, et al. Need for additional calcium to reduce the risk of hip fracture with vitamin D supplementation: Evidence from a comparative meta-analysis of randomized controlled trials. *J Clin Endocrin Metab* 2007;92(4):1415–1423.

Chambers EC, Heshka S, Gallagher D, et al. Serum magnesium and type-2 diabetes in African Americans and Hispanics: a New York cohort. *J Am Coll Nutr* 2006;25(6):509–513.

Cockayne S, Adamson J, Lanham-New S, et al. Vitamin K and the prevention of fractures: Systematic review and meta-analysis of randomized controlled trials. *Arch Intern Med* 2006;166:1256–1261.

Cohen HW, Alderman MH. Sodium, blood pressure, and cardiovascular disease. *Curr Opin Cardiol* 2007;22:306–310.

Cohen HW, Hailpern SM, Fang J, et al. Sodium intake and mortality in the NHANES II follow-up study. *Am J Med* 2006;119:275.e7–275.e14.

Cole P, Rodu B. Epidemiologic studies of chrome and cancer mortality: A series of meta-analyses. *Regul Toxicol Pharmacol* 2005;43:225–231.

Denic S, Agarwal MM. Nutritional iron deficiency: an evolutionary perspective. *Nutrition* 2007;23(7–8):603–14.

Department of Health and Human Services. Bone Health and Osteoporosis. A Report of the Surgeon General. US DHHS. Rockville, MD. Office of the Surgeon General. 2004.

Dhingra R, Sullivan LM, Fox CS, et al. Relations of serum phosphorus and calcium levels to the incidence of cardiovascular disease in the community. *Arch Int Med* 2007;167:879–885.

Duffield-Lillico AJ, Dalkin BL, Reid ME, et al. Selenium supplementation, baseline plasma selenium status and incidence of prostate cancer: an analysis of the complete treatment period of the Nutritional Prevention of Cancer Trial. *BJU Int* 2003;91:608–12.

Fadyl H, Inoue S. Combined B12 and iron deficiency in a child breast-fed by a vegetarian mother. *J Pediatr Hematology/Oncology* 2007; 29(1):74.

Fleming DJ, Jacques PF, Tucker KL, et al. Iron status of the free-living, elderly Framingham Heart Study cohort: an iron-replete population with a high prevalence of elevated iron stores. *Am J Clin Nutr* 2001;73:638–646.

Food and Nutrition Board, Institute of Medicine, *Dietary Reference Intakes for Vitamin A, Vitamin K, Arsenic, Boron, Chromium, Copper, Iodine, Iron, Manganese, Molybdenum, Nickel, Silicon, Vanadium, and Zinc.* Washington, DC: National Academies Press, 2001.

Food and Nutrition Board, Institute of Medicine, *Dietary Reference Intakes: Vitamin C, Vitamin E, Selenium, and Carotenoids.* Washington, DC: National Academies Press, 2000.

Food and Nutrition Board, Institute of Medicine, *Dietary Reference Intakes for Thiamin, Riboflavin, Niacin, Vitamin B6, Folate, Vitamin B12, Pantothenic Acid, Biotin, and Choline.* Washington, DC: National Academies Press, 1998.

Food and Nutrition Board, Institute of Medicine, *Dietary Reference Intakes for Calcium, Phosphorus, Magnesium, Vitamin D, and Fluoride.* Washington, DC: National Academies Press, 1997.

Food and Nutrition Board, Institute of Medicine, *Dietary Reference Intakes for Water, Potassium, Sodium, Chloride, and Sulfate.* Washington, DC: National Academies Press, 2004.

Frassetto LA, Morris RC, Sellmeyer DE, et al. Adverse effects of sodium chloride on bone in the aging human population resulting from habitual consumption of typical American diets. *J Nutr* 2008;138:419S–422S.

Garland CF, Gorham ED, Mohr SB, Grant WB, Giovannucci EL, Lipkin M, Newmark H, Holick MF, Garland FC. Vitamin D and prevention of breast cancer: pooled analysis. *J Steroid Biochem Mol Biol* 2007;103(3–5):708–711.

Gass M, Dawson-Hughes B. Preventing osteoporosis-related fractures: an overview. *Am J Med* 2006;119(4S1):S3–S11.

Geleijnse JM, Witterman JCM, Stijnen T, Kloos MW, Hofman A, Grobbee DE. Sodium and potassium intake and risk of cardiovascular events and all-cause mortality: the Rotterdam Study. *Eur J Epidemiol* 2007;22:763–770.

Giannini A, Mirra N, Patria MF. Health risks for children raised on vegan or vegetarian diets. *Pediatr Crit Care Med* 2006;7(2):188.

Goh YI, Bollano E, Einarson TR, et al. Prenatal multivitamin supplementation and rates of congenital anomalies: a meta-analysis. *J Obstet Gynaecol Can* 2006;28(8):680–689.

Gorham ED, Garland CF, Garland FC, et al. Optimal vitamin D status for colorectal cancer prevention: a quantitative meta analysis. *Am J Prev Med* 2007;32(3):210–216.

Green MH, et al. Changes in hepatic parenchymal and nonparenchymal cell vitamin A content during vitamin A depletion in the rat. *J Nutr* 1988;118(11):1331–1335.

Greer FR, Krebs NF for the American Academy of Pediatrics Committee on Nutrition. Optimizing bone health and calcium intakes of infants, children, and adolescents. *Pediatrics* 2006;117(2):578–585.

Griffith LE, Guyatt GH, Cook RJ, et al. The influence of dietary and nondietary calcium supplementation on blood pressure: an updated metaanalysis of randomized controlled trials. *Am J Hypertens* 1999;12(1 Pt 1):84–92.

Guyton JR. Niacin in cardiovascular prevention: mechanisms, efficacy, and safety. *Curr Opin Lipidol* 2007;18:415–420.

Hathcock JN, Shao A, Vieth R, Heaney R. Risk assessment for vitamin D. *Am J Clin Nutr* 2007;85:6–18.

He FJ, Markandu ND, Coltart R, Barron J, MacGregor GA. Effect of short-term supplementation of potassium chloride and potassium citrate on blood pressure in hypertensives. *Hypertension* 2005;45(4):571–574.

Heaney RP. Role of dietary sodium in osteoporosis. *J Am Coll Nutr* 2006;25(3S):271S–276S.

Heilberg IP, Schor N. Renal stone disease: causes, evaluation and medical treatment. *Arq Bras Endocrinol Metabol* 2006;50(4):823–831.

Holick MF. Resurrection of vitamin D deficiency and rickets. *J Clin Invest* 2006;116(8):2062–2072.

Huerta MG, Roemmich JN, Kington ML, et al. Magnesium deficiency is associated with insulin resistance in obese children. *Diabetes Care* 2005;28(5):1175–1181.

Hummel M, Standl E, Schnell O. Chromium in metabolic and cardiovascular disease. *Horm Metab Res* 2007;39(10):743–751.

Iannotti LL, Tielsch JM, Black MM, Black RE. Iron supplementation in early childhood: health benefits and risks. *Am J Clin Nutr* 2006;84:1261–1276.

Iannotti LL, O'Brien KO, Chang SC, et al. Iron deficiency anemia and depleted body iron reserves are prevalent among pregnant African–American adolescents. *J Nutr* 2005;135(11):2572–2577.

Institute of Medicine, Food and Nutrition Board. *Dietary Reference Intakes for Thiamin, Riboflavin, Niacin, Vitamin B6, Folate, Vitamin B12, Pantothenic Acid, Biotin, and Chlorine.* Washington, DC. National Academies Press, 1998.

Johnson A, Munoz A, Gottlieb J, Jarrard D. High dose zinc increases hospital admissions due to genitourinary complications. *J Urology* 2007;177(2):639–643.

Kleefstra N, Gans ROB, Houweling ST, et al. Chromium treatment has no effect in patients with type 2 diabetes in a western population. *Diabetes Care* 2007;30:1092–1096.

Lanham-New SA. The balance of bone health: tipping the scales in favor of potassium-rich, bicarbonate-rich foods. *J Nutr* 2008;138(1):172S–177S.

Larsson SC, Wolk A. Magnesium intake and risk of type 2 diabetes: a meta–analysis. *J Int Med* 2007;262:208–214.

Lengg N, Heidecker B, Seifert B, Trüeb RM. Dietary supplement increases anagen hair rate in women with telogen effluvium: results of a double-blind, placebo-controlled trial. *Therapy* 2007;4(1):59–65.

Lippman SM, Goodman PJ, Klein EA, et al. Designing the selenium and vitamin E cancer prevention trial (SELECT). *J Natl Cancer Inst* 2005;97(2):94–102.

Lonsdale D. A review of the biochemistry, metabolism and clinical benefits of thiamin(e) and its derivatives. *Evid Based Complement Alternat Med* 2006;3(1):49–59.

Meyers DG, Jensen KC, Menitove JE. A historical cohort study of the effect of lowering body iron through blood donation on incident cardiac events. *Transfusion* 2002;42(9):1135–1139.

Milman U, Blum S, Shapira C, et al. Vitamin E supplementation reduces cardiovascular events in a subgroup of middle-aged individuals with both type 2 diabetes and the haptoglobin 2-2 genotype. *Arter Thromb Vasc. Biol* 2008;28:341–347.

Mittal MK, Florin T, Perrone J, et al. Toxicity from use of niacin to beat urine drug screening. *Ann Emerg Med* 2007;50:587–590.

Mizón C, Ruz M, Csendes A, et al. Persistent anemia after Roux-en-Y gastric bypass. *Nutr* 2007; 23(3):277–280.

Neogi T, Booth SL, Zhang YQ, et al. Low vitamin K status is associated with osteoarthritis in the hand and knee. *Arthritis Rheum* 2006;54(4):1255–1261.

Njar VCO, Gediya L, Purushottamachar P, et al. Retinoic acid metabolism blocking agents (RAM-BAs) for treatment of cancer and dermatological diseases. *Bioorg Med Chem* 2006;14:4323–4340.

Office of Dietary Supplements. *Vitamin Fact Sheets.* National Institute of Health. Washington, DC. Available from http://ods.od.nih.gov/factsheets/chromium.asp

Omenn GS, Goodman GE, Thornquist MD, et al. Effects of a combination of beta carotene and vitamin A on lung cancer and cardiovascular disease. *NEJM* 1996;334(18):1150–1155.

Penniston KL, Tanumiharjo SA. The acute and toxic effects of vitamin A. *Am J Clin Nutr* 2006;83;191–201.

Pieracci FM. Barie PS. Diagnosis and management of iron-related anemias in critical illness. *Critical Care Medicine* 2006; 34(7):1898–1905.

Pizzo G, Piscopo MR, Pizzo I, Giuliana G. Community water fluoridation and caries prevention: a critical review. *Clin Oral Investig* 2007;11(3):189–193.

Reid ME, Duffield-Lillico AJ, Sunga A, et al. Selenium supplementation and colorectal adenomas: An analysis of the nutritional prevention of cancer trial. *Int J Cancer* 2006;118:1777–1781.

Rimm EB; Willett WC; Hu FB. Folate and vitamin B6 from diet and supplements in relation to risk of coronary heart disease among women. *JAMA* 1998;279(5):359–364.

Saglam H, Buyukuysal L, Koksal N, Ercan I, Tarim, O. Increased incidence of congenital hypothyroidism due to iodine deficiency. *Pediatr Int* 2007;49:76–79.

Sanyal S, Karas RH, Kuvin JT. Present-day uses of niacin: effects on lipid and non-lipid parameters. *Expert Opin Pharmacother* 2007;8(11):1711–1717.

Schneider JM, Fujii ML, Lamp CL, et al. Anemia, iron deficiency, and iron deficiency anemia in 12–36-mo-old children from low-income families. *Am J Clin Nut* 2005;82(6):1269–1275.

Smith AH. Hexavalent chromium, yellow water, and cancer: A convoluted saga. *Epidemiol* 2008;19:24–26.

Solomon LR. Disorders of cobalamin (vitamin B12) metabolism: Emerging concepts in pathophysiology, diagnosis, and treatment. *Blood Rev* 2007;21:113–130.

Stranges A, Marshall JR, Ntarajan R, et al. Effects of long-term selenium supplementation on the incidence of type 2 diabetes. *Ann Intern Med* 2007;147:217–223.

Sung KC, Kang JH, Shin HS. Relationship of cardiovascular risk factors and serum ferritin with C-reactive protein. *Arch Med Res* 2007;38(1):121–125.

Tang BMP, Eslick GD, Nowson C, Smith C, Bensoussan A. Use of calcium or calcium in combination with vitamin D supplementation to prevent fractures and bone loss in people aged 50 years and older: a meta-analysis. *Lancet* 2007;370:657–666.

The Heart Outcomes Prevention Evaluation (HOPE) 2 Investigators Homocysteine lowering with folic acid and B vitamins in vascular disease. *NEJM* 2006;354(15):1567–1577.

Todd T, Caroe T. Newly diagnosed iron deficiency anaemia in a premenopausal woman. *BMJ* 2007;3;334(7587):259.

van Oijen MGH, Vlemmix F, Laheij RJF, Paloheimo L, Jansen JBMJ, Verheugt FWA. Hyperho-mocysteinemia and vitamin B12 deficiency: The long-term effects in cardiovascular disease. *Cardiology* 2007;107:57–62.

Vieth R, Bischoff-Ferrari H, Boucher BJ, et al. The urgent need to recommend an intake of vitamin D that is effective. *Am J Clin Nutr* 2007;85:649–650.

Villar J, Abdel-Aleem H, Merialdi M, et al. Campodonico L, Landoulsi S, Carroli G, Linkheimer M, World Health Organization randomized trial of calcium supplementation in low calcium intake pregnant women. *Am J Ob Gyn* 2006;194:639–649.

Vivekananthan DP, Penn MS, Sapp SK, et al. Use of antioxidant vitamins for the prevention of cardiovascular disease: meta-analysis of randomised trials. *Lancet* 2003;361(9374):2017–2023.

Walker J, MacKenzie AD, Dunning J. Does reducing your salt intake make you live longer? *Interact Cardiovasc Thorac Surg* 2007;6(6):793–798.

Wenzel LB, Anderson R, Tucker DC, et al. for Hemochromatosis and Iron Overload Study Research Investigators. Health-related quality of life in a racially diverse population screened for hemochromatosis: results from the Hemochromatosis and Iron Overload Screening (HEIRS) study. *Genet Med* 2007;9(10):705–712.

Zasloff M. Fighting infections with vitamin D. *Nat Med* 2006;12(4):388–390.

Ziaei S, Norrozi M, Faghihzadeh S, Jafarbegloo E. A randomised placebo-controlled trial to determine the effect of iron supplementation on pregnancy outcome in pregnant women with haemoglobin ,13.2 g/dl. *J Obstet Gynaecol* 2007;114:684–688.

Zimmermann MB, Connolly K, Bozo M, Bridson J, Rohner F, Grimci L. Iodine supplementation improves cognition in iodine-deficient schoolchildren in Albania: a randomized, controlled, double-blind study. *Am J Clin Nutr* 2006;83:108–114.

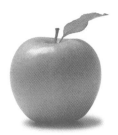

Part II
Nutrition Throughout the Life Cycle

3 Nutrition in Pregnancy and Lactation

Lisa Hark[1] and Darwin Deen[2]

[1] Jefferson Medical College, Philadelphia, PA
[2] City College of New York, New York, NY

OBJECTIVES *

- Understand the metabolic and physiologic consequences of pregnancy and lactation.
- Recognize the importance of incorporating nutrition into the history, review of systems, and physical examinations of pre-pregnant and pregnant women.
- Recognize the additional nutritional requirements for women during pregnancy and lactation.
- Determine the appropriate weight gain during pregnancy for normal-weight, underweight, and overweight pregnant women.
- Recommend dietary modifications to help alleviate common nutrition-related problems during pregnancy.
- Be prepared to counsel breastfeeding women about the nutritional requirements for lactation.

*Source: Objectives for chapter and cases adapted from the *NIH Nutrition Curriculum Guide for Training Physicians*. (www.nhlbi.nih.gov/funding/training/naa)

Introduction

While adequate nutrition is important throughout the life span, it is especially crucial for pregnant and lactating females, whose nutrient and energy demands are substantially increased during this time. By understanding the changes in nutritional requirements throughout pregnancy and during lactation healthcare providers can make informed recommendations regarding diet alterations and supplementation.

Research demonstrates that maternal nutrition affects not only the health and development of the newborn but also the subsequent health of the child as it grows, even into adulthood. Adult risk for chronic diseases is increasingly being linked to the fetal nutritional environment and it is important to recognize risk factors for deficiencies or excesses during pregnancy. Avoiding nutritional deficiencies during pregnancy promotes optimal outcomes for both mother and baby; avoiding nutritional deficiencies during lactation promotes prolonged breastfeeding, maternal health and satisfaction, and optimal infant development.

Medical Nutrition and Disease: A Case-Based Approach, 4th edition. Edited by Lisa Hark.
© 2009 Wiley-Blackwell Publishing, ISBN: 978-1-4051-8615-5.

Metabolic and Physiologic Consequences of Pregnancy

The physiological and biochemical changes that occur during pregnancy are primarily designed to accommodate and promote the growth and development of the fetus. These include the development and growth of the feto–placental unit, increased maternal blood volume, increased maternal adipose tissue, decreased gastrointestinal (GI) motility, and breast enlargement to prepare for lactation. Throughout pregnancy, hormonal alterations create maternal insulin resistance and increase the uptake of fatty acids in extra-uterine tissues, both of which promote transport of glucose to the developing fetus. In order to support the additional energy requirements of their developing fetuses, women must adjust their daily caloric intake throughout pregnancy. The requirements depend upon pre-conception body mass index (BMI), maternal developmental stage (adolescence versus adulthood), and the gestational age of the pregnancy. Additionally, as fetuses depend on maternal dietary consumption to support their nutritional as well as metabolic needs, it is crucial that pregnant women increase their intake of various nutrients to ensure that their own resources are not depleted and that fetal requirements are adequately met.

Integrating Nutrition into the Obstetric History

Ideally, every woman should meet with a healthcare provider for a pre-pregnancy physical examination and nutritional assessment; however, according to the March of Dimes, 50 percent of pregnancies are unplanned. A major objective of the obstetric healthcare team is to collect sufficient information to evaluate the pregnant woman's nutritional status and identify risk factors for the pregnancy. For each pregnant patient, a detailed obstetric history should be recorded and reviewed, as the events during and outcomes of previous pregnancies have implications for the current pregnancy. This should include the total number and dates of prior pregnancies and describe maternal and fetal outcomes and complications. The obstetric history should also include information about the women's previous deliveries of:

- low birth-weight infant (<2500 g; <5 lb 8 ounces)
- high birth-weight infant (>4000 g; >8 lb 13 ounces)
- small-for-gestational-age infant (<10th or >90th percentile for gestational age)
- stillbirth (≥20 weeks)
- spontaneous abortion (<20 weeks)
- neonatal death

Previous weight-gain patterns during pregnancy, prior history of nausea, vomiting, or hyperemesis during pregnancy, gestational diabetes, eclampsia, anemia, pica, weight status (BMI), and patterns of contraception use should also be determined. Previous breastfeeding experience should be assessed as well as the woman's preference regarding breastfeeding her infant in this pregnancy.

The medical history should also identify maternal risk factors for nutritional deficiencies and chronic diseases with nutritional implications (e.g., absorption disorders, eating disorders, metabolic disorders, infections, diabetes mellitus, PKU (phenylketonuria), sickle cell trait, or renal disease). Woman who have had closely spaced pregnancies (i.e., less than a year between pregnancies) are at increased risk of having depleted nutrient reserves. Maternal nutrient depletion may be associated with an increased incidence of preterm birth, intrauterine growth restriction (IUGR), and maternal mortality/morbidity. Caffeine, tobacco, alcohol, and recreational drug consumption should also be quantified in the medical history, as should any vitamin or herbal supplementation or alternative pharmacological therapies. A history of medication use should also be obtained to evaluate the extent to which past or present medications may affect nutrient absorption.

In addition to the medical history, questions regarding professional, social, economic, and emotional stresses and specific religious practices (including dietary restrictions and fasting) should be included to account for any impact they may have on the patient's nutritional status. Some work environments adversely impact dietary intake, as they may not provide adequate time during the day to eat proper meals or allow access to only nutritionally marginal food. For this reason, pregnant patients should be asked about the conditions of their employment, and identified limitations and potential solutions should be discussed. For women identified as lower socioeconomic status, it is important to inquire about access to nutritious food and the ability to store and prepare food and referral to food assistance programs may be appropriate (e.g. Women, Infants and Children).

Nutrition Assessment in Pregnancy

The purpose of a nutrition assessment is to identify those women with nutritional risk factors that could jeopardize their health or the health of their fetus. A thorough evaluation of a woman's nutritional status prior to or during pregnancy includes clinical, dietary, and laboratory components. Both patient interviews and written questionnaire formats are appropriate for gathering information about current and past dietary practices. Pertinent dietary information includes appetite, meal patterns, dieting regimens, cultural or religious dietary practices, vegetarianism, food allergies, cravings and/or aversions. Information about abnormal eating practices, such as following food fads, bingeing, purging, laxative or diuretic use, or pica (eating non-food items: e.g. ice, detergent, starch, chalk, clay, or rocks, etc.) is essential. Other relevant information includes the habitual use of caffeine-containing beverages (more than 200 mg/day), sugar substitutes and other special "diet" foods, vitamins, minerals, and herbal supplements. Dietary supplements may not be volunteered and their use may be inappropriate or dangerous during pregnancy. A woman's current dietary practice can be assessed using the 24-hour recall, usual intake, or food frequency questionnaire discussed in Chapter 1.

Some women are receptive to nutrition counseling just prior to or during pregnancy, making this an opportune time to encourage the development of good nutritional and physical activity practices aimed at preventing future medical problems such as obesity, diabetes, hypertension, and osteoporosis. Pregnant and lactating women found to have nutritional risk factors may benefit from a referral to a registered dietitian (See Table 3-1).

Table 3-1 Medical Conditions Where Consultation With a Registered Dietitian is Advisable

- Pregnancy involving multiple gestations (twins, triplets)
- Frequent gestations (less than a three month inter-pregnancy interval)
- Use of tobacco, alcohol, or chronic medicinal or illicit drug use
- Severe nausea and vomiting (hyperemesis gravidarum)
- Eating disorders, including anorexia, bulimia, and compulsive eating
- Inadequate weight gain during pregnancy
- Adolescence
- Restricted eating (vegetarianism, macrobiotic, raw food, vegan)
- Food allergies or food intolerances
- Gestational diabetes mellitus (GDM) or history of GDM
- Prior history of low-birth-weight babies or other obstetric complications
- Social factors that may limit appropriate intake (e.g., religion, poverty)

Source: Lisa Hark, PhD, RD. Used with permission.

Physical Examination

An essential part of the clinical evaluation is assessing pre-pregnancy weight for height by calculating the BMI or using BMI tables (Figure 1-2). The BMI is used to evaluate weight status and should be explained to the patient to help her set appropriate weight-gain goals. Whenever possible, pre-pregnancy weight should be ascertained from clinical records obtained just prior to pregnancy. Current weight should be measured and rate of weight gain assessed at each visit.

Maternal Weight-Gain Recommendations

Maternal weight gain is attributable both to increases in the mother's tissue (increased circulating blood volume, breast mass, uterine size) and feto–placental growth within the uterus (increased size of the fetus, placenta, and amniotic fluid volume). During the first half of gestation, weight gain primarily reflects changes in maternal stores and fluid status. In the second half of gestation, weight gain is the result of a continued increase in maternal stores and fluid, as well as fetal growth. Rapid weight gain near the end of gestation, after approximately 32 weeks, usually represents the accumulation of tissue edema.

The rate of weight gain during pregnancy is important because maternal weight gain and infant birth weight are correlated. Most weight gain should occur in the second and early third trimesters (18 to 30 weeks). Adequate weight gain in the second trimester of pregnancy appears to be predictive of fetal and neonatal weight, even if weight gain is inadequate during the remainder of the pregnancy.

The Institute of Medicine (Table 3-2) recommendations state that women with low pre-pregnancy body mass indices (BMI <19.8 kg/m^2) should increase their caloric intake substantially to attain a weight gain between 28 and 40 pounds during the course of pregnancy. Women with normal pre-pregnancy BMI (19.8–26.0 kg/m^2) should increase their caloric intake moderately to gain between 25 and 35 pounds during the course of pregnancy, and women with high BMI (>26.0 to 29.0 kg/m^2) should increase their caloric intake in a limited fashion, to gain

Table 3-2 Recommended Weight Gain During Pregnancy

BMI	Weight Gain (kg)	Weight Gain (pounds) or lbs not ibs
Underweight BMI <18.5	12.7-18.2	28-40
Normal Weight BMI 18.5–24.9	11.4-15.9	25-35
Overweight BMI 25–29.9	6.8-11.4	15-25
Obese BMI >30.0	6.8	15
Twin Gestation	15.9-20.4	35-45

Source: *Recommended Weight Gain During Pregnancy.* Institute of Medicine.

between 15 and 25 pounds during the course of pregnancy. An area of controversy is the weight gain needs of obese women. Women with a BMI greater than 30 kg/m^2 are considered obese and should gain 15 pounds during the pregnancy. Women who are short (<62 inches) should strive for weight gain patterns similar to those recommended for women with high pre-pregnancy BMI to avoid excess fetal weight gain, which can lead to the potential for cephalo–pelvic disproportion, one of the most prevalent indications for cesarean section delivery.

Low Pre-conception BMI (underweight)

Women with low pre-conception BMI (<19.8 kg/m^2) are at risk for delivering low birth weight infants and/or developing toxemia. If a woman who was underweight before conception does not gain adequate weight during her pregnancy, these risks are increased. As with general nutritional assessment and treatment, the optimal time for evaluating and treating underweight women is prior to conception, however, this is an unrealistic option in many cases. A woman with a BMI of less than 19.8 kg/m^2 who is considering pregnancy should be encouraged to gain weight before conceiving. If an underweight woman has conceived without gaining adequate weight, she should be encouraged to gain between 28 and 40 pounds over the course of her pregnancy. Protein–calorie supplementation may assist in correcting preconception nutritional deficits and provide adequate nutrients for fetal development.

Inadequate weight gain (<2 lb/month during the second and third trimesters) is associated with low-birth-weight infants, IUGR, and fetal complications. Inhibited fetal growth usually correlates with inadequate weight gain. Discrepancy in gestational age versus uterine size or biparietal diameter of the fetal head, as measured by sonography, are signs of IUGR. Women with inadequate weight gain or weight loss should have repeated and thorough nutritional evaluations. Careful diet histories should be taken to determine the adequacy of dietary intake, supplementation should be provided as necessary, and referral to a registered dietitian is advised.

Overweight and obesity

Women with high preconception BMIs (>26 kg/m^2) are at risk for developing diabetes, hypertension, and thromboembolic events, and for delivering macrosomic infants (>4000 g or 8 pounds, 13 ounces). Although there is considerable controversy regarding the management of pregnancy in obese women, the current guidelines call for limited maternal weight gain of up to 15 pounds. Despite pre-conception obesity, severe caloric restriction during pregnancy should not be considered, as caloric restriction is linked to inadequate intake of important micro- and macronutrients. Even in severe obesity carbohydrate recommendations are 175 g/day. Adequate consumption of calcium, iron, folate, B vitamins, and protein are particularly crucial during pregnancy, regardless of maternal weight. If caloric intake is inadequate, ingested proteins are catabolized for energy needs and are therefore unavailable for maternal/fetal protein synthesis. An estimated 32 kcal/kg/day is necessary for optimal use of ingested protein. Severe restriction of caloric intake, paired with severe restriction of carbohydrate intake, can result in ketosis, which in studies of diabetic women has been shown to be detrimental for the developing fetus. Studies have also suggested an association between ketosis and reduced uterine blood flow. Ketone bodies are concentrated in amniotic fluid and absorbed by the developing fetus.

The mental development of children whose mothers have had ketonuria during pregnancy has been shown to be stunted, although the direct causal link between fetal ketosis and inhibited mental development has yet to be definitively established. To avoid inadequate intake of crucial nutritional components, which can adversely impact both mother and fetus, pregnant women with a high pre-conception BMI should limit their weight gain during the course of their pregnancies. However they should not severely restrict their caloric intake such that the nutrients required to sustain a healthy pregnancy are insufficient. Rapid, excessive weight accumulation is usually the result of fluid retention, which is associated with, but does not cause, toxemia. Fluid retention in the absence of hypertension or proteinuria is not an indication for salt restriction or diuretic therapy, but women who retain fluid should be monitored for other signs of toxemia. Edema in the lower extremities is caused by the accumulation of interstitial fluid secondary to obstruction of the pelvic veins and commonly occurs during the later stages of pregnancy. Edema can be treated by elevating the legs and wearing support hose.

Excessive weight gain during pregnancy may also be caused by fat deposition. As excessive weight gain is associated with both maternal and fetal morbidities, weight gain that exceeds the recommendations appropriate for pre-conception BMI should be monitored. A careful dietary history should be taken to determine the source of excess weight gain and recommendations for dietary changes should be offered accordingly.

Adolescence

It is helpful for the healthcare team to stress the importance of good, life-long nutritional habits, as well as the nutritional changes necessary for optimal pregnancy outcome. Young adolescents, in particular, may still be growing and may need to gain additional weight to accommodate normal growth during the 40 weeks of the average gestation.

The pattern of weight gain, as well as the total weight gain during pregnancy, has been shown to be particularly important in the adolescent population. Inadequate weight gain prior to 24 weeks, even if total pregnancy weight gain is adequate, is associated with low-birth-weight deliveries in the adolescent population. Pregnant adolescents should strive for weight gain patterns similar to those recommended for women with low pre-pregnancy BMI. Adolescents need to fulfill the energy requirements of their developing fetuses as well as the nutritional requirements of their own continued growth and development. However, adolescents are more likely to consume diets that are low in micronutrients, such as iron, zinc, folate, calcium, and vitamin A, B_6, and C, and higher in energy from macronutrients including total fat, saturated fat, and sugar.

Recent research on adolescents suggests that the components of the diet are also important determinants of birth weight. Adolescents whose diets are higher in total carbohydrates appear to have lower overall risks of delivering a low birth weight baby or having a preterm delivery compared to adolescents with diets lower in carbohydrates.

Laboratory Evaluation

Routine tests related to the nutritional status of pregnant women should be performed at the beginning of pregnancy and intermittently as appropriate including screening for anemia (hemoglobin, hematocrit) and for gestational diabetes, the latter at 24 to 28 weeks gestation. When iron stores are low, serum ferritin and MCV levels should be checked. The clinician must be aware of ethnic or racial differences when interpreting these laboratory studies. For example, African-American women are more likely to have higher levels of ferritin than Caucasian women. Patients of African-American, Southeast Asian, and Mediterranean descent are also at increased risk for having sickle cell disease, sickle cell trait, and/or one of the thalassemias. They should be evaluated for these inherited disorders if their initial screen shows anemia in the presence of normal iron stores. Urinary screening for the presence of glucose and protein, as a screen for diabetes and renal disease, respectively, should also be conducted.

Maternal Nutrient Needs: Current Recommendations

Energy and Protein

The total maternal energy requirement for a full-term pregnancy is estimated at 80,000 calories. Basal requirements can be determined based on maternal age, stature, activity level, pre-conception weight, BMI, and gestational weight gain goals.

During the first trimester, total energy expenditure does not change greatly and weight gain is minimal; therefore, additional energy intake is recommended only in the second and third trimesters. An additional 340 kcal/day is recommended during the second trimester and 452 kcal/day during the third trimester. Additional protein is needed during pregnancy for fetal, placental, and maternal tissue development. Protein recommendations are therefore increased from 46 g/day for an adult, non-pregnant woman to 71 g/day during pregnancy.

Vitamin and Mineral Supplementation Guidelines

Routine vitamin/mineral supplementation for women reporting appropriate dietary intake and demonstrating adequate weight gain (without edema) is not mandatory. However, most healthcare providers prescribe a prenatal vitamin and mineral supplement because many women do not consume an adequate diet to meet their increased nutritional requirements during the first trimester of pregnancy, especially with regard to folic acid.

Folic Acid

Folic acid deficiency is the most common vitamin deficiency during pregnancy, with well-known associations with birth defects. Severe folate deficiency manifests as megaloblastic anemia. The increased demand for folic acid during pregnancy is the result of increased maternal erythropoesis, which increases most significantly during the second and third trimesters. However, since embryonic neural tube closure is complete by 18 to 26 days after conception, it is especially crucial that pregnant women consume adequate folic acid before and during the first four weeks of pregnancy. In 1992, the Centers for Disease Control and Prevention (CDC) recommended that all women of childbearing age take 400 µg/day of supplemental folic acid, in order to ensure adequate levels of folate are present when pregnancy occurs, whether intended or not. The RDA for folate in women of childbearing age is currently 400 µg/day, and for pregnant women is 600 µg/day. Women with a history of neural tube defects should be advised to consume higher doses.

Typically, the diet in the United States has lacked folate-rich food sources and patients might have been deficient in folate. For this reason, the United States government began the folic acid fortification program in 1997. Grains, such as cereals, pastas, rice, and breads, are now fortified with folic acid. Good dietary sources of natural folate include dark green leafy vegetables, green beans and lima beans, orange juice, fortified cereals, yeast, mushrooms, pork, liver, and kidneys. (See Appendix F: Food Sources of Folate.)

Dietary folate is dramatically influenced by food storage and preparation; for instance, it is destroyed by boiling or canning. Folate stores are likely to be easily depleted among women who have folate-deficient diets, are alcoholic, or are of lower socioeconomic status. Additionally, evidence exists to suggest that the long-term use of oral contraceptives inhibits folate absorption and enhances folate degradation in the liver. Therefore, folate stores may be more rapidly depleted in women who have used oral contraceptives, which may lead to a higher incidence of folate deficiency in such women if they become pregnant.

Calcium

In contrast to maternal iron and folate stores, which are relatively small and therefore easily depleted, maternal calcium stores are large and are mostly stored skeletally, allowing for easy mobilization as needed. Over the course of pregnancy, a single fetus requires between 25 and 30 grams of calcium, which represents a mere 2.5 percent of total maternal stores. In the first half of pregnancy, calcium requirement is only an additional 50 mg/day above the 1000 mg/day required of non-pregnant women. Most of the additional calcium requirement during pregnancy occurs during the third trimester, during which the fetus absorbs an average of 300 mg/day. Evidence has shown that calcium supplementation reduces the risk of developing hypertension during pregnancy, in women who did not have adequate calcium intake.

The RDA for calcium in women 19 to 50 years old is 1000 mg/day; for the adolescent female age 9 to 19, calcium requirements are 1300 mg/day. Obtaining adequate intake of dietary calcium presents no problem for women who consume at least 3 servings of dairy foods every day. Even in women who limit their intake of dairy foods because of lactose intolerance seem to be able to tolerate yogurt and cheese on a daily basis. At least 3 servings/day of low-fat dairy foods should be encouraged. Additionally, many vegetables also contain calcium, and products fortified with calcium, such as soymilk, orange juice, cereal and bread, may also be suggested (See Appendices G and H: Food Sources of Calcium).

If increased intake is not possible or effective, supplementation may be needed. Calcium carbonate, gluconate, lactate, or citrate may provide 500 to 600 mg/day of calcium to account for the difference between the amount of calcium required and that consumed. The tolerable upper intake for calcium during pregnancy is 2500 mg/day. The standard prenatal vitamin contains 250 mg/serving. Multivitamins marketed to the non-pregnant population generally have less than 200 mg/serving. Calcium is thought to be absorbed in doses of 600 mg at one time making it unlikely that pregnant women would reach the upper tolerable limit.

Iron

Iron deficiency anemia during pregnancy has been associated with an increased risk of maternal and infant death, pre-term delivery, and low-birth-weight babies; and has negative consequences for normal infant brain development and function. The prevalence of iron deficiency in pregnancy is higher in African-American women, low-income women, teenagers, women with less than a high school education, and women who have had two or three prior pregnancies. *Healthy People 2010* goals include reducing anemia among pregnant females in their third trimester from 29 to 20 percent and reducing ethnic and income disparities. Women, Infant, and Children's (WIC) Programs have been successful in reducing the prevalence of iron deficiency anemia during pregnancy and postpartum.

According to the CDC, screening for anemia should take place prior to pregnancy, as well as during the first, second, and third trimester in high-risk individuals as

Table 3-3 Diagnosis of Anemia in Pregnancy

Lab test	1st Trimester	2nd Trimester	3rd Trimester
Hemoglobin (g/dL)	<10	10.5	<10
Hematocrit (%)	<37	35	<33

Source: Centers for Disease Control and Prevention.

shown in Table 3-3. Since hemoglobin levels normally decline during pregnancy due to the significant increase in maternal blood volume, ferritin and mean corpuscular volume should be measured as diagnostic criteria, since these values remain constant. Serum ferritin is useful in assessing the post-gastric bypass pregnant patient. A serum ferritin level of less than 15 ng/mL warrants aggressive treatment and may require intramuscular injection rather than oral supplementation in these patients.

A total iron increase of over 1000 mg is required during pregnancy. Throughout pregnancy, maternal blood volume increases 20 to 30 percent, and erythropoeisis under such conditions requires that an additional 450 mg of iron be delivered to the maternal marrow. The fetus and the placenta require 350 mg of iron, and approximately 250 mg of iron is lost in blood during delivery. It is difficult for many women to meet the iron requirements of pregnancy by diet alone. Healthcare providers generally recommend iron supplementation in the form of a daily supplement of 30 mg of elemental iron in the form of simple salts, beginning around the twelfth week of pregnancy for women who have normal pre-conception hemoglobin measurements.

The RDA for iron is 27 g/day in pregnancy and 9 g/day for lactating women. For women who are pregnant with multiple fetuses or those with low pre-conception hemoglobin measurements, a supplement between 60 and 100 mg/day of elemental iron is recommended until hemoglobin concentrations are normal. Once previously anemic women's hemoglobin concentrations become normal, they may decrease their supplemental iron intake to 27 mg/day. Iron supplementation can have gastrointestinal side effects such as constipation, and a stool softener or natural laxative should be prescribed with iron supplementation. (See Appendix L: Food Sources of Iron.)

Vitamin D

In order to ensure proper absorption of calcium, adequate vitamin D intake is essential; however, vitamin D supplementation during pregnancy has been questioned and based on new data may be advised. The Adequate Intake (AI) for vitamin D during pregnancy is 200 IU/day, which is the same for non-pregnant and lactating women. Supplementation at this level of 200 IU/day can be considered for strict vegetarians or women who avoid sunlight or fortified milk. (See Appendix B: Food Sources of Vitamin D.)

Vitamin A

The RDA for vitamin A is 770 μg/day in pregnancy and 1300 μg/day during lactation. Severe vitamin A deficiency is rare in the United States and an adequate intake of vitamin A is readily available in a healthy diet. Women with lower socioeconomic status, however, may consume diets with inadequate amounts of vitamin A. Increasing dietary intake of vitamin A is possible and should be encouraged in lieu of supplementation to avoid excessive intake, which has been reported to be teratogenic (leading to abnormal fetal development). Over-the counter multivitamin supplements may contain excessive doses of vitamin A and thus should be discontinued during pregnancy. Additionally, topical creams that contain retinol derivatives commonly used to treat acne should be discontinued during pregnancy and in women trying to get pregnant.

Dietary Fiber

There are no specific recommendations for dietary fiber intake during pregnancy. However, increased intake of high-fiber foods, such as vegetables, whole grains, and fruits, is recommended for the prevention and treatment of constipation, a common problem during pregnancy. Always advocate adequate fluid intake when increasing dietary fiber. (See Appendix O: Food Sources of Dietary Fiber.)

Fluids

Pregnancy represents a unique state where circulating blood volume increases by 50 percent. Tissue fluid also increases, while blood pressure generally decreases in the second trimester before recovering to pre-pregnant levels near term. This is the result of vasodilation of the capacitance venous blood vessels, requiring substantial fluid intake during pregnancy in order to maintain blood pressure and blood flow to vital organs. The increase in circulating blood volume begins in the early part of pregnancy and the failure of this to occur has been associated with preterm delivery, intrauterine growth restriction, and hypertensive disorders of pregnancy. General recommendations are to drink at least 64 ounces (1920 mL) of water per day. In areas where the water supply is suspected to contain lead, women should be encouraged to drink bottled water. Excessive lead intakes may result in spontaneous abortion, decreased stature, and impaired neuro-cognitive development of the baby.

Food Contamination

Food contaminated by contact with heavy metals or pathogenic bacteria can produce devastating effects on the developing fetus, and most heavy metals are considered teratogenic. In particular, case reports of teratogenicity or embryotoxicity have been reported involving methyl mercury, lead, cadmium, nickel, and selenium. In addition, heavy metals can have neurotoxic effects on the fetus. Mercury can be removed from vegetables by peeling or washing well with soap and water. Consumption of raw fish products and highly carnivorous fish (including tuna, shark, tilefish, swordfish, and mackerel) should be limited or avoided during pregnancy. All foods should be handled in a sanitary and appropriate manner to prevent bacterial contamination. All dairy foods and juices consumed during pregnancy should be pasteurized. *Listeria monocytogenes* contamination results in food poisoning during and outside of pregnancy. In pregnancy, however, it can develop into a blood-borne, transplacental infection that can cause chorioamnionitis, premature labor, spontaneous abortion, or fetal demise. To avoid listeriosis, pregnant women should wash vegetables and fruits, cook meats, and avoid processed, pre-cooked meats (cold cuts) and soft cheeses (brie, blue cheese, Camembert, and Mexican caso-blanco).

Alcohol

Alcohol is a known teratogen. Excessive consumption of alcohol by pregnant women can result in fetal alcohol syndrome (FAS) which manifests in such deformities as microcephaly, cleft palate, and micrognathia. While it is certain that heavy maternal drinking is harmful to developing fetuses, the issue of whether more modest amounts of alcohol consumption are acceptable during pregnancy remains controversial. Heavy alcohol consumption during pregnancy is also associated with low neonatal weight, deficiencies in B vitamins and protein. Maternal alcoholism contributes to fetal nutritional deficiencies because it inhibits maternal absorption of nutrients, and poses a toxic threat to the developing fetus.

There is no known safe level of alcohol consumption during pregnancy, therefore, it is currently recommended that alcohol intake be avoided by pregnant women and women attempting to become pregnant. According to the American College of Obstetrics and Gynecology, no amount of alcohol consumption can be considered safe during pregnancy. Alcohol should be avoided entirely throughout the first trimester. Although the debate remains as to whether mild-to-moderate drinking affects fetal development in the latter trimesters of pregnancy, the Council on Scientific Affairs of the American Medical Association recommends abstinence from alcohol throughout pregnancy. The CDC recommends that clinicians identify women at risk in the preconception period and provide education and support for cessation of alcohol use.

Cigarette Smoking

Nicotine consumption during pregnancy has been consistently associated with low neonatal weight. If women who smoke become pregnant, they should be advised to discontinue cigarette use for the sake of their fetuses.

Caffeine

According to the March of Dimes, women who are pregnant or trying to become pregnant should limit their caffeine intake to no more than 200 mg per day, which is equivalent to about one 12-ounce cup of coffee. A recent study by Weng et al. found that women who consume 200 mg of caffeine or more a day are twice as likely as women who consume no caffeine to have a miscarriage. The U.S. Food and Drug Administration's recommendation is for pregnant women to reduce their intake of caffeine from all sources. Since caffeine is present in teas, hot cocoa, chocolate, energy drinks, coffee ice cream, and soda, it is best to advise decaffeinated beverages for women who are pregnant or trying to become pregnant.

Exercise During Pregnancy

Many studies support the benefits of moderate exercise in women whose pregnancies are considered low-risk. According to the American College of Obstetricians and Gynecologists (ACOG) most pregnant women should participate in 30 minutes or more of moderate exercise on most, if not all, days. Safe activities include walking, swimming, dancing, and yoga. Regular physical activity reduces constipation, backache, fatigue, and sleep disturbances; improves posture; promotes muscle tone, strength, endurance, energy level and mood; and reduces varicose veins. It may help reduce the risk of diabetes and high blood pressure during pregnancy and help women cope better with labor and recover faster after delivery.

Pregnant women should be advised to avoid contact sports and any activities that can cause even mild trauma to the abdomen, such as ice hockey, kickboxing, soccer, and basketball; activities with a high risk for falling, such as gymnastics, horseback riding, downhill skiing, and vigorous racquet sports; scuba diving; exercising at high altitudes (more than 6000 feet); and jumping on a trampoline. They should be advised to drink plenty of fluids before, during, and after exercise and avoid hot tubs, saunas, and Jacuzzis. Warning signs to stop exercising include vaginal bleeding, uterine contractions, decreased fetal movement, fluid leaking from the vagina, dizziness or feeling faint, increased shortness of breath, chest pain, headache, muscle weakness, and calf pain or swelling.

Common Nutrition-related Problems During Pregnancy

Discomforts of pregnancy such as nausea and vomiting, constipation, and heartburn may generally be improved by implementation of the guidelines summarized below.

Nausea and Vomiting

Nausea and vomiting appear to be associated with increased levels of the pregnancy hormone human chorionic gonadotropin. Human chorionic gonadotropin doubles every 48 hours in early pregnancy and peaks at about 12 weeks gestation. Nausea is experienced by 60 percent of pregnant women and, of these, only a small percent require hospitalization for severe hyperemesis gravidarum.

Heartburn and Indigestion

Heartburn and indigestion are usually caused by gastric content reflux that results from both lower esophageal pressure and decreased motility. Limited gastric capacity, secondary to a shift of organs to accommodate the growing fetus, contributes to these symptoms in the third trimester of pregnancy. Strategies for managing heartburn or indigestion are the same as those suggested for managing nausea and shown in Table 3-4.

Table 3-4 Strategies for Managing Nausea, Vomiting, Heartburn, and Indigestion in Pregnancy

- Eat small, low-fat meals and snacks (fruits, pretzels, crackers, non-fat yogurt) slowly and frequently.
- Avoid strong food odors by eating room temperature or cold foods and using good ventilation while cooking.
- Drink fluids between meals, rather than with meals.
- Avoid foods that may cause stomach irritation such as spearmint, peppermint, caffeine, citrus fruits, spicy foods, high-fat foods, or tomato products.
- Wait 1 to 2 hours after eating a meal before lying down.
- Take a walk after meals.
- Wear loose-fitting clothes.

Source: Lisa Hark, PhD, RD. Used with permission.

Constipation

Constipation during pregnancy is associated with an increase in water reabsorption from the large intestine. In addition, smooth muscle relaxation with resultant slower gastrointestinal tract motility occurs during pregnancy. The pregnant woman often notes overall gastrointestinal discomfort, a bloated sensation, an increase in hemorrhoids and heartburn, and decreased appetite. Strategies for managing constipation during pregnancy are shown in Table 3-5.

Table 3-5 Strategies for Managing Constipation in Pregnancy

- Increase fluid intake to 2 or 3 quarts per day (water, herbal teas, non-caffeinated beverages)
- Increase daily fiber intake (high-fiber cereals, whole grains, legumes, bran)
- Use psyllium fiber supplement (Metamucil)
- Increase consumptions of fruits and vegetables (fresh, frozen, and dried)
- Participate in moderate physical activity (walking, swimming, yoga)

Source: Lisa Hark, PhD, RD. Used with permission.

Gestational Diabetes Mellitus

Gestational diabetes mellitus (GDM) is defined as glucose intolerance with onset or first recognition during pregnancy. It occurs in approximately 4 percent of all pregnancies, resulting in more than 135,000 cases annually. GDM is usually diagnosed during the second or third trimester, at which time insulin-antagonist hormone levels increase and insulin resistance occurs. After delivery, approximately 90 percent of all women with GDM become normoglycemic but they are at increased risk of developing type 2 diabetes.

The goal of treatment is to prevent the maternal and fetal complications associated with GDM. These complications include fetal macrosomia and its attendant fetal and maternal injury associated with delivery (increased risk of cesarean section, operative vaginal delivery, and shoulder dystocia). Additional fetal complications include a possible increased incidence of fetal death and ketonemia, which has been associated with lower intelligence scores at 2 to 5 years of age.

Because fetal morbidity may be increased, it is currently recommended that all pregnant women be screened for GDM at 24 to 28 weeks of gestational age, as the use of risk factors alone may fail to identify up to 50 percent of patients with GDM. For high-risk patients, screening by 16 weeks is recommended. High-risk patients are those with a personal history of abnormal glucose tolerance, obesity, a first-degree relative with type 2 diabetes, ethnic groups with a high prevalence of gestational diabetes (African-American, Native American, Southeast Asian, Pacific Islander, Hispanic), glucosuria, or prior obstetric history consistent with diabetes (e.g., macrosomia, fetal anomalies, neonatal hypoglycemia).

The main screening tool for GDM is a 150 mL, 50-gram glucose load with a one-hour serum glucose blood test. A result greater than or equal to 130 to 140 mg/dL for the one-hour screen is abnormal. For the roughly 20 percent of patients who test positive, a three-hour 100-gram glucose load test is performed.

The diagnosis of GDM is made when two or more serum glucose values are met or exceeded. The diagnosis of GDM is an excellent predictor of type 2 diabetes developing later in life. According to the Diabetes Prevention Program (DPP), this risk is at least 40 percent over the 3 years following the pregnancy. It is recommended that a patient with GDM be re-screened for type 2 diabetes after pregnancy.

Medical Nutrition Therapy for Gestational Diabetes

The goals of medical nutrition therapy for GDM are to provide appropriate calories for gestational weight gain, achieve and maintain normoglycemia, and avoid ketonemia and ketonuria. Individualization of the meal plan is recommended as the ideal percentage and type of carbohydrate are uncertain. Monitoring blood glucose, urine or blood ketones, appetite, and weight gain is essential for individualizing the meal plan and for adjusting the meal plan throughout pregnancy.

Generally, 40 to 45 percent of total energy intake should be from carbohydrate, which is distributed throughout the day into three small-to-moderate sized meals and two to four snacks. An evening snack is usually needed to prevent accelerated ketosis overnight. Carbohydrate is not as well tolerated at breakfast as it is at other meals, possibly due to the associated increased levels of cortisol and growth hormones. Therefore, the initial meal plan may limit carbohydrate to 30 grams at breakfast with adjustments made later based on blood glucose monitoring results. To satisfy hunger, protein foods, can be added.

Patients with serum glucose values persistently above the thresholds require the addition of insulin therapy in order to achieve adequate glycemic control. Recent data evaluating the use of second-generation sufonylureas, like glyburide, are encouraging but require more study.

Lactation

Metabolic and Physiologic Changes During Lactation

Breast enlargement begins early in pregnancy due to the hormones generated by the pituitary gland and the corpus luteum. The lacteal cells also differentiate in preparation for milk production that begins when the infant is born. As the breast undergoes these preparatory changes, the areola (the pigmented area surrounding the nipple) becomes darker and more prominent, and the skin over the nipple becomes more elastic and more erect in order to facilitate suckling.

Lactogenesis is believed to be initiated by the abrupt decrease in progesterone and estrogen following parturition (giving birth). As the infant begins to suckle, stimulating the receptors in the nipple and areola, nerve impulses are sent to the hypothalamus. The hypothalamus, in turn, stimulates the release of the hormones oxytocin and prolactin from the posterior pituitary gland. Prolactin stimulates milk production in the breast, and oxytocin stimulates myoepithilial cells around ducts to contract and eject milk from the alveolus. Milk accumulates in the lactiferous sinuses under the areola and is released when the areola is compressed between the baby's tongue and palate.

Benefits of Breastfeeding

Breast milk contains leukocytes (specifically, macrophages), immunoglobins (secretory IgA, IgG, IgM, and antiviral antibodies), bifidus factor (to support *Lactobacillus bifidus*), lysozymes (to promote bacterial lysis), interferon, lactoferrin (to bind whey protein and inhibit *E. coli* colonization), lactadherin (to protect against symptomatic rotavirus infections), growth factors and cytokines (bFGF, EGF, NGF, TGF, G-CSF, interleukins, TNF-alpha and others), prostaglandins, hormones (pituitary, hypothalamic and steroid), gastrointestinal peptides (VIP, gastrin, GIP), and other unique components (e.g., complement factors, glutamine, oligosaccharides, nucleotides, and long-chain polyunsaturated fatty acids). Many of these components work alone or in combination to minimize risk of infection in the nursing infant.

Breastfed infants are hospitalized less frequently during the first six months of life. Significant healthcare cost savings from the decreased incidence of lower respiratory infections, otitis media, and gasteroenteritis are associated with breastfeeding. Strong evidence suggests that human milk also decreases the incidence and severity of diarrhea, bacteremia, bacterial meningitis, urinary tract infections, and necrotizing enterocolitis. Many studies have demonstrated the protective effect of breast milk against immune- or autoimmune-related diseases (e.g. chronic and inflammatory bowel diseases, type 1 diabetes, allergic diseases). Breast milk may also prevent sudden infant death syndrome (SIDS) and cancers such as leukemia and lymphoma. Breastfeeding promotes jaw and tooth development in the infant, and enhances maternal–fetal bonding.

Breastfeeding mothers experience earlier return to pre-gravid weight, decreased accumulation of adipose tissue, delayed return of ovulation with increased pregnancy spacing, improved bone remineralization upon resumption of menses, and reduced risk of ovarian and premenopausal breast cancer. Breast milk also offers the added benefit of convenience; it is at the proper temperature, and requires neither preparation nor storage.

Types of Breast Milk

The composition of breast milk changes from colostrum, to transitional, to mature milk. Colostrum is produced during the later stages of pregnancy and is present in highest concentration during the first few days of lactation. It is high in protein, immunoglobins, beta-carotene, sodium, potassium, chloride, fat-soluble vitamins, minerals, and unique hormones. Colostrum promotes growth of bifidus flora and maturation of the gastrointestinal tract and meconium passage. Transitional milk is produced 7 days to 2 weeks post-partum. It is higher in fat and lactose and lower in protein and minerals than colostrum. Mature milk is usually produced by the fifteenth day of lactation through the termination of lactation. It is composed of emulsified fat and lactose, it provides 20 to 22 calories/ounce and is nutritionally optimal.

Breast milk is rich in nutrients and other substances essential to growth and development during the first six months of life. When breastfeeding, women should encourage their infants to suckle on each breast for as long as the infant shows signs of hunger; usually this is 10 to 15 minutes per breast. It is important to teach nursing mothers early signs of hunger. Crying is a very late sign. If a child makes sucking movements, brings his/her hands to their mouth, displays rapid eye movements, makes soft cooing or sighing sounds, or is restless, the baby is probably hungry. Mothers should be encouraged to feed at least 8 times in each 24-hour period, as breast milk is easily digested and clears the gut faster than formula. The emptying time of breast milk from the infant's stomach is, on average, 1.5 hours, compared with 3 hours for formula-fed infants.

Breast Milk Composition

Fat Breast milk is rich in most nutrients required to sustain the newborn's appropriate growth during the first 6 months of life. The total amount of fat in breast milk is constant, but its composition varies with the duration of the feeding. Initially, breast milk has a relatively low fat content. Following the first let-down reflex, breast milk becomes higher in fat and calories. The fat content of breast milk provides 50 percent of the infant's total energy requirements in readily absorbable form. Therefore, it is essential that the infant be allowed to nurse on each breast until he or she is satisfied to derive the fat calories from the feeding. Encouraging the infant to suckle on each breast for 10 minutes or more ensures adequate calorie consumption.

Protein Breast milk contains whey and casein proteins. Whey accounts for roughly 70 percent of the total protein in breast milk, mainly in the form of alphalactalbumin, lactoferrin, and secretory IgA. Casein accounts for the remaining 30 percent of breast milk's total protein composition and forms micelles that enhance the absorption of calcium, phosphorous, iron, zinc, and copper. The total protein concentration is relatively low, but it is the optimal concentration for infant nutrition.

Carbohydrate The primary carbohydrate source in breast milk is the disaccharide lactose. Small amounts of glucose and immunologically active oligosaccharides and glycoproteins are also present.

Vitamin D Some breastfed infants are at risk for rickets caused by vitamin D deficiency because breast milk contains only small quantities of this nutrient. The risk is enhanced for dark-skinned infants of mothers with decreased vitamin D levels resulting from dietary deficiencies and/or minimal sun exposure. Currently, the

American Academy of Pediatrics recommends that all exclusively breastfed infants receive 400 IU of vitamin D daily by two months of age regardless of skin color.

Vitamin K Breast milk contains only small traces of vitamin K. However, supplementation is generally unnecessary, as most infants receive vitamin K injections immediately following delivery to prevent hemorrhagic disease of the newborn. All breastfed infants should receive 1.0 mg of vitamin K oxide intramuscularly after the first feeding is completed. This should be within the first 6 hours of life.

Nutritional Recommendations for Lactating Women

Energy and Protein

Approximately 85 kcal are required to produce 100 mL of breast milk. Stored energy from maternal fat reserves provides 100 to 150 kcal/day, but this may not be sufficient. Therefore, current recommendations advise that the daily caloric intake of lactating women be increased by 500 kcal/day for the first 6 months and 400 kcal/day for 7 to 9 months. This may not be necessary for all women. Postpartum women should avoid diets and medications that promise rapid weight loss. Weight loss should always be gradual, particularly for lactating women, who require more calories than non-lactating women to support breast milk production. Protein requirements for lactating women are recommended at 71 g/day.

Calcium

Normally 2 to 8 percent of total body calcium is mobilized for breast milk production during lactation which will be restored following the onset of menses. Diets of adults of low socioeconomic status are often low in calcium.

Iron

Iron requirements are lower during lactation (9 mg/day) than during pregnancy (27 mg/day) until menstruation resumes (18 mg/day). In the United States, studies of lactating women consuming 2700 kcal/day suggest that they are not likely to meet the RDAs for calcium and zinc. Diets that contain less than 2700 kcal/day may also be low in magnesium, vitamin B_6, and folate. Adolescent mothers' diets may be particularly low in iron.

Vitamin Supplements

Prenatal vitamin supplements are routinely prescribed to lactating women to ensure adequate intake. However, lactating women should be encouraged to obtain their nutrients from a well-balanced, varied diet. Also, they should continue to drink to thirst or about 2 to 3 quarts of fluids per day to prevent dehydration. New guidelines from the American Academy of Pediatrics advise supplementation with 400 IU of vitamin D should be initiated within days of birth for all breast fed infants.

Common Problems Experienced While Breastfeeding

Healthcare providers can readily manage most of the common problems associated with breastfeeding; however, referral to a mother-to-mother support group can be very helpful for many common problems and referral to a Certified Lactation Consultant can ensure continued lactation when problems are more complex.

Mastitis Mastitis is an infection of the breast tissue that up to 30 percent of lactating women may experience. Symptoms include breast pain, swelling, flu-like symptoms, headache, and fever. Mastitis is caused by bacteria that enter the breast through a break or crack in the skin of the areola or through the opening to the milk ducts. Bacteria from the skin or the infant's mouth enter the milk duct and can multiply, leading to pain, redness, and swelling of the breast as the infection progresses. Clogged milk ducts, cracked nipples, feeding on one breast only, wearing a tight bra, wet breast pads, infrequent feeding, anemia, fatigue, and stress can also increase the risk of developing mastitis. It is important to advise women to nurse frequently, feeding on the unaffected breast first. Antibiotics are typically prescribed and should be taken for 10 to 14 days. Getting plenty of rest, wearing a comfortable bra, and changing breast pads often can help prevent the development of mastitis.

Contraindications to Breastfeeding Infectious Disease Women with active, untreated tuberculosis, typhoid, active herpes in the area of the breast, rubella, mumps, or human immunodeficiency virus (HIV) should not breastfeed their infants. In some developing countries, the infant mortality risks of not breastfeeding may override the morbidity and mortality risks associated with the possible acquisition of such maternal infections. The main route of transmission of HIV from mother to child is breastfeeding; transmission of the virus can be prevented by encouraging use of commercial infant formulas and discouraging breastfeeding for infants of HIV-positive mothers. Other common infections, such as influenza, should not interfere with breastfeeding.

Other contraindications for breastfeeding in the United States are infants with classic galactosemia, mothers who are positive for human T-cell lymphotropic virus type I or II, mothers receiving exposure to radioactive isotopes, mothers on specific antimetabolite or chemotherapeutic agents, and mothers using drugs of abuse. It is important to note that there are many conditions for which mothers have been told to avoid breastfeeding that are indeed compatible with breastfeeding. Cytomegalovirus (CMV) is not a contraindication for breastfeeding in the term baby. The clinician must weigh the risk benefit of breastfeeding in the premature infant born to a mother with CMV. Neither Hepatitis B or C is a contraindication to breastfeeding.

Medications As in pregnancy, some medications, herbal remedies, nutritional supplements, and alternative therapies should be avoided during lactation. Several drugs, including nicotine and estrogen-containing oral contraceptives, can decrease milk supply and interfere with milk production. Medications can pass through human milk to the infant. It is best to evaluate each medication individually before making a decision about use. Considerations include the molecular weight of the drug, peak concentration, protein binding, half life, relative infant dose (RID), infant age, maternal dose, risk/benefit to mother and baby, and alternative medication options. Drugs pass into human milk if they are highly lipid soluble, have a low molecular weight (<500), low protein binding, or are in high concentration in maternal plasma.

There are several resources available, to help make decisions about medication use. The American Academy of Pediatrics, position statement entitled The Transfer of Drugs and Other Chemicals Into Human Milk is included in the *Breastfeeding Handbook for Physicians*. Discussion about contraception should include the risk of milk supply depletion with all hormone-related forms of birth control. Medications that are contraindicated for breastfeeding women include bromocriptine, tetracycline, cyclophosphamide, cyclosporine, doxorubicin, ergotamine, lithium, methotrexate, phencyclidine (PCP), and phenindione.

Substance Abuse Substance abuse and the use of recreational drugs should be actively discouraged during lactation. Illegal substances, such as amphetamines, cocaine, heroin, or marijuana, as well as nicotine pass into breast milk when ingested by the mother and should be discouraged. Addicted women should be encouraged to enter appropriate treatment programs and should be drug free before lactation is initiated. Lactating women should be advised to quit smoking because in addition to the long-term health risks, smoking decreases breast milk volume and is associated with shortened exclusive and total breastfeeding duration. Modest consumption of coffee and alcohol (i.e., less than one to two cups/drinks daily) is not known to adversely affect lactation or the infant's health. Alcohol does pass readily into breast milk so its intake should be limited.

Promotion and Support of Breastfeeding

As healthcare professionals, it is our ethical and professional responsibility to promote, protect, and support breastfeeding. Women should be informed of not only the benefits of breastfeeding but the inherent risks of not breastfeeding. Position papers published by the American Academy of Pediatrics, American Dietetic Association, and the International Lactation Consultants Association provide guidance for clinicians in supporting breastfeeding efforts. The American Academy of Family Physicians also has excellent guidelines on the clinical management of breastfeeding. Breastfeeding infants should be monitored closely for their growth and observation of the mother infant dyad should be a routine part of postpartum care. Breast milk is the optimal food source for infants.

Case 1 **Prevention of Neural Tube Defects**

Frances Burke[1] and Ann Honebrink[2]

[1] University of Pennsylvania School of Medicine, Philadelphia, PA
[2] University of Pennsylvania Health System, Radnor, PA

OBJECTIVES

- Define the prevalence, etiology, and pathogenesis of neural tube defects.
- Describe the association between folate levels and prevention of neural tube defects in the developing fetus.
- Given a pre-pregnant woman's detailed medical, obstetric, dietary, and social history, evaluate the risk of having a child with a neural tube defect.
- Evaluate the nutritional adequacy of a pre-pregnant woman's diet.

PL is a 32-year-old married Puerto-Rican-American woman who has missed her period and discovers that she is pregnant. This was an unplanned pregnancy and PL presents for her first prenatal visit at 5 weeks of gestation (normal gestation period is 40 weeks). She is a gravida 3 para 1011.

The term para has four components that describe the number of pregnancies: *n* full-term births; *n* preterm births; *n* early pregnancy losses, including miscarriages, elective terminations, and ectopic pregnancies; and *n* live children. Thus, as a para 1011, PL has had one full-term birth, no preterm births, one miscarriage, and has one living child.

Past Medical/Surgical and Obstetric History

PL's previous delivery was by cesarean section. This was performed for arrest of the normal progress of labor at 39 weeks gestation. Her infant weighed 7.5 pounds (3.4 kg) at birth. She is not hypertensive and has no history of pregnancy-induced hypertension during her previous gestation. Her one-hour glucose tolerance test at 28 weeks was normal in her prior pregnancy. She has no chronic medical problems and has had no surgeries other than the cesarean section and a dilation and evacuation at the time of her miscarriage. PL currently takes no medications, vitamins, minerals, or herbal supplements. She denies any allergies or food sensitivities to medications or foods.

Social History

PL stays at home to care for her 2-year-old daughter. She reports having little free time to exercise. She does not smoke or drink alcohol. She denies any history of sexual abuse or domestic violence. She lives at home with her husband and daughter.

Medical Nutrition and Disease: A Case-Based Approach, 4th edition. Edited by Lisa Hark.
© 2009 Wiley-Blackwell Publishing, ISBN: 978-1-4051-8615-5.

Family History
PL has a sister-in-law (her husband's sister) who had a 24-week loss of a baby found to have anencephaly. Her parents, siblings, and other nieces and nephews are all in good health and free from chronic diseases. Both of her paternal grandparents had heart disease prior to their deaths in their mid sixties. Her maternal grandmother has type 2 diabetes mellitus controlled on oral hypoglycemic agents and her maternal grandfather had a myocardial infarction and died at 54 years of age.

Physical Examination
Vital Signs
Temperature: 98.4 °F (37 °C)
Heart Rate: 80 BPM
Respiration: 18 BPM
Blood Pressure: 120/70 mm Hg
Height: 5′6″ (168 cm)
Current/Usual weight: 145 lb (66 kg)
BMI: 23.5 kg/m^2

Exam
General: Tired-looking, pale, in no acute distress
Heart: Regular rate and rhythm with no murmurs, rubs, or gallops
Resp: Lungs clear to auscultation and percussion
Abdomen: Soft and non-tender without any masses
Pelvic: External genitalia normal, cervix clear on speculum exam, uterus soft and top-normal size (consistent with 5 week pregnancy) with no adnexal masses on bimanual exam, no tenderness
Extremities: Varicose veins with no clubbing, cyanosis or edema, veins non-tender and not inflamed

PL's 24-Hour Dietary Recall:
Breakfast (home)

Bagel	1 each
Cream cheese	1 Tbsp
Coffee	1 cup
2 percent low-fat milk	1 ounce (30 mL)

Lunch (home)

Turkey breast lunchmeat	3 ounces (85 g)
Potato bread	2 slices
Mayonnaise	1 Tbsp
Diet Coke	12 ounces (360 mL)

Snack (home)

Pretzels	1 ounce (28 g)

Dinner (home)

Fried Flounder	5 ounces (142 g)
Corn on the cob	1 ear

Margarine	1 Tbsp
Diet Coke	12 ounces (360 mL)
Low-fat frozen yogurt	1 cup

Total Calories: 1521 kcal
Protein: 80 grams (21% of total calories)
Fat: 54 grams (32% of total calories)
Carbohydrate: 179 grams (47% of total calories)
Calcium: 608 mg
Iron: 10 mg
Folate: 238 μg

Case Questions

1. What is the physiologic basis for the increased folate requirements for normal neural tube development during pregnancy?
2. What is the prevalence of neural tube defects (NTD) in the United States and who is at higher risk of having a child with an NTD?
3. What is the evidence that folic acid supplementation reduces the risk of neural tube defects?
4. How can an individual develop a folate deficiency? Which populations are at risk for low folate intake?
5. Describe the rationale for the food fortification program and its potential benefits.
6. List food sources high in folate. Based on the nutrition assessment of PL's diet history, what dietary modifications would you suggest?
7. Should a vitamin and mineral supplement be considered for this patient? Why or why not?

Answers to Questions: Case 1
Part 1: Physiology and Prevalence

1.What is the physiologic basis for the increased folate requirements for normal neural tube development during pregnancy?

Folate, and its metabolically active form tetrahydrofolate, are cofactors for the enzymes involved in one-carbon transfer reactions that include the synthesis of nucleic acids and several amino acids (Chapter 7: Case 7.1). Therefore, adequate levels are particularly important at times of rapid cell growth, such as in fetal and placental development. Women are thought to have pregnancies affected by neural tube defects (NTD) for two reasons, and frequently for a combination of these two reasons. The first is an increased folate demand in pregnancy and decreased dietary intake and the second is a genetic defect in the production of enzymes involved in folate metabolism.

The neural tube is formed very early in pregnancy, between 18 and 30 days post-conception. This means that formation is initiated even before the woman may know she is pregnant, since the missed period would generally occur at 14 days post-conception. Since the neural tube goes on to form the spine and brain, defects in the formation of the neural tube can include the absence of formation of most of the brain (anencephaly) as well as defects in the closure of the lower tube (spina bifida) to the open neural tube defects (meningoceles, and myoceles). This early formation, and the detrimental effects of folate deficiency on neural tube formation, form the basis for the recommendation that folic acid supplementation should be begun prior to conception and continued at least through the first trimester of pregnancy.

2. What is the prevalence of NTD in the United States and who is at risk of having a child with an NTD?

Spina bifida and anencephaly, the two most common types of NTDs, occur in approximately 3000 pregnancies (0.76 per 1000 births) each year in the United States. Prevalence varies according to race and ethnicity, with Hispanic women demonstrating the highest rates, while the lowest rates are found among black and Asian women. Women who have had a previous pregnancy affected by an NTD or who are personally affected by an NTD are at a higher risk (2 to 3 percent) in a current pregnancy. A family history of a close family member (sibling, niece, or nephew) with an NTD raises a woman's risk of an affected pregnancy to approximately 1 percent, as does a maternal history of diabetes or the consumption of certain anti-seizure medications such as valproic acid or carbamazepine. A higher risk of NTDs is also associated with increased maternal weight. Since PL'S sister-in-law lost a baby at 24 weeks gestation with anencephaly, her risk increases. However, 95 percent of children with NTDs are born to couples without any family history of NTDs.

In women with a history of a previously affected pregnancy, it has been shown that supplementation with 4 milligrams (4000 micrograms) of folic acid per day, initiated one month prior to attempting to conceive and continued throughout the first trimester of pregnancy, reduced the risk of a repeat NTD by 72 percent. While there is not yet definitive evidence that other high risk groups (such as close family members of affected individuals, diabetics, or women on anti-seizure medications) will benefit from higher levels of supplementation, many experts feel that women in these high-risk groups should be prescribed a higher dose of a folic acid supplement, at least 1000 micrograms per day, prior to conception and in early pregnancy. When recommending higher levels of supplementation to patients, it is important to emphasize that a separate folic acid supplement and NOT multiple doses of multivitamins (MVI) be utilized. Additional daily MVI consumption could lead to toxicity of other vitamins, particularly vitamin A, which is teratogenic to the developing fetus.

Part 2: Folate and Neural Tube Defects

3. What is the evidence that folic acid supplementation reduces the risk of NTD?

Several controlled and observational trials have shown that periconceptional and early pregnancy consumption of folic acid supplements can reduce a woman's risk for having an infant with an NTD by as much as 50 to 70 percent. To increase folic acid consumption by women of childbearing age, the United States Food and Drug Administration (FDA) mandated folic acid fortification of grain products beginning January 1998. Since that time the Centers for Disease Control (CDC) has evaluated the impact of folic acid fortification on the prevalence of NTDs.

Using data from eight population-based birth defect surveillance systems with prenatal diagnosis of NTDs, the CDC reported that the prevalence of NTDs in the United States declined by an estimated 1000 cases from 4000 (1995–1996) to 3000 (1999–2000). This 26 percent decrease in NTD-affected pregnancies since mandatory folic acid fortification began highlights the success of this public health policy. A recent study completed in Canada where the level of folate fortification is similar, showed a 46 percent reduction in the prevalence of NTDs. The higher baseline rate of NTDs compared to the United States might explain the greater risk reduction.

4. How can an individual develop a folate deficiency? Which populations are at risk for low folate intake?

The term folate includes all compounds that have the vitamin properties of folic acid – including folic acid and naturally occurring compounds in food. Folate deficiency in humans is attributed to sub-optimal dietary intake of folate, behavioral and environmental factors, and genetic defects. Humans cannot synthesize folate from other sources and are therefore entirely dependent on dietary sources or supplements to meet their folate requirements.

Folate deficiency is common today since most adults frequently consume diets high in fat and processed foods, with less than the daily recommended servings of fresh fruit and vegetables. Minority women from low socioeconomic and educational backgrounds have been found to have poor folate intakes due to limited use of folate rich foods. In pregnancy the increased demand for folate is not met by self-selected diets.

Folate functions as a methyl donor for the enzyme methylenetetrahydrofolate reductase (MTHFR), which is involved in the conversion of homocysteine to methionine. Folate deficiency results in an elevated serum homocysteine level. It is estimated that two-thirds of hyperhomocysteinemia is due to a folate deficiency. Mutations in the MTHFR gene that have been linked to an increased risk of NTD increase the metabolic requirement for folate and also result in elevated serum homocyteine levels. These levels can be normalized by additional folate intake. However, genetic defects appear to account for only a small percentage of cases of folate deficiency.

5. Describe the rationale for the food fortification program and its potential benefits.

In September 1992, the United States Public Health Service (PHS) recommended that all women of childbearing age consume 400 µg of folate daily (600 µg during pregnancy) to lower their risk of having a child with a NTD. The PHS indicated that this could be achieved by (1) improving dietary habits, (2) fortification of the food supply, and (3) daily consumption of a folic acid supplement. However, most women were not getting this amount from their diets and were not taking folic acid supplements. Data from the third National Health and Nutrition Examination Survey (1989 to 1991) showed that mean folate intake was 230 +/− 7.8 μg/day for non-pregnant woman ages 20 to 29 and 237 +/− 9.0 μg/day for ages 30 to 39, levels below the Dietary Reference Intakes (DRI).

Bentley et al. analyzed food and supplement data since the mandatory folate fortification and found that the median daily total folate intake (from food and supplements) for all women of childbearing age increased by at least 100 μg. Although this is significant, only 39 percent of non-Hispanic whites, 28 percent of Hispanics, and 26 percent of non-Hispanic black women are reported to consume the recommended 400 μg per day, which falls far short of the FDA's target goal of 50 percent.

The March of Dimes has conducted public education campaigns encouraging women of childbearing age to consume an adequate daily intake of folate. Since 1995, The Gallup Organization has been commissioned by the March of Dimes to conduct surveys on national samples of women ages 18 to 45 to measure changes in behavior, knowledge, and awareness relative to folate consumption. In 2007, 40 percent of women reported taking a daily folic acid supplement, which is an increase from 28 percent in 1995. Only 12 percent of women, however, were aware that folic acid should be taken before pregnancy and only one in five women knew that folic acid prevented birth defects. Efforts to educate young women (18 to 24 years) on the importance of folic acid supplementation should be increased since this group demonstrated the least awareness, knowledge, and practice of all age groups surveyed.

Folic acid, also known as pteroylmonoglutamic acid, is the synthetic compound used in dietary supplements and fortified foods. Since January 1, 1998, FDA has required fortification of all enriched grain products (flour, breads, rolls and buns, corn, grits, cornmeal, farina, rice, and noodle products) with 140 μg of folic acid per 100 grams (3.5 ounces) of grain product. To not exceed the DRI's "tolerable upper level" of 1000 μg per day for adults, higher levels were not recommended. Although folic acid is a water-soluble B-complex vitamin with no known toxicity, higher doses of folic acid might mask a vitamin B_{12} deficiency. Folic acid would correct anemia (pernicious, megaloblastic, or macrocytic anemia) but does not prevent the neurological consequences associated with a vitamin B_{12} deficiency.

Folate fortification of foods has been associated with decreased prevalence of NTDs and possible improvement in first-year survival rates among infants with spina bifida. Folate status, as measured by mean serum and red blood cell folate concentrations, has also improved in non-pregnant women across all population groups in the United States since mandatory fortification. A recent report by Pfeiffer et al., however, looking at NHANES survey data from 1999 to 2000 through 2003 to 2004 suggests a decline in blood folate concentrations particularly among non-Hispanic whites. This underscores the need to continue monitoring the changes in folic acid intake and folate status in American women of childbearing age to evaluate, revise, and implement new and existing policies and programs aimed at reducing cases of NTDs.

Part 3: Medical Nutrition Therapy

6. List food sources high in folate. Based on the nutrition assessment of PL's diet history, what dietary modifications would you suggest?

Major sources of dietary folate include dark green leafy vegetables, dried beans, citrus fruits, and fortified cereals. Orange juice is the largest single source of folate consumed by Americans, and it is estimated that it contributes approximately ten percent of one's daily intake of dietary folate. (See Appendix F: Dietary Sources of Folate.)

Folate occurs in dietary sources as polyglutamate, a conjugated form that is less absorbed than free folate. Foods containing 55 μg folate per serving are considered to be excellent sources of folate. When assessing dietary folate intake, it is important to ask very specific questions since there are wide variations in folate content within each food group. For example, eight ounces of orange juice contains approximately 100 μg of folate as compared to negligible amounts in apple juice.

An analysis of PL's intake shows that she consumed only 238 μg of folate, well below her recommended intake. An individual can easily consume 400 to 500 μg of folate daily by following the Food Guide Pyramid guidelines that suggest 3 to 5 servings of vegetables (2.5 cups), 2 to 4 servings of fruits (2 cups), and 6 to 11 servings of grain daily (with at least one-half coming from whole grain sources). PL's diet is deficient in fruits and vegetables. Recommended dietary modifications could include either adding orange juice or a fresh orange or grapefruit to breakfast, carrots sticks to lunch, and a green vegetable, such as broccoli or asparagus, to dinner. In addition to these naturally occurring sources of folate, a ready-to-eat fortified breakfast cereal could contribute significantly to PL's folate intake. Folate is also contained in whole grains and whole grain products such as oatmeal or oat bran cereals, wheat germ, whole grain breads and brown rice, that could easily be incorporated into PL's diet.

7. Should a vitamin and mineral supplement be considered for this patient? Why or why not?

In the United States at least 50 percent of all pregnancies are unplanned. Therefore, the American Academy of Pediatrics, along with the United States PHS, recommends that women of childbearing age consume 400 μg folic acid per day. This is the amount contained in an over-the-counter multivitamin supplement. Since PL is at a slightly higher risk for a NTD affected birth she should consult with her doctor at her 5-week pre-natal visit to discuss the amount of supplemental folic acid she should take. Pre-natal supplements generally contain 1000 μg of folic acid.

There is currently insufficient evidence to provide a recommendation to use dietary folate as the sole method to reduce the risk of NTDs; however, women still should be advised to consume a high folate diet. Folic acid is the most active form of this vitamin and the form used in vitamin preparations and food fortification. When synthetic folic acid is consumed as a supplement in the fasting state, it is nearly 100 percent bioavailable. In contrast, when folic acid is consumed with food, as in fortified cereal grain products, its absorption is reduced to approximately

85 percent. Naturally occurring food folate is only 50 percent absorbed, because the polyglutamate side chain must be cleaved before absorption can occur. Thus, supplemental folic acid taken on an empty stomach is approximately two times more bioavailable than dietary folate, and folic acid taken with food (including folic acid in fortified foods) is approximately 1.7 times more bioavailable than dietary folate. These are only estimates and may be revised over time as more data are gathered and analyzed. Future research should also be aimed at the dose–response relationship of folate and NTD prevention and quantifying, more precisely, the dose needed to prevent recurrences.

Case 2 **Encouraging Breastfeeding**

Ruth Lawrence[1] and Catherine Sullivan[2]

[1] University of Rochester School of Medicine and Dentistry, Rochester, NY
[2] Nutrition Services Branch, Raleigh, NC

OBJECTIVES

- Identify the documented advantages of breastfeeding for both mothers and infants.
- Effectively encourage pregnant women to initiate and continue breastfeeding their infants for at least the first year of life.
- Effectively counsel women regarding techniques and positioning in order to successfully breastfeed their infants.
- Provide appropriate nutritional recommendations for breastfeeding women.
- Compare and contrast the growth patterns of breastfed and formula-fed infants.

LW is a 26-year-old Korean woman who is gravida 1, para 0, in her thirty-seventh week of gestation. She is 5'6" (168 cm) tall and weighed 160 pounds (72.7 kg) prior to becoming pregnant (pre-pregnancy BMI: 25.8 kg/m^2). She now weighs 190 pounds (86 kg), and her pregnancy has been uncomplicated. LW is considering breastfeeding and questions her child birth provider about it and whether she can continue after she returns to work 8 weeks postpartum. LW had been trying to lose weight before she got pregnant. LW plans to lose her pregnancy weight quickly and fears dieting will keep her from producing enough breast milk to feed the baby adequately.

Go to questions 1–4

Follow-up

LW, who has been breastfeeding her infant, returns at 6 weeks postpartum for her checkup. She has lost 20 pounds (9 kg) and currently weighs 170 pounds (77 kg) (BMI = 27.4 kg/m^2). She reports that she is even hungrier than she was during her pregnancy, but cannot find time to eat. She is afraid that she is not producing enough milk because the baby always appears hungry and is not as chubby as her friend's formula-fed baby. She reports that her mother told her she should avoid eating vegetables and chocolate because they will upset the baby's stomach and produce gas. A friend told her that it was not safe for her to try to lose weight while breastfeeding, saying she might get "too skinny." LW is also concerned about how to feed the baby when she returns to work in 2 weeks. A 24-hour recall is as follows.

Medical Nutrition and Disease: A Case-Based Approach, 4th edition. Edited by Lisa Hark.
© 2009 Wiley-Blackwell Publishing, ISBN: 978-1-4051-8615-5.

LW's 24-Hour Dietary Recall
Breakfast (home): She reports that she often skips breakfast

Corn flakes	1 cup
Skim milk	1/2 cup

Lunch (home)

Whole-wheat bread	2 slices
Peanut butter	2 Tbsp.
Jelly	1 Tbsp.
Orange juice	8 ounces (240 mL)

Snack (home)

Snickers candy bar	1–2 ounces (57 g)
Water	1 cup

Dinner (home)

Baked chicken	2 thighs (6 ounces)(170 g)
Baked potato	1 medium
Margarine	2 Tbsp.
Apple sauce	1/2 cup
Diet cola	12 ounces (360 mL)

Snack (home)

Ice cream	1 cup

Total Calories: 2035 kcal
Protein: 78 g (15% of calories)
Fat: 95 g (41% of calories)
Carbohydrate: 228 g (44% of calories)
Calcium: 505 mg
Iron: 8.4 mg

Case Questions

1. What advice can be given to LW to help her decide to breastfeed her infant?
2. How quickly can a postpartum woman expect to lose weight?
3. What dietary recommendations should be given to LW to ensure that her baby will receive adequate nutrition?
4. What are the guidelines regarding frequency and length of time to breastfeed an infant?
5. How will LW know if her breast-fed baby is getting enough to eat? Compare the growth patterns of breast-fed and formula-fed infants.
6. How should LW's weight loss and dietary intake be assessed?
7. How can breastfeeding women prepare to return to work?

Answers to Questions: Case 2
Part 1: Encouraging Breastfeeding

1. What advice can be given to LW to help her decide whether to breastfeed her infant?

According to the Institute of Medicine, American Academy of Pediatrics (AAP), American Academy of Family Physicians (AAFP), American College of Obstetrics and Gynecology (ACOG), and the American Dietetic Association (ADA), breast-feeding is the recommended way to feed infants in the United States. Exclusive breastfeeding is the preferred method for normal full-term infants from birth to six months because of the documented advantages for both the baby and the mother. Breastfeeding, complemented by appropriate introduction of solid foods after 6 months of age, is recommended for the remainder of the first year, and longer if desired (AAP, AAFP, ACOG, ADA). To achieve this goal, it is important to learn how to breastfeed during the early months and after returning to work. For that reason, LW should be encouraged to contact a licensed International Board Certified Lacta-tion Consultant (IBCLC) and only if no IBCLC is available, a leader from a mother-to-mother support group such as La Leche League or a peer counselor program.

It is important that a mother receive social and emotional support for her decision to breastfeed. Women are most likely to succeed at breastfeeding when encouraged by their health care provider(s) during pregnancy, and outside sources for support and assistance (husband or significant other, patient's mother or mother-in-law, mother-to-mother support groups).

2. How quickly can a postpartum woman expect to lose weight?

A woman should not expect to return to her pre-pregnancy weight immediately after delivery. On average, a new mother loses 15 pounds (6.8 kg) within the first week after delivery. Many mothers are concerned about their weight gain during pregnancy and worry that they may not return to their pre-pregnancy weight since many women retain 5 to 10 pounds (2.3 to 4.5 kg) per pregnancy. Lactating women eating nutritionally balanced diets typically lose 1 to 2 pounds (0.45 to 0.9 kg) per month during the first 4 to 6 months of lactation, a rate more rapid than if they were bottle-feeding their infants. A weight loss of more than 1.5 pounds (0.68 kg) per week, even in women with excess fat stores, can decrease breast milk production and jeopardize the nutritional status of both the mother and the baby. However, not all women lose weight during lactation. Some studies suggest that approximately 20 percent of women maintain or gain weight during this time and may lose the additional weight after they wean their infants.

3. What dietary recommendations should be given to LW to ensure that her baby will receive adequate nutrition?

The Institute of Medicine makes the point that breast milk will be ideal even if the diet is not ideal. Lactating women should be encouraged to obtain their nutrients from a well-balanced, varied diet to meet their nutritional needs while lactating, as they have an increased need for essentially all nutrients, especially protein, calcium, and vitamins A, C, and D, compared with non-lactating women. Pregnant and lactating women have been noted to have sub-normal vitamin D levels contributing to an increased incidence of sub-clinical rickets in breastfeeding infants. The specific needs of individual women vary depending on the volume of milk produced daily, the age and size of their infants, their individual metabolism, and their postpartum nutritional status. Supplementing vitamin D (1000 IU per day) is an acceptable recommendation.

During pregnancy, most women store approximately 2 to 4 kilograms of body fat, which can be mobilized to supply a portion of the additional calories used for lactation. Body fat supplies an estimated 200 to 300 kcal per day during the first 3 months of lactation. An additional 500 kcal per day, which is needed for lactation, must come from the diet.

4.What are the guidelines regarding frequency and length of time to breastfeed an infant?

Breastfeeding should ideally be initiated within the first hour after birth. Skin-to-skin contact is essential for getting breastfeeding off to a good start. Feeding the baby on demand, frequent suckling, and completely emptying milk from the breasts helps to increase the mother's milk supply. The duration of a feeding should not be limited during the first few days. In the beginning, it may take 2 to 3 minutes of suckling to stimulate the release of oxytocin (a hypothalamic hormone produced in the posterior pituitary gland). Oxytocin initiates "let-down," the term for the process by which the milk begins to empty from the breast due to the contraction of myoepithelial cells. Prolactin, a hormone produced in the anterior pituitary gland, stimulates milk production. Early and frequent feeding reduces the risk of engorgement. Removing the infant from the breast prior to let-down does not stimulate milk supply and may frustrate both the mother and infant.

The infant should be encouraged to suckle the first breast until the milk flows. When the infant stops suckling and pulls away from the breast the baby should be placed on the other breast after burping for as long as the infant suckles. Although the duration of feeding may vary among infants, feeding should be infant-led and not clock-led.

The composition and volume of breast milk change during each feeding. The milk provided after about 5 to 10 minutes is the richest in fat and therefore caloric content. It is called the "hind milk." Infants need to nurse long enough to become satiated and to obtain sufficient calories from the breast milk for appropriate growth and development. Mothers should be instructed that the infant will get 75 percent of the milk volume in the first 5 to 10 minutes after the "let-down," but only 50 percent of the calories because breast milk becomes higher in fat and calories after the first five minutes.

Once lactation is established, an infant who suckles vigorously usually empties the breast 10 to 20 minutes after let-down has occurred. It may take up to an hour to "empty" both breasts. Infants will suckle until satisfied and should alternate starting breasts with each feeding in order to ensure even milk production. A full-term newborn infant should feed eight to twelve times during 24 hours. Human milk is easily digested and empties from the infant's stomach in 90 minutes, while formula empties in 3 to 4 hours.

Read the Follow-up at beginning of case.

5. How will LW know if her breastfed baby is getting enough to eat? Compare the growth patterns of breast fed and formula fed infants.

The best way to be sure that babies are receiving adequate amounts of breast milk is to monitor their growth and development. Milk production generally works on the principle of supply and demand. That is, the more a baby feeds, the more milk is produced. In the first few days of life, it is not uncommon for a full-term newborn to feed every 1 to 3 hours during each 24-hour period; this helps to stimulate initial milk production. About six weeks postpartum, feeding frequency will diminish to about 8 times in 24 hours once the milk supply has been established. Full-term newborns experience an initial weight loss. This weight loss should not exceed 7 percent of their birth weight. It is very important to monitor weight gain in the first few days of life. A return to birth weight should occur by day 10. If weight gain is not achieved then the patient should be referred to the physician and a lactation professional. A baby who has at least six wet diapers and a minimum of three stools per day and is gaining weight appropriately (at least 7 ounces per week) is usually consuming enough milk.

Breast-fed and formula-fed infants have slightly different growth patterns. In the first two to three months human milk-fed infants gain weight more rapidly. After the first few months of life, the weight gain is similar to formula-fed infants and then begins to slow down. The current Centers for Disease Control and Prevention growth charts are based on NHANES data of only a few healthy breastfed and formula fed children. It is an average of fat and thin not a standard. The WHO also has developed growth charts based on breastfeeding infants in good health and represent how infants should grow. They are the new international standard.

Although breast fed infants consume less milk over a 24-hour period and there-fore have a lower energy intake, they are more energy efficient than formula-fed infants. By their third birthday, breast-fed infants have a lower percentage of body fat and are rarely obese. Data from the Darling Study have shown that breast-fed infants are less likely to be overfed and have a decreased risk of becoming overweight or obese later in life compared to formula-fed children, which may be because they learn to stop eating when they are satisfied. Breast-feeding is one suggestion experts are advocating as a way to prevent obesity in children (see Chapter 4).

Part 2: Follow-up

6. How should LW's weight loss and dietary patterns be assessed?

Although LW desires to lose weight, the goal should be for her to achieve slow and steady weight loss so that she does not compromise her own health or milk supply. Currently, her dietary intake is slightly below what is recommended to support lactation. Her calorie requirements for lactation are estimated to be

2225 to 2325 kcal/kg/day, calculated on the basis of 25 kcal/kg/day (based on BMI >25 kg/m^2) plus an additional 300 to 400 kcal per day for lactation. Extra calories for lactation should be adjusted based on the BMI, activity level, and age of the woman. Her diet does not provide adequate amounts of iron, calcium, vitamin A, vitamin D, vitamin B$_{12}$, vitamin D, folate, and zinc. To enhance her nutrient intake she should be encouraged to follow the " My Pyramid for Lactation" (http://www.mypyramid.gov/mypryamidmoms) and to increase her intake of whole grain or enriched breads and cereals, lean proteins, fruit and vegetables, low-fat vitamin D enriched milk or yogurt, and include an iron-rich snack, such as raisins or dried fruit in the morning. She should limit her intake of concentrated sweets. She should also be advised to continue to take her prenatal vitamin. She may also need to consider taking a vitamin D supplement. The AAP recommends that exclusively breastfed infants receive oral vitamin D drops of 400 IU shortly after birth. This would be the ideal time to encouraged LW to start her baby on vitamin D. In addition, her fluid intake is low and she should be encouraged to drink more nutritious fluids (up to 2 liters per day), such as skim milk fortified with vitamin D, 100 percent juices, and water.

7. How can breastfeeding women prepare to return to work?

A mother returning to work can continue to breast feed by renting or purchasing a breast pump to remove milk during the day for use at home while she is working. The advantages of pumping the breast at least every four hours are to ensure that the baby will receive breast milk when the mother is at work and to promote the continued supply of breast milk even though the baby is not feeding during the day. It is important for the mother to pump to avoid engorgement and mastitis. Breastfeeding exclusively whenever the woman is not working will help milk production to continue. Breast milk can be stored in the refrigerator for less than 4 days, in the freezer for less than 3 months, and in a deep freezer ($-18°$ to $-20\,°C$) for less than 12 months for term infants (Human Milk Banking Guidelines).

The father or a caretaker should offer the bottle because the baby may expect to breastfeed when the mother is present. Offering one bottle of expressed breast milk about once a day, starting about two weeks before the mother returns to work, may help the infant learn how to suck from a bottle, which is different from breastfeeding. Once the mother returns to work, the baby should be given expressed breast milk during the day. When the mother returns from work, she should breastfeed as soon as possible.

Chapter and Case References

American Academy of Pediatrics, American College of Obstetricians and Gynecologists. *Breastfeeding Handbook for Physicians*. 2005.

American Academy of Pediatrics. Breastfeeding and the use of human milk. *Pediatrics* 2005;115(2);496–506.

Academy of Breastfeeding Medicine Protocol Committee. ABM Clinical Protocol #13: Contraception During Breastfeeding. *Breastfeeding Medicine* 2006;1(1):43–51.

American College of Obstetricians and Gynecologists Committee Opinion Number 315. Obesity in Pregnancy. *Am Coll Obst Gyn* 2005;106:67;1–5.

American College of Sports Medicine. Roundtable Consensus Statement: Impact of Physical Activity during Pregnancy and Postpartum on Chronic Disease Risk. *Med Sci Sports Exerc.* 2006;38(5):989–1006.

American Diabetes Association. Standards of medical care in diabetes – 2008. *Diabetes Care.* 2008;31Suppl 1:S12–54.

American Diabetes Association. Position statement: gestational diabetes mellitus. *Diabetes Care* 2004; 27(Suppl. 1):S88–S90.

American Dietetic Association, Position of the American Dietetic Association: Promoting and Supporting Breastfeeding. *J Amer Dietet Assoc.* 2005;105(5):810–18.

Armstrong E, Harris LH, Kukla R, Kuppermenn M, Little MO, Lyerly AD, Mitchell LM. Maternal caffeine consumption during pregnancy and the risk of miscarriage. *Am J Obstet Gynecol.* 2008;198(3):279.e1–8.

Artal R, Catanzaro RB, Gavard JA, Mostello DJ, Friganza JC. A lifestyle intervention of weight-gain restriction: diet and exercise in obese women with gestational diabetes mellitus. *Appl Physiol Nutr Metab.* 2007;32(3):596–601.

Barker DJ. The developmental origins of adult disease. *Eur. J Epid* 2003;18(8):733–6.

Basile L, Taylor S, Taylor SN, et al. The effect of high-dose vitamin D supplementation on serum vitamin D levels and milk calcium concentration in lactating women and their infants. *Breastfeeding Medicine* 2006;1:27–35.

Bentley TG, Willett WC, Weinstein MC, Kuntz KM. Population-level changes in folate intake by age, gender, and race/ethnicity after folic acid fortification. *Am J Public Health.* 2006;96(11):2040–7.

Burstein E, Levy A, Mazor M, Wiznitzer A, Sheiner E. Pregnancy outcome among obese women: a prospective study. *Am J Perinatol.* 2008;195(6):S220–S220.

Carlson S, Aupperle P. Nutrient requirements and fetal development: recommendations for best outcomes. *J Fam Prac;* 2007;56(11 Suppl Womens):S1–6.

Chang MW, Nitzke S, Guilford E, Adair CH, Hazard DL. Motivators and barriers to healthful eating and physical activity among low-income overweight and obese mothers. *J Am Diet Assoc.* 2008;108(6):1023–8.

Cox JT, Phelan ST. Nutrition during pregnancy. *Obstet Gynecol Clin North Am.* 2008;35(3):369–83.

Food and Nutrition Board, Institute of Medicine. *Dietary Reference Intakes for Energy, Carbohydrate, Fiber, Fat, Fatty Acids, Cholesterol, Protein, and Amino Acids.* National Academies Press, Washington, DC, 2002.

Giglia RC, Binns CW. Alcohol, pregnancy and breastfeeding; a comparison of the 1995 and 2001 National Health Survey data. *Breastfeed Rev.* 2008;16(1):17–24.

Hadden DR. Prediabetes and the big baby. *Diabet Med.* 2008;25(1):1–10.

Hale, Thomas. *Medications and Mother's Milk.* Pharmasoft Publishing, 2006.

Hamprecht K, Maschmann J, Jahn G, et al. Breastfeeding and cytomegalovirus infections. *J Chemother.* 2007;19 Suppl 2:49–51.

Healthy People 2010. Department of Health and Human Services. Washington, DC. www.healthypeople.gov.

International Lactation Consultant Association. *Clinical Guidelines for the Establishment of Exclusive Breastfeeding,* 2005.

Institute of Medicine. *Nutrition During Pregnancy: Weight Gain, Nutrient Supplements.* National Academies Press, Washington, DC, 1990.

Johansson S, Iliadou A, Bergvall N, et al. The association between low birth weight and type 2 diabetes: contribution of genetic factors. *Epidemiology.* 2008;19(5):659–65.

Lawrence R, Lawrence R. *Breastfeeding: A Guide for the Medical Profession.* 6th edition Elsevier Mosby, 2005.

Lee H, Jang HC, Park HK, Metzger BE, Cho NH. Prevalence of type 2 diabetes among women with a previous history of gestational diabetes mellitus. *Diabetes Res Clin Pract.* 2008;81(1):124–9.

Mahomed K. Iron supplementation in pregnancy. *Cochrane Database of Systematic Reviews.* 2005;1.

Mehta SH. Nutrition and pregnancy. *Clin Obstet Gynecol.* 2008;51(2):409–18.

Morris SN, Johnson NR. Exercise during pregnancy: a critical appraisal of the literature. *J Reprod Med.* 2005 Mar;50(3):181–8.

Mottola MF. The role of exercise in the prevention and treatment of gestational diabetes mellitus. *Curr Diab Rep.* 2008;8(4):299–304.

Pfeiffer CM, Caudill SP, Gunter EW, Osterloh J, Sampson EJ. Biochemical indicators of B vitamin status in the US population after folic acid fortification: results from the National Health and Nutrition Examination Survey 1999–2000. *Am J Clin Nutr.* 2005;82(2):442-50.

Poulton A, Nanan RK. Effects of prolonged and exclusive breastfeeding on childhood behavior and maternal adjustment: evidence from a large randomized trial. *Pediatrics.* 2008;122(2):474.

Rasmussen KM, Kjolhede CL. Maternal obesity: a problem for both mother and child. *Obesity.* 2008;16(5):929–31.

Saloojee H. HIV and exclusive breastfeeding: Just how exclusive and when to stop? *Prev Med.* 2008l;47(1):36–7.

Savitz DA, Chan RL, Herring AH, Howards PP, Hartmann KE. Caffeine and miscarriage risk. *Epidemiology.* 2008;19(1):55–62.

Shearer WT. Breastfeeding and HIV infection. *Pediatrics.* 2008;121(5):1046–7.

Stotland NE, Chang YW, Hopkins LM, Caughey AB. Gestational weight gain and adverse neonatal outcomes among term infants. *Obstet Gyncol* 2006; 108(3):635–43.

Stuebe AM, Rich-Edwards JW, Willett WC. Manson JE. Michels KB. Duration of lactation and incidence of type 2 diabetes. *JAMA* 2005;294(20):2601–10.

Thomas AM, Gutierrez YM. *American Dietetic Association Guide to Gestational Diabetes Mellitus.* American Dietetic Association, Chicago, IL, 2005.

US Preventive Services Task Force. *The Guide to Clinical Preventive Services 2005.* Department of Health and Human Services. Washington, DC.

Weng X, Odouli R, Li DK. Maternal caffeine consumption during pregnancy and the risk of miscarriage: a prospective cohort study. *Am J Obstet Gynecol* 2008;198(3):279.

Wieringa FT, Dijkhuizen MA, van der Meer JW. Maternal micronutrient supplementation and child survival. *Lancet.* 2008;371(9626):1751–2.

4 Infants, Children, and Adolescents

Elizabeth B. Rappaport[1], Jennifer Thorpe[2], and Andrew M. Tershakovec[3]

[1] Jefferson Medical College, Philadelphia, PA
[2] The Children's Hospital of Philadelphia, Philadelphia, PA
[3] Merck Research Laboratories, North Wales, PA

OBJECTIVES*

- Take an appropriate pediatric history relating to the nutritional assessment and management of children and adolescents.

- Evaluate growth parameters of an infant, child, or adolescent using the appropriate growth charts published by the US Centers for Disease Control and Prevention (CDC).

- Select laboratory tests and diagnostic procedures appropriate to assess, support, and manage the nutrition of infants, children, and adolescents.

- Summarize the current recommendations (proposed by relevant health-professional organizations and government agencies) for healthy nutrition and activity level of infants, children, and adolescents by age and sex.

*Source: Objectives for chapter and cases adapted from the *NIH Nutrition Curriculum Guide for Training Physicians.* (www.nhlbi.nih.gov/funding/training/naa)

Assessment of Nutritional Status and Dietary Intake in Children

Good nutrition during infancy, childhood, and adolescence supports normal growth and development and provides a foundation for adult health. Historically, childhood malnutrition was equated with undernutrition, weight loss, stunted growth, and impaired development. Poor nutrition in childhood now also encompasses "over-nutrition" and obesity, which can also be associated with specific micronutrient deficiencies, significant co-morbidities, and increased risk of disease and disability in adulthood. In addition, children and adolescents with certain medical conditions are at risk for nutritional deficiencies that require attention and proactive management. Healthcare professionals taking care of infants, children, and adolescents can profoundly influence their immediate and long-term health and longevity. Therefore, clinicians must become adept in assessing the nutritional status of children, in developing an appropriate nutritional management plan, and in counseling caregivers as well as children to foster healthful eating habits.

Medical Nutrition and Disease: A Case-Based Approach, 4th edition. Edited by Lisa Hark.
© 2009 Wiley-Blackwell Publishing, ISBN: 978-1-4051-8615-5.

Assessing Growth and Development

Evaluation of growth and development is the cornerstone of pediatric nutrition assessment. Updated growth charts were released in 2000 by the Centers for Disease Control and Prevention (CDC), based on National Health and Nutrition Examination Survey (NHANES) data collected from 1971 to 1994. These charts represent the combined growth patterns of breast-fed and formula-fed infants in all racial and ethnic groups and include graphs depicting BMI-for-age and sex. Children and adolescents should be measured without shoes using a wall-mounted stadiometer and weighed wearing light clothing. A length board should be used for infants. For infants and children less than 2 years of age, weight-for-length should be assessed. Once the child can stand, weight-for-height should be substituted. For children and adolescents 2 to18 years, BMI (kg/m^2) can be calculated or determined using standard charts or web-based tools such as those available at www.cdc.gov/growthcharts as shown in Figures 4-1 and 4-2.

Height (length), weight, and weight-for-length or BMI should be plotted on a sex specific growth chart kept with the child's medical records so that the individual values and a longitudinal record of the child's growth can be examined and evaluated. Plotted values of all three of these growth parameters should be assessed to determine:

- whether they are following consistently along a particular percentile line,
- the degree to which particular plotted values deviate from the child's prior pattern of growth,
- where these values fall relative to the norms in the growth charts.

For children less than 2 years of age, the growth assessment should include a measure of head circumference. Note also that measurements of length and height differ slightly so standard growth curves for evaluating length and height should not be used interchangeably. Children who are underweight (BMI <5th percentile), losing weight, or whose linear growth has slowed or ceased should be assessed for nutritional deficiencies and for medical conditions that could impair growth or nutritional status. Similarly, children observed to be gaining weight rapidly or to have an increasing BMI percentile should be evaluated. Classification of BMI for children and adolescents is shown in Table 4-1.

Children who are overweight or obese are at substantially increased risk for type 2 diabetes, hypertension, and other cardiovascular disease risk factors. The Fourth Report on the *Diagnosis, Evaluation and Treatment of High Blood Pressure in Children and Adolescents* provides guidelines for the measurement, evaluation, and treatment of high blood pressure in youth and is available on the National Heart, Lung, and Blood Institute web site (www.nhlbi.nih.gov).

Beyond assessing growth, relative weight, blood pressure, and physical examination should be part of the nutritional assessment of any child. Gross micronutrient deficiencies are rare in the United States, but the risk of deficiencies may be increased in certain situations. For example, deficiencies of fat-soluble vitamins may occur with intestinal malabsorption, thus xeropthalmia (vitamin A) and peripheral neuropathy (vitamin E) may occur. Signs and symptoms associated with vitamin deficiencies are described in Chapters 1 and 2.

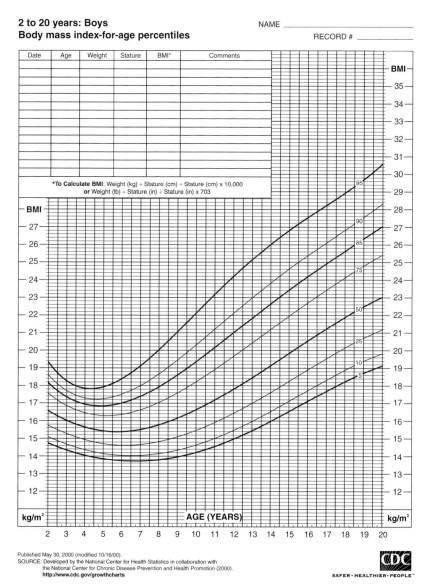

2 to 20 years: Boys
Body mass index-for-age percentiles

NAME _____

RECORD # _____

*To Calculate BMI: Weight (kg) ÷ Stature (cm) ÷ Stature (cm) x 10,000
or Weight (lb) ÷ Stature (in) ÷ Stature (in) x 703

Published May 30, 2000 (modified 10/16/00).
SOURCE: Developed by the National Center for Health Statistics in collaboration with
the National Center for Chronic Disease Prevention and Health Promotion (2000).
http://www.cdc.gov/growthcharts

Figure 4.1 2 to 20 Years: Boys' Body Mass Index-for-Age Percentiles
Source: http://www.cdc.gov/nchs/data/nhanes/growthcharts/set1clinical/cj41l023.pdf

Laboratory Assessment

As part of a regular nutritional evaluation, broad screening using laboratory tests is generally not recommended. General assessments can include a complete blood count (CBC), serum electrolytes, creatinine, and albumin. Serum albumin is commonly used as an assessment of general nutritional and protein status. Evaluation

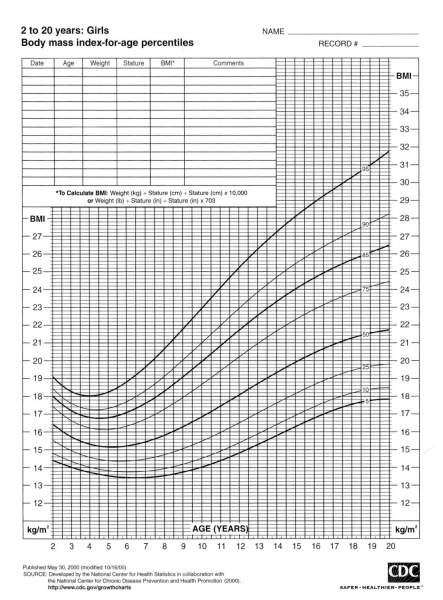

Figure 4.2 2–20 Years: Girls' Body Mass Index-for-Age Percentiles.
Source: http://www.cdc.gov/nchs/data/nhanes/growthcharts/set1clinical/cj41l024.pdf

of the CBC, including white blood cell morphology and red blood cell size, can provide evidence of deficiencies in iron, folate, and vitamin B_{12}. Blood chemistries can indicate electrolyte and mineral imbalances, though blood levels are not always good indicators of whole body balance.

Table 4-1 BMI Classification for Children and Adolescents

BMI Category	Recommended terminology
<5th percentile	Underweight
5th–84th percentile	Healthy weight
85th–94th percentile	Overweight
95th–97th percentile	Obesity
98th–99th percentile	Moderately obese
>99th percentile	Severely obese

Source: Center for Disease Control and Prevention Used with permission.

Fasting glucose

Data from a nationally representative sample indicate that approximately 0.5 percent of US adolescents have diabetes. Seventy percent of these youth have type 1 diabetes and 30 percent have type 2 diabetes. An estimated 39,000 US adolescents have type 2 diabetes and nearly 2.8 million have impaired fasting glucose ($\geq$100 mg/dL; 5.6 mmol/L). In selected high-risk groups, glucose intolerance and type 2 diabetes occur more frequently. In a predominantly Hispanic and African-American cohort of over 1700 eighth grade students in which 29 percent had BMIs $\geq$95th percentile for age and sex, elevated fasting glucose ($\geq$100 mg/dL) was present in 40 percent of the cohort. Impaired glucose tolerance (glucose $\geq$140 mg/dL 2-h postglucose challenge) occurred in 2.3 percent. The frequency of impaired glucose tolerance was nearly twice as high (4.1 percent) in the heaviest subset, those with BMI $\geq$95th percentile. Rates of impaired glucose tolerance were also higher in Hispanic (3.2 percent) and Native American (7.3 percent) youth than in the overall cohort. Among children in a weight management clinic, impaired glucose tolerance was reported in 14 of 55 (25 percent) severely obese children (4 to 10 years of age) and in 23 of 112 (21 percent) of severely obese adolescents (11 to 18 years of age). In severely obese youth, the progression from impaired glucose tolerance to type 2 diabetes may be rapid, particularly in those with continuing weight gain. Adolescence is a period of particularly high risk for the onset of type 2 diabetes.

Overweight children and adolescents, particularly those with a family history of type 2 diabetes, are at increased risk of developing glucose intolerance and eventually type 2 diabetes. The recommended screening test is fasting plasma glucose. The American Diabetes Association criteria for type 2 diabetes screening in children and adolescents are shown in Table 4-2. In the evolution of type 2 diabetes, post-prandial glucose increases earlier than fasting glucose; some experts therefore recommend determining plasma glucose two hours after a standard glucose load or two hours after a meal.

Lipids

Screening for hypercholesterolemia should start at the age of 2 years, and target children with a positive family history of early atherosclerotic vascular disease (AVD) or hypercholesterolemia. A positive family history of early AVD is defined

Table 4-2 Testing for Type 2 Diabetes in Asymptomatic Children and Adolescents

---

- Overweight (BMI >85th percentile for age and sex, weight for height >85th percentile, or weight 120% of ideal for height)

Plus any two of the following risk factors:

- Family history of type 2 diabetes in first- or second-degree relative.
- Race/ethnicity (American Indian, African-American, Hispanic, Asian American, Pacific Islander).
- Signs of insulin resistance or conditions associated with insulin resistance (acanthosis nigricans, hypertension, dyslipidemia, PCOS, or small-for-gestational-age birthweight).

Age of initiation: age 10 years or at onset of puberty, if puberty occurs at a younger age.

Frequency: every 3 years.

Test: Fasting plasma glucose (FPG) preferred

*Clinical judgment should be used to test for diabetes in high-risk patients who do not meet these criteria.

Source: Standards of medical care in diabetes–2009. *Diabetes Care* 2009, 32 Suppl 1:S15.

as a parent or grandparent with a heart attack, sudden death thought to be related to AVD, angina, angioplasty, peripheral vascular disease, or cerebrovascular disease before age 55. Alternatively, some suggest using a sex-specific age cut point of 55 years for men and 65 for women. Children with high cholesterol levels tend to become adults with high cholesterol levels. However, as tracking of lipid levels over time is not perfect, not all the hypercholesterolemic children will become hypercholesterolemic adults. Also, there are concerns that with universal screening, more children may be placed on inappropriate, nutritionally inadequate diets. Current recommendations focus on screening children and adolescents at high risk for hypercholesterolemia, in order to identify those who should receive focused and aggressive intervention.

Iron Status

Iron deficiency, a relatively common problem, is usually due to inadequate dietary intake of iron and occurs most commonly during times of rapid growth or increased blood loss, such as infancy and early childhood and during adolescence (especially for girls). As specific measures of iron stores (e.g., serum ferritin, transferrin, iron binding capacity, free erythrocyte protoporphyrin) are costly and not widely available, hemoglobin and red blood cell indices are the laboratory parameters most commonly used to evaluate children for iron deficiency. These are, however, insensitive measures; data from the National Health and Nutrition Examination Survey (NHANES) III indicated that iron deficiency with anemia accounted for 11 to 26 percent of all children and adolescents with iron deficiency. Data from NHANES 2002 indicate that the overall prevalence of iron deficiency in US children under 5 years still exceeds the *Healthy People 2010* target of 1 to 5 percent. Of 4.5 million low-income children under 5 years old participating in federally funded maternal and child health programs in 2006, 14 percent had anemia.

An analysis of nationally representative cross-sectional data on children 2–16 years of age from NHANES III (1988–1994) revealed the prevalence of iron deficiency to be 2.3 percent, 1.8 percent, and 4.7 percent in children 2 to 5, 6 to 11, and 12 to 16 years of age respectively. In addition, these analyses identified a substantially increased risk of iron deficiency with and without anemia in overweight and obese children compared to normal weight children with iron deficiency prevalence of 15 percent in obese adolescent girls. A later examination of data from toddlers (1 to 3 years old) surveyed during NHANES IV (1999 to 2002) revealed an iron deficiency prevalence of 20 percent among obese toddlers compared to a prevalence of 7 to 8 percent among overweight and normal weight toddlers. A study of children (mean age 11.3 ± 3.6 years) referred to a university-affiliated endocrinology clinic showed a significant inverse relationship between BMI and serum iron levels; iron deficiency was noted in 39 percent, 12 percent, and 4 percent of obese, overweight, and normal weight children, respectively. Even in the absence of anemia, iron deficiency is associated with poor growth and neuro-cognitive development in infants and behavioral and learning problems in older children and adolescents. Iron deficiency and iron-deficiency anemia are also associated with decreased exercise capacity and physical endurance and therefore may contribute to the diminished exercise capacity observed in obese children and adolescents. Thus, it is important to evaluate overweight and obese children regardless of age for the presence of iron deficiency and/or iron-deficiency anemia.

Vitamin D

Vitamin D deficiency is a common and poorly recognized condition that occurs in infants, children, adolescents, and adults. Supplementation with 400 IU of vitamin D should be initiated within days of birth for all breastfed infants, and for nonbreastfed infants and children who do not ingest at least 1 L of vitamin D–fortified formula or milk daily.

Premature infants, dark-skinned infants and children, and children who reside at higher latitudes (particularly above 40°) may require larger amounts of vitamin D supplementation, especially in the winter months, and consideration should be given to supplementing with up to 800 IU of vitamin D per day. A high index of suspicion for vitamin D deficiency should be maintained for these infants and children. Vitamin D levels vary by race, season, and latitude and may be affected by diet and body mass index. Chronic, severe, vitamin D deficiency in young children results in rickets, due to poor bone mineralization and abnormal maturation of growing bone cells (chondrocytes). Despite existing recommendations regarding vitamin D supplementation in infants, severe vitamin D deficiency with rickets, occasionally accompanied by hypocalcemic tetany, is still observed and reported. Most affected children are dark skinned and have limited exposure to UV light, are fed unfortified "health food" milk alternatives, or are breast-fed without vitamin D supplementation by mothers with vitamin D insufficiency or deficiency. Recent studies indicate that compared to white children, African-American and Hispanic youth are at greater risk for vitamin D deficiency and that obese children are at increased risk for vitamin D deficiency. Less severe forms of vitamin D insufficiency may prevent children and adolescents from attaining optimal peak bone mass and place them at increased risk for development of osteoporosis and fractures during adulthood. Inadequate intake of calcium rich foods such as dairy products, now commonly observed in children and adolescents, may further increase these risks.

Although the role of vitamin D in bone and mineral metabolism has long been recognized, emerging epidemiologic, biochemical, and animal model data indicate that vitamin D also affects extra-skeletal health. The vitamin D receptor (VDR), a steroid hormone nuclear receptor that binds the active form of vitamin D, $1,25(OH)_2D$, regulates gene transcription, and is present in many tissues including heart, stomach, pancreas, brain, skin, and cells of the immune system. Many of these tissues may be affected by circulating $1,25(OH)_2D$, while others may produce the active hormone locally from circulating $25(OH)D$.

The principal source of vitamin D is solar UV-B (wavelengths of 290–315 nm) irradiation. Dietary sources of vitamin D other than vitamin supplements are limited and include oily fish, some fish oils, and egg yolks. Although some foods in the United States are vitamin D fortified, including milk, some cereals, orange juice, some yogurts, and margarine, most US children do not eat sufficient quantities of vitamin D-containing foods to provide adequate vitamin D intake. Supplementation with 400 IU of vitamin D should be initiated within days of birth for all breast-fed infants, and for non breast-fed infants and children who do not ingest at least 1 L of vitamin D fortified formula or milk daily. Premature infants, dark-skinned infants and children, and children who reside at higher latitudes (particularly above 40°) may require larger amounts of vitamin D supplementation, especially in the winter months, and consideration should be given to supplementing with up to 800 IU of vitamin D per day. A high index of suspicion for vitamin D deficiency should be maintained for these infants and children. (See Appendix B: Food Sources of Vitamin D).

Evaluating Dietary Adequacy in Children

Dietary intake is difficult to assess accurately in an out-patient setting, as it is based on recall and requires that both the health care provider and the patient or caregiver understand portion sizes and content of a variety of foods. Infants, children, and adolescents being evaluated for abnormal growth or development should generally be assessed by a pediatric nutrition professional such as a registered dietitian. Nevertheless, with the high prevalence of overweight and obesity in the pediatric population, primary care providers must make a general assessment of eating behavior and estimate calorie and nutrient intake in order to counsel patients and their caregivers.

Pediatric Calorie and Nutrient Requirements

Nutrient requirements are largely determined by lean body mass and activity level. Therefore, body composition, which changes during the course of growth and development, must be considered when estimating nutrient needs of children and adolescents. Percent body fat, or fat mass, is high in infants and toddlers and decreases as children enter their elementary school years. During puberty, percent

Table 4-3 Energy and Protein Requirements in Children and Adolescents

Age	Energy (kcal/day) Males	Energy (kcal/day) Females	Protein (Grams/day) Males	Protein (Grams/day) Females
0–6 months	570	520	9.1	9.1
7–12 months	743	676	11	11
1–2 years	1046	992	13	13
3–8 years	1742	1642	19	19
9–13 years	2279	2071	34	34
14–18 years	3152	2368	52	46

Source: Institute of Medicine, *Dietary Reference Intakes for Energy and protein.* National Academy of Science, National Academy Press, Washington, DC: 2008.

body fat increases in both boys and girls. Lean body mass (LBM) also increases, approximately tripling in boys and doubling in girls. As they reach adulthood, females retain a higher percentage body fat and lower lean body mass than males. Pubertal changes in body composition drive changes in nutrient requirements and the difference in lean body mass between men and women accounts for differences in calorie and nutrient requirements.

Various recommended energy and nutrient allowances have been formulated for growing children based on the changing nutritional needs associated with growth and development. For the general population, the USDA has developed the My Pyramid system based on the *Dietary Guidelines for Americans* (www.mypyramid.gov). This guidance system is intended to provide a framework for adults and children for determining what and how much to eat each day, and provides an individualized approach to formulating intake and activity goals. Dietary Reference Intake (DRI) values developed by the Food and Nutrition Board, Institute of Medicine, National Academy of Sciences provide another useful tool for determining specific energy and protein requirements as shown in Table 4-3.

Adjustments for Activity and Illness

In pediatric acute care settings, specific adjustments are made for special circumstances such as differing activity levels and illness. For example, fever increases energy needs by 7 percent for each degree above 98.6°F of body temperature (or 12 percent for each degree above 37°C). Illness, trauma, major surgery, extensive burns, or recovery from undernutrition can double energy requirements. Chronic under-nutrition with loss of lean body mass can decrease energy needs by 20 to 30 percent. However, energy needs may increase rapidly in the malnourished child who is being repleted. For example, with significant malnutrition, a child may be dehydrated and in a state of slowed metabolism, an adaptation that decreases calorie and nutrient requirements. Laboratory assessments may appear relatively normal. However, refeeding causes anabolism and a rapid increase in metabolic processes, greatly increasing caloric and nutrient needs. These changes, along with rehydration, can unveil significant electrolyte and micronutrient deficiencies (e.g., potassium, magnesium). Overly aggressive refeeding without adequate nutrient supplementation can be associated with serious morbidity, including cardiac dysfunction, arrhythmias, congestive heart failure, and even death. Therefore, a significantly malnourished child must be repleted slowly, under close monitoring and supervision (see Chapter 4: Case 4.2).

Infant Feeding
Breast or Bottle (Lactation discussed in Chapter 3)
Except for special formulas, manufacturers of infant formulas generally try to approximate the composition of human breast milk. Recently, formula manufacturers have begun to add omega-3 and omega-6 fatty acids, DHA (docosahexaenoic acid), and ARA (arachidonic acid) to infant formulas. These fatty acids are found in breast milk and are required for normal brain and eye development. There has been a proliferation of private-label formulas or "generic" formulas in the retail market in recent years. Although there may be differences in ingredient formulations, private label infant formulas are considered safe for use in infants, as they are subject to the same FDA regulations as major brands of infant formula (see Table 4-4).

Weaning Babies from Breast Milk or Formulas
Infants should remain on breast milk or formula until the age of 1 year. Most health care providers feel that cow's milk is an important source of calories, protein, and calcium for children over 1 year of age. The American Academy of Pediatrics (AAP) recommends that cow's milk not be given to children under 1 year of age. Earlier introduction of cow's milk is associated with gastrointestinal blood loss due to milk protein-induced inflammatory reaction in the small bowel. This blood loss may be sufficient to deplete iron stores and to produce anemia. In addition, cow's milk has a higher protein and phosphorus content than breast milk or infant formula. These components present a solute load that exceeds the capacity of the immature kidney and may precipitate dehydration and electrolyte imbalance.

Iron Supplementation
Even though breast milk is lower in iron than cow's milk, the iron in breast milk is more readily absorbed. As the fetus gains a significant proportion of its iron stores during the third trimester, babies born prematurely are at higher risk for iron deficiency than full-term infants. Pre-term infants who are fed with human milk should be provided with iron at 2 (mg/kg)/day at 1 month of age and through 12 months of age. Pre-term infants who are formula-fed may benefit from supplemental iron provided at 1 (mg/kg)/day in addition to the iron present in pre-term and transitional formulas, also continued through the first year of life. Encouraging consumption of iron-fortified solid foods or foods naturally high in iron is further recommended for older infants and children (see Appendix L: Food Sources of Iron).

Table 4-4 Indications and Types of Infant Formulas

Formula	Indications	Unique properties	Examples
Milk-based	Breast milk substitute for term infants	+/− Iron Ready to feed, powder, or liquid concentrate Variable whey: casein 20 kcal/ounces May contain DHA/ARA	Enfamil Lipil, Similac Advance Enfamil Lactofree Lipil Similac Sensitive, Similac Sensitive RS Enfamil Gentlease Lipil Enfamil AR Lipil Good Start Supreme DHA & ARA Good Start Supreme
Soy-based	Breast milk substitute for infants with lactose intolerance or milk protein allergy*	Lactose-free, may contain sucrose May contain DHA/ARA May contain fiber	Enfamil Prosobee Lipil, Similac Isomil Advance Similac Isomil DF Good Start Soy DHA & ARA
Premature	Breast milk substitute for Low birth weight, hospitalized Preterm infants	Low lactose Whey: casein 60:40 High calcium and phosphorus 20 and 24 cal/ounces	Enfamil Premature Lipil Similac Special Care Advance
Premature Transitional	Breastmilk substitute for preterm Infants >2.5 kg or discharge Formula for preterm infants	22 kcal/ounces RTF or powder w/ ARA / DHA	Enfamil Enfacare Lipil Similac Neosure Advance
Human Milk Fortifier	Add to breast milk for premature Or low birth weight babies	Increases calorie, protein and Vitamin/mineral content of breast milk	Similac Human Milk Fortifier Enfamil Human Milk Fortifier
Older Infant	Older babies (>9 mos.) and Young toddlers (<24 mos.)	Varies	Good Start 2 DHA & ARA Good Start 2 Soy DHA & ARA Enfamil Next Step Lipil, & w/ Soy Enfamil Next Step Prosobee Lipil Similac Go & Grow Similac Go & Grow Soy

(Continued)

Table 4-4 (*Continued*)

Formula	Indications	Unique properties	Examples
Hypoallergenic	Milk or soy protein allergy	Hydrolyzed protein Sucrose-free, Lactose-free May contain DHA/ARA	Nutramigen Lipil
Predigested	Malabsorption Short bowel syndrome Allergy	Lactose-free Hydrolyzed protein or free Amino acids May contain DHA/ARA	Similac Alimentum, Pregestimil Lipil Nutramigen AA Lipil Elecare, Neocate
Fat-modified	Defects in digestion, absorption, or transport of fat	Contains increased % of kcals as MCT	Monogen Portagen (no longer recommended for infants) Similac Alimentum Pregestimil Lipil
Carbohydrate-modified	Simple sugar intolerance	Requires addition of complex carbohydrate to be complete	RCF 3232 A
Amino acid-modified	Inborn errors of metabolism	Low or devoid of specific amino acids that cannot be metabolized	Multiple products
Electrolyte-modified	Renal or cardiac disease or other disease state requiring low renal solute load	Decreased potassium content Decreased calcium and Phosphorus content	Similac PM 60/40

Source: Department of Clinical Nutrition, The Children's Hospital of Philadelphia, 2009. Used with permission.

*Children allergic to milk protein may also be allergic to soy protein.

DHA – Docosahexaenoic acid
ARA – Arachidonic acid
RTF – Ready-to-Feed

Introducing Solid Food

Recommendations concerning the introduction of solid food have changed considerably over the years. In the past, many children ate a wide variety of foods as early as the first month of life. Now, the consensus among health care providers is to delay the introduction of solid foods until the child is at least four months old. The American Academy of Pediatrics and The World Health Organization both recommend breast milk as the sole nutrient source until six months of age.

Infants are not physiologically ready to accept solid foods from a spoon until they are at least four months of age. It is around this time that the oral extrusion reflex becomes extinguished and infants develop sufficient head and neck control and coordination of the oral musculature to begin taking solid foods.

The introduction of solid foods marks the beginning of a critical period during which the infant learns to master eating from a spoon and to accept different tastes and textures. Not coincidentally, an infant's readiness for these experiences generally corresponds to a physiologic need to supplement the amounts of calories and nutrients available from breast milk or formula. However, breast milk, formula, or a combination should still continue to be the major source of calories and nutrients during the remainder of the infant's first year. As Table 4-5 shows, most solid foods have lower caloric density than breast milk or formula and therefore should not be the major nutrient source.

Preventing and Managing Food Allergies

Introducing solid foods earlier in an infant's life may stimulate the development of food allergies. Infants from families with known food allergies are most at risk. Food allergies – actually, food hypersensitivity reactions – occur in 2 to 8 percent of children less than 3 years of age. Approximately 90 percent of food allergies are associated with the following group of eight foods: peanuts, tree nuts (such as walnuts or cashews), eggs, milk, fish, shellfish, soy, and wheat. Approximately 2.5 percent of infants will experience allergic reactions to cow's milk in the first three years of life, 1.5 percent to egg, and 0.6 percent to peanuts. Many children outgrow food allergies during the first few years of life. Approximately 85 percent

Table 4-5 Comparison of the Relative Caloric Densities of Common Infant Foods and Beverages

Food/Beverage	Caloric density
Whole cow's milk	19 kcal/ounces
Infant formula	20–24 kcal/ounces
Human milk	20 kcal/ounces*
Baby food vegetables	9–19 kcal/ounces
Baby food fruits	14–20 kcal/ounces

Source: Andrew Tershakovec MD. Merck. Used with permission.
*This value represents an average, as the fat content of breastmilk varies somewhat between individuals and the stage of feeding.

of children with reactions to milk and eggs become tolerant to them by five years of age. Even peanut allergy may remit in up to 20 percent of children.

The following terms, suggested by the American Academy of Allergy and Immunology Committee on Adverse Reactions to Foods, more clearly define food reactions:

- *Adverse reaction*: clinically abnormal response believed to be caused by an ingested food or food additive.
- *Food hypersensitivity* (*allergy*): immunologic reaction resulting from the ingestion of a food or food additive.
- *Food anaphylaxis*: classic allergic hypersensitivity reaction to food or food additives involving IgE antibody and release of chemical mediators.
- *Food intolerance*: general term describing an abnormal physiologic response to an ingested food or food additive; can include idiosyncratic, metabolic, pharmacologic, or toxic response.

General Guidelines for Introducing New Foods

Most experts agree that new foods should be introduced gradually, with an interval of at least three days between successive new food introductions. Following this procedure makes it easier to detect a child's inability to tolerate a newly introduced food. Table 4-6 summarizes how to feed an infant during the first year of life and is often very helpful to hand out to parents of infants.

Cereals For formula-fed infants, iron-fortified cereals are the first recommended solid food. Generally offered first at 6 months of age, rice cereal is fortified with iron, is generally non-allergenic, and is usually well-tolerated. Begin with 1 to 2 tablespoons in the morning, mixed with formula or breast milk. The cereal should be mixed to a consistency similar to that of applesauce. Cereal can be thickened as the child grows older. Feeding cereal from a spoon helps the baby learn this new skill, which takes a few weeks. Parents should be advised to avoid putting cereal in a bottle, as it does not, as commonly believed, help children to sleep through the night. Furthermore, the need to make a larger hole in the nipple to prevent clogging may cause a rapid intake of this viscous mixture and lead to choking.

Fruits/Fruit Juice Cooked and strained or pureed fruits, either homemade or purchased baby food without added sugar, may be started after rice cereal. Fresh, mashed bananas also may be introduced at this time. Peeled, soft fruits such as peaches and pears may be cut into small pieces and started at 8 to 10 months of age. Foods that are harder to chew, such as apples, should be deferred until the child has a greater capacity to chew. Juices made from 100 percent fruit, such as apple juice, may also be offered at this time. According to the American Academy of Pediatrics (AAP), no juice should be given to babies younger then 6 months of age. Juice intake should be limited to less than 4 ounces per day for children over six months to ensure adequate intake of other foods. Encourage parents to dilute juice with water and to only offer 100 percent juice without added sugars.

Table 4-6 How to Feed Your Infant During the First Year of Life

Age in months	Breast milk or iron fortified infant formula *	Cereals and breads	Fruits & fruit juices **	Vegetables	Protein foods	Dairy foods
0–4 Months	5–10 feedings/day 17–24 fluid ounces a day (510–720 mL)	None	None	None	None	None
4–6 Months	4–7 feedings/day 24–32 fluid ounces/day (720–960 mL/day)	First food for formula-fed infants: Rice or barley infant cereals (iron fortified). Mix cereal with formula until thin. Start with 1 tbsp. at each feeding for a few days, and increase to 3–4 tbsp. per day. Feed with small baby spoon (don't expect baby to eat much at first).	None	None	First food for breast-fed or partially breast-fed infants: smooth preparations of single meats (beef, veal, lamb, turkey, chicken) in small quantities of up to 2 tbsp/day.	None

(Continued)

Table 4-6 (Continued)

Age in months	Breast milk or iron fortified infant formula *	Cereals and breads	Fruits & fruit juices **	Vegetables	Protein foods	Dairy foods
7–8 Months	4–5 feedings/day 24–32 fluid ounces/day (720–960 mL/day)	Single grain infant cereals–rice, oatmeal, barley (iron fortified) in the morning. 3–9 tbsp/day, mixed with breast milk or infant formula. Two feedings a day. Oven-dried toast or teething biscuits, crackers, or toast strips.	Strained or mashed fruits (fresh or cooked), mashed bananas, applesauce. Infant 100% fruit juices. Less than 4 ounces /day mixed with water and served in a cup.	Strained or mashed, well-cooked: dark yellow or orange (not corn), dark green vegetables. Start with mild vegetables such as green beans, peas, or squash. 1/2–1 jar or 1/4–1/2 cup/day.	Smooth preparations of single meats: beef, veal, lamb, turkey, chicken in small quantities (up to 2 tbsp/day)	Cottage cheese, yogurt
8–9 Months	3–4 feedings/day 24–32 fluid ounces/day (720–960 mL)	Infant cereals or plain hot cereals mixed with breast milk or formula. Toast, bagels, crackers, teething biscuits. Small pieces of cooked noodles, potatoes.	Peeled soft fruit wedges: bananas, peaches, pears, oranges, apples (skin removed). 100% fruit juices including orange and tomato juices. 4–6 ounces/day. (120–180 mL)	Cooked, mashed vegetables.	Well cooked, strained, ground, or finely chopped chicken, fish, and lean meats: 2–3 tbsp/day (remove all bones, fat, skin). No peanut butter until 1 year. Cooked dried beans. Egg yolks and whites.	Cottage cheese, yogurt, bite-size cheese strips.

Table 4-6 (*Continued*)

Age in Months	Breast Milk or Iron Fortified Infant Formula *	Cereals and Breads	Fruits & Fruit Juices **	Vegetables	Protein Foods	Dairy Foods
10–12 Months	3–4 feedings a day 24–32 fluid ounces/day (720–960 mL) by cup or bottle	Infant or cooked cereals mixed with breast milk or formula. Unsweetened cereals, white/wheat breads. Mashed potatoes, rice, noodles, spaghetti.	All fresh fruits peeled and seeded or canned fruits packed in water. 100% fruit juices 4–6 ounces/day (120–180 mL).	Cooked vegetable pieces. Some raw vegetables: tomatoes, cucumbers.	Small tender pieces of chicken, fish or lean meat. Cooked beans, pasta.	Cottage cheese, yogurt, bite-size cheese strips.

Source: Lisa Hark, PhD, RD and Diane Barsky, MD. Used with permission.
*These are general guidelines. Feeding schedules vary somewhat between children
**There is no specific need for juice in an infant's diet.

Vegetables Cooked, strained vegetables, without added salt, either homemade or as commercially prepared baby food, are appropriate to start at six to eight months of age. The importance of avoiding salt should be stressed. Infants do not require extra sodium, and adding salt may encourage a greater salt intake later in life. Raw vegetables that are soft or cooked (steamed) may be introduced at 1 year of age. Hard vegetables such as raw carrots should not be introduced until the child's top and bottom molars have erupted and she can adequately chew and swallow these items without choking. Parents who do not themselves eat a wide range of fruits and vegetables may hesitate to offer such foods to their infants. Research suggests that taste preferences are inherited, so if a parent does not like broccoli, there is an increased chance that the child will also not like it. However, as noted below, repeated offering of a new food may overcome a child's initial resistance or rejection of an unfamiliar taste or texture.

Eggs In the past, experts recommended that cooked egg yolks be introduced to infants over the age of 6 months, but that the introduction of egg whites should be delayed until the child reaches one year of age because of the potential risk of inducing an allergy to eggs in younger infants. However, recent recommendations from the AAP state that there is no convincing evidence that delaying the introduction of highly allergenic foods, such as eggs, beyond 6 months of age has a significant protective effect on the development of atopic disease.

Meat Red meat can be an important source of iron. For breast-fed and partially breast-fed infants, smooth preparations of single meat (beef, veal, lamb, turkey, chicken) are suggested as the first solid food. Recent research indicates that the early consumption of meats improves the iron and zinc status of the older infant. Meats should be well puréed to avoid the risk of choking. Iron supplementation of vegetarian breast-fed babies who will not be given meat should be considered (elemental iron 1 mg/kg/day) if dietary sources of iron are not adequate.

Starch/Carbohydrates Children tend to like pasta, spaghetti, noodles, and dry cereal. However, other essential foods with higher nutrient density should be introduced first during the meal to ensure that the child's diet is complete and balanced. Introducing whole grains early-on may help children to acquire a life-long taste for them.

Fats Diets limited in saturated fat are clearly beneficial for the prevention of chronic disease in adults. Unfortunately, cases have been reported of failure to thrive, in which young children were fed a very low-fat, calorically inadequate diet. On the other hand, a longitudinal study has reported normal growth and development over more than ten years in a group of children whose parents were counseled to follow a lower fat, nutritionally adequate diet starting in infancy. To be prudent, the AAP recommends that dietary fat should not be limited before age 2. However, children should not eat high-fat foods such as whole milk, french fries, chicken nuggets, pizza, macaroni and cheese, hot dogs, fried foods, or ice cream every day.

Beverages Soft drinks such as soda (regular and diet) are highly acidic and contribute to dental caries in children by demineralizing and eroding tooth enamel. In addition, the sugar content of these beverages sustains bacterial growth, which also produces acidic by-products that demineralize teeth and cause cavities. Soda and other sweetened beverages, such as juice drinks, iced teas, and sports drinks, can contribute to excess calorie intake. They should not be given to young children and only provided in limited amounts to older children.

Choking Hazards Parents and caregivers should be warned not to feed infants foods that pose a hazard for choking or aspiration. These include nuts, popcorn, grapes, raisins, raw carrots or celery, and hot dogs.

Psychosocial and Behavioral Implications and Recommendations

Eating habits formed in the first 2 years of life are thought to persist for several years, if not for a lifetime. Therefore, healthy eating patterns should be established as early as possible. New foods may need to be introduced 5 to 10 times before a child will accept them. Children imitate the eating behaviors that they observe, so parental role-modeling exerts a strong influence on a child's development of healthy eating patterns. Children's appetites vary with their growth rate and may fluctuate from day to day. Studies have shown that when children are allowed to determine on their own how much they eat, their intake may vary considerably from meal to meal, but over a period of several days, it will in almost all cases be appropriate to their needs.

Potential Feeding Problems

Children begin expressing personal preferences at an early age and simultaneously develop mechanisms for self-control. Parents must therefore take care to strike a balance between helping guide a child's food choices to develop healthy eating habits and providing sufficient opportunities for experimentation and control. Over-controlling parental behaviors have been associated with a child's decreased ability to appropriately control his/her own caloric intake. Parents should provide children with a healthy selection of food and children should be allowed to determine how much food they need to eat. Children who consume a variety of foods over time and demonstrate appropriate growth are likely to be consuming an adequately balanced diet. Parents who worry that their child is not eating enough and allow the child to eat anything and at any time of the day simply to ensure that he or she eats something may be promoting poor eating habits.

Problems also surface when parents engage in power struggles with their children over eating issues. Two-year-old children may want to eat the same food for days at a time. Meeting the child's request may be a better response than turning mealtime into a battle. Left on their own, children eventually will tire of the same food, but if winning each mealtime struggle is in the balance, these episodes may worsen.

Confusion and rushing at mealtimes, as well as distractions such as television at mealtimes, may also disrupt the formation of appropriate eating habits. Sitting at the table and having a family meal on a regular basis is associated with significantly better psychosocial functioning in children and adolescents.

Nutrition During Adolescence

Adolescents undergo major physical and psychological changes that affect their behavior and nutritional status. Issues of autonomy and rebellion, testing and searching behaviors, and the development of formal operational thought (logical reasoning) are all normal characteristics of adolescents that must be considered when addressing their nutritional needs and behavior.

Requirements for Growth

Adolescents' energy and nutrient needs increase as they enter their pubertal growth spurt. However, the energy needs of adolescents, on a per kilogram basis, are much lower than those of infants and children. Infants double their body weight over a few months, whereas older children and adolescents may double their weight over a period of 6 to 9 years. Adolescent girls' iron requirements also increase as they begin to menstruate.

Lifestyle Issues

Adolescence marks a time of psychological, physical, and social changes that may influence eating habits. In particular, adolescents commonly have (1) a tendency to skip meals (especially breakfast and lunch); (2) sufficient money and opportunities to purchase foods (including fast foods) on their own outside the home or school environment; (3) increased consumption of "junk food" and sweetened beverages (adolescent males in particular); (4) a tendency to diet, particularly adolescent girls; (5) changes in physical activity including increased activity among adolescents participating in competitive sports or, conversely, decreased physical activity such as with non-athletic adolescents.

Some adolescents also explore restrictive dietary practices, fad diets, or vegetarianism that may put them at risk for vitamin, mineral, and trace element deficiencies. Eating disorders such as anorexia nervosa and bulimia nervosa also become a concern in adolescence. They occur across all major ethnic groups and all socio-economic levels, and teen athletes may be at higher risk of developing an eating disorder. Common features of eating disorders include dysfunctional eating habits, body image misperception, and rapid weight loss. Eating disorders are generally classified as mental health problems, therefore a team approach to treatment that includes medical management, psychological interventions, and nutritional counseling is recommended (see Chapter 4: Case 4.3).

Malnutrition in Childhood and Adolescence

For millennia, custom, ancestral teaching, seasonal availability and climate, and the luck of the hunter governed what was put on the table to nurture and sustain families, tribes, and societies. Travel, trade, agriculture industrialization, and now a global marketplace have altered the forces that govern available foods and diet. Few people still raise their own food or obtain it by hunting and gathering. People eat what is available and affordable. Choices of when, where, and how much to eat may still follow culture and custom, but they are also influenced by education, marketing, and socioeconomic status. Biological mechanisms that control eating and metabolism evolved in this historic context but now interact with a modern environment in which Western-style calorie-dense foods are widely available and intensely promoted. High-energy-density foods such as fats and sweets are generally less expensive than low-energy-density foods such as fruits and vegetables. Furthermore, the cost of foods high in fat and simple carbohydrates rises little even during economic inflation while the cost of fruits, vegetables, dairy products, meat, and fish increases substantially. Despite our relative affluence, many US children and adolescents are poorly nourished.

Undernutrition in Children

Undernutrition may be the result of a poor or sub-optimal diet; total calorie intake may be inadequate or excessive and specific nutrient intake may be inadequate or unbalanced. Adequate and appropriate nutrition during childhood and adolescence promotes normal growth and development. Furthermore, nutrition and physical activity during childhood and adolescence may influence disease risk, productivity, and quality of life during childhood and during adulthood. Inadequate calorie and nutrient intake may impair linear growth, neuro-cognitive development, and specific organ system development, and may increase mortality.

The prevalence of underweight (defined as <5th percentile for age and sex-specific norms) in US children and adolescents is below the expected rate of 5 percent. Among low-income children from birth to age 5 years, the overall prevalence of underweight decreased from 6 percent in 1995 to 4.7 percent in 2004. Although it is important to identify, evaluate, and treat underweight children, acute undernutrition is not currently considered a major public health concern. Much of the underweight and undernutrition observed in children occurs in those with medical conditions associated with altered metabolism, intestinal malabsorption, or decreased caloric intake (e.g., congenital heart disease, cystic fibrosis, inflammatory bowel disease, poorly controlled type 1 diabetes, and significant food allergy and intolerance).

Treatment of deficiencies

As part of the evaluation for a suspected nutritional deficiency, it is important to also assess the cause for the deficiency, as the therapy for the deficiency will be related to the etiology. For example, milder deficiencies related to inadequate dietary intake of a nutrient may be managed with dietary modification, or a relatively short term of therapeutic supplementation followed by long-term dietary modification. In patients with significant malabsorption due to cystic fibrosis or short bowel syndrome, long-term high dose supplementation may be necessary. Non-enteral

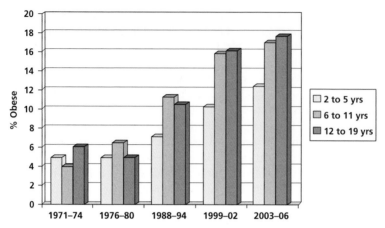

Figure 4.3 Increases in Obesity Prevalence in Children and Adolescents, 1971–2006
Source: Adapted from Ogden CL. *JAMA* 2006;295(13):1549-55. Ogden CL, Carroll MD, Flegal KM. *JAMA*. 2008;299(20):2401-2405.

avenues of delivery of the supplement may also be considered. In cases of deficiency that require active therapeutic supplementation, it is also important to judge the appropriate rate of rehabilitation. For example, xerophthalmia due to vitamin A deficiency is a medical emergency requiring immediate and aggressive vitamin A supplementation to prevent blindness. On the other hand, with significant vitamin D deficiency, overly aggressive and rapid supplementation of vitamin D without adequate calcium supplementation may precipitate severe hypocalcemia.

Overweight and Obesity in Children

Overweight and obesity affect one-third of US children and represent major threats to their current and future health. The prevalence of obesity is inversely proportional to educational attainment and income and is higher among African-Americans and Hispanics than among Caucasians in the United States as shown in Figure 4-4.

Disorders associated with obesity in youth include hypertension, cardiovascular disease, type 2 diabetes, asthma, sleep apnea, depression, and poor psycho-social

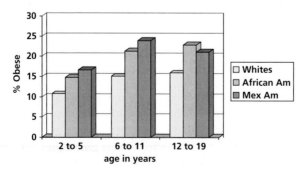

Figure 4.4 Prevalence of Obese Children and Adolescents by Race/Ethnicity
Source: Adapted from Ogden CL, Carroll MD, Flegal KM. *JAMA*. 2008;299(20):2401-2405.

adjustment. These have substantial impact on the lives of children and adolescents, on their utilization of health care services, and on their ability to attend school and engage in activities that support healthy growth and development. Children and adolescents exhibit features of the metabolic syndrome including dyslipidemia, insulin resistance, and glucose intolerance, and show evidence of endothelial dysfunction and increased carotid intima-media thickness – factors associated with an increased risk of cardiovascular disease in adulthood.

In contrast to their normal weight peers, individuals who were obese during adolescence and young adulthood have diminished academic achievement, lower household incomes, and higher rates of household poverty. In adults, obesity increases the risk of injury, illness, and absence from work. Compared to their normal weight peers, overweight children and adults utilize more health care resources and the cost of their care is greater. The costs of overweight and obesity to individuals, to families, and to society at large are staggering and are predicted to increase over the coming decades. Obesity appears to be both a cause and a consequence of increasing social inequalities in the United States.

Genetics and Environment

Considerable attention has been given to the complex interplay of genetic and environmental factors contributing to the contemporary surge in obesity prevalence. The "thrifty gene hypothesis" postulates a survival advantage for individuals able to store energy efficiently during times of plenty and utilize it during times of scarcity. Exposed to an environment with abundant food, these individuals would continue to store excess calories as fat and to become obese. Based upon this theory, racial and ethnic groups newly introduced into environments where food is abundant after generations of living in areas of food scarcity would be particularly susceptible to the development of obesity. Pima Indians of the Southwestern United States and immigrants from Mexico to the United States – groups with high frequencies of obesity and insulin resistance – provide supporting evidence for this hypothesis.

Conversely, in regions such as Western Europe, where food has been relatively abundant for generations, selective pressures may have favored individuals who remained relatively lean (i.e., do not efficiently store calories as fat) over those who developed obesity, insulin resistance, and cardiovascular disease. This would potentially contribute to the observed racial/ethnic disparities in obesity prevalence. Nevertheless, even individuals without a "thrifty metabolism" need only have an energy imbalance of 100 kcal per day to gain 10 pounds in one year. (One 20 ounce can of sugar sweetened soft drink contains approximately 200 calories and briskly walking or jogging one mile consumes approximately 100 calories.) Indeed, as eating habits have changed and high caloric density foods have become more available, obesity rates in Western Europe have also increased.

Epigenetic modifications of the genome have been postulated as a mechanism whereby the metabolic environment may affect or alter gene expression. This could potentially occur *in utero* or during postnatal life. Although the molecular mechanism is not clear, the intrauterine environment affects the risk of obesity, insulin resistance, and cardiovascular disease. Children born to mothers who were obese prior to and during pregnancy or those who had hyperglycemia, glucose intolerance, or diabetes during pregnancy are at increased risk of obesity, insulin resistance, and cardiovascular disease, as are low birth weight infants, whether they were born prematurely or were small for gestational age.

Time spent engaged in physical activity or exercise and time spent in sedentary pursuits affect energy expenditure. Children and adolescents should have no more than two hours of screen time daily (e.g. watching television or playing computer games) and should engage in at least 60 minutes of moderate to vigorous physical activity daily and half of that activity should occur during the school day. Many children with chronic illness are also at increased risk of obesity. This may be attributed, at least in part, to real or imagined limitations in their ability to pursue an active lifestyle.

Low-family income and food insecurity or insufficiency are associated with under nutrition in some children and with increased prevalence of overweight and obesity in others. Obtaining foods needed to support adequate and appropriate calorie and nutrient intake may be difficult for families with limited income. In order to prevent hunger, these families may choose foods that provide the highest energy content at the lowest cost. Thus they would select calorie dense foods, high in fat and sugar, over more costly nutrient rich foods such as fruits, vegetables, and low-fat dairy products. These food choices may predispose children and adolescents to develop overweight and obesity and could put them at risk of having inadequate intake of essential nutrients including iron, calcium, and vitamin D. Furthermore, child poverty and food insecurity during childhood can foster later eating patterns that predispose to the development of childhood overweight and obesity and to maintenance of obesity during adulthood. Family income and socioeconomic status – both past and current – may affect dietary habits and preferences. Therefore, information regarding food insecurity, food insufficiency, and hunger should be part of the medical and diet history as they may influence therapeutic and social service interventions directed toward preventing or ameliorating nutritional deficiencies, underweight, and overweight or obesity.

Childhood Nutritional Factors in Preventing Adult Cardiovascular Disease

The association between elevated cholesterol levels and heart disease has been well documented in adults. Several studies suggest that adult atherosclerosis has its roots in childhood, and link early atherosclerosis and vascular dysfunction in children with childhood dyslipidemia. Furthermore, lifestyle factors, such as diet and physical activity, have been linked to lipoprotein levels and other CVD risk factors in children and adults. This is especially important to consider given the association between obesity and dyslipidemia (including increased triglycerides and decreased HDL-cholesterol). The rapidly rising prevalence of childhood obesity accounts at least in part for the increasing prevalence of lipid abnormalities in children.

The original recommendations relating to hypercholesterolemia in children and adolescents were released by the National Cholesterol Education Panel (NCEP) in

1992, and later endorsed and updated by the American Academy of Pediatrics and the American Heart Association over the last several years.

Vascular Disease and Dysfunction in Children and Adolescents

The atherosclerotic process has been noted to begin in childhood and adolescence. The earliest atherosclerotic lesion is the fatty streak, a collection of lipid-laden macrophages in the intima of an artery. Autopsy studies of children and young adults from the Bogalusa Heart Study who died of various causes, principally trauma, have shown a correlation between pre-morbid cholesterol levels and early atherosclerotic changes, and the prevalence of changes was positively associated with age, blood pressure, and BMI. Other studies have demonstrated an association between atherosclerotic disease and other factors, such as age, smoking, BMI, and elevated blood pressure, and the extent of vascular lesions rises exponentially with an increasing number of risk factors in young adults. Studies of young American men killed during the Korean and Vietnam wars found evidence of even more significant vascular disease in some cases. In one survey, almost half of the men (mean age 22 years) had some degree of coronary atherosclerosis and 5 percent had severe coronary artery disease.

Imaging and functional studies have also identified the onset of vascular disease and dysfunction in childhood. Carotid intima-media thickness, assessed by ultrasound as a surrogate marker for atherosclerosis, has been observed to be increased in adolescents and young adults with hypercholesterolemia, and in those with a positive family history of premature heart disease. Arterial stiffness and distensibility, also assessed by ultrasound, are associated with familial and non-familial hypercholesterolemia, elevated blood pressure, decreased cardiovascular fitness, and obesity.

Dietary and Lifestyle Recommendations for Hypercholesterolemia

In addition to the focus on children at risk, a healthy lifestyle and diet are recommended for all children as part of population-based prevention. Though a low fat diet is not recommended for children less two years of age, a healthy well balanced diet is appropriate at all ages. The recommended diet would include at least 20 percent and no more than 30 percent of calories from fat, less than 10 percent of calories as saturated fat, and less than 300 mg cholesterol per day. This Therapeutic Lifestyle Changes (TLC) diet is recommended as initial therapy for children with hypercholesterolemia over the age of 2 years as well as for the population-based prevention. Children under the age of two require a higher fat diet to maintain normal growth and central nervous system development. Greater dietary modification is recommended for children with hypercholesterolemia whose LDL-C remains greater than 130 mg/dL after an adequate period of compliance with the TLC diet (see Chapter 6: Cardiovascular Disease). Drug therapy can be considered for severely elevated LDL-C levels (LDL-C >190 mg/dL or >160 mg/dL with other CVD risk factors) after dietary intervention in children 10 years or older.

Though the initial NCEP dietary recommendations did not focus on caloric intake, given the rising prevalence of obesity, and the interaction between obesity and lipid levels, these dietary recommendations for the general population and for hypercholesterolemic children have evolved to aim for caloric intake that maintains or achieves a healthy weight as a priority. Consistent with this, dietary intervention must be viewed as one component of a comprehensive program to reduce cardiovascular disease risk. Exercise, blood pressure, sedentary/physical activities, smoking (active and passive), relative weight and excessive weight gain, and risk factors for the development of diabetes are all factors that should be assessed in the general population and especially in children and adolescents with hyperlipidemia.

For children and adolescents with mixed dyslipidemia, dietary management should focus on limiting the intake of simple carbohydrates, and a special focus on weight management, in addition to the TLC diet.

Overweight and Obesity
Prevention and Management Issues

Health care professionals should play an integral role in the prevention and treatment of obesity. Given the limited success in treating obesity, efforts to prevent excessive weight gain in children and adolescents should be a priority. As part of normal clinical care, relative weight and BMI, growth patterns and blood pressure should be monitored and results communicated regularly to parents. Primary care providers should assess the child's overall lifestyle and give parents information regarding these factors. Such assessments should be undertaken for all children, but especially those who are overweight or obese, or who are gaining excess weight, and for those at risk for excessive weight gain (e.g., children of obese parents).

Parents should be instructed that they have the responsibility to serve as role models, authority figures, and as behavior modification agents for their children. Difficulties arise if parents do not perceive the poor lifestyle issues as problematic, or are unwilling to make changes to alter family practices and behaviors. In such settings, the primary care provider should help parents to understand and accept the importance of the issue, and then work to find acceptable steps to address the issue. Motivational interviewing – a process in which assessment and intervention are interwoven, and information gained from the interview allows for collaborative assessment of priorities and the setting of goals – has been recommended for use in primary care settings to address weight and lifestyle management.

The healthy lifestyle recommendations in Table 4-7 can also form the initial outline for an obesity intervention. As noted above, providers can interact with the family using a motivational interviewing paradigm to identify the issues of importance. For many children and families, adopting a stepwise approach to identify targeted behaviors and to advance the degree of change and the number of behaviors over time is useful. As appropriate, a more structured program, which

Table 4-7 Healthy Lifestyle Recommendations to Maintain or Achieve Healthy Weight

- Limit consumption of sugar-sweetened and fruit juice beverages to 0–1 serving (6 ounces)/day
- Adequate consumption of fruits and vegetables, generally ≥5 servings/day (see USDA guidelines- www.mypyramid.gov)
- Limit TV and other screen time to <2 hours/day (none before 2 years of age)
- Greater than 1 hour/day physical activity
- Incorporate physical activity (e.g., walking, bike riding) into normal routine
- Remove TVs and other screens from child's primary sleeping area
- Eat a healthy breakfast daily
- Limit eating out at restaurants
- Encourage family meals together at the table
- Involve the whole family in lifestyle changes
- Provide age-appropriate portion sizes
- Avoid the imposition of overly restrictive control on eating

Source: Andrew Tershakovec, MD. Merck. Used with permission.

includes such things as keeping a log or a diary of dietary intake and of physical and sedentary activities, can be considered. With guidance from a dietitian, a formal eating plan can also be considered. Contracting with parents and children for goal setting and achievement may be useful. Such a structured program requires frequent follow-up. Counseling to aid parents with parenting skills and motivation, and in cases of significant family conflict or dysfunction, may be helpful or necessary. When the resources are available, group meetings, separately for children and families, have been shown to be effective. Experience suggests that the degree of weight loss is proportional to the amount of contact between the provider/program and the child and his family. Structured weight management programs commonly start with interactions every 1 to 2 weeks, and over time extend the time interval between meetings.

Such intensive intervention efforts may be beyond the resources of a primary healthcare provider, and thus require appropriate referral. Also, environmental change and support for lifestyle intervention should include the school and community to recruit multiple aspects of the child and family's environment. Though this is a long-term effort, primary care providers can advocate for adequate physical education and recess, appropriate nutritional guidelines for meals and vending machines in schools, access to safe parks and recreation facilities, and sources of affordable, healthy food choices in the community as part of an overall obesity prevention and treatment program. However, the primary care provider should still implement and support intervention and preventive efforts as much as is possible within the office setting as part of a comprehensive intervention and prevention effort. At a minimum, assessment and education related to relative weight and growth patterns and overall lifestyle should be completed.

There is limited experience with very-low-calorie weight loss diets in children and adolescents. Such restrictive diets should be undertaken only with appropriate supervision and guidance, be maintained over a limited time, and be employed only in patients with severe degrees of obesity associated with concurrent morbidity. Though weight loss can generally be induced with such a dietary program, experience suggests most people regain much of the lost weight after transitioning off the very-low-calorie diet. Therefore, a coordinated program to manage this transition and to maintain the new weight must be considered.

Medications
Sibutramine, a serotonin reuptake inhibitor, is approved in the United States for use in adolescents 16 years or older. Orlistat, an enteric lipase inhibitor, is approved for those 12 and older. The limited experience with adolescents suggests these medications can be used relatively safely, but the effects on weight gain (in growing adolescents) or weight loss have been modest. If medications are utilized, this should be as part of a comprehensive weight management and lifestyle/behavior modification program.

Bariatric Surgery
Bariatric surgery, including gastric bypass or gastric banding, is being utilized with increasing frequency in adults, and is generally associated with significant weight loss and improvements in obesity related co-morbidities. However, the surgery itself and the longer term post-operative period are associated with a moderate rate of complications and adverse events. The experience with children and adolescents is relatively limited. Bariatric surgery should be considered only in cases of severe obesity, or in the presence of significant obesity related co-morbidities, after an adequate trial of aggressive non-surgical weight loss. Surgery should generally be considered only for older adolescents who are physically mature, and can better understand the lifelong implications of the surgical intervention. Just as adults who undergo bariatric surgery require medical and psychosocial support prior to and following the intervention, adolescents undergoing bariatric surgery should receive long-term specialized follow-up to prevent nutritional deficiencies and to minimize other post-surgical morbidity. (See Chapter 1, Case 1.2.)

Conclusion
In conclusion, nutrition during childhood and adolescence has both immediate and long-term effects on growth, development, health, and quality of life. Therefore all young patients should have a careful and comprehensive evaluation of physical growth, nutrient intake, and energy balance. Physical examination and selected laboratory tests may be needed to identify specific nutrient deficiencies, biochemical abnormalities, or modifiable risk factors for disease (e.g. dyslipidemia, iron-deficiency anemia, vitamin D deficiency) that could be managed with nutritional counseling and dietary modification. Health-care providers must identify nutritional inadequacies and counsel parents and children regarding appropriate food intake and levels of physical activity to support optimal growth and development and to prevent disease and disability.

Case 1 **Overweight Child with Insulin Resistance**

Andrew M. Tershakovec[1], Lisa Hark[2], and Elizabeth B. Rappaport[2]

[1] Merck Research Laboratories, North Wales, PA
[2] Jefferson Medical College, Philadelphia, PA

OBJECTIVES

- Take an appropriate dietary and medical history including family history of overweight or obesity, and social history regarding physical activity, sedentary activity, and other lifestyle issues.

- Perform an appropriate physical examination for an overweight or obese child or adolescent; and evaluate the patient for other signs and symptoms of chronic diseases associated with obesity (e.g. hypertension, insulin resistance, dyslipidemia, sleep apnea, orthopedic problems, etc.).

- Identify factors responsible for increasing weight in order to recommend suitable dietary or lifestyle changes.

- Recognize the importance of the patient and patient's family involvement in making changes; and the social, emotional, and psychological factors that may support the development of obesity and may influence the response to intervention.

TR is an 11-year-old boy who comes to see his physician for a health maintenance visit. His parents note that he has gained a lot of weight since last year, but feel that he "does not eat that much" and is an active boy. They are at a loss to explain his weight gain.

Past Medical History

TR was a full-term infant (birth weight 3950 g). His mother notes he has always had a good appetite, and grew rapidly as a young child (she says he is "big boned"). In kindergarten, he was a head taller than most of the other children. TR's mother notes his weight gain had been relatively stable until he reached the age of 7, when his rate of weight gain increased steadily over the next 4 years.

TR had recurrent ear infections, and was a loud snorer as a toddler. A tonsillectomy and adenoidectomy (T&A) was performed when TR was 2 years old. TR was diagnosed with asthma at the age of 9. He currently uses an Albuterol inhaler and inhaled steroids as needed for preventive care. He has never been admitted to the

---

Medical Nutrition and Disease: A Case-Based Approach, 4th edition. Edited by Lisa Hark.
© 2009 Wiley-Blackwell Publishing, ISBN: 978-1-4051-8615-5.

hospital for an asthma attack, but his mother says she does not want him running too much as he easily gets short of breath.

Family History

TR's family history is positive for type 2 diabetes, obesity, and heart disease. His mother had gestational diabetes during her pregnancy with TR. She is 35 years old and has a BMI of 35 kg/m^2 (obesity class II) and was recently told she has an elevated blood glucose level indicative of pre-diabetes. His father (age 36) has a BMI of 28 kg/m^2 (overweight). His maternal grandmother (age 65) is obese (BMI 32 kg/m^2) and has hypertension and type 2 diabetes; his maternal grandfather (age 67) had a myocardial infarction (MI) at age 53.

Social/Development/Puberty

TR's development is described as normal. He walked at age 15 months, was toilet trained at 2 $^1/_2$ years. He is described as an average student, who keeps mostly to himself. He admits that the kids at school have been teasing him about his weight for several years and call him "tubby." He has few friends and spends most of his free time alone. TR denies smoking, alcohol, drugs, or sexual activity.

Social History

TR's mother works from 9:00 am to 5:00 pm daily in food service. TR's father works the night shift in maintenance at a local refinery (10:00 pm to 6:00 am). TR goes to his grandmother's house directly after school. He is an only child.

Diet/Physical Activity History

TR's parents state that he "does not eat that much." When asked what he eats during the day (24-hour recall), the parents reveal that he enjoys eating breakfast with his father when he arrives home at 7:00 am (usually scrambled eggs, toast and juice), a sandwich for lunch at school (peanut butter and jelly with 2 cookies, juice or chocolate milk), and a healthy dinner (baked chicken, potatoes, green beans, and milk), which they all eat together when mom arrives home from work. TR's parents state that he is active with soccer (goalie position) and baseball during the year. TR is described as a restless sleeper. He reports feeling tired during the day and his parents report he frequently falls asleep while watching TV.

Review of Systems

Skin: No history of rashes
Neurologic: No headaches, tremors, seizures.
Endocrine: No polyphagia, polydipsia, or polyuria
Pulmonary: Snoring remitted after the tonsils and adenoids removed, but has recurred over the last few months.
Joints: No swelling; complains that his legs hurt if has to walk for a long distance.

Physical Examination
Vital Signs
Temperature: 99°F (37°C)
Heart rate: 95 BPM
Respiratory rate: 26 BPM
Blood pressure: 135/85 mm Hg (>99th percentile for age, sex, and height)
Current weight: 82 kg (180 lb) (>95th percentile for age)
Current height: 162 cm (63.8 inches) (>95th percentile for age)
BMI: 30.9 kg/m² (>95th percentile for age)
Weight history:
8 *y/o*: 40 kg (>95th percentile for age)
9 *y/o*: 55 kg (>95th percentile for age)
10 *y/o*: 70 kg (>95th percentile for age)

Exam:
General: Overweight boy in no acute distress, no hirsutism, no edema, no Cushingoid features
HEENT: Wrinkled, hypertrophied skin with increased pigmentation at base of neck, non-palpable thyroid
Eyes: EOMI, PERRL, normal disc margins
Abdomen: BS (+), soft, no masses or organomegaly palpable, liver span by percussion 8 cm, stretch marks noted
Cardiac: Regular rate and rhythm, S1, S2, no murmurs
Chest: Clear
Genitalia: Tanner I boy, phallus largely obscured by fat pad, testes normal
Neurologic: Alert, strength 5/5, DTR +2 upper and lower extremities, normal tone
Orthopedic: Wide-based gait without a limp, mild bowing of lower aspect of legs bilaterally, full range of motion in hips.

Laboratory Data

Patient's Fasting Values	Normal Values
Glucose: 87 mg/dL	70–99 mg/dL
Insulin: 28 μU/mL	<20 μU/mL
HbA1C: 4.3%	<3-6%
Total Cholesterol: 212 mg/dL	desirable <200 mg/dL
Triglycerides: 145 mEq/L	desirable <120 mg/dL
LDL-C: 105 mg/dL	desirable <130 mg/dL
HDL-C: 38 mg/dL	desirable ≥40 mg/dL
ALT: 37 U/L	10-30 U/L
AST: 55 U/L	10-30 U/L
TSH: 2.3 μU/L	0.5-5.0 μU/L

Case Questions
Part 1: Diagnosis

1. Describe methods that can be used to assess TR's weight.
2. Describe the risk factors and health consequences associated with being an overweight child or adolescent.
3. What additional information should be asked regarding TR's increasing weight over the past 4 years?
4. Prior to recommending treatment, how can TR and his family's readiness to change be assessed and how should this treatment process be explained?
5. What are the appropriate medical nutrition therapy and physical activity recommendations for TR and his family?
6. What type of behavior modification techniques can be used to help TR and his family implement these dietary and lifestyle suggestions?

Answers to Questions: Case 1
Part 1: Diagnosis

1. Describe methods that can be used to assess TR's weight.
In the current CDC growth charts, which include BMI growth curves for children and adolescents, overweight is defined as a BMI between the 85th and 95th percentile, and obesity is defined as BMI greater than the 95th percentile. However, BMI is only a screening tool and the patient's degree of overweight can be confirmed on physical examination. Such screening is necessary to identify those who require intervention. The goal of intervention may be weight loss, or weight stabilization depending on the specific circumstances. Decreasing the rate of weight gain while a child is growing will help decrease ultimate gain in relative weight. TR's BMI of 31.2 kg/m^2 puts him at the 97th percentile for BMI for his age and sex. This places him in the obese category (see Table 4-1).

It is apparent from his weight history that TR was always a large child, but began to gain weight rapidly over the last few years. It is common that overweight pre-pubertal children are taller than their normal weight counterparts. These overweight children tend to enter puberty earlier, have their growth spurt earlier, and then attain a normal adult height.

2. Describe the risk factors and health consequences associated with being an overweight child or adolescent.
Overweight children and adolescents are at risk for similar health problems as adults who are overweight or obese, including type 2 diabetes, hypertension, dyslipidemia, sleep apnea, asthma, gall bladder disease, orthopedic problems, and non-alcoholic fatty liver disease. TR was diagnosed with asthma at age 9. It is not known if the asthma limits his activity and thus contributes to his weight gain, or if the asthma itself somehow contributes to the development of obesity. TR's dyspnea on exertion may be due to asthma or to his poor cardiovascular fitness. If TR's asthma

is not well controlled, this should be addressed. Similarly, some assessment of TR's cardiovascular fitness should be completed. If he is found to have limited exercise capacity an appropriate program for his fitness level should be recommended with the goal that he may eventually be able to participate in normal physical activity without restriction.

Sleep Apnea Upon further questioning about his sleep patterns, TR and his parents indicate that he is a restless sleeper, has daytime sleepiness, and snores loudly. These symptoms may be consistent with sleep apnea. TR should be referred to a pulmonary specialist for further evaluation and possibly a formal sleep study.

Diabetes Recently, there has been a dramatic increase in the prevalence of type 2 diabetes in children and adolescents, especially in African-American and Hispanic populations. This may be explained, in part, by the parallel increase in the prevalence of overweight among children and teenagers. A positive family history of type 2 diabetes is associated with an increased risk of insulin resistance (insulin resistance is thought to be part of the etiology of type 2 diabetes). TR's grandmother has diabetes already, and the mother's history of gestational diabetes and current elevated glucose level suggest she has insulin resistance and is at risk of developing type 2 diabetes. The increased skin pigmentation that TR demonstrates could be acanthosis nigricans, which is associated with insulin resistance. Thus a fasting serum glucose, insulin, and hemoglobin A1c were obtained. The normal glucose (87 mg/dL) and hemoglobin A1c (4.3 percent), with an elevated insulin level (28 mIU/mL), is consistent with insulin resistance. Since TR is obese, has a strong family history of type 2 diabetes and cardiovascular disease, and has acanthosis nigricans and prehypertension, he meets the criteria for screening for diabetes. His fasting glucose is in the normal range. However, in the evolution of type 2 diabetes, post-prandial glucose increases earlier than fasting glucose. Therefore, some experts recommend determining plasma glucose two hours after a standard glucose load or 2 hours after a meal.

Heart Disease/Hypertension Due to the fact that TR has multiple risk factors for adult cardiovascular disease (family history of heart disease, obesity, elevated blood pressure), a fasting lipid panel was ordered. These results, when compared to the age appropriate percentiles, indicate that TR has elevated triglyceride levels, and a reduced HDL-C level. Hypertriglyceridemia and low HDL-C are the most common lipid abnormalities associated with insulin resistance. TR's blood pressure is in the range for prehypertension (>120/80) and should be re-checked in 6 months.

Non-alcoholic fatty liver disease Overweight children may present with increased liver enzymes [alanine amino transferase (ALT) and aspartate amino transferase (AST)], which may be indicative of hepatic fatty infiltration. Abnormal liver function tests have been described in 6 to 10 percent of obese adolescents. This condition, know as non-alcoholic fatty liver disease (NAFLD), has been described to progress to cirrhosis and liver failure in adults and in children. Obesity-associated

NAFLD is commonly associated with insulin resistance. Other than weight loss, there is currently no accepted therapy for NAFLD.

3. What additional information should be asked regarding TR's increasing weight over the past 4 years?

TR's 24-hour recall looks "healthy" upon first glance. Although TR's parents feel he is "not a big eater" it is important to probe for excess calories, such as sodas and juices, as well as high-fat foods. Dietary information provided for obese individuals tends to be grossly under-reported. Studies suggest that obese adolescents under-report their caloric intake by as much as 40 to 60 percent, and that obese individuals under-report to a greater degree than non-obese individuals.

Further questioning reveals TR eats breakfast with his father at 7:00 a.m. and then again with his mother at 8:00 a.m. (bowl of Cocoa Puffs cereal with whole milk and a 16 ounce (480 mL) glass of orange juice). He eats his lunch from home, but also has access to the soda machine, where he buys a 20 ounce (600 mL) bottle of soda everyday with lunch. After school he spends most days with his grandmother, who serves him a hamburger, fries, and a 16 ounce soda or another sandwich with chocolate milk at 3:30 p.m. for a snack. He eats dinner at 6:00 p.m. when he arrives home. TR also enjoys either ice cream and a few chocolate chip cookies or an 8 ounce (240 mL) glass of whole milk with peanut butter crackers before bed.

TR's parents stated that he is active with soccer in the fall and baseball in the spring. He usually has one game each week and plays goalie or a defensive position where there is very little running involved. As both teams have many players, TR never plays more than half a game or about 25 minutes. Following the game TR's family often go to a fast food restaurant to celebrate. TR is sedentary during the winter months.

Further questioning about TR's television, video, and computer game usage reveals that on weekdays, on average, he watches three hours of television per day. On weekends TR watches television, plays video or computer games, or "surfs the web" for up to 6 hours per day.

4. Prior to recommending treatment, how can TR and his family's readiness to change be assessed and how should this treatment process be explained?

Prior to recommending any dietary or lifestyle suggestions, it is very important to assess both TR's and his family's interest in making changes. It is best to directly address the motivation and willingness to change with TR and his parents. Some families may express significant interest in changing, yet will be unable to identify concrete changes they are willing to undertake. It is also important to assess other potential environmental obstacles (e.g. uncooperative family members like TR's grandmother).

TR's parents stated in the initial work-up that he has gained a lot of weight since last year; they seem to realize that there may be a problem with his weight. However, the fact that they do not recognize his sedentary lifestyle and increased caloric intake as a problem suggests some denial, or lack of willingness to change. Because TR says he dislikes the teasing, he may have some interest in changing. However, the fact that TR is becoming more and more withdrawn may suggest depression or other psychosocial issues that may be necessary to address before weight management interventions can be successful.

When explaining the process of weight management and the implications of excessive weight gain, it is useful to show the family the child's growth curve. The specific medical issues affecting the child should also be discussed. In TR's case, his asthma, insulin resistance, acanthosis nigricans, restless sleep and snoring, prehypertension, and dyslipidemia are likely related to his obesity. The family history of insulin resistance, diabetes, and premature heart disease should also be noted as additional reasons for increased vigilance. Explaining to parents and other family members that improved diet and activity patterns with weight stabilization or weight loss can decrease TR's risk of developing diabetes and cardiovascular disease may motivate them to support him and potentially to join him in these changes.

In general, the initial goals of a pediatric weight management program are to decrease the rate of weight gain. Keeping weight stable while a child grows decreases relative weight. With significant obesity, as in this case, weight loss may be appropriate.

5. What are the appropriate medical nutrition therapy and physical activity recommendations for TR and his family?

The most important dietary change that should be recommended for TR is to establish a regular eating pattern. Most days, TR is eating two breakfasts, lunch, two dinners, and an evening snack. The first step would be to eliminate one of his breakfast meals and to reduce the amount of juice he is drinking to about 6 ounces (180 mL) per day. He could also try a low-sugar cereal with at least 3 grams of fiber, such as Multigrain Cheerios and change to two percent reduced fat milk to be later changed to one percent low-fat or fat-free milk, all of which will considerably reduce his carbohydrate, saturated fat, and caloric intake. He may also enjoy a slice of low calorie whole wheat toast with peanut butter. Lunch could remain the same, with the substitution of fresh fruit and carrot sticks as a dessert. Purchasing soda with lunch should be discouraged and eliminating all soda and sugar containing drinks should be considered. Maybe he could bring a bottle of water or purchase one from the vending machines, now available in most schools.

TR's grandmother should be included in any discussions since she is his after-school caregiver. Because she has type 2 diabetes, she may be receptive to the idea of prevention in her grandson. Healthy after-school snack suggestions for TR include fruit, low-fat yogurt, low-fat granola bar, bowl of cereal with low fat milk, microwave "lite" popcorn, or a frozen fruit bar. Snacks are a normal and important part of a child's diet; however, choices should not be high in calories. Given that TR was eating a full meal as an afternoon snack, providing guidance regarding an appropriate serving size for a snack would be important.

Beverage choices are another common problem with overweight children. Efforts should be made to limit the intake of all sugar containing beverages including juices. Many families feel that since juices are "natural," their intake should not be limited.

It is not unusual to see a child ingest 500 to 1000 calories a day in juice, soda, and other sugar-sweetened beverages. Eliminating or significantly limiting juice, soda, and sports drinks, and switching to low-fat milk will likely reduce weight gain. Dinner meals seem to be the healthiest and could remain the same, except for the whole milk. In addition to healthy food choices and meals, children and families should be instructed on proper serving sizes for children for meals and snacks.

TR's family should provide ample opportunities for him to eat fruits and vegetables and low-fat dairy products. They should limit availability of salty snacks and prepared foods as these are sources of excess sodium intake, which has been linked to blood-pressure elevation and to increased consumption of sugar-sweetened beverages.

Parents and families should assess and plan opportunities for increased physical activity. Find activities that the child enjoys (i.e., do not expect a child to regularly use a treadmill). Parents need to provide an environment where being active several times a week is normal and expected. Parents should be role models and participate in activities with their children. They should not assume children are active during school recess as physical education has been consistently decreased and often eliminated from school curriculum. Parents should also monitor and set daily limits for sedentary activities, such as watching TV and playing computer and video games, as less than 2 hours per day is suggested by the American Academy of Pediatrics. According to the Centers for Disease Control and Prevention (CDC), children and adolescents should engage in at least one hour of physical activity every day.

6. What type of behavior modification techniques can be used to help TR and his family implement these dietary and lifestyle suggestion?

It is important to assess the child and family's psychosocial well-being before initiating a behavior modification program. For example, if the child is depressed, the depression will probably make weight management more difficult. In some cases, it may be best to defer the weight management program until the psychological or psychiatric issues are directly addressed. Similarly, significant family difficulties, such as a family member with anorexia or a substance abuse problem, should be identified and addressed.

The issues surrounding eating and weight are complex and frequently emotionally charged. As few families will have the insight to address these issues as part of a "self-help" program without outside assistance, it is important to institute a behavior modification program with the guidance of a behavior specialist. Little research has directly assessed the efficacy of different behavioral components of a weight management program. However, there are several factors that are commonly included in most weight management programs. These include the following:

Motivation It is important to assess the child's and family's motivation to participate in the weight management program. Experience suggests that in addition to an interested and motivated participant, children do better in the program when a parent is also an active and supportive participant in the program. Using the theoretical concept of the transtheoretical model and the stages of change to assess a family's potential to change and to plan an appropriate intervention program can be considered.

Stepwise approach Even motivated children and families should not be overwhelmed with too much change at once. Initial goals should be chosen as ones that can be achieved relatively easily to allow the child and family to experience early success and build self-esteem. Additional and more challenging goals should then be added over time.

Stimulus control and environmental modification Provide an environment that includes only healthy choices. Trying to restrict a child from eating certain foods in the home (e.g. chips, soda) while these foods are still in the house may be counterproductive.

Role modeling It is important to have as many people as possible, and hopefully the whole family, act as role models in all aspects of the behavior modification program. Though all family members may not have a weight problem, the environmental and lifestyle changes recommended for the targeted child are part of an overall healthy lifestyle appropriate for all family members.

Positive reinforcement and parenting skills Parents should be instructed in appropriate parenting skills, including methods of positive reinforcement and appropriate limit setting.

Self-monitoring Parents and children should be instructed in methods of self monitoring (keeping a diet diary, keeping an activity log), generally focusing on dietary intake and physical activity. Experience suggests that persons who self monitor significantly decrease caloric intake and generally do much better in weight management programs.

Case 2 **Malnutrition and Refeeding Syndrome in Children**

John A. Kerner[1] and Jo Ann T. Hattner[2]

[1] Lucile Packard Children's Hospital/Stanford University, Palo Alto, CA
[2] Stanford University School of Medicine, Palo Alto, CA

OBJECTIVES

- Describe the physiologic and metabolic adaptations that occur during starvation.
- Describe the physiologic processes that occur when refeeding an undernourished patient.
- Identify potential clinical manifestations of the refeeding syndrome and explain the most common laboratory abnormalities that may occur during refeeding.
- Summarize the clinical recommendations for minimizing or avoiding the complications associated with refeeding.

RD is an 8-year-old boy of Liberian descent who lives in the United States with his parents. In October, RD and his family flew to Liberia to spend a few months with their extended family. Several weeks after his arrival, political unrest erupted. RD and his family were forced from their homes at gunpoint, taken to a university, and held against their will in overcrowded, unsanitary conditions. Medical and food supplies were scarce. Food was provided by soldiers outside the camp who lowered buckets of rice and occasionally fish over the barbed-wire fences. Daily tea was also provided. Many of the hostages died from starvation. RD and his family escaped after 3 months of captivity and sought refuge in the American Embassy. From there, they were airlifted to a neighboring country. Shortly thereafter, RD returned to the United States.

Vital Signs (US Embassy)

Temperature: 97 °F (36 °C)
Heart rate: 45 BPM
Respiratory rate: 18 BPM
Blood pressure: 100/80 mm Hg

After 3 months of virtual starvation, the family reported that RD ate "everything he could get his hands on." Upon follow-up with his local physician in the United States, RD was immediately referred to the local emergency room for evaluation of undernutrition.

Medical Nutrition and Disease: A Case-Based Approach, 4th edition. Edited by Lisa Hark.
© 2009 Wiley-Blackwell Publishing, ISBN: 978-1-4051-8615-5.

Anthropometric Data

Date	Height			Weight			BMI	
	(cm) (in)	Percentile		(kg)(lb)	Percentile		kg/m²	Percentile
1/7*	127 (50″)	50th		19 (42)	<5		11.8	<5th
1/10	127 (50″)	50th		22 (48)	10-25		13.6	<5th

*At initial presentation to the emergency room.

Past Medical History

RD tested positive for malaria in the past; no other problems were noted. On admission, he was not taking any medications or vitamins. RD has no known food allergies. He was having 4 to 5 loose stools per day.

Social/Diet History

By report, prior to his imprisonment in the refugee camp, RD's food supply met 100 percent of his needs. While in the refugee camp, his estimated intake amounted to only 250 to 300 kcal/day, with 30 grams of protein per week. Four days after he escaped, his intake rose to an estimated 2500 to 3000 kcal/day, with 80 to 90 grams of protein per day.

Further evaluation in the hospital produced the following clinical picture.

Physical Examination
Vital Signs
Temperature: 101.8°F (38°C)
Heart rate: 120 BPM
Respiratory rate: 30 BPM
Blood pressure: 80/50 mm Hg

Exam
General: Eight-year-old boy who appears apathetic and emaciated
Skin: Dry, scaly dermatitis
Head: Alopecia, thinning hair lacking in luster
Abdomen: Mildly distended
Extremities: Bipedal edema; and muscle wasting

Laboratory Data

Date	Ca (mg/dL)	PO4 (mg/dL)	Mg (mg/dL)	K (mEq/L)	Albumin (g/dL)
1/7*	8.0	3.0	1.8	3.6	2.7
1/10	6.3	1.0	0.9	2.0	2.4
Normal	(9–11)	(2.5–4.6)	(1.8–2.9)	(3.5–5.3)	(3.5–5.8)

*At initial presentation to the emergency room.

Case Questions

1. What nutrition-related changes in body function probably occurred during the past 3-month period of starvation?
2. Based on the physical examination and laboratory data, what clinical and biochemical manifestations of undernutrition does RD exhibit?
3. What metabolic and physiologic changes occur as RD begins to eat again? Why are his electrolyte abnormalities of primary concern?
4. Based on RD's physical examination and laboratory data, what complications of refeeding does he exhibit?
5. How could the complications of refeeding that RD experienced have been minimized or avoided?

Answers to Questions: Case 2
Part 1: Physiology

1. What nutrition-related changes in body function probably occurred during the past 3-month period of starvation?

The body's systems adapt to calorie and protein deficits in a complex manner. Chronic nutritional deprivation results in a mildly catabolic state. The body's compensatory mechanisms involve changes in energy metabolism and hormone regulation. Fat from adipose tissue and protein from muscle mass are mobilized and converted to energy via glucose and ketones. The brain increases its use of free fatty acids replacing glucose as an energy source. The catabolism of fat and protein result in a loss of lean body mass, electrolytes, and water. The basal metabolic rate (BMR) decreases to conserve energy; the body becomes hypothermic, hypotensive, and bradycardic; and physical activity decreases. Growth hormone and thyroid hormone regulation decrease or stop growth, which helps to lower the BMR. Production of insulin, which promotes anabolism of catecholamines, cortisol, and glucagon, also decreases. The net effect facilitates survival by decreasing the BMR and promoting conservation of protein and organ function.

Overall decreases in cellular mass may eventually result in functional loss of vital organs. Respiratory muscle loss may lessen respiratory efficiency. Myocardial atrophy may reduce cardiac output. Decreased intravascular fluid volume results in decreased cardiac output.

Gastrointestinal (GI) atrophy slows motility and gastric acid secretion and causes thinning of the mucosa, villous atrophy, and decreased production of digestive enzymes. These effects reduce GI function and can result in malabsorption and diarrhea, further exacerbating the malnutrition and increasing susceptibility to infection. Liver wasting causes altered metabolism and decreased protein synthesis. The kidney's ability to concentrate urine decreases, causing diuresis.

2. Based on the physical examination and laboratory data, what clinical and biochemical manifestations of undernutrition does RD exhibit?

Specific manifestations include wasting and apparent emaciation (depleted somatic protein and subcutaneous fat stores) due to protein-energy undernutrition. Though protein status may be depleted at initial presentation, serum albumin and protein values are commonly normal due to the decreased blood volume (hemoconcentration). However, as the child is refed, the total blood volume increases, and albumin and protein concentrations may decrease (hemodilution). The changes in calcium, phosphate, magnesium, and potassium levels may be associated with his undernutrition as well as his rapid refeeding. Bradycardia, hypothermia, and a decreased respiratory rate are common bodily defense mechanisms in undernutrition that result in decreased energy needs. In addition, RD exhibited signs and symptoms of vitamin and mineral deficiencies, such as dry scaly dermatitis (essential fatty acids, vitamin A, niacin); alopecia (protein, biotin); and thinning, lusterless hair (essential fatty acids, zinc, protein). Non-specific manifestations include decreased growth rate and physical activity. The child generally appears apathetic with a flat affect.

RD presents with severe wasting demonstrated by his low body mass index (BMI) and weight change, suggesting acute undernutrition. If RD's starvation had continued, he would have manifested stunted or slowed height growth. His low serum albumin level suggests depleted visceral protein status as well, although most children with marasmus will have normal albumin levels.

Part 2: Initiating Refeeding

3. What metabolic and physiologic changes occur as RD begins to eat again? Why are his electrolyte and mineral abnormalities of primary concern?

Refeeding syndrome is a term used to describe the broad range of metabolic abnormalities and physiologic consequences that can occur during nutrition repletion with rapid reinstitution of feeding in a severely malnourished person. These changes can lead to significant pathologic consequences, including death. Awareness of the physiologic adaptation and metabolic changes with fluid and electrolyte shifts with refeeding is of primary concern. It is important to note that these changes can occur, to a greater or lesser degree, in every pediatric or adult patient who has been deprived of adequate nutrients. Pediatric patients with the conditions listed in Table 4.8 are at particular risk for refeeding syndrome.

When refeeding is initiated in the undernourished patient, anabolism begins almost immediately. A rapid alteration in hormonal levels – primarily an increase

Table 4-8 Conditions of Pediatric Patients at Risk for Refeeding Syndrome

- Protein-calorie malnutrition (e.g. refugees or famine victims)
- Chronic conditions causing under-nutrition: cancer, congenital heart disease, cystic fibrosis, Crohn's disease, chronic liver disease, neglect
- Morbid obesity with massive weight loss of 10% within the past two months
- IV hydration without provision of sufficient calories and protein for 10–14 days
- Anorexia nervosa
- Patients <80% of ideal body weight (defined as 50% weight for stature)
- Dysphagia caused by neuromuscular diseases (e.g., cerebral palsy)

Source: John A. Kerner and Jo Ann T. Hattner. Used with permission.

in insulin production – occurs, as the shift from fat to carbohydrate metabolism occurs and glucose becomes the predominant fuel. The glucose load with corresponding insulin release results in cellular uptake of glucose, phosphate, potassium, magnesium, and water, as well as protein synthesis. At this time the basal metabolic rate increases. Anabolism requires energy, nutrients, and enzymes as intermediate compounds to act as building blocks for regrowth. Increased requirements for anabolism may cause or unmask deficiencies, including life-threatening imbalances, thus inhibiting anabolism.

The cardiovascular adaptations of undernutrition, including myocardial atrophy and volume contraction, must also be considered when refeeding an undernourished patient. A rapid alteration in calories, fluid, and particularly sodium intake may cause fluid shifts and intravascular volume overload, causing the patient to go into congestive heart failure.

The most common laboratory abnormalities encountered when refeeding undernourished patients involve serious deficiencies in potassium, phosphate, magnesium, and calcium. The etiologies of each of these abnormalities include the following:

Potassium Insulin, secreted in response to the increased glucose load during refeeding, causes glucose and potassium to enter the intracellular space. This may result in a rapid fall in serum potassium. Hypokalemia may alter nerve and muscle function resulting in cardiac arrhythmias, hypotension, and cardiac arrest. A potassium concentration of less than 3.0 mEq/L is considered severe hypokalemia.

Phosphate Hypophosphatemia is the predominate feature of the refeeding syndrome. As anabolism increases, the need for phosphorylated intermediates also increases. Phosphate bound to these compounds is, in effect, "trapped" intracellularly. The resulting imbalance may cause severe hypophosphatemia, which may lead to cardiac, neuromuscular, hepatic, hematologic, and respiratory dysfunction and, ultimately, organ failure.

Because phosphorus plays such a major role in the metabolic consequences of refeeding, hypophosphatemia is known as the "hallmark sign" of refeeding syndrome.

Magnesium Refeeding syndrome is associated with hypomagnesemia and the mechanism is probably multifactorial. Intracellular movement of magnesium into cells with carbohydrate feeding, and preexisting magnesium status, are two of the possible factors. Magnesium is also a cofactor for many enzyme systems and many biochemical reactions, including those involving ATP. As the metabolic rate increases, magnesium requirements rise. Magnesium is also required for normal parathyroid function. Thus, hypomagnesemia may cause hypokalemia likely due to impaired sodium/potassium-ATPase activity. In addition, hypomagnesemia may cause hypocalcemia likely due to impaired parathyroid function.

Calcium As growth is initiated, calcium requirements increase. Maintenance of calcium levels may be affected if hypomagnesemia is present. Serum levels of calcium are maintained in such cases at the expense of bone deposits. Thus, chronic undernutrition alters bone mineralization. Hypocalcemia may also alter muscle and myocardial function, causing tetany and cardiac arrhythmias.

4. Based on RD's physical examination and laboratory data, what complications of refeeding does he exhibit?

RD exhibits fluid overload, as evidenced by the edema. This condition could be exacerbated by his low albumin level as fluid leaks from the capillaries because of decreased oncotic pressure. In addition, he may be in congestive heart failure because of his decreased cardiac output secondary to loss of heart muscle function from protein catabolism. The stress of a restored blood volume on a depleted cardiac muscle could result in cardiac decompensation. Furthermore, his myocardial function may be altered by electrolyte imbalances, putting him at greater risk for cardiac arrhythmia.

RD demonstrated dangerously low serum calcium, phosphate, magnesium, and potassium levels after refeeding due to rapid utilization of depleted mineral stores to initiate anabolism.

5. How could the complications of refeeding that RD experienced have been minimized or avoided?

The following treatment recommendations will help to avoid or minimize the complications of refeeding in children and adults:

- Refeed slowly, with gradual increases in fluid, salts, and calories. Begin with 50 to 75 percent of resting energy expenditure (predicted or measured). Increase calories 10 to 20 percent each day until calorie goal is met while closely monitoring lab values, specifically calcium, phosphate, sodium, glucose, potassium, and magnesium, and the patient's overall clinical state. Consider stopping or slowing the advancement of calories if fluid overload, congestive heart failure, or electrolyte imbalance develops.
- Provide multivitamin and mineral supplements.
- Provide additional thiamin supplementation over and above the multivitamin supplement with the initiation of carbohydrate feedings. Thiamin is an important cofactor in carbohydrate metabolism and undernutrition can result in depleted stores.
- Correct electrolyte abnormalities prior to initiation of enteral or parenteral nutrition support and monitor serum levels.
- Monitor vital signs closely during refeeding to detect changes in cardiorespiratory function early. Continuous electrocardiographic monitoring may be appropriate.
- Monitor fluid intake and output carefully to avoid stressing the undernourished cardiorespiratory system and to avoid potential fluid overload.
- Monitor daily weight gain. Excessive weight gain suggests fluid retention.

Case 3 **Eating Disorders in Adolescent Athletes**

Diane Barsky

The Children's Hospital of Philadelphia, Philadelphia, PA

OBJECTIVES

- Recognize how rapid growth during puberty alters adolescents' nutritional requirements.
- Identify teenagers at risk for eating disorders and determine appropriate interventions.
- Assess the nutrient intake of adolescent athletes and their risk of developing nutritional deficiencies.
- Outline the time sequence of the adolescent growth spurt and the stages of pubertal development described by Tanner.

AB is a 15-year-old female who has been a member of her school's cross-country running team for the past 2 years. She presents to her physician after an episode of fainting while she was competing in a 5-kilometer race. Prior to fainting she felt dizzy, but she has denied heart pounding, shortness of breath, or visual changes. She reports drinking water prior to starting the race. AB has experienced episodes of muscle cramping and headaches over the past 2 weeks.

History of Present Illness

Six months ago she reported abdominal pain and a burning sensation in her chest. Her symptoms subsequently improved with the use of antacids and a change in her eating pattern by consuming smaller, more frequent meals. According to her medical records, AB was at the 50th percentile for her weight-for-age on the growth charts until last year. She has lost 15 pounds (6.8 kg) during the past year and is currently at the 5th percentile for weight-for-age.

Past Medical History

AB's history is negative for heart disease, asthma, epilepsy, or diabetes. She has no previous history of fainting. AB takes antacids occasionally, but she is not taking any over-the-counter supplements, medications, vitamins, or minerals. She has no known allergies.

Social/Development

AB is a high achieving student. Her current circle of friends includes mostly school athletes. Upon further questioning, AB expresses concern over recent changes in

---

Medical Nutrition and Disease: A Case-Based Approach, 4th edition. Edited by Lisa Hark.
© 2009 Wiley-Blackwell Publishing, ISBN: 978-1-4051-8615-5.

her body, such as breast development and widening hips. She wants to maintain a trim, muscular physique and fears excessive weight gain will affect her speed and athletic agility. She denies smoking, alcohol, drugs, or sexual activity.

Diet History

To prepare herself for the race, AB had been consuming a high-protein (80 to 100 g/day), low-fat, low-carbohydrate diet for the past few weeks. Twenty-four hours prior to the race, she consumed two high-carbohydrate meals.

AB states that she enjoys eating, but follows a low-fat regimen to minimize weight gain. On occasion, she indulges in high-fat or high-sugar foods. She admits to small weight fluctuations during the past year, but she increases the intensity of her exercise routine to keep her weight at 90 pounds (41 kg). She denies vomiting or abuse of laxatives, enemas, or diuretics. AB frequently skips meals and compensates by snacking. During the interview, she frequently expresses concern that she is overweight and not muscular enough for long-distance running. Based on a 24-hour dietary recall, AB consumes approximately 900 to 1000 kcal per day.

Menstrual History

Menses started when AB was 12 years of age. She reports a normal cycle every 30 days until 8 months ago, when menses abruptly ceased.

Physical Examination
Vital Signs

Temperature: 96°F (35.6°C)
Heart rate: 68 BPM
Respiratory rate: 14 BPM
Blood pressure: 90/62 mm Hg
Height: 162 cm (64 inches) (50th percentile for age)
Current weight: 41 kg (90 lb) (5th percentile for age)
Ideal weight: 53 kg (117 lb) (50th percentile for age)
BMI: 15.6 kg/m^2

Exam

General: Thin, muscular female appearing sad, anxious, and younger than her age.
HEENT: Pale face, pale conjunctiva; no palpable goiter, dental erosions, gag reflex somewhat diminished. Enlarged salivary glands
Cardiac: Normal rate and rhythm
Breasts: Elevation of breast mound with areola, Tanner 3
Genitalia: Coarse pubic hair with sparse distribution, Tanner 3
Neurologic: Reflexes slightly decreased in upper and lower extremities
Extremities: Dry, coarse skin at dorsum of hand

Laboratory Data

Patient's Lab Values	Normal Values
Sodium: 142 mEq/L	133–143 mEq/L
Potassium: 2.5 mEq/L	3.5–5.3 mEq/L
CO_2: 32 mmol/L	24–32 mmol/L
Calcium: 8.2 mg/dL	9–11 mg/dL
Phosphate: 4.2 mg/dL	2.5–4.6 mg/dL
Albumin: 3.5 g/L	3.5–5.8 g/L
Hemoglobin: 11.2 g/dL	11.8–15.5 g/dL

Case Questions

1. What clues in AB's medical history and physical examination indicate that she may have an eating disorder?
2. Based on AB's laboratory values, what are the possible causes of her fainting spell, muscle cramps, and headaches?
3. Is AB's Tanner staging appropriate for her age?
4. Is AB's current diet appropriate for her age and physical activity level?
5. What nutrient deficiencies is AB at risk for developing?
6. What treatment recommendations are appropriate for AB at this time?

Answers to Questions: Case 3
Part 1: Diagnosis

1. What clues in AB's medical history and physical examination indicate that she may have an eating disorder?

There are several clues in AB's past medical history that may lead the clinician to suspect she has an eating disorder. The history of a burning sensation in her chest and abdominal pain that responded to antacids signals possible esophagitis, which may be secondary to self-induced vomiting, or purging. Purging behavior may be associated with both anorexia nervosa and bulimia nervosa. The hallmark of anorexia nervosa is an altered perception of body image with resulting restriction of calories and body weight maintained significantly below normal weight for age and height (less than 85 percent expected weight) (Tables 4-9 and 4-10). Bulimia nervosa is a disorder characterized by frequent episodes of binge eating followed by purging (self-induced vomiting or ingestion of laxatives or cathartics to induce vomiting). Patients with bulimia nervosa tend to be of normal or increased weight.

AB's presentation is consistent with anorexia nervosa, purging type. She is preoccupied with her body image, expressing an intense fear of gaining weight, and exercises vigorously to maintain herself at a low weight. Her fears about the body changes of puberty, and using her exercise to control her weight are also clues. Despite her degree of undernutrition, AB views herself as overweight, unable to acknowledge the seriousness of her condition. These symptoms are typical of the anorexia nervosa diagnosis. Her physical examination with BMI of 15.6 kg/m^2, current weight in the 5th percentile for age, loss of dental enamel, enlarged salivary glands, along with the coarse skin on the dorsum of her hand are consistent with the purging.

Table 4-9 Diagnostic Criteria for Bulimia Nervosa

Recurrent episodes of binge eating. An episode of binge eating is characterized by both of the following:

1. Eating, in a discrete period of time (e.g., within any 2-hour period), an amount of food that is definitely larger than most people would eat during a similar period of time in similar circumstances; and
2. A sense of lack of control over eating during the episode (e.g., a feeling that one cannot stop eating or control what or how much one is eating).

Recurrent inappropriate compensatory behavior in order to prevent weight gain, such as self-induced vomiting; misuse of laxatives, diuretics, or other medications; fasting; or excessive exercise.

The binge eating and inappropriate compensatory behaviors occur, on average, at least twice a week for 3 months.

Self-evaluation is unduly influenced by body shape and weight.

The disturbance does not occur exclusively during episodes of anorexia nervosa.

TYPES

Purging type: The person regularly engages in self-induced vomiting or the misuse of laxatives or diuretics.

Non-purging type: The person uses other inappropriate compensatory behaviors, such as fasting or excessive exercise, but does not regularly engage in self-induced vomiting or the misuse of laxatives or diuretics.

Source: American Psychiatric Association: Diagnostic and Statistical Manual of Mental Disorders, Fourth Edition. Washington, DC, American Psychiatric Association, 1994. Reprinted with permission Copyright 1994 American Psychiatric Association.

Table 4-10 Diagnostic Criteria for Anorexia Nervosa

Refusal to maintain body weight over a minimal normal weight for age and height (e.g., weight loss leading to maintenance of body weight 15 percent below that expected; or failure to make expected weight gain during period of growth, leading to body weight 15 percent below that expected).

Intense fear of gaining weight or becoming fat, even though underweight.

Disturbance in the way in which one's body weight or shape is experienced, undue influence of body shape and weight on self-evaluation, or denial of the seriousness of current low body weight.

In females, absence of at least three consecutive menstrual cycles when otherwise expected to occur (primary or secondary amenorrhea). (A woman is considered to have amenorrhea if her periods occur only following hormone, e.g., estrogen, administration).

TYPES

Restricting type: During the episode of anorexia nervosa, the person does not regularly engage in binge eating or purging behavior (i.e., self-induced vomiting or the misuse of laxatives or diuretics).

Binge eating/purging type: During the episode of anorexia nervosa, the person regularly engages in binge eating or purging behavior (i.e., self-induced vomiting or the misuse of laxatives or diuretics).

Source: American Psychiatric Association: Diagnostic and Statistical Manual of Mental Disorders, Fourth Edition. Washington, DC, American Psychiatric Association, 1994. Reprinted with permission. Copyright 1994 American Psychiatric Association.

AB's medical problems could be explained by her eating disorder. Although she denied vomiting, her possible esophagitis and electrolyte abnormalities (hypokalemia and alkalosis) suggest vomiting in an effort to keep her weight down. It is not unusual for patients who purge food to deny vomiting or laxative abuse.

AB's low body weight and therefore low body fat cannot support normal menstrual cycles, resulting in secondary amenorrhea, defined as an absence of menses for 6 months or for three usual cycle intervals following previous normal menstruation. Amenorrhea is more common among female athletes than in the general population; however, unless women with amenorrhea meet the other diagnostic criteria for eating disorders as shown in Tables 4-9 and 4-10, amenorrhea does not confirm an eating disorder.

Eating disorders primarily occur in adolescents and college-aged women. Eating disorders are more often found in industrialized cultures, and occur in all socioeconomic levels and across all major ethnic groups. Given the emphasis on weight, certain athletes are at higher risk for the development of eating disorders. Those especially at risk include dancers, long-distance runners, figure skaters, actors, models, wrestlers, gymnasts, and jockeys.

2. Based on AB's laboratory values, what are the possible causes of her fainting spell, muscle cramps, and headaches?

Electrolyte abnormalities are probable causes of AB's fainting spells, dizziness, and muscle cramps. AB's low potassium level and metabolic alkalosis, indicated by an elevated carbon dioxide level (characteristic of base excess), are probably due to losses of potassium and hydrogen ions during self-induced vomiting. Low serum potassium and/or low serum calcium levels can lead to muscle cramps, headaches, dizziness, and abnormal heart rhythms. Her low serum calcium level may be secondary to insufficient intake of calcium or vitamin D deficiency.

AB is at risk for dehydration if she has been inducing vomiting without orally replacing her fluid loss. During a race, she will lose additional free water, sodium, and potassium from sweating. Dehydration can cause headaches and weakness. Also, depletion of glycogen reserves, due to inadequate consumption of energy and carbohydrates, may result in poor muscle endurance and cramping. AB's low hemoglobin level, which may be indicative of iron deficiency anemia, may also contribute to her early fatigue and muscle weakness due to her diminished capacity to transport oxygen (Table 4-11).

3. Is AB's Tanner staging appropriate for her age?

AB demonstrates an arrest of her pubertal development. Puberty starts in girls at an earlier age than in boys. Girls usually demonstrate acceleration of linear growth at the onset of puberty and reach peak growth velocity early, at Tanner stage two or three, whereas boys reach peak growth velocity when genital and pubic hair are at Tanner stage four or five. In healthy females, menarche usually occurs one year after their growth peak after the rise in estrogen stimulated closure of their growth plates. Females typically reach their maximal growth velocity (a rate of 9.0 centimeters per year) at a mean age of 12.5 years. AB's height is already at the 90th percentile for her age, and she has experienced menarche. Therefore, her Tanner stage should be

Table 4-11 Medical Complications of Anorexia Nervosa and Bulimia Nervosa

Anorexia nervosa	Bulimia nervosa
Physical Signs and Symptoms	
Cachexia, body fat depletion	Ulceration or scarring of knuckles (due to abrasions received while inducing vomiting)
Bradycardia, hypotension, hypothermia	
Salivary gland hypertrophy	Salivary gland hypertrophy
Lanugo hair	Dental enamel erosion, tooth decay
Amenorrhea	Oligomenorrhea or amenorrhea
Edema	Enlarged parotids
Constipation	Loss of gag reflex
Polyuria	Esophagitis
	Constipation/diarrhea
	Peripheral edema
	Irregular menses
Laboratory Findings	
Anemia, leukopenia	Electrolyte abnormalities (hypokalemic alkalosis)
Elevated liver enzymes	Elevated serum amylase
Hypoglycemia	Metabolic alkalosis/acidosis
Increased serum cholesterol	Hypoglycemia
Hypothalamic/pituitary/endocrine	Hypocalcemia
gland abnormalities	Dehydration
Delayed gastric emptying	
Cortical atrophy on computed tomography	
Complications	
Sudden death possibly related to the presence of prolonged QT interval	Pancreatitis
	Ipecac-induced cardiomyopathy
Acute gastric dilatation	Esophageal or gastric rupture
Osteoporosis	Pneumomediastinum
	"Cathartic colon"

Source: Reprinted with permission from Devlin MJ, Walsh T. Anorexia nervosa and bulimia nervosa. In Obesity. Bjorntorp P, Brodoff BN, eds. Philadelphia: Lippincott, 1992.

more advanced, but being undernourished and having a reduced amount of body fat prevents an appropriate hormonal milieu to support the progression of puberty.

Part 2: Nutrition Assessment

4. Is AB's current diet appropriate for her age and physical activity level?

No. AB's diet is inadequate to meet her needs, as she is consuming less than 1000 kcal per day and frequently skips meals. A sufficient diet would not normally maintain an adolescent at only 90 pounds (41 kg). Growing adolescents have increased energy requirements to support their rapid growth (calories per kg). In addition, vigorous exercise, such as running, further increases energy requirements 30 to 50 percent above basal metabolic needs. Her restriction of the variety and quantity of food she consumes places her at risk for several vitamin and mineral deficiencies as described below.

5. What nutrient deficiencies is AB at risk for developing?

AB is at risk for developing a calcium deficiency. The highest requirements for calcium are during infancy and adolescence. Adolescent's high calcium requirements are due to increased bone modeling with calcium deposition, promoted by the hormonal changes associated with puberty and the associated growth peak (1300 mg/day). Maximal bone mass during skeletal maturation is achieved by adolescence or early adulthood and provides the best protection against bone loss after menopause (osteoporosis). However, according to the NHANES III, only 20 percent of teenage girls meet the RDA for calcium. AB intentionally avoids dairy products such as cheese and ice cream because they are high in fat, but she could eat low-fat or fat-free sources and calcium fortified foods or drinks.

AB also most likely has iron-deficiency anemia. Adolescents also require increased dietary iron to support growth. Foods rich in iron, which include liver, red meat, legumes, dried fruits, and green vegetables, are often lacking in an adolescent's diet.

6. What treatment recommendations are appropriate for AB at this time?

A team approach that combines medical management, cognitive–behavioral intervention, and nutritional counseling is important in the treatment of patients with eating disorders. Eating disorders are viewed as psychiatric conditions but these patients must be followed medically since there is a significant morbidity and mortality associated with these conditions. There are many potential medical complications that include delayed gastric emptying, heart failure, pancreatitis, diarrhea, osteopenia, and life-threatening electrolyte disturbances. Patients with anorexia may also experience cognitive deficits secondary to undernutrition or the subsequent refeeding process.

Psychotherapeutic assessment and intervention are crucial in establishing a diagnosis, evaluating the risk of suicide, and assessing the severity of the psychological symptoms as well as other co-morbid conditions such as depression, anxiety, substance abuse, or personality disorders. If AB's prognosis is to improve, she needs to recognize her problem, improve her perceived body image, and set and achieve nutritional and weight goals. In addition to psychiatric/psychological and medical intervention, a dietitian should provide guidance for nutritional rehabilitation and education.

The initial goals of medical nutrition therapy for AB should be to gain control over her purging behavior, stop her caloric restriction, and support steady weight gain. Increases in caloric intake should be gradual to avoid refeeding syndrome. Efforts to help AB accept a healthier weight goal should be undertaken. If purging continues despite psychological intervention, medication may reduce her binging and purging. Psychopharmacologic interventions (antidepressants and neuroleptics) have been less successful with anorexia nervosa than with bulimia nervosa.

Treatment for eating disorders can usually be initiated as outpatient therapy as long as the patient is medically and psychiatrically stable. Those who are 25 to 30 percent below their ideal weight are often hospitalized because the severity of their undernutrition is life-threatening. Since AB is only 90 pounds (41 kg), she will require close monitoring by her physician, and she may need to be hospitalized if her weight does not increase in the next few weeks.

Chapter and Case References

Alaimo K, Olson CM, Frongillo EA Jr. Low family income and food insufficiency in relation to overweight in US children: is there a paradox? *Arch Pediatr Adolesc Med.* 2001;155(10):1161–1167.

American Diabetes Association, Type 2 diabetes in children and adolescents. American Diabetes Association. *Diabetes Care.* 2000;23(3):381–389.

Azumagawa K, Kambara Y, Kawamura N, et al. Anorexia nervosa and refeeding syndrome. A case report. *Sci World J.* 2007;9(7):400–3.

Avis HJ, Vissers MN, Stein EA, et al. A systematic review and meta-analysis of statin therapy in children with familial hypercholesterolemia. *Arterioscler Thromb Vasc Biol.* 2007 27(8):1803–10.

Barlow SE, Expert committee, Expert committee recommendations regarding the prevention, assessment, and treatment of child and adolescent overweight and obesity: summary report. *Pediatrics.* 2007;120 Suppl 4:S164–92.

Berenson GS, Srinivasan SR, Bao W, et al. Association between multiple cardiovascular risk factors and atherosclerosis in children and young adults. *N Engl J Med.* 1998;338(23):1650–1656.

Brotanek JM, Gosz J, Weitzman M, et al. Iron deficiency in early childhood in the United States: risk factors and racial/ethnic disparities. *Pediatrics.* 2007;120(3):568–75.

Casey PH, Simpson PM, Gossett JM, et al. The association of child and household food insecurity with childhood overweight status. *Pediatrics.* 2006;118(5):1406–13.

Centers for Disease Control. 2006 Pediatric Nutrition Surveillance, *Growth and Anemia Indicators by Race/Ethnicity and Age.* Available from http://www.cdc.gov/pednss/pednss_tables/tables_numeric.htm.

Centers For Disease Control, *Youth Risk Behavior Surveillance - United States 2005. MMWR,* 2006. 55(SS-5): pp. 1–108.

Daniels SR, Arnett DK, Eckel RH, et al. Overweight in children and adolescents: pathophysiology, consequences, prevention, and treatment. *Circulation.* 2005;111(15):1999–2012.

Davis MM, Gance-Cleveland B, Hassink S, et al. Recommendations for prevention of childhood obesity. *Pediatrics.* 2007;120 Suppl 4:S229–53.

Duncan GE. Prevalence of diabetes and impaired fasting glucose levels among US adolescents: National Health and Nutrition Examination Survey, 1999–2002. *Arch Pediatr Adolesc Med.* 2006;160(5):523–8.

Duncan GE, Li SM, Zhou XH. Prevalence and trends of a metabolic syndrome phenotype among U.S. Adolescents, 1999–2000. *Diabetes Care.* 2004;27(10):2438–43.

Dunn RL, Stettler N, Mascarenhas MR. Refeeding syndrome in hospitalized pediatric patients. *Nutr Clin Pract.* 2003;18:327–332.

Estabrooks PA, Shetterly S. The prevalence and health care use of overweight children in an integrated health care system. *Arch Pediatr Adolesc Med.* 2007;161(3):222–227.

Expert Committee Recommendations on the Assessment, Prevention, and Treatment of Child and Adolescent Overweight and Obesity. 2007. Available from http://www.ama-assn.org/ama/pub/category/11759.html.

Expert panel on the identification evaluation and treatment of overweight in adults. clinical guidelines on the identification, evaluation, and treatment of overweight and obesity in adults: executive summary. *Am J Clin Nutr.* 1998;68(4):899–917.

Falkner B, Gidding SS, Ramirez-Garnica G, et al. The relationship of body mass index and blood pressure in primary care pediatric patients. *J Pediatr.* 2006;148(2):195–200.

Gidding SS, Nehgme R, Heise C, et al. Severe obesity associated with cardiovascular deconditioning, high prevalence of cardiovascular risk factors, diabetes mellitus/hyperinsulinemia, and respiratory compromise. *J Pediatr.* 2004;144(6):766–9.

Gordon CM, Feldman HA, Sinclair L, et al. Prevalence of vitamin D deficiency among healthy adolescents. *Arch Pediatr Adolesc Med.* 2004;158(6):531–7.

Greer, GR, Sicherer SH, Burks W. Effects of early nutritional interventions on the development of atopic disease in infants and children: the role of maternal dietary restriction, breastfeeding, timing of introduction of complementary foods, and hydrolyzed formulas. Pediatrics. 2008;121(1):183–191.

Hampl SE, Carroll CA, Simon SD et al. Resource utilization and expenditures for overweight and obese children. *Arch Pediatr Adolesc Med.* 2007;161(1):11–4.

Heller KE, Burt BA, Eklund SA. Sugared soda consumption and dental caries in the US. *J Dental Res.* 2001;80(10):1949–53.

Hofman PL, Regan F, Cutfield WS. Premature birth and later insulin resistance. *N Engl J Med.* 2004;351(21):2179–86.

Huh SY, Gordon CM. Vitamin D deficiency in children and adolescents: epidemiology, impact and treatment. *Rev Endocr Metab Disord.* 2008;9(2):161–170.

Institute of Medicine, *Food Marketing to Children and Youth, Threat or Opportunity?* The National Academies Press. Washington, DC: 2006.

Joseph A, Ackerman D, Talley JD, et al. Manifestations of coronary atherosclerosis in young trauma victims – an autopsy study. *J Am Coll Cardiol.* 1993;22(2):459–467.

Khakoo GA, Lack A. Introduction of solids to the infant diet. *Arch Dis Child.* 2004;89(4): 295.

Khardori R. Refeeding syndrome and hypophosphatemia. *J Intensive Care Med.* 2005 20(3):174–5.

Kraft MD, Btaiche IF, Sacks GS. Review of the refeeding syndrome. *Nutr Clin Pract.* 2005 Dec;20(6):625–33.

Kleinman R, (editor). *Pediatric Nutrition Handbook, 5th ed.*, American Academy of Pediatrics, 2004.

Krebs NF, Himes JH, Jacobsen D, et al. Assessment of child and adolescent overweight and obesity. *Pediatrics.* 2007;120 Suppl 4:S193–228.

Kuczmarski RJ, Ogden CL, Guo SS, et al. 2000 CDC growth charts for the united states: methods and development. *Vital Health Stat.* 2002;11(246):1–18.

Institute of Medicine (IOM), Committee on Prevention of Obesity in Children and Youth, and Food and Nutrition Board. *Preventing childhood obesity: Health in the balance.* National Academies Press, Washington, DC, 2005.

Misra M, Pacaud D, Petryk A, et al. Drug and Therapeutics Committee of the Lawson Wilkins Pediatric Endocrine Society. Vitamin D deficiency in children and its management: review of current knowledge and recommendations. *Pediatrics* 2008;122(2): 398-417.

Monsivais P, Drewnowski A. The rising cost of low-energy-density foods. *J Am Diet Assoc.* 2007;107(12):2071–6.

Nead KG, Halterman JS, Kaczorowski JM, et al. Overweight children and adolescents: a risk group for iron deficiency. *Pediatrics.* 2004;114(1):104–8.

Olson CM, Bove CF, Miller EO. Growing up poor: long-term implications for eating patterns and body weight. *Appetite.* 2007;49(1):198.

Ogden CL, Carroll MD, Flegal KM. High body mass index for age among US children and adolescents, 2003–2006**.** *JAMA.* 2008;299(20):2401–2405.

Palesty JA, Dudrick SJ. The goldilocks paradigm of starvation and refeeding. *Nutr Clin Pract.* 2006;21(2):147–54.

Pittas AG, Lau J, Hu FB, et al. The role of vitamin D and calcium in type 2 diabetes. A systematic review and meta-analysis. *J Clin Endocrinol Metab.* 2007;92(6):2017–29.

Polhamus B, Thompson D, Dalenius K, et al. *Pediatric Nutrition Surveillance 2004 Report.* Atlanta: U.S. Department of Health and Human Services, Centers for Disease Control and Prevention; 2006.

Rosenbloom AL. Implications for Primary Care of Diabetes and Impaired Fasting Glucose Prevalence in Adolescents. *Arch Pediatr Adolesc Med.* 2006;160(5):550–552.

Schwimmer JB, Burwinkle TM, Varni JW. Health-related quality of life of severely obese children and adolescents. *JAMA.* 2003;289(14):1813–9.

Sinha R, Fisch G, Teaque B, et al. Prevalence of Impaired Glucose Tolerance among Children and Adolescents with Marked Obesity. *N Engl J Med.* 2002;346(11):802–810.

Smotkin-Tangorra M, Purushothaman R, Gupta A, et al. Prevalence of vitamin D insufficiency in obese children and adolescents. *J Pediatr Endocrinol Metab.* 2007;20(7):817–23.

Spear BA, Barlow SE, Ervin C, et al. Recommendations for treatment of child and adolescent overweight and obesity. *Pediatrics.* 2007;120 Suppl 4:S254–88.

Standards of medical care and diabetes 2009. *Diabetes Care* 32 Suppl 1: S13–61.

The STOPP-T2D prevention study group, presence of diabetes risk factors in a large U.S. eighth-grade cohort. *Diabetes Care.* 2006;29(2):212–217.

The Fourth Report on the Diagnosis, Evaluation, and Treatment of High Blood Pressure in Children and Adolescents (NHLBI). National Heart Lung and Blood Institute. Available from http://www.nhlbi.nih.gov/health/prof/heart/hbp/hbp_ped.pdf.

Wang G, Dietz WH. Economic burden of obesity in youths aged 6 to 17 years: 1979–1999. *Pediatrics.* 2002;109(5):E81–1.

Weiss R, Taksali SE, Tamborlane WV, et al. Predictors of changes in glucose tolerance status in obese youth. *Diabetes Care.* 2005;28(4):902–909.

Weiss R, Dziura J, Burgert TS, et al. Obesity and the metabolic syndrome in children and adolescents. *N Engl J Med.* 2004;350(23):2362–74.

Wieckowaka AA, Feldstein AE. Nonalcoholic fatty liver disease in the pediatric population: a review. *A Curr Opin Pediatr.* 2005;17:636–641.

Woolford SJ, Gebremariam A, Clark SJ, et al. Incremental hospital charges associated with obesity as a secondary diagnosis in children. *Obesity.* 2007;15(7):1895–1901.

5   Older Adults

Jane V. White and Ronald H. Lands

Graduate School of Medicine, University of Tennessee, Knoxville, TN

OBJECTIVES [*]

- Recognize the physiological changes associated with aging and describe their impact on nutrient requirements, absorption, and metabolism.
- List common risk factors associated with poor nutritional status in older Americans.
- Understand the tools used to assess nutritional, functional, cognitive, and emotional status in older adults and the impact that alterations in any one or more of these parameters has on health and quality of life.

*Source: Objectives for chapter and cases adapted from the *NIH Nutrition Curriculum Guide for Training Physicians.* (www.nhlbi.nih.gov/funding/training/naa)

The older adult population is rapidly expanding in the United States and in most Western nations. By the year 2030, an estimated 71.5 million Americans will be 65 years of age or older, which is double the current elder population. Of these, approximately 9.6 million Americans will be 85 years of age or older. Women continue to outnumber men as age increases. Minority populations (Hispanics, Asians/Pacific Islanders, Native Americans, and African Americans) are projected to represent approximately 25 percent of the elderly population by 2030. Nutrition programs and services for older Americans need to become more diverse and flexible to meet the needs of this increasingly heterogeneous population.

Health status and ability for self-care in older people are determined by multiple factors: age-related physiological changes, presence or absence of acute/chronic medical conditions, polypharmacy, isolation, grief, poverty, and a decline in cognitive/functional status. Information on the health and nutritional status of older Americans suggests that diet plays a major role in the health of adults aged 65 years and older. According to the Healthy Eating Index, only 21 percent of older Americans had diets that were rated "good" when compared to younger adults; approximately 14 percent reported diets rated "poor," and 67 percent consumed diets that "need improvement." Nutrient intake tends to decline as age increases and regulation of energy intake in response to over- or underfeeding is less precise. Total calories, fluid, fiber, and intakes of calcium and vitamins D, B_{12}, and folate generally fall below those suggested by the Recommended Dietary Allowances (RDAs) and the Dietary Reference Intakes (DRIs), especially in older people with limited economic resources (Tables 5-1, 5-2).

Medical Nutrition and Disease: A Case-Based Approach, 4th edition. Edited by Lisa Hark.
© 2009 Wiley-Blackwell Publishing, ISBN: 978-1-4051-8615-5.

Table 5-1 Dietary Reference Intakes for Adults Aged ≥ 51 Years: Macronutrients and Minerals

Gender Age (y)	Protein[1] (g)	Carbohydrate (g)	Fiber (total)[2] (g)	Calcium[2] (mg)	Magnesium (mg)	Iron (mg)	Zinc (mg)	Copper (µg)	Chromium[2] (µg)	Selenium (µg)
Men										
51–70 y	56	130	30	1,200	420	8	11	900	30	55
>70 y	56	130	30	1,200	420	8	11	900	30	55
Women										
51–70 y	46	130	21	1,200	320	8	8	900	20	55
>70 y	46	130	21	1,200	320	8	8	900	20	55

All values represent the RDA unless otherwise noted.

[1] 0.80 g/kg/day

[2] Adequate Intakes (AIs) represent the recommended average daily intake level based on observed or experimentally determined approximations. AIs are used when there is insufficient information to determine an RDA.

Source: Institute of Medicine of the National Academies, Food and Nutrition Information Center (FNIC) Dietary Reference Intakes (DRI) and Recommended Dietary Allowances (RDA): http://www.nal.usda.gov/fnic/etext/000105.html# q2.

Table 5-2 Dietary Reference Intakes for Adults Aged ≥ 51 Years: Vitamins

Gender Age (y)	Vitamin A (μg RAE)[1]	Vitamin D[2] (μg)/(IU)	Vitamin E (mg)/(IU)	Vitamin K[2] (μg)	Vitamin C (mg)	Thiamin (mg)	Riboflavin (mg)	Niacin (mg)	Folacin (μg)	Vitamin B6 (mg)	Vitamin B12 (μg)
Men											
51–70 y	900	10/400	15/22	120	90	1.2	1.3	16	400	1.7	2.4
>70 y	900	15/600	15/22	120	90	1.2	1.3	16	400	1.7	2.4
Women											
51–70 y	700	10/400	15/22	90	75	1.1	1.1	14	400	1.5	2.4
>70 y	700	15/600	15/22	90	75	1.1	1.1	14	400	1.5	2.4

All values represent the RDA unless otherwise noted.

[1] RAE – retinol activity equivalents

[2] Adequate Intakes (AIs) represent the recommended average daily intake level based on observed or experimentally determined approximations. AIs are used when there is insufficient information to determine an RDA.

Source: Institute of Medicine of the National Academies, Food and Nutrition Information Center (FNIC) Dietary Reference Intakes (DRI) and Recommended Dietary Allowances (RDA): http://www.nal.usda.gov/fnic/etext/000105.html# q2.

Inadequate physical activity is also a health risk in older people, with only 22 percent of older adults reporting engaging in regular leisure time activity. Strength training is recommended as part of a comprehensive conditioning program to improve balance and decrease falls. Yet only 13 percent of older Americans report engaging in strength training.

Physiologic Changes Associated with Aging

Recognition of the physiological changes that usually occur with the aging process is essential to evaluating diet and health. Physiological decline escalates in the fifth decade, with some functional measures changing very little (e.g. conduction velocity of cardiac myocytes) and others undergoing substantial alteration (e.g. renal plasma flow). Not all organs age in the same manner or at the same rate. Table 5-3 highlights age-related physiological changes and their potential consequences.

Table 5-3 Age-Related Physiologic Changes with Potential Nutrition-Related Outcomes

Organ system	Change	Potential outcome
Body composition	↑ Fat	↓ Basal metabolic rate
		↑ Fat-soluble drug storage, with prolonged half-life
	↓ Body water	↑ Concentration of water-soluble drugs
Gastrointestinal	↓ Gastric acid secretion	↓ Absorption of folate, protein-bound vitamin B_{12}
	↓ Gastric motility	↓ Bioavailability of minerals, vitamins, protein
	↓ Lactase activity	Avoidance of milk products, with reduced intake vitamin D and calcium
Hepatic	↓ Size and blood flow	↓ Albumin synthesis rate
	↓ Activity drug-metabolizing enzymes	Poor or delayed metabolism of certain drugs
Immune	↓ T-cell function	Energy
		↓ Resistance to infection
Neurologic	Brain atrophy	↓ Cognitive function
Renal	↓ Glomerular filtration rate	Reduced renal excretion of metabolites, drugs
Sensory-perceptual	↓ Taste buds, papilla on tongue	Altered taste threshold, reduced ability to detect sweet/salt, increased use of salt/sugar
	↓ Olfactory nerve endings	Altered smell threshold, reduced palatability causing poor food intake
Skeletal	↓ Bone density	↑ Fractures

Source: Nutrition Screening Initiative. 2626 Pennsylvania Ave. NW, Suite 301, Washington, DC 20037. Used with permission.

Total body water decreases by approximately 20 percent, and thirst perception declines with age making older people more susceptible to dehydration. Older people are also less likely to exhibit the classic signs and symptoms of dehydration. In one study, dehydration was diagnosed in 6.7 percent of community dwelling elders admitted to the hospital. In long-term care facilities, dehydration was estimated to occur in 50 percent of febrile episodes and in 27 percent of those admitted to the hospital. The mortality of elders with untreated dehydration exceeds 50 percent. Dehydration is associated with the development of impaired cognition, kidney stones, infectious diseases, constipation, and increased risk of thrombo–embolic complications. Fluid intake should be carefully monitored and adjusted to accommodate each individual's medical status and fluid tolerance. Generally, six cups of fluid per day will meet the hydration needs of most older people.

With age, body fat increases and basal metabolic rate (BMR) decreases due to reductions in lean body mass and increases in adipose tissue. Moderate exercise helps to preserve lean body mass, thereby slowing the rate at which this process occurs. Among individuals of the same age and gender, however, body fat content is much more variable than is lean body mass. The health risk associated with overweight (BMI: 25 to 30 kg/m^2) declines as age increases, although obesity (BMI >30 kg/m^2) is still a health risk.

Digestion and absorption of macronutrients appear to be well preserved as aging occurs because of the large and efficient reserve of the gastrointestinal tract. However, reductions in gastric acid secretion and gastric motility may contribute to decreased absorption of critical nutrients such as folate, vitamin B_{12}, vitamin D, and calcium. The etiology of gastroesophageal reflux disease, constipation, diarrhea, and/or fecal incontinence may be physiologic, induced by drugs, poor fiber, and/or fluid intake and can be difficult to analyze and address.

Although an independent effect of age on taste and smell has been demonstrated, it is highly variable among individuals, and its impact on food intake and diet quality is uncertain. Chronic disease, medication use, poor oral hygiene, dentures, smoking, and poor nutritional status itself are significant contributors to age-related changes in taste and smell. Changes in the sleep cycle often lead to poor sleep quality, insomnia, daytime drowsiness, reduced participation in activities, and depression. These factors may limit access to a healthy diet.

Risk Factors for Poor Nutritional Status in Older Adults
Acute and Chronic Diseases or Disorders

Most older adults have at least one chronic disease or condition and many have several. The prevalence of chronic disease increases with advancing age and varies according to gender and race. The most common are hypertension (48 percent), arthritis (47 percent), heart disease (29 percent), cancer (20 percent), diabetes (16 percent), and sinusitis (14 percent). Hearing impairment is estimated to affect one-half of older men and one-third of older women. Approximately 17 percent of older adults report blindness in one or both eyes. Approximately 9 percent report problems with vision and hearing. Leading causes of death among those 65 years of age and older include heart disease, cancer, and stroke, respectively.

The presence of a chronic disease or condition often results in a prescribed or self-imposed modification in food intake. Such modifications frequently limit variety and result in decreased total nutrient intake.

Oral Health Problems

Approximately 26 percent of the older population in the United States is edentulous. Edentulism is higher among minorities and among those who smoke, are uninsured, have less formal education, and reside in a nursing home. Nearly one-third of older Americans with natural teeth have untreated root or crown cavities, while 41 percent have periodontal disease. The incidence of periodontal disease is higher in those with cardiovascular disease or diabetes. Patients who have loose, decaying, or missing teeth, difficulty chewing, ill-fitting dentures, or who fail to wear their dentures are at increased risk for poor nutritional status due to a decreased or modified food intake.

Cognitive and Emotional Impairment

Changes in the level of cognitive function that are associated with normal aging are difficult to quantify but can significantly impact health. Memory loss, which is estimated to occur in about 13 percent of Americans aged 65 and older, makes it difficult to obtain a history, identify health or nutrition problems that need to be addressed, and assess whether prior interventions have been implemented, and their efficacy. The limited data from longitudinal sources suggest that short-term memory (20 seconds or less) declines with age. Progressive dementia is characterized by a gradual decline in multiple cognitive functions that cause losses of the ability to make choices, to initiate activities (such as shopping and food preparation), and to simply remember to eat appropriately. Dementia is a major risk factor for undernutrition; there is extensive evidence that patients with dementia often become undernourished.

Grief or mourning is viewed as a normal part of life, yet the elderly confront it more often because they are more likely to experience loss/death of friends, spouses, or loved ones. In individuals of all ages, grief may dramatically disrupt memory and can result in a general sense of confusion and disorganization. Disease processes for which mourners may be at increased risk include myocardial infarction, gastrointestinal cancer, hypertension, neurodermatitis, rheumatoid arthritis, diabetes, thyrotoxicosis (women in particular), depression, alcohol/drug abuse, undernutrition, headaches, low back pain, colds/flu, excessive fatigue, impotence, and sleep disorders. Although the symptoms of grief such as insomnia, changes in appetite, difficulty in decision-making, and problems in cognition can mimic those of a depressive disorder, it is important to distinguish between these conditions. Older adults may need more frequent contact with their physician during the first two years following a grief-inducing incident.

In older people, depression can present as cognitive impairment with memory and concentration being particularly affected. However, change in appetite (usually a reduction but sometimes a pathological increase) is a defining feature of "major depression" – a depression that may require treatment with antidepressant drugs.

The depressed individual may become undernourished with decreased food intake as a result of feelings of poor self-esteem, lack of motivation, and negativity. New onset of reduced food intake should always lead to consideration of depression as a cause.

Isolation

Nineteen percent of men and 38 percent of women aged 65 years and older live alone. The likelihood of living alone increases as age advances. A sense of loneliness is greatest among those who are widowed, childless, physically disabled, and those who live alone and have few contacts. Other individuals who feel lonely are those who subjectively feel that their health is poorer, or that their economic condition is inadequate, and those with hearing or visual impairments.

Elderly people who have limited social interaction or infrequent contact with family, friends, or neighbors on an individual level, and who are unable or unwilling to access social support systems on a broader level, may experience decreased food intake, lack of appetite, and limited motivation to shop and prepare meals as a result. Eating is a social event that is often enhanced by the presence of others. Loneliness, and in particular, the lack of a companion at mealtimes, tends to have a negative impact on food intake.

Alcohol/Drug Use

The potential benefits of moderate alcohol use (1 to 2 drinks/day) in older individuals include mood enhancement, stress reduction, sociability, social integration, maintenance of long-term cognitive functioning, improved cardiovascular health, and enhanced bone mineral density. The American Geriatrics Society defines risky drinking for people age 65 and older as more than 7 drinks/week or more than 3 drinks/day. Studies of elderly Medicare beneficiaries suggest that while 65 percent report no alcohol consumption in a typical month, about 26 percent reported drinking within guidelines and 9 percent reported drinking in excess of these guidelines. Prevalence of excess was higher for men (16 percent) and those ages 65 to 70 (13 percent). Early-onset alcoholics frequently have a family history of alcoholism and higher prevalence of antisocial behavior. Poverty and family estrangement are common in this group. Late-onset drinkers usually have higher education and income levels, and smoke. They are more likely to have greater resources, family support, and better treatment outcomes. Depression, loneliness, and lack of social support are the most frequent reasons given for late-onset drinking by the elderly.

The typical daily amount of alcohol/drug consumed, and the duration and frequency of consumption, should be ascertained using a brief questionnaire validated in older populations as shown in Table 5-4. Interviewing family members may also be helpful. Remember when screening for alcohol abuse that denial or understatement of amount or frequency of alcohol consumption is common. Ascertain the presence of anxiety, depression, or other psychiatric/personality disorders and look for isolation, falls, accidents, or other clues for intoxication. Remind patients that use of prescription or over-the-counter medications may be a contraindication to alcohol consumption.

Table 5-4 AUDIT Questionnaire and Scoring

Questions	0	1	2	3	SCORES
How often do you have a drink containing alcohol?	Never	Monthly or less	2–4 times a month	2–3 times a week	4 or more times a week
How many standard drinks containing alcohol do you have on a typical day when drinking?	1 or 2	3 or 4	5 or 6	7 to 9	10 or more
How often do you have six or more drinks on one occasion?	Never	Less than monthly	Monthly	Weekly	Daily
During the past year, how often have you found that you were not able to stop drinking once you had started?	Never	Less than monthly	Monthly	Weekly	Daily or almost daily
During the past year, how often have you failed to do what was normally expected of you because of drinking?	Never	Less than monthly	Monthly	Weekly	Daily or almost daily
During the past year, how often have you needed a drink in the morning to get yourself going after a heavy drinking session?	Never	Less than monthly	Monthly	Weekly	Daily or almost daily
During the past year, how often have you has a feeling of guilt or remorse after drinking?	Never	Less than monthly	Monthly	Weekly	Daily or almost daily
During the past year, how often have you been unable to remember what happened the night before because you had been drinking?	Never	Less than monthly	Monthly	Weekly	Daily or almost daily
Have you or someone else been injured as a result of your drinking?	Never		Yes, but not in the past year		Yes, during the past year
Has a relative or friend, or doctor or other health worker been concerned about your drinking or suggested you cut down?	Never		Yes, but not in the past year		Yes, during the past year

Source: Saunders JB, Aasland OG, Babor TF, et al. Development of the alcohol use disorders identification test (AUDIT): WHO Collaborative project on early detection of persons with harmful alcohol consumption-II. *Addiction.* 1993;88:791-803.

Scoring the AUDIT:
- Scores for each question range from 0 to 4 , with the first response for each question (Never) scoring 0, the second (e.g., less than monthly) scoring 1, the third (e.g., monthly) scoring 2, the fourth (e.g., weekly) scoring 3, and the last response (e.g., daily or almost daily) scoring 4. For questions 9 and 10, which only have three responses, the scoring is 0, 2, and 4 (from left to right).
- **A score of 8 or more is associated with harmful or hazardous drinking, a score of 13 or more in women and 15 or more in men, is likely to indicate alcohol dependence.**

Socioeconomic Status

Approximately 9 percent of the older US population lived below the poverty level in 2006 and another 4 percent were classified as near poor (125 percent of the poverty level). Women, minorities, elders living in central cities, rural areas, and in the South had higher than average poverty rates. Elders living alone or with non-relatives were more likely to be poor than those living in families. Hispanic and African–American women living alone experience highest poverty rates, 40.5 percent and 37.5 percent, respectively.

Many older individuals are reluctant to use food stamps or similar feeding programs because of embarrassment and "welfare stigma." Many do not know how to access federal programs, are uncomfortable going to a congregate dining site, do not qualify for home-delivered meals, or are placed on a long waiting list. Food/meals provision activities sponsored by churches or other non-governmental agencies are often the type of help that elders find acceptable. Consideration of the older person's socioeconomic status and knowledge of available social service options are essential to reducing nutritional risk in elders.

Functional Capacity

In 2005, 42 percent of older Americans reported some degree of disability, with 26 percent reporting difficulty in the performance of one or more Activities of Daily Living (ADLs). ADL's reflect an individual's capacity for self care, and Instrumental Activities of Daily Living (IADLs) reflect more complex tasks that enable a person to live independently in the community as shown in Table 5-5. The percent of individuals experiencing disability with both ADLs and IADLs increases with both ADLs and IADLs as people age.

Even after controlling for demographic, socioeconomic, gender, and racial factors, the level of disability predicts increased mortality risk. It is imperative that when

Table 5-5 Commonly Used Measures of Functional Capacity

Activities of daily living (ADLs)	Instrumental activities of daily living (IADLs)
Bathing	Telephone use
Dressing	Walking
Toileting	Shopping: groceries/clothes
Transferring	Meal preparation
Continence	Housework/laundry
Feeding	Home maintenance/repair
	Take medicines
	Manage money

ADLs reflect capacity for self-care
AIDLs reflect capacity for independent living

taking a medical history in older individuals questions regarding functional capacity, including the ability to access, purchase, prepare, and consume an adequate diet be included.

Polypharmacy

A recent survey of adult Americans showed that in those age 65 and older, 89 percent report that they are currently taking a prescription drug on a regular basis. Many average taking four prescription drugs a day. Women are more likely to say they are taking a prescription drug than men. Cost is the major factor cited by those failing to fill a prescription. The classes of drugs most commonly used by older persons include proton pump inhibitors, statins, antihypertensives, antidepressants, anti-inflammatory agents, antihistamines, and oral hypoglycemic agents. The use of several concurrent medications is the standard of care for an increasing number of conditions. So although multiple medications are often necessary in elders, those prescribing the drugs rarely consider the potential detriment to nutritional health of each and every prescription. Elderly people in poor health and taking multiple medications are at highest risk for undernutrition.

Vitamin and mineral supplement use varies by ethnicity, with approximately 54 percent of non-Hispanic white, 31 percent of black, and 38 percent of Hispanic elderly reporting use. Use of herbal preparations is reported by approximately 13 percent of non-Hispanic white, 16 percent of black, and 5 percent of Hispanic elderly. Females are more likely to use herbal products than males. It is also increasingly clear that some complementary and alternative medicines are pharmacologically active substances, and their potential impact needs to be considered (i.e. St. John's wort See Chapter 2: Case 2.2).

Nutrition Screening and Assessment Tools

There is no single physical or biochemical parameter that accurately measures nutritional status. Thus, a number of tools have been developed in an attempt to provide relevant information that clinicians can use in the identification of poor nutritional status in the elderly. The Nutrition Screening Initiative's (NSI) Determine Checklist and Level 2 Screen are shown in Figure 5-1. The Subjective Global Assessment, The Meals on Wheels mnemonic, the Mini Nutritional Assessment, the NSI Care Alerts, and the Health Care Financing Administration (Centers for Medicare and Medicaid Services) Nutrition and Hydration Care are examples of structured approaches to nutrition screening and assessment in the elderly. Almost all contain assessment of involuntary weight loss and lack of appetite – the two parameters that are most consistently correlated with poor nutritional status. Regardless of the tool used, a structured approach to nutrition screening and assessment must become an integral component of the care of each older person, either free living or institutionalized.

The Warning Signs of poor nutritional health are often overlooked. Use this Checklist to find out if you or someone you know is at nutritional risk.

DETERMINE YOUR NUTRITIONAL HEALTH

Read the statements below. Circle the number in the "yes" column for those that apply to you or someone you know. For each "yes" answer, score the number in the box. Total your nutritional score.

	YES
I have an illness or condition that made me change the kind and/or amount of food I eat.	2
I eat fewer than 2 meals per day.	3
I eat few fruits or vegetables or milk products.	2
I have 3 or more drinks of beer, liquor, or wine almost every day.	2
I have tooth or mouth problems that make it hard for me to eat.	2
I don't always have enough money to buy the food I need.	4
I eat alone most of the time.	1
I take 3 or more different prescribed or over-the-counter drugs a day.	1
Without wanting to, I have lost or gained 10 pounds in the last 6 months.	2
I am not always physically able to shop, cook and/or feed myself.	2
TOTAL	

Total Your Nutritional Score. If it's –

0–2   **Good!** Recheck your nutritional score in 6 months.

3–5   You are at **moderate nutritional risk.** See what can be done to improve your eating habits and lifestyle. Your office on aging, senior nutrition program, senior citizens center or health department can help. Recheck your nutritional score in 3 months.

6 or more   You are at **high nutritional risk.** Bring this Checklist the next time you see your doctor, dietitian or other qualified health or social service professional. Talk with them about any problems you may have. Ask for help to improve your nutritional health.

Remember that Warning Signs suggest risk, but do not represent a diagnosis of any condition. Turn the page to learn more about the Warnings Signs of poor nutritional health.

These materials are developed and distributed by the Nutrition Screening Initiative, a project of:

AMERICAN ACADEMY OF FAMILY PHYSICIANS

THE AMERICAN DIETETIC ASSOCIATION

THE NATIONAL COUNCIL ON THE AGING, INC.

The Nutrition Screening Initiative • 1010 Wisconsin Avenue, NW • Suite 800 • Washington, DC 20007
The Nutrition Screening Initiative is funded in part by a grant from Ross Products Division of Abbott Laboratories, Inc.

Figure 5-1 Determine Your Nutrition Health
Source: Nutrition Screening Initiative Washington, D.C.

Nutritional Needs of Older Adults

The nutritional needs of older adults are difficult to quantify due to "physiological diversity and heterogeneity" and the prevalence of chronic disease. Deficiency signs and symptoms are uncommon in elderly who live in the community, but are occasionally seen in people who are frail, homebound, and who must rely on others to meet basic needs. They are also more common among those in institutional care. In general, nutrient needs in older adults appear to be similar to those for

The Nutrition Checklist is based on the Warning Signs described below.
Use the word <u>DETERMINE</u> to remind you of the Warning Signs.

DISEASE

Any disease, illness or chronic condition which causes you to change the way you eat, or makes it hard for you to eat, puts your nutritional health at risk. Four out of five adults have chronic diseases that are affected by diet. Confusion or memory loss that keeps getting worse is estimated to affect one out of five or more of older adults. This can make it hard to remember what, when, or if you've eaten. Feeling sad or depressed, which happens to about one in eight older adults, can cause big changes in appetite, digestion, energy level, weight, and well-being.

EATING POORLY

Eating too little and eating too much both lead to poor health. Eating the same foods day after day or not eating fruit, vegetables, and milk products daily will also cause poor nutritional health. One in five adults skip meals daily. Only 13% of adults eat the minimum amount of fruit and vegetables needed. One in four older adults drink too much alcohol. Many health problems become worse if you drink more than one or two alcoholic beverages per day.

TOOTH LOSS/MOUTH PAIN

A healthy mouth, teeth, and gums are needed to eat. Missing, loose, or rotten teeth or dentures which don't fit well, or cause mouth sores, make it hard to eat.

ECONOMIC HARDSHIP

As many as 40% of older Americans have incomes of less than $6,000 per year. Having less -- or choosing to spend less -- than $25-30 per week for food makes it very hard to get the foods you need to stay healthy.

REDUCED SOCIAL CONTACT

One-third of all older people live alone. Being with people daily has a positive effect on morale, well-being, and eating.

MULTIPLE MEDICINES

Many older Americans must take medicines for health problems. Almost half of older Americans take multiple medicines daily. Growing old may change the way we respond to drugs. The more medicines you take, the greater the chance for side effects such as increased or decreased appetite, change in taste, constipation, weakness, drowsiness, diarrhea, nausea, and others. Vitamins or minerals, when taken in large doses, act like drugs and can cause harm. Alert your doctor to everything you take.

INVOLUNTARY WEIGHT LOSS/GAIN

Losing or gaining a lot of weight when you are not trying to do so is an important warning sign that must not be ignored. Being overweight or underweight also increases your chance of poor health.

NEEDS ASSISTANCE IN SELF CARE

Although most older people are able to eat, one of every five have trouble walking, shopping, buying and cooking food, especially as they get older.

ELDER YEARS ABOVE AGE 80

Most older people lead full and productive lives. But as age increases, risk of frailty and health problems increase. Checking your nutritional health regularly makes good sense.

The Nutrition Screening Initiative • 1010 Wisconsin Avenue, NW • Suite 800 • Washington, DC 20007
The Nutrition Screening Initiative is funded in part by a grant from Ross Products Division of Abbott Laboratories, Inc.

Figure 5-1 (*Cont.*) Nutrition Screening Initiative: Warning Signs

middle-aged adult populations. However, for some nutrients, clear evidence of increased need exists.

The recently revised Dietary Reference Intakes (DRIs) (Table 5-2) represent quantitative estimates useful in planning and assessing diets for healthy people. To date, DRIs have been established for the vitamins and minerals essential for maintenance of bone health, for the B-complex vitamins, and for choline. Those nutrients for which clear evidence of increased need in older adults has been established include:

Calcium

Osteoporosis is major health risk for older women and men. There were 20 million hospitalizations for osteoporotic hip fractures in 2005. Calcium recommendations were set at levels associated with maximum retention of body calcium since bones that are calcium rich are known to be less susceptible to fracture. For males and females age 51 years and older including those over age 70, the RDA for calcium is 1200 mg/day and the tolerable upper intake level (UL) for calcium is 2500 mg/day. Supplements should be considered for those whose dietary intake of calcium is poor.

Vitamin D

For vitamin D, the RDA for men and women ages 51 to 70 years is 400 IU/day, and for those over age 70 it is 600 IU/day. A recent meta-analysis of the dose of vitamin D needed to prevent hip and non-vertebral fractures in older people suggests that a daily intake of 700–800 IU is optimal, although in clinical practice considerably higher doses may be prescribed without apparent or reported undue side effects. The tolerable upper intake level (UL) for vitamin D for adults is 2000 IU/day; however, this level was established in 1997 and thus newer data regarding the role of vitamin D were not considered in its formulation. Although supplements have been routinely recommended for frail homebound or institutionalized elderly, whose exposure to sunlight is limited, or in those in whom evidence of osteomalacia or osteoporosis is documented, recent studies suggest that 61 percent of white and 91 percent of black Americans have vitamin D insufficiency. A minimal serum level of $25(OH)_2D$ of 32 ng/mL (80 nmol/L) is needed for optimal intestinal absorption of calcium and maintenance of bone health. However, vitamin D is increasingly viewed as important to immune function, maintenance of normal blood pressure, and cancer prevention. Vitamin D status should be routinely assessed and supplements prescribed when food intake is inadequate to maintain optimal status.

Folate

The RDA for folate for adults age 51 years and older is 400 μg/day. Since folate fortification of grain products is now widespread in the United States (generally at 100 μg/serving), it is felt that most older people can obtain an adequate folate intake from their diet. The upper intake limit for folate has been set at 1000 μg/day (1 mg/day). Caution should be exercised when recommending large amounts of folate fortified foods or supplements. Excessive consumption of folic acid may mask a vitamin B_{12} deficiency, allowing the neurologic sequelae to progress even though the anemia associated with this deficiency resolves. Folate has a theoretical dual effect on cancer, protecting against cancer initiation but facilitating progression and growth of pre-neoplastic cells and subclinical cancers that are common in older populations. High blood folate levels may reduce response to anti-folate drugs used in the treatment of rheumatoid arthritis, psoriasis, malaria, and some forms of cancer, thus, higher folic acid intakes may not benefit some people.

Vitamin B$_{12}$

The RDA for vitamin B$_{12}$ for individuals over age 50 is 2.4 µg/day. Although most Americans who consume animal products can get sufficient vitamin B$_{12}$ from food, it is estimated that between 10 to 30 percent of older people have lost the ability to adequately absorb protein-bound vitamin B$_{12}$. Thus the Food and Nutrition Board recommends that people over age 50 meet most of their dietary requirement for vitamin B$_{12}$ with synthetic B$_{12}$ from fortified foods or supplements. Most oral supplements currently on the market contain free, as opposed to protein-bound B$_{12}$. Intrinsic factor and HCL (needed to cleave B$_{12}$ from its protein carrier) are not needed for the digestion/absorption of this form of B$_{12}$ versus the food form of B$_{12}$. Widespread use of vitamin B$_{12}$ injections is no longer necessary if the free form of B$_{12}$ is given as an oral supplement in amounts of 2000 micrograms daily. Vitamin B$_{12}$ is available over the counter in the form of tablets and lozenges. Patients who are taking Metformin for the treatment of diabetes have been shown to also have poor vitamin B$_{12}$ absorption. Check serum and red blood cell vitamin B$_{12}$ levels and prescribe vitamin B$_{12}$ supplements as described above when levels are borderline-low or below normal.

Vitamin B$_6$

The RDA for vitamin B$_6$ in adults above age 50 is 1.5 mg/day. It has been suggested that adequate intake of vitamin B$_6$ helps to reduce homocysteine levels and thus the risk of cardiovascular disease; however, this theory remains unproven. The upper intake for vitamin B$_6$ has been set at 100 mg/day. Adults who take doses of vitamin B$_6$ above this level are at increased risk of developing progressive, crippling neurologic damage.

Conclusion

Poor nutritional status is a common, yet frequently overlooked problem in old age. It is a potential sign of treatable illness, which must be evaluated. It has medical consequences, both short- and long-term, including being a major factor in the prevention, treatment, and ability to recover from acute/chronic illness. It is a contributor to morbidity in the majority of frail, dependent elders. By considering nutrition in all aspects of medical decision-making (e.g., diagnosis, medication prescription, surgery, rehabilitation, referral, placement), quality of life can be improved and successful aging can be the outcome for a higher proportion of our nation's adults.

Case 1 **Malnutrition and Depression**

Katherine Galluzzi

Philadelphia College of Osteopathic Medicine, Philadelphia, PA

OBJECTIVES

- Identify common risk factors for poor nutritional status in older adults.
- Describe the effects of undernutrition on physiologic function in geriatric patients.
- Develop a nutritional care plan for an older adult with poor nutritional status and weight loss secondary to altered living situation.
- Provide nutritional counseling appropriate to the physiologic, emotional, social, and financial changes that occur with aging.
- Recognize the unique contribution of different members of a health care team including social workers, home health aides, and community volunteers in the effort to improve the nutritional status of older people.

ML is an 80-year-old African-American widow who was brought to her primary care physician's office by the local Older Americans Transportation Service. She had missed two prior scheduled office visits due to the recent death of her husband and a subsequent fall, which resulted in an intertrochanteric fracture of her right hip.

On presentation, ML appeared withdrawn and much more frail than on previous visits. She answered in a monotone with terse, non-spontaneous speech, and she lacked expression. Her chief complaint, aside from pain with ambulation, is nocturnal leg cramps (which she calls "charlie-horses"). When asked about how she has been coping after the loss of her husband, she became tearful. She admitted that in addition to the loss of companionship, the loss of his pension has caused tremendous financial hardship.

Past Medical History

ML tripped on the steps in her house two months ago and fractured her right hip. She underwent an open reduction/internal fixation surgery to repair the fracture and the operation went well. There were no serious operative complications, but she lost approximately 350 cm^3 of blood during the procedure (1 unit $= 500$ cm^3). ML underwent inpatient rehabilitation for 10 days after discharge from the surgical service and then returned home, where she lives alone. She ambulates slowly with a cane and can climb stairs only with difficulty.

During her inpatient rehabilitation stay, she was diagnosed with depression and was started on a selective serotonin reuptake inthibitor (SSRI) antidepressant. She has a history of hypertension, Stage 2 chronic kidney disease, and osteoporosis,

---

Medical Nutrition and Disease: A Case-Based Approach, 4th edition. Edited by Lisa Hark.
© 2009 Wiley-Blackwell Publishing, ISBN: 978-1-4051-8615-5.

the latter discovered at the time of her hip fracture two months ago. ML had an appendectomy at age 46 and bilateral cataract surgeries three years ago. She has no previous history of pneumonia, tuberculosis, hepatitis, or urinary tract infection.

Medications

ML currently takes hydrochlorothiazide 25 mg daily for hypertension, fluoxetine (Prozac) 20 mg daily for depression, and an iron supplement for anemia three times per day. She also self-medicates with over-the-counter preparations of acetaminophen 500 mg three times a day, and frequently uses over-the-counter laxatives and glycerin suppositories for her constipation, which she attributes to her iron tablets. Due to her kidney disease, she has been warned to avoid over-the-counter analgesics that might contain non-steroidal anti-inflammatory medications, but she nevertheless takes occasional doses of ibuprofen 200 mg for pain. She does not take a multi-vitamin, calcium, or vitamin D supplement. She has no known food allergies.

Social History

ML lives alone in the small three-story row-home she has occupied since she married 58 years ago. Her son and daughter both live out of state. Although they call her every few weeks, they have not visited since her husband's death. ML states that she used to attend church and visit the local senior center regularly with her husband, but has not been to either lately. ML explains that she has no energy to "get up and go" anymore and she falls asleep in front of the television. She also reports being constipated and that her food does not have much taste. She avoids alcohol and tobacco and drinks one cup of coffee and two cups of tea daily.

Review of Systems

General: Weakness, fatigue, weight loss, and depression.
Mouth: Food lacks taste (hypogeusia); dry, "thick-feeling" tongue; sores in corners of mouth.
GI: Poor appetite, constipation.
Extremities: Hip pain when climbing stairs, some tenderness at old incision site, chronic low back pain, and troublesome episodes of nocturnal leg cramps that awaken her from sleep.

Physical Examination
Vital Signs
Temperature: 97.0 °F (36 °C)
Heart rate: 88 BPM
Respiration: 18 BPM
Blood pressure: 130/80 mm Hg
Height: 5′6″ (168 cm)
Current weight: 110 lb (50 kg)
Usual weight: 140 lb (64 kg)
BMI: 18 kg/m²
Weight 6 months ago prior to surgery: 125 lb (57 kg)
Percent weight change: 12% [(125 − 110/125) × 100]

Exam

General: Thin, frail-appearing elderly African-American woman who is appropriately conversant but withdrawn. She is well groomed, but her clothes are loose fitting, suggesting weight loss.

Skin: Warm to touch, "ashy"-appearing patches of dryness and flaking to elbows and lower extremities

HEENT: Temporal muscle wasting, no thyroid enlargement

Mouth: Ill-fitting dentures, sore beneath bottom plate; cracks/fissures at corners of mouth (angular chelitis), tongue is dry and pale without ulcers or plaques

Cardiac: Regular rhythm at 88 beats per minute, soft systolic murmur

Abdomen: Well-healed appendectomy site scar, no enlargement of liver or spleen, diffusely diminished bowel sounds

Extremities: Well-healed cicatrix overlying right hip with slight surrounding erythema, no sores on feet, trace pretibial edema to both lower extremities

Rectal: Hard stool in vault, stool test for occult blood negative

Neurologic: Alert, good memory, no evidence of sensory loss, slight psychomotor retardation evident

Gait: Slightly wide-based with decreased arm swing, antalgic and tentative but with safe, appropriate use of cane

Laboratory Data

Patient's Lab Values	Normal Values
Albumin: 2.5 g/dL	3.5–5.8 g/dL
Hemoglobin: 11.0 g/dL	11.8–15.5 g/dL
Hematocrit: 33.0%	36–46%

ML's 24-Hour Dietary Recall

At her physician's request, ML provided the following 24-hour dietary recall, stating that this represents her usual daily intake:

Breakfast (home)

Jelly doughnut	1 whole
White toast	1 slice
Jelly	2 Tbsp.
Coffee	1 cup

Lunch (home)

Butter cookies	2 each
Chicken and rice soup	1 cup
Saltine crackers	6 each
Tea	2 cups

Dinner (home)

White bread	1 slice
Jelly	2 Tbsp.
Peanut butter	2 Tbsp.
Butter cookies	2 each

Total calories: 1270 kcal
Protein: 25 g/day (8% of calories)
Fat: 42 g (30% of calories)
Carbohydrate: 201 g (63% of calories)
Calcium: 153 mg
Iron: 6 mg

Case Questions

1. What information from the case history would cause you concern over ML's functional status?
2. Based on that information, what medical, environmental, and social factors could lead to nutritional problems in this patient?
3. What do ML's BMI and percent weight change indicate about her nutritional status?
4. What are ML's calorie and protein requirements for repletion? What general conclusions can you draw regarding ML's diet?
5. How can ML's diet be improved to meet her increased requirements, achieve weight gain, and relieve her constipation?
6. What specific recommendations would you offer to improve ML's nutritional status?

Answers to Questions: Case 1
Part 1: Assessing Activities of Daily Living

1. What information from the case history would cause you concern over ML's functional status?

ADLs: Although ML can feed herself, she has trouble chewing because of her loose dentures and a sore in her mouth. She has insufficient money for a visit to the dentist. ML also exhibits poor mobility; she walks with a cane, has difficulty with stairs, and fears falling since her hip fracture. Although she is mobile, she reports pain with movement and moves slowly about the house. Finally, ML dislikes eating alone, which may negatively impact her food intake.

IADLs: Since her injury, ML has been afraid to go outside, which may be secondary to fear of falling or lack of energy from exertion. Because she does not drive and is unaccustomed to using public transportation, she has difficulty shopping for food and other necessities. ML reports a very limited social life; since her husband's death she has avoided church, community programs, and the senior center. Her reported dislike of cooking for one person most likely will have a negative effect on the quality and quantity of her food intake. She denies difficulty with dressing, grooming, or toileting, and feels that if her husband were alive she would resume cooking meals.

2. Based on that information, what medical, environmental, and social factors could lead to nutritional problems in this patient?

ML's ill-fitting dentures and hypogeusia may lead to decreased intake and under-nutrition. Depression over the loss of her husband may decrease her appetite. The prevalence of depression in community-dwelling elders was noted by Sachs-Ericsson et al. to range from 8 to 16 percent. A study by Cabrera et al. found depression in 24.3 percent of elderly subjects, and noted a significant association (p <0.001) between depression and nutritional deficit even after adjusting for variables such as low educational and socio-economic level, and smoking.

ML lives alone in a three-story row-home and is not interested in cooking for herself since her husband died. Her impaired ambulatory function and lack of money for assistance with household tasks have negatively impacted her dietary intake. She is also homebound, and therefore at risk of vitamin D deficiency due to inadequate sunlight exposure. Furthermore, she no longer participates in community activities that could provide support, meals, and social interaction. Her children have not visited recently or provided any assistance. Finally, the loss of her husband's pension has significantly reduced her income.

Part 2: Nutrition Assessment

3. What do ML's BMI and percent weight change indicate about her nutritional status?

Note that in this case the value used for ML's usual weight is 125 pounds (57 kg), as it was 6 months earlier prior to surgery (rather than her usual weight of 140 lbs prior to her husband's death). Her percent weight change greater than 10 percent in a period of 6 months represents a clinical indicator for undernutrition. Weight loss is not a normal part of aging and frequently represents an underlying disease process, such as depression, pulmonary or renal disease, or occult malignancy. Most nutrition experts currently consider satisfactory weight for those aged 65 and older as BMI between 24 and 27 kg/m^2. ML's BMI of 18 kg/m^2 clearly indicates that she is underweight and based on the overall assessment, she is at risk for undernutrition.

4. What are ML's calorie and protein requirements for repletion? What general conclusions can you draw regarding ML's diet?

ML's total estimated daily calorie requirements, based on the DRI, are calculated using the equation below (as described in Chapter 1, Table 1-7):

$$354 - (6.91 \times age) + physical\ activity\ coefficient \times (9.36 \times weight\ in\ kg) + (726 \times height\ in\ meters)$$

$$354 - (6.91 \times 80) + 1.12 \times (9.36 \times 50\ kg) + (726 \times 1.68\ m) = 1545\ kcal/day.$$

The estimated total daily protein requirements are 1.5 grams per kg of weight: (50 kg) $\times$ (1.5 g/kg) = 75 g/day.

ML's usual daily intake provides 1270 calories and 25 grams of protein. Her diet is low in calories due to her poor appetite. ML's limited consumption of meats and poultry products, resulting in a poor overall protein and iron intake, is probably due to her low-income status and poor dentition. Because ML stopped drinking milk many years ago and does not shop for dairy foods regularly, her diet is deficient in calcium and vitamin D. Fruits, vegetables, and fluids also appear to be below acceptable limits in ML's diet.

Part 3: Medical Nutrition Therapy

5. How can ML's diet be improved to meet her increased requirements, achieve weight gain, and relieve her constipation?

Constipation, which is very common in older adults, can often be corrected by increasing fiber and fluid intake and physical activity. Examples of high-fiber foods include fruits, vegetables, bran cereals, and whole-grain products such as whole-wheat bread and brown rice. One bowl of raisin bran cereal or oatmeal every day would most likely be sufficient to achieve bowel regularity. If these measures are not sufficient, fiber supplements can be recommended. She should be advised to drink at least 6 glasses (8 ounces each) of water daily, and preferably more if tolerated to help alleviate constipation. The elderly, however, are prone to hypodypsia (blunted thirst response), which leads to inadequate fluid intake. Older adults may require prompting or frequent reminders to ensure adequate fluid intake. In light of her weight loss and inadequate dietary intake, ML's diet clearly needs to be higher in calories, protein, and calcium to fulfill her current requirements. She should also be asked whether she is taking her iron supplements, as older adults tend to discontinue these if constipation occurs.

High-Calorie, High-Protein Dietary Recommendations

Breakfast (home)

Coffee	8 ounces (240 mL)
Instant oatmeal	1 package
Lactose-free 2% milk	6 ounces (180 mL)
Orange juice	4 ounces (120 mL)

Lunch (senior center)

Chicken drumstick	3 ounces (85 g)
Baked potato	1 medium
Margarine	2 Tbsp.
Green beans	1/2 cup

Snack (senior center)

Lactose-free 2% milk or yogurt	8 ounces (240 mL)
Canned peaches	1/2 cup

Dinner (home)

Tuna salad	4 ounces (113 g)
Saltine crackers	6 each
Tomatoes	3 slices
Vanilla pudding	1/2 cup

Snack (home)

Applesauce	1/2 cup

Total Calories: 1540 kcal
Protein: 72 g (19% of calories)
Fat: 57 g (33% of calories)
Carbohydrate: 190 g (49% of calories)
Calcium: 974 mg
Iron 15 mg

Table 5-6 Council on Nutrition Appetite Questionnaire

A.My appetite is:	**B. When I eat, I feel full after:**
1. Very poor	1. Eating only a few mouthfuls
2. Poor	2. Eating about a third of a plate/meal
3. Average	3. Eating over half of a plate/meal
4. Good	4. Eating most of the food
5. Very good	5. Hardly ever
C. I feel hungry:	**D. Food tastes:**
1. Never	1. Very bad
2. Occasionally	2. Bad
3. Some of the time	3. Average
4. Most of the time	4. Good
5. All of the time	5. Very good
E. Compared to when I was 50, food tastes:	**F. Normally, I eat:**
1. Much worse	1. Less than one regular meal a day
2. Worse	2. One meal a day
3. Just as good	3. Two meals a day
4. Better	4. Three meals a day
5. Much better	5. More than three meals a day (including snacks)
G. I feel sick or nauseated when I eat:	**H. Most of the time my mood is:**
1. Most times	1. Very sad
2. Often	2. Sad
3. Sometimes	3. Neither sad nor happy
4. Rarely	4. Happy
5. Never	5. Very happy

Scoring:
Total the score by adding the numbers associated with the patient's response. A score of less than 28 is cause for concern. If the total is

8–16 The patient is at risk for anorexia and needs nutrition counseling.
17–28 The patient needs frequent reassessment.
>28 The patient is not at risk at this time.
Source: Wilson MM et al. *Am J Clin Nutr* 2005;82:1074–81.

6. What specific recommendations would you offer to improve ML's nutritional status?

In addition to the recommended dietary modifications, ML and/or her primary care physician should take the following steps to ensure her continued well-being:

- Contact her children and other family members for support and to help her arrange to move to an apartment or a smaller, single-story home.
- Contact her other health care providers, specifically her psychiatrist or psychologist, regarding recommended changes in medications and make arrangements to have her dentures properly adjusted. Consider utilizing the Council on Nutrition Appetite Questionnaire (CNAQ - Table 5-6) at quarterly evaluations to assess ML's appetite. Wilson et al. have shown the the CNAQ is a short, simple appetite assessment tool that predicts weight loss in community dwelling adults and long-term care residents.

- Drink high-calorie, high-protein liquid supplements or suggest adding non-fat powdered milk to puddings to increase her intake of calories, protein, vitamins, and minerals.
- Prescribe a multivitamin and mineral supplement with 100 percent of the RDA for older adults and calcium (600 mg BID) with at least 1000 IU vitamin D.
- Use a microwave oven to prepare convenience foods and decrease cooking time.
- Contact a social worker to help ML get in touch with the area Council on Aging, Meals on Wheels, and other community resources.
- Consider a home health aide to monitor ML's weekly weight and food intake and assess whether her ambulatory status is improving or whether she is at increased risk of falling again.
- Utilize church, synagogue, and community volunteers to shop for food or contact a grocery store that delivers.
- Undergo further rehabilitation and exercise therapy to increase her diminished mobility.
- Contact a neighbor with whom ML could share meals or travel to the senior center daily for a hot lunch.

Chapter and Case References

Baker H. Nutrition in the elderly: diet pitfalls and nutrition advice. *Geriatrics.* 2007;62(10):24–6.

Baker H. Nutrition in the elderly: nutritional aspects of chronic diseases. *Geriatrics.* 2007;62(9):21–5.

Baker H. Nutrition in the elderly: hypovitaminosis and its implications. *Geriatrics.* 2007;62(8):22–6.

Baker H. Nutrition in the elderly: An overview. *Geriatrics.* 2007;62(7):28–31.

Barrett LL. *Prescription drug use among midlife and older Americans.* American Association of Retired Persons, 2005, Washington, DC.

Bischoff-Ferrari HA, Willett WC, Wong JB, et al. Fracture prevention with vitamin D Supplementation. A meta-analysis of randomized controlled trials. *JAMA* 2005;293:2257–2264.

Buvat DR. Use of metformin as a cause of vitamin B_{12} deficiency. *Am Fam Physician.* 2004;69:264–266.

Cabrera MA, Mesas AE, Garcia AR, de Andrade SM. Malnutrition and depression among community-dwelling elderly people. *J Am Diet Assoc.* 2007;8(9):582–584.

Callen B, Wells TJ. Screening for nutritional risk in community-dwelling old-old. *Pub Health Nurs.* 2005;22(2):138–148.

CNAQ: Council on Nutrition Appetite Questionnaire. Available from medschool.slu.edu/agingsuccessfully/pdfsurveys/appetitequestionnaire.pdf.

DHHS. Substance Abuse and Mental Health Services Administration. Office of Applied Studies. 2006 National Survey Data on Drug Use and Health: National Results. University of Michigan, Monitoring the Future Study, 2006.

Donini LM, Savina C, Rosano A, Cannella C. Systematic review of nutrition status evaluation and screening tools in the elderly. *J Nutr Health Aging,* 2007;11(5):421–32.

Federal Interagency Forum on Aging-Related Statistics. 2008 *Older Americans. Key Indicators of Well-Being.* Federal Interagency Forum on Aging-Related Statistics. US Government Printing Office. Washington, DC 2008.

Feldbaum I, German L, Castel H, et al. Characteristics of undernourished older medical patients and the identification of predictors for undernutrition status. *Nutr J.* 2007;6:37.

Fritz K, Elmadfa I. Quality of nutrition of elderly with different degrees of dependency: elderly living in private homes. *Ann Nutr Metab.* 2008;52 Suppl 1:47–50.

Khazai N, Judd SE, Tangpricha V. Calcium and vitamin D: skeletal and extraskeletal health. *Curr Rheumatol Rep.* 2008;10(2):110–117.

Kripke C. Is oral vitamin B12 as effective as intramuscular injection? *Am Fam Physician.* 2006;73:65.

Kuzminski AM, Del Giacco EJ, Allen RH, et al. Effective treatment of cobalamin deficiency with oral cobalamin. *Blood.* 1998;92(4):1191–1198.

Martin C, Kayser-Jones J, Stotts N, Porter C, Froelicher E. Risk for low weight in community-dwelling, older adults. *Clin Nurs Spec.* 2007;21(4):203–211.

Merrick EL, Horgan CM, Hodgkin D, et al. Unhealthy drinking patterns in older adults: prevalence and associated characteristics. *J Am Geriatr Assoc.* 2007;56:214–223.

Raji MA, Kuo Y-F, Snih SA, Sharaf BM, Loera JA. Ethnic differences in herb and vitamin/mineral use in the elderly. *Ann Pharmacother.* 2005;39:1019–1023.

Rivlin RS. Keeping the young-elderly healthy: is it too late to improve our health through nutrition? *Am J Clin Nutr.* 2007;86(5):1572S–6S.

Rosenzweig A, Progerson H, Miller MD, Reynolds CF. Bereavement and late-life depression: grief and its complications in the elderly. *Annu Rev Med.* 1997;48:421–428.

Sachs-Ericsson N, Joiner T, Plant EA, Blazer DG. The influence of depression on cognitive decline in community-dwelling elderly persons. *Am J Geriatr Psychiatry.* 2005 May;13(5):402–8.

Smith AD, Young-In K, Refsum H. Is folic acid good for everyone? *Am J Clin Nutr.* 2008;87:517–533.

Tariq SH. Gastroenterology. *Clinics Ger Med.* 2007;23(4):xi–xiii.

The Joint Comission. *Improving and Measuring Osteoporosis Management.* The Joint Commission; Oakbrook Terrace, IL 2007.

Vargas CM, Yellowitz JA, Hayes KL. Oral health status of older rural adults in the United States. *J Am Diet Assoc.* 2003;134:470–486.

Wells JL, Dumbrell AC. Nutrition and aging: assessment and treatment of compromised nutritional status in frail elderly patients. *Clin Interv Aging.* 2006;1(1):67–79.

Wilson MM, Thomas D, Rudenstein L, Chibnall J, Anderson S, Baxi A, Diebold M, Morley J. Appetite assessment: simple appetite questionnaire predicts weight loss in community-dwelling adults and nursing home residents. *Am J Clin Nutr.* 2005;82:1074–81.

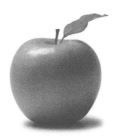

Part III
Integrative Systems and Disease

6 Cardiovascular Disease

Jo Ann S. Carson and Scott M. Grundy

University of Texas Southwestern Medical Center, Dallas, TX

OBJECTIVES [*]

- Identify patients at risk for coronary heart disease including identification of risk factors, assessment of abdominal obesity by waist circumference, and use of a nutrition history that targets dietary components relevant to atherosclerosis, hypertension, and/or heart failure.

- Given a patient's medical history and laboratory data, propose an optimal set of goals for nutritional risk factor reduction using the NCEP and AHA guidelines for nutrition and exercise.

- Describe the parameters of the National Cholesterol Education Program's Therapeutic Lifestyle Changes (TLC) Diet.

- Discuss issues related to vitamin supplementation for prevention or treatment of cardiovascular disease.

- Summarize the dietary parameters of the DASH diet for the hypertensive patient.

- Prioritize nutritional goals for the patient with heart failure.

[*]Source: Objectives for chapter and cases adapted from the NIH Nutrition Curriculum Guide for Training Physicians. (www.nhlbi.nih.gov/funding/training/naa)

According to the National Center for Health Statistics and the American Heart Association (AHA), about one third of Americans have cardiovascular disease (CVD). Nutrition plays a key role in the prevention and treatment of various types of cardiovascular disease, particularly the most common forms in the American population – coronary heart disease (CHD) and hypertension.

The importance of nutrition in CHD has heightened with growing awareness of metabolic syndrome, in which elevated triglyceride and reduced high-density-lipoprotein cholesterol (HDL-C) levels, insulin resistance, and hypertension combined with abdominal obesity increase the potential for morbidity and mortality from heart disease. The positive association between dietary fat, particularly saturated fat, and the risk for developing CHD is irrefutable. This association is presumed to reflect the increased serum cholesterol and low-density-lipoprotein cholesterol (LDL-C) levels that result from a high intake of saturated fat. The association of obesity with the development of hypertension, type 2 diabetes, and consequent CVD further heightens the need for all health care workers to be educated in the role of nutrition in health promotion and disease prevention.

Medical Nutrition and Disease: A Case-Based Approach, 4th edition. Edited by Lisa Hark.
© 2009 Wiley-Blackwell Publishing, ISBN: 978-1-4051-8615-5.

Evidence Base for Diet and Heart Disease

This is strong evidence that diet, largely through its effect on serum lipids, influences the incidence of heart disease. Intake of saturated fat increases LDL-C levels, thereby increasing the risk for CHD. Large-scale clinical trials have shown conclusively that reducing serum LDL-C levels reduces the number of acute cardiac events and deaths from CHD both in patients with existing disease and those at risk due to elevated lipids. Angiographic studies have demonstrated that LDL-C reduction slows the progression of atherosclerosis in patients with known disease. Atherosclerosis is now viewed not simply as the deposition of lipid in the artery, but as a complex inflammatory response to damage to the endothelial lining of arteries.

Dietary Lipids

An understanding of the basic biochemistry of fat and fatty acids is needed to address the role of dietary fat in the prevention and treatment of heart disease. Dietary fats are composed chiefly of three fatty acids attached to a glycerol molecule. All fats are a combination of saturated, monounsaturated, and polyunsaturated fatty acids. Fat is the most calorically dense nutrient, supplying nine calories per gram. Therefore, a diet high in fat is generally high in calories. Reducing total fat intake and adhering to an exercise program can help an individual lose weight. The effects of different types of fats on serum lipids are discussed below and summarized in Table 6-1.

Saturated Fats

Saturated fats are fatty acids with no double bonds. With the exception of palm and coconut oil, foods high in saturated fat are solid at room temperature and are primarily from animal sources. Major contributors of saturated fat include fatty meats, such as cold cuts, sausage, and bacon, and regular fat dairy products, including whole or two percent milk, cheese, and ice cream. According to the NHANES data (2003 to 2004), approximately 11 percent of the calories in the American diet comes from saturated fat. Saturated fatty acids, when contrasted with unsaturated fatty acids, decrease synthesis and activity of LDL-C receptors, promoting an increase in serum LDL-C, thereby contributing to atherogenesis. An increase of 1 mg/dL in serum LDL-C increases CHD risk by one percent. A meta-analysis of dietary studies concluded that for every one percent increase in calories from saturated fat, serum LDL-C increases approximately two percent.

Polyunsaturated Fats

Two major categories of polyunsaturated fats (PUFA) are omega-3 and omega-6 fatty acids. Vegetable oils such as corn, canola, sunflower, safflower, and soybean contain omega-6 fatty acids. Omega-6 fatty acid (linoleic acid), an essential fatty acid, cannot be synthesized by the body and is required in the diet. Arachidonic acid, which is synthesized from linoleic acid, is the major omega-6 fatty acid found in cell membranes and the precursor of prostaglandins. The Dietary Reference Intake

Table 6-1 Summary of Dietary Changes to Impact Serum Lipids

Lipid goal	Dietary manipulation	Dietary advice
To lower LDL-C	Decrease saturated fat	Limit portion size of meats; Use lean meats and fat-free dairy products
	Replace saturated fat with MUFA and/or PUFA	Use canola or olive oil for MUFA; can use safflower or corn oil for PUFA
	Limit *trans* fatty acids	Use soft, *trans*-free margarine
		Limit baked goods with partially hydrogenated oils
	Limit cholesterol	Limit egg yolks, organ meats, butterfat, and high-fat meats
To lower triglycerides	Include MUFA	Use olive or canola oil, peanuts, pecans
	Include omega-3	Have cold water fish weekly
	Eliminate alcohol	
	Lose weight if overweight	
To raise HDL-C	Use MUFA in place of PUFA	Use canola or olive oil
	Lose weight if overweight	
	Limit *trans* fatty acid intake	
	Avoid high carbohydrate diets	

Source: Jo Ann S. Carson, PhD, RD. Used with permission.

for linoleic acid is an Adequate Intake of 17 g/day for men and 12 g/day for women. Substitution of PUFA for saturated fat in the diet lowers LDL-C and HDL-C and reduces risk for CHD.

Omega-3 fatty acids include the very long chain eicosapentanoic acid (EPA) and docosahexenoic acid (DHA), as well as the 18-carbon alpha-linolenic acid, another essential fatty acid. The long-chain fatty acids have been shown to decrease serum triglycerides, platelet aggregation, and inflammation and may therefore provide cardiac benefits. Dietary sources include flax seed, salmon, sardines, tuna, swordfish, and herring. Epidemiologic studies suggest that healthy individuals who consumed seven ounces of fish per week are 30 to 40 percent less likely to die from a cardiac event than those who do not regularly consume fish. The AHA and the American Dietetic Association advise consumption of fish at least twice a week to reduce cardiovascular risk.

In patients with heart disease, some studies indicate the benefit of omega-3 fatty acids, but the evidence is very preliminary. Some clinical trials suggest an intake of approximately 1 g/day of EPA/DHA can reduce death from cardiac events. Other studies indicate a trend toward less restenosis after angioplasty for patients receiving omega-3 dietary supplements. Doses of 3 to 4 g/day can be prescribed to lower serum triglyceride in hypertriglyceridemic patients. Although omega-3 fatty acids lower triglycerides, they also slightly increase LDL-C. As research continues, it is appropriate to encourage a dietary pattern that incorporates omega-3 fatty acids, especially from fatty fish, but the long-term benefit of omega-3 supplementation is unclear.

Monounsaturated Fats

Monounsaturated fats (MUFA) contain one double bond; oleic acid is the most common dietary form. Oils high in oleic acid include canola and olive oil. Other dietary sources of MUFA include avocados, peanuts, and pecans. Epidemiologic evidence from the Mediterranean region, where diets are rich in MUFA, have demonstrated a lower incidence of CHD. This finding was corroborated by a clinical trial, the Lyon Diet Heart Study. Shorter-term clinical trials of a Mediterranean style diet have shown improvement in a number of risk factors, including lowering serum triglyceride and reduction of inflammatory markers, such as C-reactive protein. Substitution of oleic acid for saturated fatty acids reduces LDL-C levels. A diet high in MUFA lowers LDL-C and serum triglycerides without lowering HDL-C. Provision of some calories from MUFA, which might otherwise be provided from carbohydrate, can lower LDL-C without lowering HDL-C or raising triglyceride levels.

Trans Fatty Acids

Hydrogenation – the addition of hydrogen atoms to an unsaturated fat – can change a fatty acid double bond from a *cis* to *trans* configuration. The major source of *trans* fatty acids is partially hydrogenated vegetable oils. Food manufacturers have used this process to prolong the shelf-life of foods such as crackers, cookies, potato chips, and puddings. Randomized clinical trials indicate that *trans* fatty acids raise LDL-C levels when compared with naturally occurring *cis* fatty acids; they also decrease HDL-C. The structural similarity of *trans* fat to saturated fat may explain the detrimental effects.

Although margarines contain *trans* fatty acids, use of a soft or liquid margarine maintains a lower LDL-C than does a comparable diet containing butter (a source of saturated fat and cholesterol). There are *trans*-free tub margarines available that should be recommended. Since the requirement to include *trans* fatty acid information on food labels, many food processors have substituted either a healthier vegetable oil, a specially produced interesterified fat that has less *trans* fat, or a saturated fat blends (such as palm and canola oils). It is anticipated that these actions have reduced the *trans* fat intake in the United States.

Dietary Cholesterol

Although saturated fat is perhaps the major dietary factor responsible for raising serum LDL-C levels, a high intake of cholesterol in the diet can also increase serum LDL-C. Animal foods are sources of cholesterol, with the highest being egg yolk and organ meats. Meat and dairy sources of saturated fat, such as cheese, cream, and fatty meats, also contain substantial amounts of cholesterol.

Table 6-2 Major Risk Factors That Modify LDL Goals (Exclusive of LDL Cholesterol)

- Cigarette smoking
- Hypertension (BP ≥140/90 mm Hg or on anti-hypertensive medication)
- Low HDL-C (<40 mg/dL)[†]
- Family history of premature CHD (CHD in male first-degree relative <55 years; CHD in female first-degree relative <65 years)
- Age (men ≥45 years; women ≥55 years)

[†] HDL-C ≥60 mg/dL counts as a "negative" risk factor; its presence removes one risk factor from the total count.
Source: National Cholesterol Education Program. Adult Treatment Panel (ATP) III Guidelines.

Hyperlipidemia

Hyperlipidemia, the clinical term used to describe elevated cholesterol, LDL-C, or triglyceride levels, increases the risk of atherosclerosis. When atherosclerosis proceeds to occlusion or rupture of a blood vessel, myocardial infarction, stroke, or peripheral vascular disease results (depending upon the affected site). Various lipoproteins transport cholesterol and triglycerides in the blood. The majority of cholesterol is carried in the blood by LDL-C and transported into the cells via LDL-C receptors. Low-density lipoproteins are the major atherogenic lipoproteins. In contrast, cholesterol carried by HDL-C represents cholesterol being released by the cells. The majority of serum triglyceride is present in very low-density lipoproteins (VLDL). Rather than an earlier clinical approach of assessing total cholesterol, a fasting lipid profile of the patient's LDL-C, HDL-C, and triglyceride levels is now recommended by the National Cholesterol Education Program, Third Adult Treatment Panel (NCEP ATP III).

Assessment of the Hyperlipidemic Patient (Framingham Data)

The clinical approach to the hyperlipidemic patient is well outlined in the NCEP ATP III guidelines. Key steps include the assessment of risk factors that allows determination of lipoprotein goals and delineation of the need for lifestyle change and, if needed, the addition of pharmacologic treatment. Individuals with existing evidence of CHD or diabetes should aim for a goal LDL-C of 100 gm/dL or less. Individuals without either diagnosis, but with two or more risk factors (Table 6-2) are further stratified as to their risk of a coronary event within the next 10 years based on Framingham data. This estimate of risk takes into account age, gender, total cholesterol, smoking, HDL-C, and blood pressure.

Metabolic Syndrome

Recent attention regarding risk for CHD has focused on a constellation of characteristics termed metabolic syndrome. Metabolic syndrome includes (1) insulin resistance, (2) hypertension, (3) dyslipidemia that can include elevated serum triglycerides, low HDL-C, and small, dense LDL-C, (4) a prothombotic state, and (5) a proinflammatory state. Although sophisticated laboratory analyses – such as determination of C-reactive protein or measurement of insulin resistance – can

Table 6-3 Diagnosing Metabolic Syndrome: 3 or More of the Following 5 Criteria

Abdominal obesity	Waist circumference Men >40 inches Women >35 inches
Pre-Hypertension	BP ≥130/≥85 mm Hg
Glucose intolerance	FBG ≥100 mg/dL
High triglycerides	≥150 mg/dL
Low HDL-C	Men <40 mg/dL Women <50 mg/dL

Source: National Cholesterol Education Program. Adult Treatment Panel (ATP) III Guidelines and AHA/NHLBI Scientific Statement on Diagnosis and Treatment of Metabolic Syndrome (or to use the same amount of space, could just cite the AHA/NHLBI statement rather than ATP III.

strengthen the diagnosis of metabolic syndrome, a series of simple measurements shown in Table 6-3 provide a reliable means of clinical identification of individuals at risk for metabolic syndrome. The presence of abdominal obesity is a valuable clue to metabolic syndrome. It can easily be assessed via the patient's waist circumference, which is described in detail in Chapter 1.

Medical Nutrition Therapy for Hyperlipidemia and Metabolic Syndrome

Diet and exercise are cornerstones of the effective treatment of hyperlipidemia. The NCEP ATP III Guidelines enumerated four essential components of the Therapeutic Lifestyle Changes Diet (TLC) for achievement of LDL-C goals. They encompass the following:

- LDL-C-raising nutrients should be minimized.
  - ○ Keep dietary intake of saturated fat to less than 7 percent of total calories.
  - ○ Keep *trans* fat as low as possible (<1% of total calories).
  - ○ Keep dietary cholesterol intake less than 200 mg per day.
  - ○ Total fat is allowed within the range of 25 to 35 percent of calories.
- Therapeutic options may be added for further LDL-C lowering.
  - ○ Include 2 grams of plant stanol/sterol esters/day.
  - ○ Increase viscous fiber intake to 10 to 25 grams per day.
- Total calories should be adjusted to maintain desirable body weight and prevent weight gain.
- Physical activity should include enough moderate exercise to expend at least 200 calories per day.

For patients with hypertriglyceridemia, the proportion of dietary carbohydrate and fat can be shifted such that dietary fat is at the upper end of the allowed range (about 35 per cent of calories), while calorie intake is provided for either weight loss or weight maintenance. The ATP III recommended distribution for macronutrients is shown in Table 6-4 and specific food-based guidance is provided in Table 6-5. Adopting lifestyle changes that incorporate new long-term dietary habits demands an investment of time and family support. Referral to a registered dietitian for

Table 6-4 Macronutrient Recommendations for the Therapeutic Lifestyle Changes (TLC) Diet

Component	Recommendation
Saturated fat	Less than 7% total calories
Polyunsaturated fat	Up to 10% of total calories
Monounsaturated fat	Up to 20% of total calories
Total fat	25–35% of total calories*
Carbohydrate†	50–60% of total calories*
Dietary fiber	20–30 grams per day
Protein	Approximately 15% of total calories

Source: National Cholesterol Education Program. Adult Treatment Panel (ATP) III Guidelines.
*ATP III allows an increase of total fat to 35 percent of total calories and a reduction in carbohydrate to 50 percent for persons with the metabolic syndrome. Any increase in fat intake should be in the form of either polyunsaturated or monounsaturated fat.
† Carbohydrate should derive predominantly from foods rich in complex carbohydrates including grain – especially whole grains, fruits, and vegetables.

medical nutrition therapy provides a comprehensive assessment of nutritional status, development of negotiated, tailored behavior change goals, and strategies to achieve these goals. The dietitian can assist patients with problem areas such as portion size, eating out, and tips for food purchasing and preparation. Continued reinforcement and monitoring of behavior change by health care professionals is important for achieving and maintaining lifestyle changes. Many lipid centers have full-time or part-time dietitians on staff who routinely counsel patients and work closely with the health care team.

Other Nutritional Components
Stanol/Sterol Esters
Plant sterols and their chemically modified counterpart, plant stanols, have been esterified and incorporated into a growing number of products, such as margarine, yogurt, and orange juice. Consuming two tablespoons per day of sterol fortified spread can provide two to three grams of sterol/stanol esters per day and lower LDL-C levels by 7 to 15 percent. In the gastrointestinal tract, sterol/stanol esters compete with cholesterol for incorporation into micelles and thus absorption. Two possible concerns regarding use of plant sterol/stanol fortified margarines are (1) if margarine use is increased, some means of caloric adjustment is needed to maintain energy balance; (2) concurrent reduced absorption of dietary carotenoids suggests the need for attention to consume adequate intake of fruits and vegetables.

Dietary Fiber
Inclusion of viscous or soluble fiber in the diet can decrease LDL-C levels. Based on evidence from a meta-analysis of over 50 clinical trials, ATP III recommends inclusion of at least 5 to 10 grams of viscous fiber daily, with the option of greater intakes in the range of 10 to 25 grams daily. The 5 to 10 gram per day has been

Table 6-5 Food Based Advice for Therapeutic Lifestyle Changes (TLC) Diet

Food Items to Choose More Often	Food Items to Choose Less Often
Breads and Cereals	
≥6 servings per day, adjusted to caloric needs	Many bakery products, including doughnuts, biscuits, butter croissants, Danish, pies, cookies
Breads, cereals, especially whole grain; pasta; rice; potatoes; dry beans and peas; low-fat crackers and cookies	Many grain-based snacks, including chips, cheese puffs, snack mix, regular crackers, buttered popcorn
Vegetables and Fruits	
3–5 servings vegetables per day fresh, frozen, or canned, without added fat, sauce, or salt	Vegetables fried or prepared with butter, cheese, or cream sauce
2–4 servings fruits per day fresh, frozen, canned, dried	Fruits fried or served with butter or cream
Dairy Products	
2–3 servings per day fat-free, $\frac{1}{2}$%, 1% milk, buttermilk, yogurt, cottage cheese; fat-free & low-fat cheese	Whole milk/2% milk, whole-milk yogurt, ice cream, cream, cheese
Eggs	
≤2 egg yolks per week	Egg yolks, whole eggs
Egg whites or egg substitute	
Meat, Fish & Poultry	
≤5 ounces per day	Higher fat meat cuts: ribs, t-bone steak,
Lean cuts loin, leg, round; extra lean hamburger; cold cuts made with lean meat or soy protein; skinless poultry; fish	regular hamburger, bacon, sausage; cold cuts: salami, bologna, hot dogs; organ meats: liver, brains, sweetbreads; poultry with skin; fried meat; fried poultry; fried fish
Fats and Oils	
Amount adjusted to caloric level: Unsaturated oils; soft or liquid margarines and vegetable oil spreads, salad dressings, seeds, and nuts	Butter, shortening, stick margarine, chocolate, coconut

Source: National Cholesterol Education Program. Adult Treatment Panel (ATP) III Guidelines.

shown to reduce LDL-C by about 5 percent. The hypocholesterolemic effect of soluble fiber results from its ability to form a gel-like substance in the gut, which binds and removes bile acids from the body through the stool before they are reabsorbed. Hepatic conversion of cholesterol into new bile acids reduces serum cholesterol. Some of the best dietary sources that provide 2 to 4 grams of viscous fiber per serving include dried beans (lima, pinto, kidney), oatmeal, oat bran, citrus fruits, pears, and Brussels sprouts.

Soy

The benefit of soy in lowering cholesterol is not as well substantiated as the nutritional approaches discussed above. The Food and Drug Administration has approved a health claim for soy foods that 25 grams of soy protein per day, as part of a diet low in saturated fat and cholesterol, may reduce the risk of heart disease. Studies indicate wide variation in effects on LDL-C levels (4 to 24 percent). The AHA has concluded that the major benefit of soy protein is its use as a substitute for less heart-healthy fatty animal products, rather than substantial benefit inherent in the soy itself.

Supplemental Vitamins

Although supplementation with antioxidants and B vitamins was common in the 1990s as a strategy to reduce atherosclerosis, clinical trials have failed to demonstrate significant benefit. In fact, use of an antioxidant "cocktail" of vitamins C and E, beta-carotene, and selenium actually lowered the beneficial sub fraction HDL_2 cholesterol in patients receiving simvastatin and niacin treatment; it also reduced the stenosis lowering effect of the medical treatment. Beyond use of a daily multi-vitamin supplement, patients should be encouraged to obtain antioxidants and other vitamins from a diet rich in colorful fruits and vegetables and grains, rather than through supplements.

Medical Nutrition Therapy for CHD (Chapter 6: Case 6.1)

Nutrition issues should be addressed with patients who have hyperlipidemia, CHD, or a family history of heart disease during most routine primary care visits. One quick reminder of nutrition issues to consider is the use of WAVE, an acronym suggesting consideration of the patient's Weight, Activity, and diet in terms of Variety and Excess. (See http://outside.utsouthwestern.edu/chn/naa/wave/wave_info.htm) Specific to hyperlipidemia, it is valuable to address the excesses in the diet that would contribute saturated fat and cholesterol.

Weight Control

Attention to calorie balance is important for most patients. Fostering control of caloric intake and encouraging increased physical activity are key to weight main-tenance and weight reduction. Weight reduction in overweight patients improves parameters associated with metabolic syndrome, including reducing LDL-C and triglycerides, increasing HDL-C, reducing blood pressure, and normalizing elevated serum glucose levels. In many cases, as little as 7 to 10 percent weight reduction alone can eliminate the need for drug therapy in these clinical syndromes.

Conversely, it is possible that initiation of a lipid-lowering medication prompts patients to feel attention to diet is no longer needed. Failure to follow appropriate diet with use of drugs can necessitate higher doses of drugs, increasing any potential for side effects. Therefore, physicians should continue to emphasize the underlying benefit of a calorically balanced, low saturated fat diet when lipid-lowering drugs are used.

Alcohol

In addition to the general lifestyle issues of diet and exercise, a specific issue often raised in patient conversations regarding heart disease is consumption of alcohol.

Alcohol, in relation to heart disease, has both positive and negative effects. A first step in advising patients regarding alcohol is to obtain an adequate alcohol intake history.

Although light-to-moderate intake of alcohol may reduce the risk of CHD, intake over 30 grams per day (more than 2 drinks) is associated with an increased mortality due to hypertension, pancreatitis, hypertriglyceridemia, gastrointestinal malignancies, stroke, cardiomyopathy, cirrhosis, accidents, and breast cancer. Moderate alcohol intake is defined as no more than 2 drinks per day for men and 1 drink per day for women. A drink is defined as 5 ounces of wine, 1.5 ounces of 80-proof liquor, or 12 ounces of beer.

In terms of benefits, alcohol may have cardioprotective effects by increasing HDL-C levels and reducing LDL-C oxidation via the antioxidant polyphenols (catechin, quercetin, resveratrol). A CHD patient can continue to drink alcohol in moderation if free of other medical, psychiatric, or social problems. However, it is *not* appropriate to recommend alcohol intake to a non-drinker or an at-risk drinker for its cardioprotective effect, as there are many other effective non-pharmacological therapies.

Hypertension (Chapter 6: Case 6.2)

Hypertension affects over 50 million people in the United States and is a major risk factor for the development of CHD, cardiomyopathy, and stroke. Diet and other lifestyle factors have enormous potential for the prevention and treatment of hypertension and in some cases can obviate the need for drug therapy or lower the dose required. This is particularly evident in patients with prehypertension (blood pressure: 120/80 to 130/89 mm Hg).

Nutritional factors that may contribute to the development of essential hypertension include obesity, high sodium intake, low potassium, and calcium intake, and excessive alcohol consumption. The Dietary Approaches to Stop Hypertension (DASH) trial and the subsequent DASH-sodium trials and the PREMIER study have substantiated the benefit of a comprehensive dietary approach in prevention and treatment of hypertension.

The DASH diet, outlined in Table 6-6, provides for a substantial intake of potassium and calcium through the inclusion of fruits and vegetables and low-fat dairy products. In addition, meat portions are limited and nuts are used to provide magnesium and additional fiber. The diet limits saturated fat and cholesterol comparable to the dietary parameters of the TLC diet of ATP III. Clinical trials have demonstrated that the DASH diet reduced diastolic blood pressure by as much as 5 mm Hg, regardless of age, gender, ethnicity, or preexisting hypertension. The diet was more effective among African-American and hypertensive individuals. For patients with Stage 1 hypertension (blood pressure: 140/90 to 159/99 mm Hg) the diet's effectiveness in lowering blood pressure was similar to that of a single-agent anti-hypertensive therapy.

After the original trial, the DASH-sodium trial investigated the effect of the DASH diet combined with three different levels of sodium (3300 mg, 2400 mg, and

Table 6-6 DASH Diet

Food Group	Daily Servings	Serving Sizes
Grains & grain products	7–8	1 slice bread 1 cup dry cereal* $\frac{1}{2}$ cup cooked rice, pasta, or cereal
Vegetables	4–5	1 cup raw leafy vegetable $\frac{1}{2}$ cup cooked vegetable 6 ounces vegetable juice
Fruits	4–5	6 ounces fruit juice 1 medium fruit $\frac{1}{4}$ cup dried fruit $\frac{1}{2}$ cup fresh, frozen, or canned fruit
Low-fat or fat-free dairy foods	2–3	8 ounces milk 1 cup yogurt 1 $\frac{1}{2}$ ounces cheese
Meats, poultry, and fish	2 or less	3 ounces cooked meats, poultry, or fish
Nuts, seeds, and dry beans	4–5 per week	1/3 cup or 1 $\frac{1}{2}$ ounces nuts 2 Tbsp or $\frac{1}{2}$ ounces seeds $\frac{1}{2}$ cup cooked dry beans
Fats and oils**	2–3	1 tsp soft margarine 1 Tbsp low fat mayonnaise 2 Tbsp light salad dressing 1 tsp vegetable oil
Sweets	5 per week	1 Tbsp sugar 1 Tbsp jelly or jam $\frac{1}{2}$ ounces jelly beans 8 ounces lemonade

This DASH eating plan is based on 2,000 calories daily. The number of servings may vary from those listed depending on caloric needs.
*Serving sizes may vary between $\frac{1}{2}$ and 1 $\frac{1}{4}$ cups.
**Fat content changes serving counts for fats and oils: (1 Tbsp of regular salad dressing equals $\frac{1}{2}$ serving; 1 Tbsp of fat-free dressing equals 0 servings).
Source: National Heart, Lung, and Blood Institute.

1500 mg). Reductions in blood pressure were proportional to the level of sodium restriction. Thus, optimum medical nutrition therapy for hypertension provides a diet that includes:

- reduced sodium intake
- generous amounts of potassium and calcium
- abstinence from or moderation of alcohol intake
- continued weight control.

Obesity and Hypertension

Obesity is a major risk factor in the development of hypertension. It has been estimated that 60 percent of the hypertensive population are more than 20 percent overweight. A linear relationship exists between the degree of obesity and the severity of hypertension. The beneficial effect of weight reduction in hypertensive individuals has been clearly documented. Controlled dietary intervention trials estimate that a mean reduction in body weight of 20 pounds (9.2 kg) is associated with a 6.3 mm Hg reduction in systolic blood pressure and a 3.1 mm Hg reduction in diastolic blood pressure. The exact mechanism of obesity-induced hypertension is unclear, but increased cardiac output, sodium retention, and increased sympathetic activity in response to elevated insulin levels are all thought to be significant contributors. Weight reduction should be the primary goal for the overweight hypertensive patient, since even a ten percent change in body weight is sufficient to reduce blood pressure.

Dietary Sodium Intake

Population studies have repeatedly demonstrated a relationship of hypertension to higher sodium intakes. However, not all individuals respond the same way to dietary sodium. Depletion and loading studies indicate that up to 50 percent of hypertensive patients are salt-sensitive. Salt sensitivity appears to be associated with several demographic variables such as obesity, African-American race, and older age. Unfortunately, there is no simple way to determine salt sensitivity in the clinical setting.

The Joint National Committee on Prevention, Detection, Evaluation and Treatment of High Blood Pressure (JNC VII) recommends limiting sodium to 2400 mg daily for patients with hypertension. The typical American diet contains approximately 4 to 8 grams of sodium per day. Table salt and foods high in sodium – such as salted, smoked, canned, and highly processed foods – should be limited. The use of convenience foods, fast foods, and eating out frequently all contribute to higher sodium intakes among Americans. Key questions for patients with hypertension are:

- Do you use a salt shaker at the table or in cooking?
- Do you read labels for sodium content? (Recommend <400 mg/serving.)
- How often do you eat canned, smoked, frozen, and processed foods?

Dietary Potassium Intake

Epidemiologic and observational studies have reported an inverse correlation between potassium intake and blood pressure, especially among African-Americans and individuals consuming a high-sodium diet. More recently, several small intervention studies have shown that potassium supplementation results in a modest hypotensive effect. Although the exact mechanism remains unclear, effects of potassium supplementation include naturesis, inhibition of renin release, and decreased thromboxane production. For practical purposes, increasing dietary intake of potassium may have a beneficial effect on blood pressure. Foods high in potassium include oranges, orange juice, potatoes (especially with the skins), and bananas. To maintain a high potassium intake, the DASH diet includes 8 to 10 servings of fruits and vegetables daily. Certain diuretic therapy, specifically loop diuretics, frequently induces potassium wasting. Increasing dietary intake in these patients may obviate the need for synthetic potassium supplements, which require close monitoring.

Dietary Calcium Intake

Calcium intake may be lower among hypertensive patients than among normotensive individuals. Increased dietary intake may reduce the incidence of hypertension and calcium supplements may produce a hypotensive effect in some patients. Although dietary calcium has been correlated with blood pressure, calcium supplementation has not been shown to significantly lower blood pressure. On the other hand, the inclusion of low-fat dairy food within the framework of the DASH diet did provide additional blood pressure lowering, as outlined in Table 6-6, which advises two to three servings per day of fat-free or low-fat dairy food. (See Appendices G and H: Dietary Sources of Calcium.)

Alcohol Intake

Individuals who drink three or more alcoholic beverages per day account for 5 to 7 percent of those diagnosed with hypertension. Evidence shows that two or more drinks per day can lead to an increase in blood pressure. Although alcohol acts as a vasodilator, chronic alcohol ingestion is associated with increased formation of the vasoconstrictor thromboxane. Chronically increased levels of this prostaglandin metabolite may be partially responsible for the hypertensive effect of chronic alcohol ingestion. In controlled studies, reducing alcohol consumption in this population has been associated with a modest reduction in blood pressure.

Heart Failure

Heart failure (HF), which affects nearly 5 million adults in the United States, is characterized by decreased cardiac output, venous stasis, sodium and fluid retention, and undernutrition. Reduced function of the left ventricle and accompanying neurohormonal changes promote accumulation of sodium and water. Shortness of breath, fatigue, and inactivity result. The dearth of clinical trials regarding medical nutrition therapy for HF provides a much weaker evidence-base than the basis for nutritional intervention for hyperlipidemia or hypertension. Nevertheless, attention to medical nutrition therapy in the management of patients with HF is critical.

Causes of Undernutrition in Heart Failure

Cardiac cachexia is the wasting and undernutrition seen in patients with long-standing HF. As myocardial function progressively deteriorates, patients present with loss of adipose tissue and lean body mass secondary to poor nutritional intake and decreased activity. Upper-body and temporal wasting with lower-extremity edema are the hallmark features of this condition. The proposed mechanisms to explain cardiac cachexia include:

- impaired cellular oxygen supply
- increased nutrient losses
- increased nutritional requirements
- decreased nutritional intake.

Impaired cellular oxygen supply Decreased cardiac output reduces oxygen delivery to cells, resulting in inefficient substrate oxidation and inadequate synthesis of high-energy intermediary metabolites.

Increased nutrient losses Hypoxemia and increased venous pressure may cause bowel edema with subsequent fat and protein malabsorption. Decreased synthesis of hepatic bile salts and pancreatic enzymes caused by oxygen deprivation to the liver and pancreas may further contribute to this. Proteinuria is also a feature of HF secondary to the reduced renal blood flow characteristic of this disorder.

Increased nutritional requirements Patients with HF can be hypermetabolic and therefore have increased nutritional requirements. This hypermetabolic state is caused by the increased work required for breathing, the mechanical work of the heart, and oxygen consumption related to alterations in neuroendocrine activity. If additional calories are not ingested to meet these increased demands, weight loss ensues.

Decreased nutritional intake Factors that may result in an inadequate food intake in patients with HF include one or all of the following:
- hepatomegaly and ascites reduce functional gastric volume causing early satiety
- dyspnea and fatigue induced by eating
- unpalatable low-sodium diets
- anorexia, nausea, or vomiting from medications used to treat CHF.

Medical Nutrition Therapy for Heart Failure

Medical nutrition therapy for patients with HF should be aimed at controlling sodium and fluid retention, restoring and maintaining body weight, providing adequate energy, protein, vitamins, and minerals, and repletion of protein stores in patients who have lost lean body mass.

Dietary Sodium Intake

Patients with HF retain sodium and fluid and therefore, dietary sodium restriction is a cornerstone of treatment. The level of sodium restriction may be individualized according to the severity of the HF. It is recommended that patients with symptomatic HF reduce dietary sodium intake to 2 to 3 grams (2000 to 3000 mg) per day. The American Dietetic Association Evidence Analysis Library reports fair evidence for restricting sodium intake to 2 grams per day. Sodium restriction supports the effectiveness of diuretic agents in achieving negative sodium balance. One-fourth or more of hospital re-admissions for patients with HF are due to non-compliance with dietary advice. Patients need more than to be told "stay away from salt." They need to be able to state their recommended level of dietary sodium, use values on the nutrition label to guide their intake, and distinguish between very high and very low sources of sodium.

A recent study in an urban heart failure clinic linked knowledge of dietary sodium sources with consumption of fewer high sodium foods. Another report indicated that one hour of education before hospital discharge decreased likelihood of rehospitalization by 35 percent and saved $ 2823 per patient. Whether the patient is seen in the acute care or ambulatory care setting, referral to the registered dietitian for assessment of their nutritional status and assistance in achieving the skills needed to manage a sodium restricted diet at home is appropriate for cost-effective management of HF. Salt substitutes are available to flavor foods, but many of them substitute potassium for sodium. Patients with renal failure or those taking potassium-sparing diuretics should avoid these products. (See Appendix I: Dietary Sources of High Sodium Foods.)

Fluid

Heart failure associated with dilutional hyponatremia may require restricting fluid intake to 1500 to 2000 mL per day. The fluid may be restricted slightly more in the hospital setting. Some suggest limiting daily fluid intake to an amount equal to the 24-hour urine output volume plus 500 mL. Traditional nutrition assessment parameters, such as actual body weight or weight change, may not accurately reflect nutritional status in HF patients. For example, cardiac cachexia may go undetected if body weight is normal or elevated because of sodium and water retention. In addition, serum protein levels, such as albumin, may be decreased secondary to either undernutrition or artificially as a result of fluid overload. When HF appears well controlled with no evidence of edema or ascites, and low serum BNP (B-type natriuretic peptide) levels, increase in weight is more likely actual dry weight gain.

Calories and Protein

Daily caloric intake should be adequate to promote weight gain (if needed) in patients with HF. Research indicates HF patients generally need higher calories than a healthy control subject, but research to date does not provide an accurate definition of how many calories most HF patients need. Some practitioners estimate dietary calories at 1.5 times the basal energy expenditure. Another set of recommendations suggests 28–30 kcal/kg of ideal body weight for weight maintenance and 32–35 kcal/kg actual weight for the undernourished patient. Provision of 1.5 g/kg/day of protein can promote anabolism and achieve positive nitrogen balance in a patient with cardiac cachexia. High-protein, high-calorie supplements are often necessary to achieve this calorie requirement, especially when the patient has a poor appetite. Nutritional supplements, both liquid and pudding forms, are available and provide a high concentration of calories and protein in a relatively small volume. The sodium and fluid content of HF supplements must be considered in the total daily sodium and fluid allowance. Small, frequent meals also may help HF patients achieve an adequate dietary intake. Patients who cannot meet their caloric and protein requirements orally may require enteral tube feeding (Chapter 12). Enteral feeding in a HF patient can be precarious as it can result in overfeeding, which will aggravate the primary condition.

For some patients, obesity places additional strain on an already compromised heart. Thus, careful assessment of nutritional status and monitoring of dietary intake are valuable in providing for optimum nutritional support.

Other Nutrients and Supplements

Reduced food intake can not only reduce caloric intake, but also intake of various nutrients. Thiamin deficiency has been noted more frequently among heart failure patients. Daily intake of a multi-vitamin can improve intake of micronutrients and reduce the possible detrimental effects of thiamine deficiency on the heart. Although a number of additional supplements have been tested for benefit, there is limited evidence of benefit to date. A few small trials have shown improved exercise tolerance and quality of life for heart failure patients receiving coenzyme Q10.

Case 1 **Disorders of Lipid Metabolism**

Wahida Karmally and Henry Ginsberg

Columbia University, New York, NY

OBJECTIVES

- Identify cardiac risk factors for coronary artery disease in obese patients without known disease.

- Describe other physical examination findings and screening and laboratory measurements relevant in a patient with disorders of lipid metabolism.

- Describe the science-based nutritional and lifestyle recommendations for patients with disorders of lipid metabolism.

- Apply the current National Cholesterol Education Program Guidelines for screening, evaluation, and treatment of disorders of lipid metabolism.

- Recognize the importance of medical nutrition therapy and lifestyle recommendations for treatment and prevention of cardiovascular disease.

JT is a 52-year-old Puerto Rican man who consults a new physician for a routine physical examination because his employer has recently changed their health insurance plan. He has not seen a physician for the past 3 years.

Past Medical History

JT has no prior history of hospitalizations or chronic illnesses. He is not taking any medications or over-the-counter dietary or herbal supplements, and he has no known food allergies.

Family History

JT's family history is positive for heart disease. His father had a fatal heart attack at age 54, and his father's brother had a heart attack at age 55. JT's uncle is currently being treated for hypercholesterolemia. There is no family history of hypertension, diabetes, or obesity.

Social History

JT works as an accountant and reports a high stress level both at work and at home. His work commitments do not allow him much free time so he frequently orders lunch in and eats at his desk. After a long day at work and his 45-minute commute home, JT feels too tired to exercise. Over the past 3 years he has experienced a 12 pound weight gain. JT attributes this to his sedentary, high-stress lifestyle, and to

---

Medical Nutrition and Disease: A Case-Based Approach, 4th edition. Edited by Lisa Hark.
© 2009 Wiley-Blackwell Publishing, ISBN: 978-1-4051-8615-5.

dining out with clients on average 2 to 3 nights per week. JT is a non-smoker. He drinks a 20 ounce (600 mL) cup of regular coffee every morning and two alcoholic beverages every evening. JT is married and has one daughter who is currently in her junior year of college.

Dietary Intake Using the 24-hour recall method, JT's physician obtained the following information about his typical diet.

Breakfast (office)

Bagel	1 large (4 ounces/113 g)
Cream cheese	2 Tbsp.
Coffee	20 ounces (600 mL)
Half-and-half	2 ounces (60 mL)

Lunch (restaurant)

Pizza with cheese	2 slices
Soda (cola)	12 ounces (360 mL)

Snack (office)

Jelly beans	1 ounce (28 g)

Evening (restaurant)

Hamburger	6 ounces (170 g)
Bun	1 large
French fries	1 cup
Vanilla ice cream	1 cup
Beer	24 ounces (720 mL)

Total calories: 2730 kcal
Protein: 106 g (16% of total calories)
Fat: 108.5 g (33.5% of total calories)
Saturated fat: 47 g (15.5% of total calories)
Monounsaturated fat: 36 g (12% of total calories)
Polyunsaturated fat: 10 g (3% of total calories)
Trans fat: 6.0 g (2% of total calories)
Cholesterol: 313 mg
Carbohydrate: 299 g (44% of total calories)
Dietary fiber: 11 g
Soluble fiber: 5 g
Sodium: 2680 mg

Review of Systems Noncontributory

Physical Examination
Vital Signs:
Temperature: 98 °F (37 °C)
Heart Rate: 76 BPM
Respiration: 20 BPM
Blood pressure: 139/88 mm Hg (High-normal 130–139/85–89 mm Hg)
Height: 5'10" (178 cm)
Current weight: 212 lb (96 kg)
BMI: 30.3 kg/m^2
Weight 2 years ago: 200 lb (91 kg)
Waist circumference: 42 inches (107 cm)

Exam
General: Obese male in no acute distress
Remainder of physical examination was normal and unremarkable

Laboratory Data
JT's lipid profile, after a 12-hour overnight fast, provided the following laboratory values:

Patient's Lab Values	Normal Values
Total cholesterol: 260 mg/dL	desirable <200 mg/dL
HDL-C: 32 mg/dL	desirable ≥40 mg/dL
LDL-C: 158 mg/dL	desirable <130 mg/dL
Triglycerides: 350 mg/dL	desirable <150 mg/dL
hsCRP: 4.5 mg/L	<3.0 mg/L
Homocysteine: 8 mol/L	<12 mol/L
Lp(a): 11 mg/dL	<20 mg/dL
Plasma glucose: 95 mg/dL	70 to 99 mg/dL

Framingham Point Score: 10-year risk for Coronary Heart Disease (CHD) is 16 percent based on total cholesterol level.

Case Questions

1. What additional questions should be asked of all patients during the general health maintenance screening?
2. What physical examination findings should one look for in a patient suspected of having disorders of lipid metabolism?
3. How should JT's lipid profile, waist circumference, and blood pressure be interpreted, based on the ATP III Guidelines? What about his hsCRP results?
4. Based on JT's medical history, physical examination, and laboratory data, how would you classify and diagnose his lipid disorder?
5. What are the science-based lifestyle recommendations for JT's disorder of lipid metabolism?
6. Is JT's current nutrient intake within the recommended guidelines of the ATP III Therapeutic Lifestyle Changes (TLC) diet?
7. What are the best dietary approaches for this patient?
8. How can JT translate the recommended dietary guidelines into food choices?
9. Should JT receive a lipid-lowering medication at this time?

Table 6-7 Causes of Secondary Dyslipidemia

Endocrine/Metabolic	Drugs
Diabetes mellitus	Alcohol
Obesity	Cyclosporine
Hypothyroidism	Androgens
Hypogonadism	Estrogens
Hypercortisolism	Progestins

Source: Henry Ginsberg, MD and Wahida Karmally, DrPH, RD, CDE, CLS. Used with permission.

Answers to Questions: Case 1
Part 1: Screening, Risk Assessment, and Diagnosis

1. What additional questions should be asked of all patients during general health maintenance screening?

During the general health maintenance screen, a thorough history should include questions related to cardiac risk factors. Traditional risk factors for coronary artery disease in this patient include elevated total, LDL-C and triglyceride levels, age (men >45), family history of heart disease, low HDL-C, borderline hypertension, obesity (BMI ≥ 30 kg/m^2), increased waist circumference (>40″), elevated hsCRP, and smoking habits. Nutrient intake, average weekly alcohol consumption, alternative medicine (dietary supplements such as botanicals, fish oil, etc.) use, exercise habits, and stress levels are also important areas to explore. The physician should also consider in the past medical history any diseases that directly increase cardiovascular risk (e.g. diabetes) or any secondary medical disorder that could be contributing or causing the disorder of lipid metabolism (Table 6-7).

2. What physical examination findings should one look for in a patient suspected of having disorders of lipid metabolism?

In addition to general health screening, patients suspected of having dyslipidemia should undergo an examination of pulses (palpation of all pulses, and auscultation for bruits in the carotid and femoral arteries), thyroid palpation (hypothyroidism is a possible secondary cause of hypercholesterolemia), an eye examination for corneal arcus senilis, and a tendon and skin examination for xanthelasmas or xanthomas.

3. How should JT's lipid profile, waist circumference, and blood pressure be interpreted, based on the ATP III Guidelines? What about his hsCRP results?

The current National Cholesterol Education Program (NCEP) ATP III guidelines recommend a complete lipoprotein profile (total cholesterol, LDL-C, HDL-C, and triglycerides) as the preferred initial laboratory test, rather than screening for total cholesterol and HDL-C alone. In addition, ATP III's major new focus is on primary prevention of CHD in persons with multiple risk factors. Primary prevention is the treatment of high risk individuals without established cardiovascular disease.

LDL-C can be calculated using the following equation. Techniques for measuring LDL-C directly also are available:

$$\text{Total cholesterol} = \text{HDL-C} + \text{LDL-C} + \text{VLDL-C or}$$

$$\text{LDL-C} = \text{Total cholesterol} - (\text{HDL-C} + \text{VLDL-C})$$

$$\text{VLDL-C} = \frac{\text{Triglyceride level}}{5}$$

In dyslipidemic states, a triglyceride level greater than 400 mg/dL invalidates the results of this equation. In addition to the screening tests described above, plasma homocysteine, Lp(a), and hsCRP levels were measured because of JT's family history of premature heart disease.

To rule out secondary or contributory causes of dyslipidemia, fasting serum glucose should also be measured to diagnose impaired glucose tolerance, pre-diabetes, or diabetes mellitus. Thyroid-stimulating hormone should also be measured to rule out hypothyroidism. If lipid-lowering drug therapy is required, baseline liver transaminases (ALT and AST) and uric acid levels may be helpful in choosing the appropriate type of drug therapy.

Patients with abdominal obesity should be evaluated for metabolic syndrome. Each of the five clinical criteria for metabolic syndrome can be obtained via a focused medical history, brief physical examination, and fasting laboratory data (Table 6-7). Recent estimates suggest that 24 percent of the US population meets the current National Cholesterol Education Panel's (NCEP) criteria for metabolic syndrome. NCEP has identified metabolic syndrome as a secondary target of therapy in dyslipidemic patients. JT has four out of the five criteria for metabolic syndrome, including abdominal obesity, elevated triglycerides, low HDL-C, and borderline high blood pressure:

- Borderline high blood pressure: 139/88 mm Hg
- Abdominal obesity: waist circumference 42″
- Low HDL-C: 32 mg/dL,
- Elevated triglycerides: 350 mg/dL

4. Based on JT's medical history, physical examination, and laboratory data, how would you classify and diagnose his lipid disorder?

This type of lipid disorder is called dyslipidemia since both JT's total plasma triglycerides and LDL-C concentrations are elevated and HDL-C is low. Although it is likely that a variety of combinations of regulatory defects in lipid metabolism account for a significant number of individuals with this phenotype, familial forms of dyslipidemia (FCHL) have been identified in which members of the same family may have dyslipidemia, only hypertriglyceridemia, or only elevated LDL-C concentrations. In the familial disorder, which appears to be transmitted as autosomal dominant gene(s), the diagnosis must rest on the presentation of combined hyperlipidemia or the presence of various phenotypes in first-degree family members along with either isolated hypertriglyceridemia or isolated LDL-C elevation in the patient. FCHL is estimated to occur in one out of 100 Americans and is the most common familial lipid disorder found in survivors of myocardial infarction.

FCHL appears to be associated with the secretion of increased numbers of very-low-density lipoprotein (VLDL) particles. Once these individuals assemble and secrete increased numbers of large triglyceride-rich VLDL, their plasma triglyceride concentrations depend on their ability to hydrolyze VLDL triglycerides with lipoprotein lipase and, to a lesser degree, with hepatic lipase.

The ability to hydrolyze VLDL triglycerides also regulates the generation of LDLs in the plasma. Thus subjects with FCHL who have very high VLDL triglyceride concentrations (and are not able to efficiently catabolize VLDLs) might have normal or reduced numbers of LDL particles in the circulation and thus a normal LDL-C concentration. If these same individuals were able to efficiently catabolize the increased numbers of VLDL particles that were entering the plasma, they would generate increased numbers of LDL particles and have both hypertriglyceridemia and a high LDL-C levels. Patients with FCHL who synthesize only normal quantities of triglycerides and secrete increased numbers of VLDLs carrying normal triglyceride loads would generate increased numbers of LDL particles and have elevated plasma LDL-C concentrations only.

5. What is the currently recommended treatment and follow-up for JT's dyslipidemia?

According to Step 9 in the ATP III Guidelines, the first step is to set his LDL-C goal. JT's non-HDL-C goal is 160 mg/dL (LDL-C goal + 30). Because JT has the metabolic syndrome and his Framingham score is 16%, the physician may decide to be more aggressive by lowering his non-HDL-C goal to 130 mg/dL.

Second, intensify weight management, and increase physical activity. If triglycerides are 200 to 499 mg/dL, after LDL-C goal is reached, set a secondary goal for non-HDL-C (total − HDL) of 30 mg/dL higher than the LDL-C goal.

Part 2: Medical Nutrition Therapy
What is the patient's stage of behavior change? And what would you say to encourage him? What are some of his barriers to change?

HJT admitted early in his visit that he feels hopeless about his weight. Now he tells the doctor that he knows he has to lose weight and wants to know how much. He also tells his doctor that he needs to get educated on choosing low-fat foods. JT has probably already been thinking about making a change (Contemplation) – and perhaps he is now moving into the Preparation stage (Table 6-8). The role of the clinician is to confirm that weight loss would be slow, provide some guidance on how much weight loss to aim for (e.g. a loss of 10 percent of body weight is often achievable over six to twelve months). Barriers to weight loss that JT may encounter:

- Stress at work. He orders his "usual" high-fat meal without looking for opportunities to find lower fat alternatives.
- There may be social meetings two to three nights that include excessive eating and drinking.
- He may be unaware of opportunities for increased daily physical activity at work.
- He is overwhelmed with work and does not feel that he can add physical activity into his routine.
- His wife may not understand the seriousness of his health and may not be supportive by cooking healthy meals when he eats at home.

Table 6-8 Stages of Change Processes of the Transtheoretical Model

Stages of change	Appropriate advice for each stage
Precontemplation: Not interested in change.	Should receive brief advice and offer of future help.
Contemplation: Thinking about making a change.	Advise patient and assist to reduce obstacles to change.
Preparation: Is getting ready to change.	Advise and provide assistance and follow-up as needed.
Action: Is working on the change.	Follow-up, support, and encouragement as needed.
Maintenance: Trying to maintain the change.	Follow-up, support, and encouragement as needed.

Source: Finckenor MA, Byrd-Bredbenner C. *J Am Diet Assoc.* 2000;100:335–342.

6. Is JT's current nutrient intake within the recommended guidelines of the ATP III Therapeutic Lifestyle Changes (TLC) diet?

The key elements of the TLC diet include:

- Saturated fat below 7% of calories; (*trans* fat <1% of calories)
- Dietary cholesterol intake below 200 mg/day
- Increase viscous (soluble) fiber to 10–25 grams/day
- Include 2 grams/day of plant sterols / stanols daily
- Weight management
- Increased physical activity

JT's current diet is not within the recommended guidelines of the TLC diet. According to the nutritional analysis of his current intake, JT's saturated fat intake is about 16 percent of his caloric intake (recommended is less than 7 percent), *trans* fat intake is 3 percent of calories (needs to be decreased to less than 1 percent of calories) and cholesterol intake is 313 mg (recommended less than 200 mg per day).

Significant sources of saturated fat in JT's diet come from high-fat dairy foods including half and half, cream cheese, mozzarella cheese, and ice cream as well as the ground red meat. His caloric intake is approximately 2700 calories per day. This excessive calorie intake combined with his sedentary lifestyle will continue to promote weight gain unless he reduces total calories and routinely participates in some physical activity. In order to lose 1 to 2 pounds of body weight per week (which is the recommended rate of weight loss), JT must reduce his weight maintenance caloric needs by at least 500 calories and increase activity by 250 calories daily. Alternatively, JT may choose to exercise more rather than eat less to achieve the targeted weight loss.

JT's typical diet is deficient in fruit and vegetables, which are generally low in calories and are nutrient dense. The DASH diet (Table 6-6) has been found to be very effective in lowering blood pressure and can also be recommended to JT. Many of the elements are similar to the "heart healthy" TLC diet (Table 6-5) (ATP III) – but the DASH diet especially emphasizes greater intake of vegetables, fruits, and whole grains. The DASH diet includes 7 to 8 servings of whole grains; 4 to 5 servings of vegetables; 4 to 5 servings of fruits; 2 to 3 servings of non-fat dairy products; 2 or less servings of meats; 2 to 3 servings of fats/oils on a daily basis. It also includes less than 3 grams of sodium/day; 4 to 5 servings of nuts/week. JT's diet contains only 11 grams of dietary fiber/day and 5 grams of soluble fiber/day, compared to the TLC diet, which recommends 10 to 25 grams of soluble (viscous) fiber/day as adjunctive therapy to reduce LDL-C.

7. What are the best lifestyle approaches for this patient?

JT's modifiable risk factors include obesity, high saturated fat diet, sedentary lifestyle, and excessive alcohol consumption. Implementing a number of lifestyle and behavioral changes should improve JT's risk profile significantly.

The first line of therapy for all lipid and non-lipid factors associated with the metabolic syndrome is weight reduction and increased physical activity. The ATP III guidelines recognize overweight and obesity as major underlying risk factors for coronary heart disease. Regular physical activity is a component in the management of dyslipidemia.

In order to make dietary recommendations, it is necessary to first define the desired endpoint or goal for each individual. Is the goal to reduce triglycerides and LDL-C with/without weight reduction? For JT the goal is to lower total cholesterol, LDL-C, and triglycerides, raise HDL-C levels, and reduce weight. He can achieve this by adhering to the TLC diet or the DASH diet and reducing his total caloric intake. Monounsaturated fat and omega-3 fatty acids should be favored in place of both saturated and omega-6 fatty acids, while keeping total fat to a maximum of 35 percent of total calories.

The specific dietary recommendations include reducing total calories and saturated fat intake (less than 7 percent), decreasing *trans* fat to less than 1 percent of calories, increase monounsaturated fat (up to 20 percent), and reduce alcohol intake.

8. How can JT translate the recommended dietary guidelines into food choices?

A hypocaloric diet, which favors monounsaturated fat, is recommended for JT. Sources of monounsaturated fats are canola oil, olive oil, hazelnuts, almonds, unsalted peanuts, peanut butter, pistachios, pecans, avocado, and high oleic acid safflower oil and sunflower oils. The main sources of omega-3 fatty acids are fatty fish such as salmon, mackerel, herring, sardines, and plant foods such as flax seeds and walnuts. The main sources of *trans* fat are the French fries and pizza crust made with partially hydrogenated oils. He can substitute with a baked potato or brown rice or barley. JT should eat more vegetables, fruits, whole grains, and beans, only non-fat or very low-fat dairy products, and chicken without skin, fish, or lean meats limited to 5 to 6 ounces per day. If he enjoys eggs, he can include 2 large eggs per week.

His fiber intake would be significantly increased with the recommended servings of fresh fruits, vegetables, and whole grains. Therapeutic options for enhancing LDL-C reduction include increased intake of viscous (soluble) fiber (10 to 25 grams per day) from oats, psyllium, dried beans, and fruits such as strawberries, apples, and vegetables such as okra and eggplant. Fat spreads containing plant stanol/sterols (2 grams per day) could be included to further lower LDL-C in place of other spreads the patient may currently be using. Plant stanols/sterols containing products available in the supermarkets, which can be obtained from products such as "Benecol" (2 to 3 servings per day), "Promise Activ" spread (2 servings per day), or "SuperShots" (one serving per day), can reduce LDL-C by 7 to 15 percent. It is important to note that these products have calories and should be replaced with other fat sources, such as margarine or cream cheese. JT will benefit from a reduction in alcohol and sodium intake. Alcohol adds calories to JT's diet and can raise triglycerides and blood pressure.

JT's Recommended Modified Fat Diet:
Breakfast
Oat cereal	2 cups
Skim milk	1 cup
Orange, navel	1

Lunch
Tuna, canned, water pack	0.5 cup
Whole wheat bread	2 slices
Tomato	1/2 medium
Carrot	1/2 cup
Mayonnaise or olive oil	1 Tbsp.
Non-fat flavored yogurt	1 cup

Dinner
Chicken breast, baked	3 ounces (85 g)
Noodles, cooked	1 cup
Broccoli/eggplant	2 cup
Romaine lettuce	2 cups
Olive oil	1 Tbsp.
Vinegar	1 Tbsp.
Banana	1 small

Snack
Apple	1 small
Peanut butter	2 Tbsp.
Skim milk	6 ounces (180 mL)

Total calories: 1960 kcal
Protein: 107 g (22% protein calories)
Total fat: 62 g (29% fat calories)
Saturated fat: 12 g (6% SFA calories)
Polyunsaturated fat: 19 g (9% PUFA calories)
Monounsaturated fat: 27 g (12% MUFA calories)
Cholesterol: 163 mg
Carbohydrate: 229 g (47% carbohydrate calories)
Fiber: 31 g
Soluble fiber: 10 g
Sodium: 2172 mg

Part 3: Lipid Lowering Medication
9. Should JT receive a lipid-lowering medication at this time?

JT may require drug therapy at some point in the future, but only after an adequate trial of lifestyle modification has been undertaken, so the answer is no. It should be emphasized, however, that if pharmacologic intervention becomes necessary it should be thought of as an adjunct, and not as a substitute to lifestyle modification as a way to reduce his lipid levels.

The physician needs to set the stage for dietary treatment and increases in physical activity. The physician's positive attitude toward lifestyle changes can influence the patient's attitude and success toward making these changes. An explanation of the positive effects that lifestyle modification can have on JT's prognosis should be highlighted. These benefits include lower LDL-C and triglyceride levels, increased HDL-C levels (usually only modestly), decreased blood pressure, increased cardiac output, increased collateral blood supply, and stress relief. Regardless of age, patients should begin any exercise program gradually and include 5 to 10 minutes of warming up at the beginning of exercise and cooling down at the end. The ultimate goal is to increase the total workout to 30 minutes daily. JT would need a stress test (>40 years of age) before he starts an exercise program.

Referring the patient to a registered dietitian often helps to facilitate dietary changes. The patient's readiness to make behavioral changes needs to be assessed. Most patients are not ready to make dramatic changes in their lifestyle habits during the first meeting. In addition, assessment of the patient's compliance is essential to determine if the diet changes are optimal to maximize their effects on lipid metabolism. Diet instruction may require several follow-up visits. Early initial follow-up (every 4 to 6 weeks) is important because it affords opportunities to verify adherence to, and provide support for, diet and exercise changes. Later, the patient can be monitored at intervals deemed appropriate to reinforce ATP III's TLC Diet and to check lipid levels. In a patient such as JT, lifestyle changes should be attempted for 4 to 6 months before considering drug therapy, because they may bring about a significant decrease in lipid parameters, thereby obviating the need for drug therapy.

Drug Treatment

If JT's lipid profile does not respond to diet and exercise, drug treatment should be initiated. The primary goal is lowering LDL-C and secondary goals are to lower triglycerides (TG) and raise HDL-C. The following drugs may be considered:

Statin lowers LDL-C and can lower TG at higher doses.

Nicotinic Acid (Niacin) lowers LDL-C and TG levels and raises HDL-C. It can also increase insulin resistance; this would be less of a risk if JT loses weight concomitantly.

Fibric Acid Derivatives Lower TG and raises HDL-C; can have a modest (about 6 percent) LDL-C-lowering effect.

Case 2 **Hypertension and Lifestyle Modifications**

Frances Burke and Diana Fischmann

University of Pennsylvania School of Medicine, Philadelphia, PA

OBJECTIVES

- Define pre-hypertension and discuss reasons behind its introduction in the JNC 7 report.
- List the diet and lifestyle factors that may contribute to the development of hypertension.
- Describe the parameters of the DASH diet for the treatment of hypertension.
- Prioritize nutritional goals for the patient with hypertension based on the medical and social history, physical examination, and laboratory data.
- Discuss counseling strategies that may impact treatment compliance in patients with hypertension.

RF is a 36-year-old African-American male with pre-hypertension. During his last visit to his family doctor his blood pressure was elevated and he complained of occasional heartburn after meals. His physician recommended a 24-hour BP monitor, Prilosec to treat heartburn, and that he focus on his diet and lifestyle for weight reduction. RF is to return in 6 weeks to review his results.

Past Medical History

RF has no significant past medical history. He describes a gradual weight gain over the past 15 years, with his current weight being his highest. He was a college-level football player weighing around 200 pounds at the time. Following his college graduation, he slowly gained approximately 40 to 50 pounds.

Family History:

RF has a positive family history of overweight and obesity, heart disease, and hypertension. His mother and brother are obese. His mother has hypertension and is currently being treated with antihypertensive medications. Paternal grandfather had a myocardial infarction (MI) at age 62 and his father has a high cholesterol level.

Medications

RF takes no medications or over-the-counter dietary supplements.

Medical Nutrition and Disease: A Case-Based Approach, 4th edition. Edited by Lisa Hark.
© 2009 Wiley-Blackwell Publishing, ISBN: 978-1-4051-8615-5.

Social/Diet History

RF lives with his wife and two children and works as a corrections officer in a local prison. He eats three meals a day. RF typically eats fast food for breakfast and lunch and enjoys snacking after dinner. He does not engage in regular physical activity and has not done so for the last ten years. He denies any recreational drug use and drinks one beer a day with dinner. RF smoked two packs of cigarettes per day for 18 years (36 pack-year history). He quit 2 years ago.

RF's Usual Diet:

Breakfast:

Bagel	1 large
Cream cheese	2 Tbsp.
Orange juice	12 ounces

Lunch:

Roast beef hoagie	10 inch size
Russian dressing	2 Tbsp.
Potato chips	2 ounces bag
Regular soda	20 ounces

Snack:

Cheese/peanut butter crackers	1 package (6 crackers)

Dinner:

Baked chicken	1 breast and thigh with skin
Baked potato	1 large
Butter	1 Tbsp.
Green salad	2 cups
French dressing	2 Tbsp.
Beer	12 ounces bottle

Snack:

Salted nuts	4 ounces
Regular soda	12 ounces

Total calories: 4117 kcal
Protein: 158 g (15% of total calories)
Fat: 185 g (41 % of total calories)
Saturated fat: 46 g (10% of total calories)
Monounsaturated fat: 57 g (12% of total calories)
Polyunsaturated fat: 25 g (5% of total calories)
Cholesterol: 334 mg
Carbohydrate: 450 g (44% of total calories)
Dietary fiber: 23 g
Soluble fiber: 1 g
Sodium: 6319 mg
Calcium: 476 mg

Review of Systems

General: Denies sleep problems
Gastrointestinal: Occasional GERD after eating
Neurologic: No headaches, tremors, seizures, or depression
Musculoskeletal: No muscle or joint pain, no swelling or redness
Pulmonary: Short of breath when climbing stairs

Physical Examination
Vital Signs

Temperature: 98.4 °F (36.8 °C)
Heart rate: 65 beats per minute (BPM)
Respiratory rate: 12 BPM
Blood pressure: 140/92 mm Hg
Height: 5′10″ (178 cm)
Current weight: 248 lbs (110 kg)
BMI: 35.5 kg/m^2
Waist circumference: 42 inches

Exam

General: Overweight male in no acute distress
Head/neck/skin: Nonpalpable thyroid; no hirsutism or striae; no acanthosis nigricans
Cardiac: S1 and S2 normal, regular rate and rhythm; no murmurs or gallops.
Chest: Clear to percussion and auscultation
Abdomen: Obese non-tender, no masses
Extremities: No edema
Neurologic: Alert and oriented to person, place, and time, intact memory.

Laboratory Data

Patient's Fasting Laboratory Values	Normal Values
Glucose: 99 mg/dL	70–99 mg/dL
Potassium: 3.8 mEq/L	3.5–5.3 mEq/L
Serum cholesterol: 210 mg/dL	desirable <200 mg/dL
Triglycerides: 175 mg/dL	desirable <150 mg/dL
HDL-C: 41 mg/dL	desirable >40 mg/dL
LDL-C: 134 mg/dL	desirable <130 mg/dL

Follow-up Description

RF returned in 6 weeks for his follow-up doctor's appointment. His 24-hour blood pressure monitor confirmed a diagnosis of stage 1 hypertension. RF reported that the Prilosec alleviated his heartburn.

Case Questions:

1. What is the difference between pre-hypertension and clinical hypertension?
2. What are the medical risks associated with high blood pressure?
3. What role does sodium play in the pathogenesis of high blood pressure?
4. What are the effects of diet and lifestyle factors on blood pressure control?
5. How does RF's lifestyle contribute to his high blood pressure?
6. What evidence-based lifestyle recommendations would you counsel RF on given his current diagnosis?
7. What factors would help to increase adherence in hypertensive patients?

Answers to Questions: Case 2

1. What is the difference between pre-hypertension and clinical hypertension?

Pre-hypertension affects approximately 70 million people in the United States. More men than women have pre-hypertension, and the prevalence in similar in both blacks and whites. The risk of developing hypertension is 2-fold higher in pre-hypertensives as compared with those who have lower BP levels. *The Seventh Report of the Joint National Committee on the Prevention, Detection, Evaluation and Treatment of High Blood Pressure* (JNC-7) first defined pre-hypertension as a systolic blood pressure (SBP) of 120 to 139 mm Hg and/or diastolic blood pressure (DBP) of 80 to 89 mm Hg. The term was established to focus attention on those individuals who were at higher than normal risk of cardiovascular disease (CVD) and in whom lifestyle approaches to prevent or delay the onset of hypertension would be beneficial.

The decision to establish this new BP category was based on the following factors:
- BP increases with age;
- about 90 percent of individuals age 55 years or older with normal BP ultimately develop hypertension in their lifetime;
- in observational studies in adults between 40 and 80 years of age, the risk of CVD doubles with each incremental elevation in BP of 20/10 mm Hg starting at 115/75 mm Hg.

Primary or essential hypertension accounts for about 95 percent of all hypertension cases, which is defined as having a SBP of 140 mm Hg or greater, having a DBP of 90 mm Hg or greater, or taking antihypertensive medications. Both genetic and lifestyle factors play a role in an individual's risk of developing hypertension.

2. What are the medical risks associated with high blood pressure?

Hypertension is a major contributor to the burden of disease, yet it remains inadequately controlled in approximately two-thirds of patients in the United States. Elevated BP is a risk factor for cardiovascular and renal diseases including stroke, coronary heart disease, heart, and kidney failure. The relationship is both continuous and consistent. Hypertension frequently coexists with other cardiovascular disease risk factors including obesity, dyslipidemia, insulin resistance, and glucose intolerance. Antihypertensive therapy has been associated with mean reductions of 35 to 40 percent in stroke incidence, 20 to 25 percent in myocardial infarction, and more than 50 percent in heart failure in clinical trials.

3. What role does sodium play in the pathogenesis of high blood pressure?

Sodium is the nutrient most widely investigated for its effect on blood pressure. Both observational and randomized controlled studies have documented that a high sodium intake increases blood pressure. In populations where the dietary intake of sodium is less than 50 mmoL (1150 mg sodium) per day, primary hypertension and age-related increases in blood pressure are almost non-existent.

The International Study of Salt and Blood Pressure (INTERSALT), a large observational study, which included 10,079 participants from 32 countries, showed that populations with average daily sodium intakes less than 1265 mg have low blood pressure and little or no increase in blood pressure with age. This study also showed a median urinary sodium excretion level of 170 mmoL (3910 mg) per day, which is approximately 10 g of salt (sodium chloride). Several randomized controlled trials have consistently shown a reduction in blood pressure with sodium restriction. A recent meta-analysis of randomized controlled trials, at least 4 weeks in duration, showed that a reduction in sodium by 50 mmoL per day decreased SBP and DBP on average by 4.0 mm Hg and 2.5 mm Hg, respectively, in hypertensive participants and by 2.0 mm Hg and 1.0 mm Hg, respectively, in normotensive participants.

Several physiological mechanisms have been proposed to explain the relationship between sodium and hypertension. Increased cardiac output associated with extracellular fluid volume expansion is one postulated mechanism for the effect of sodium excess on blood pressure; however, increased sodium intake does not raise blood pressure in all individuals. Those that are most susceptible to dietary sodium intake are considered "salt sensitive," which is thought to be associated with several factors such as age, race, weight, and plasma renin levels. It is also believed that a high sodium intake over time may impair the structure and function of the heart and kidney leading to clinical disorders in cardiac, vascular, and renal function, such as those experienced in patients with long-standing hypertension.

The Food and Nutrition Board of the National Academy of Sciences set a daily tolerable upper limit for sodium intake of 2300 mg based on its belief that excessive sodium intake is associated with an increased risk of cardiovascular disease. The American Heart Association and JNC–7 recommendations for sodium intake are similar.

4. What are the effects of diet and lifestyle factors on blood pressure control?

Several diet and lifestyle factors have been found to strongly influence blood pressure. The Dietary Approaches to Stopping Hypertension (DASH) (Table 6-6) and the DASH-Sodium dietary patterns were developed from clinical trials to provide an eating plan that reduces blood pressure. The DASH diet emphasizes eating more fruits, vegetables, low-fat dairy products, whole grains, poultry, fish, and nuts. It limits intake of fats, red meat, sweets, and sugar-containing beverages. This dietary pattern is rich in potassium, magnesium, calcium, and fiber, and low in total and saturated fat and cholesterol. The DASH trial found that adherence to this diet led to a mean reduction for all participants in SBP of 5.5 mm Hg and 3.0 mm Hg in DBP compared to the control group following a Western-style diet. Among the hypertensive participants enrolled in the trial, the mean reduction SBP was 11.4 mmHg and 5.5 mm Hg in DBP. For hypertensive participants, the reductions in BP from following this diet were equivalent to drug therapy. The greatest change in BP was seen in African-American patients, who experienced a 13.2 mm Hg mean reduction in SBP and 6.1 mm Hg in DBP.

The subsequent DASH-Sodium trial looked at the effect of limiting dietary sodium intake and showed step-wise decreases in blood pressure. Reductions in sodium intake from 150 mmol per day (3450 mg per day) to 100 mmol per day (2300 mg per day) resulted in a 1.3 mm Hg reduction in SBP, and a further reduction to 50 mmol per day (1150 mg per day) resulted in an additional decrease of 1.7 mm Hg while following the DASH diet. The current JNC-7 recommends no more than 2400 mg per day of sodium (or 6 g per day of sodium chloride, table salt) along with adherence to the DASH diet and reports an approximate reduction in SBP of 8–14 mm Hg when followed. The *US Dietary Guidelines* advocate limiting sodium intake to less than 2300 mg per day.

Body weight is one of the strongest determinants of blood pressure. A BMI of 30 kg/m^2 or greater is significantly associated with blood pressure elevations. The results of a meta-analysis of 25 clinical trials indicate that an average weight loss of 5.1 kg results in a mean drop in SBP of 4.4 mm Hg and 3.6 mm Hg in DBP. Other studies have documented that weight loss can prevent the development of hypertension by 20 percent in individuals who are overweight and pre-hypertensive. The JNC-7 also reports a reduction in SBP of approximately 5 to 20 mm Hg for each 10 kg weight loss.

Physical activity is another lifestyle factor that affects blood pressure. Epidemiologic studies have shown an inverse relationship between physical activity and blood pressure. Participating in moderate aerobic physical activity five times a week for at least 30 minutes results in significant reductions in blood pressure, from 8 to 11 mm Hg in SBP and 7 to 8 mm Hg in DBP. The JNC-7 also reports a reduction in SBP of approximately 4 to 9 mm Hg with increased physical activity. Research has also suggested an added benefit of including resistance training, in addition to aerobic exercise, as a part of routine physical activity. Recent studies have demonstrated a reduction of as high as 13 mm Hg for both SBP and DSP in patients with previously diagnosed hypertension. Significant decreases have been found after as little as four weeks after the commencement of resistance training. The American Heart Association has prescribed three days of resistance training per week (two days for beginners) with exercises targeting a mixture of the major muscle groups.

A direct relationship between alcohol use and blood pressure has been well documented. This effect is particularly evident with alcohol intakes greater than 2 drinks per day (a drink is defined as 12 ounces beer, 5 ounces wine, or 1.5 ounces spirits). A meta-analysis of 15 randomly controlled trials found that reduction of alcohol intake resulted in a decrease in SBP of 3.3 mm Hg and DBP of 2.0 mm Hg. It was also found that the greater the reduction in alcohol intake, the greater the reduction of BP. From these studies it was suggested that for each reduction of one alcoholic drink per day, a reduction in both systolic and DBP of 1 mm Hg resulted.

5. How does RF's lifestyle contribute to his high blood pressure?

RF's current diet lacks many of the major components recommended by the DASH diet. By favoring fast food restaurants and eating foods high in salt (processed meats, cheese, and salty snacks), he is increasing his consumption of sodium significantly above the recommended limits (>6000 mg/day). His intake of fruits, vegetables, and dairy foods is low, while intake of foods high in saturated fat, including cream cheese, butter, fatty lunchmeats, and chicken skin, is high. Overall his typical dietary intake is low in both calcium (476 mg/day) and potassium, and high in sodium, fat, and calories.

RF's weight and lack of physical activity are also contributing to his high blood pressure. His current BMI of 35.5 kg/m^2 places him in the Class II obesity category, well above the recommended 24.9 kg/m^2. A weight loss of 20 pounds to start would have a significant effect on reducing his blood pressure. RF's daily intake of alcohol, fruit juice, and regular soda provides an excessive amount of calories, which can promote weight gain and prevent weight loss in a sedentary individual. RF states that he has not routinely exercised in 10 years, which is another lifestyle factor contributing to his high blood pressure.

6. What evidence-based lifestyle recommendations would you counsel RF on given his current diagnosis?

RF should be counseled to follow the lifestyle recommendations outlined in the DASH-Sodium and PREMIER studies. It has been recommended that patients with hypertension, or who are at risk for hypertension, consume diets high in fruits and vegetables (8 to 10 servings/day), low-fat dairy products (2 to 3 servings/day), and low in dietary salt. One serving of a fruit and vegetable is either a $\frac{1}{2}$ cup cooked or 1 cup fresh.

RF can increase his fruit and vegetable intake by eating a banana at breakfast with a high-fiber cereal, choosing a raw vegetable such as carrot sticks at lunch with a sandwich on whole grain bread, and preparing a large salad with dinner along with a cooked vegetable. RF should limit his morning intake of 100 percent orange juice to no more than 4 ounces per day. He can try mixing the juice with water if he finds this is not a sufficient quantity. (See Appendix O: Food Sources of Dietary Fiber.)

Snacks are an especially good place for RF to increase his intake of DASH-recommended foods; all that is required is a little advance planning. Bringing a low-fat cheese stick, a cottage cheese snack pack, a fat-free yogurt, or an apple with him to work will provide a readily accessible snack, rather than choosing an item from the vending machine. Another strategy would be for RF to purchase multiple pieces of fruit at the start of the week and keep them at his desk so that he will have a healthy snack available for the rest of the week.

Eating more fish is beneficial as it is a very low calorie source of protein when prepared by grilling or baking, low in saturated fat and contains omega-3 fatty acids, which are cardioprotective. Whole grains can be easily incorporated into dinner. Brown rice and whole-wheat pasta are two substitutions (for white rice and white flour pasta) that RF can make immediately.

These dietary changes should result in weight reduction for RF. A discussion about gradually increasing his aerobic activity to recommended levels should also occur at the physician visit. Approaching the subject with activities RF enjoys may help to get him engaged in performing this activity regularly. Given RF's background as a football player, he might be interested in resuming weight lifting and resistance training, activities that he most likely participated in as a college athlete. Combining aerobic activity with strength training is an ideal way for RF to improve his health.

The PREMIER study combined the effects of following the DASH eating plan with concurrent lifestyle interventions to lose weight (goal was at least 15 pound weight loss), increase physical activity (goal was at least 180 minutes per week of moderate-intensity physical activity), reduce sodium intake (no more than 2300 mg per day), and reduce alcohol intake (no more than 2 drinks per day for men and 1 drink per day for women). The mean reduction in blood pressure when all conditions were followed was 4.6 mm Hg in SBP and 2.1 mm Hg in DBP at 6-month follow-up, and 2.1 mm Hg SBP and 1.0 mm Hg DBP at 18-months follow-up.

7. What factors would help to increase adherence in hypertensive patients?

Dietary and lifestyle changes are successful only if they are followed. A recent study based on the 1999 through 2004 National Health and Nutrition Examination Survey (NHANES) data found that only 19 percent of patients with hypertension are actually following the DASH diet. Specifically, adherence was lowest among African-Americans and individuals with a BMI of 30 kg/m^2 or higher – two groups who could benefit the most from following the DASH diet.

Various strategies have been proposed to help increase adherence. The primary means that a patient has for receiving information about the DASH diet (both how to follow it, and why it is so important) comes from the primary care physician. Therefore, it is essential that patients be given instruction during office visits; yet one study reported that only one-third of patients with hypertension received dietary counseling during office visits. Limited time to educate patients about how to properly follow the diet may reduce the potential benefits of dietary and lifestyle interventions. Physicians should make in-office instruction a priority, or if this is not possible, the patient should be referred to a dietitian or nurse educator. Furthermore, continual follow-up support from health care providers is greatly beneficial for increasing long-term maintenance of lifestyle modification.

Lower level of education is also associated with decreased adherence to the DASH diet, and this may be linked to a lack of "functional health literacy" in certain populations. This refers to the patient's ability to understand and act on health information provided, which are necessary for the implementation of a lifestyle or dietary modification. A patient who is illiterate, for example, will be unable to follow written guidelines for the DASH eating plan. Patients should be provided with examples of specific foods that may meet requirements for the DASH diet, as well as help in learning how to implement appropriate lifestyle strategies. Lack of access to fresh fruits and vegetables may also be a significant factor in DASH adherence. In many urban areas, it may be difficult to access the recommended foods. Canned fruits and vegetables are generally more available and less expensive but also very high in sodium and sugar content. Patients need to be instructed to rinse canned foods thoroughly before eating, purchase canned fruits packed in "light" syrup, and to look for "no salt added" products whenever possible.

Case 3 **Metabolic Syndrome and Lpa Genetic Defect**

Lisa Hark[1] and Frances Burke[2]

[1] Jefferson Medical College, Philadelphia, PA
[2] University of Pennsylvania School of Medicine, Philadelphia, PA

OBJECTIVES

- Identify risk factors for coronary heart disease specific for the Asian–Indian population.
- Describe how acculturation to a Western society may affect the lifestyle of the Asian–Indian immigrant.
- Discuss why it is important to understand how cultural and ethnic factors play a role in treatment recommendations.
- Provide a nutrition and physical activity plan for an Asian–Indian patient at risk for coronary heart disease.

MG is a 32-year-old Asian–Indian man who is self-referred to the Preventive Cardiology Clinic because he is concerned about his family history of heart disease. He is seeking ways in which he can avoid developing heart disease. His Lp(a) results from several months ago are 61 mg/dL (normal <20 mg/dL) and aggressive therapy is warranted, but he states that he does not want to take medication and prefers to focus on changing his diet and lifestyle. He is evaluated and referred to the nutritionist for counseling. He says he will return for follow-up in 3 months; however, he does not. He is lost to follow-up and returns to the Preventive Cardiology Clinic 3 years later.

Past Medical History

MG has no prior history of hospitalizations or chronic illnesses. He is not taking any medications or over-the-counter dietary or herbal supplements, and he has no known food allergies.

Family History

MG's family history is positive for heart disease. His father had a heart attack at age 45 and died of heart disease last year at age 50. His mother has diabetes.

Social History

He has been living in the United States for the past 11 years when he came over for college. He is an engineer, recently married and has a 1-year-old daughter. He

---

Medical Nutrition and Disease: A Case-Based Approach, 4th edition. Edited by Lisa Hark.
© 2009 Wiley-Blackwell Publishing, ISBN: 978-1-4051-8615-5.

reports that he has been very busy with work and rarely finds time to exercise. Since his father died, his mother, who has diabetes, has been living with his family on a permanent basis and she does most of the cooking.

Diet History

The nutritionist in the Preventive Cardiology Clinic determines that MG is a vegetarian and his diet includes white rice, legumes, and whole milk dairy products. He has been eating a combination of American and Indian foods since he began living in the United States 11 years ago. The nutritionist prescribes a low-saturated fat diet and a regular exercise program, both of which are supported by the physician and nurse practitioner. His typical current diet consists of the following:

Breakfast
Skips

Lunch (work)
Cheese sandwich	2 slices white bread
American cheese	2 slices
Mayonnaise	1 Tbsp.
Potato chips	2 ounce bag
Soda (cola)	12 ounces (360 mL)

Snack (office)
Whole milk yogurt	8 ounce (240 g)

Evening (home)
Samosa (stuffed potato, fried)	1 large
Curried vegetables with lamb	2 cups
Spinach panier with cheese	$\frac{1}{2}$ cup
Chickpeas	2 Tbsp.
White rice	1 cup

Total calories: 2976 kcal
Protein: 88 g (12% of total calories)
Fat: 143 g (43% of total calories)
Saturated fat: 32 g (10% of total calories)
Monounsaturated fat: 13 g (4% of total calories)
Polyunsaturated fat: 3 g (1% of total calories)
Trans fat: 0 g
Cholesterol: 147 mg
Carbohydrate: 336 g (45% of total calories)
Dietary fiber: 8 g
Soluble fiber: 0.1 g
Sodium: 3857 mg

Review of Systems
Noncontributory

Physical Examination
Vital Signs:
Temperature: 98 °F (37 °C)
Heart Rate: 78 BPM
Respiration: 21 BPM
Blood pressure: 135/85 mm Hg (initial visit)
              150/86 mm Hg (visit two, three years later)

Weight:	Visit 1	Current Visit (3 years later)
Height: 5'6″ (168 cm)	167 lbs (76 kg)	182 lbs (83 kg)
BMI (kg/m²):	27	29
Waist circumference*:	36″	39″

Exam
General: Overweight male in no acute distress
Remainder of physical examination was normal and unremarkable

Laboratory Data

	Visit 1:	Current Visit (3 yrs later)	Normal Values
Fasting glucose:	100	122	<99 mg/dL
Total cholesterol:	190	230	desirable <200 mg/dL
Fasting triglyceride:	210	250	desirable <150 mg/dL
HDL-C:	40	35	desirable >40 mg/dL (for men)
LDL-C:	116	152	desirable <130 mg/dL
Lp(a):	61	68	<20 mg/dL

Case Questions

1. Is MG at higher risk of heart disease compared to the general population and how does his ethnic background affect his risk?
2. What other laboratory studies would be helpful in determining treatment recommendations for this patient?
3. How does MG's ethnic background affect his dietary habits and lifestyle?
4. What is the best approach to take with this patient who has not followed up as recommended?
5. Based on MG's current lab results, what is the most appropriate next step in the management of this patient?
6. What factors have contributed to the change in MG's risk factor profile?

Answers to Questions: Case 3
Part 1: Risk Factors and Laboratory Assessment

1. Is MG at higher risk of heart disease compared to the general population and how does his ethnic background affect his risk?

Yes, MG is at greater risk for coronary heart disease (CHD) because he has several cardiac risk factors, including a family history of premature heart disease and metabolic syndrome. MG was diagnosed with metabolic syndrome because he meets three of the five criteria: borderline elevated blood pressure, abnormal waist circumference, and elevated triglyceride level (Table 6-3).

Asian Indians are at higher risk for coronary artery disease (CAD) than other populations, which occurs about 5 to 10 years earlier. The increased risk appears to be due to the higher rates of metabolic syndrome, insulin resistance, and diabetes. Healthy, normal weight Asian Indians are more likely to have insulin resistance compared with age and BMI-matched whites. Furthermore, insulin resistance in Asian Indians manifests at an earlier age. Conventional criteria from the Adult Treatment Panel III underestimate the prevalence of metabolic syndrome by 25 to 50 percent in Asian Indians, because this ethnic group develops metabolic abnormalities at a lower BMI and waist circumference (WC) than other ethnic groups. Therefore, several national and international organizations have recommended using the International Diabetes Federation (IDF) ethnic and gender WC criteria for central obesity (Table 6-9).

Most studies indicate that the average BMI of Asian Indians increases with urbanization and migration but is still less than that seen in whites, Mexican-Americans and blacks. MG's BMI is 27 kg/m^2 and his WC in 36 inches. He meets the IDF criteria for increased WC in addition to having an elevated blood pressure and triglyceride level at his first visit. Therefore, he should be treated with aggressive lifestyle management.

2. What other laboratory studies would be helpful in determining treatment recommendations for this patient?

In addition to comprehensive metabolic and lipid panels, MG should also be tested for lipoprotein(a) and apolipoprotein B. Asian Indians often present with

Table 6-9 Ethnic and Gender Waist Circumference (WC) Criteria for Central Obesity

	Men (inches)	Women (inches)
European Sub-Sahara Africa Middle eastern	>37"	>32"
South Asian South/Central American Japanese Chinese	>35"	>32"

Source: International Diabetes Federation. www.idf.or

a dyslipidemia that is characterized by high serum levels of apolipoprotein B, lipoprotein(a) [Lp(a)], and triglycerides and low levels of apolipoprotein A1 and high, density lipoprotein (HDL-C) cholesterol. An elevated apo B level is a stronger risk factor for CAD than LDL-C and is found in one-third of Asian Indians.

Several studies report a strong association between Lp(a) levels and coronary heart disease risk. Lp(a) is a modified form of LDL-C. It represents a class of LDL-C particles that have, as a protein moiety, apolipoprotein B-100 linked to another protein moiety, apolipoprotein(a). Lp(a) is structurally similar to plasminogen, but has no thrombolytic activity. Excess Lp(a) may promote atherosclerosis by increasing LDL-C oxidation and smooth muscle cell proliferation and by impairing endothelium-dependent vasodilation. Plasma Lp(a) levels are determined primarily by genetic factors that regulate production by the liver. Screening for Lp(a) is recommended for patients with a strong family history of premature coronary heart disease (CHD), as in MG's case. Lp(a) measurement is useful for identifying high-risk individuals and families who may be at higher risk than what might be suggested by mildly elevated total or LDL-C levels. These patients may benefit from earlier pharmacotherapy in conjunction with diet and lifestyle changes.

The optimal level of Lp(a) should be less than 20 mg/dL. Research shows that the risk of CAD is 2- to 4-fold higher when the levels of Lp(a) are above 30 to 40 mg/dL. This risk further increases when an Lp(a) level greater than 50 mg/dL is accompanied by elevated cholesterol levels. Recent studies have indicated that CAD risk is much greater when elevated Lp(a) levels are accompanied by low HDL-C versus high LDL-C cholesterol levels.

Part 2: Nutrition Assessment and Cultural Issues

3. How does MG's ethnic background affect his dietary habits and lifestyle?

Nutrition interventions for the prevention and treatment of CAD need to be compatible with individuals' cultural values and beliefs. Developing nutrition interventions that target people from diverse backgrounds presents a variety of challenges. Health professionals must recognize the importance of specific foods within cultures, and of ethno-social influences on food choices. However, generalizations about food patterns should not be made solely on the basis of race, ethnicity, or geographic origin, because food-choice diversity is common within all cultural and racial groups. In essence, America is a melting pot of cultures. Interventions are most effective when focused on each family's unique dietary history and background, without making assumptions about food habits on the basis of cultural or racial background. Factors, such as where one lives, may determine the availability of ethnic foods and issues of acculturation play a huge role in all people's food selections.

The majority of Asian Indians follow a vegetarian diet for both cultural and religious reasons. Rice and wheat are staples of the Indian diet, whereas fruit and vegetable intake are low. Many vegetarian foods and baked goods are prepared with coconut and palm oil, butter, ghee (clarified butter), vanaspati (hydrogenated fat), and coconut milk, which are very high in saturated and *trans* fats.

Asian Indians in India consume relatively more carbohydrates ($\sim$60 to 67 percent of energy intake) compared with Asian Indians living in the United States ($\sim$56 to 58 percent of energy intake). High carbohydrate intake is associated with elevated triglyceride levels. Low dietary intake and low plasma levels of omega-3 fatty acids in Asian Indians have been reported in several studies. Since his mother now lives with him on a permanent basis and prepares most of the family meals, including her in the counseling session with the dietitian would be very helpful. It is important to question MG about the types of fats that he and his family use when preparing Indian dishes at home. His saturated fat intake should be less than 7 percent of his total calorie intake and his current diet consists of 10 percent.

Asian Indians have been shown to be less physically active compared to other ethnic groups. It is culturally unacceptable for Muslim women to participate in leisure time physical activity. MG currently leads a very sedentary lifestyle. Sedentary Asian Indians are more likely to have higher BMI values, elevated serum triglycerides, and hypertension. Physical activity patterns in Asian Indians warrant further investigation, since a sedentary lifestyle could be an important risk factor for the insulin resistance commonly seen in this population.

4. What is the best approach to take with this patient who has not followed up as recommended?

Initially patients may express the desire to change lifestyle habits and appear motivated to improve their overall health but may find it challenging to make permanent changes. Later when patients do not return for their follow-up visit, it typically means that they have not followed the medical nutrition prescription that was outlined for them. Bringing patients back frequently for follow-up visits and asking them to complete food and activity records is an effective behavioral tool to keep patients on track. The best way to discuss these issues with MG is to explain where he is in terms of his CHD risk, where he needs to be to lower his risk, and how to achieve these goals. This provides a supportive, non-judgmental approach. It is important to thank MG for returning for follow-up, rather than confronting him with disappointment that he did not follow-up with his initial visit three years ago.

Part 3: Medical Treatment and Nutrition Therapy

5. Based on MG's current lab results, what is the most appropriate next step in the management of this patient?

At this point, it is important to express concern about MG's increased weight as well as the significant increase in many of his lab values. However, focusing on the behavioral goals, rather than weight, when counseling MG would be the best approach. He should understand that he now meets five of the ATP III criteria for metabolic syndrome and because of his strong family history for premature CHD, he is at high risk for developing heart disease. In addition, because his mother has diabetes and his blood sugar is now elevated, he is also at risk of developing diabetes. MG should therefore be aggressively treated with diet, exercise, and medication(s) to reduce his risk of heart disease and diabetes.

MG would benefit from a diet low in saturated and *trans* fats and restricted in total calories to achieve weight loss. Recommend that he substitute lower fat dairy products for those that are high in saturated fat, such as cheese and whole milk yogurt. Increasing his total and soluble fiber intakes (which are currently 8 grams and less than 1 gram) by substituting whole grain starches for the white bread and white rice would also be advantageous. The predominant cooking oil used in food preparation should be high in monounsaturated fat such as olive or canola oil. In addition, MG and his mom should be counseled to avoid frying and use a limited amount of oil to sauté or stir fry foods, as oils contain 135 calories per tablespoon. Refer to Table 6-10 for healthier versions of traditional Asian cuisine.

Recommend that MG increase his intake of fruits and vegetables, which will help increase his fiber intake, decrease the energy density of his diet, and help him manage his weight. Finally, MG should be counseled to avoid drinking sugar-sweetened beverages such as regular soda and even fruit juice. These beverages, which provide refined sugars, contribute to increased calories and elevated triglyceride and glucose levels. MG is recommended to begin a physical activity program 3 to 4 times a week for at least 30 minutes, which will aid in weight control and may help to improve HDL-C levels.

In addition to recommending lifestyle changes, MG is prescribed an aspirin, an anti-hypertensive agent, and an HMG CoA reductase inhibitor. ATP III stresses LDL-C target goals, which for MG is less than 100 mg/dL. Follow-up appointments with both the physician and registered dietitian are scheduled for 6 weeks to monitor changes in serum lipids, glucose, blood pressure, and weight and to reassess his medications and dietary adherence.

6. What factors have contributed to the change in MG's risk factor profile?

By helping MG reassess his life and identify factors that have contributed to his overall health, he is more likely to come to terms with his current health problems and begin to make lifestyle changes to prevent future events. It is very important that MG maintain his cultural identity, especially related to his food intake (vegetarian). By providing culturally appropriate recommendations targeted to Asian Indian patients, this will be possible. These are the factors in MG's life:

Lifestyle He has a full-time job and a new baby, and states that he is very, very busy and does not have time to exercise. MG would greatly benefit from a regular exercise program, so discussing how he can work in time to exercise, or make exercise part of his everyday life, is critical. Write him an exercise prescription and discuss his schedule and activities he enjoys. Suggest he purchase a pedometer to help quantify his activity.

Table 6-10 Healthier Versions of Traditional Asian Indian Cuisine

Traditional food	Healthier way of eating
Meat, poultry, fish, and eggs fried in ghee, butter, coconut oil, palm kernel oil, or hydrogenated fats and oils.	Bake, roast, broil, grill, or oven-fry. Remove skin from chicken before eating. Fry with canola, olive, or corn oil instead. Limit to $1/4$ cup oil.
Legumes and vegetables prepared with oil, butter, or cream yogurt to enhance flavor.	Use almond paste or non-fat yogurt in place of cream and butter. Season with onion, garlic, spices, or low-sodium chicken broth to enhance flavor.
Rice (white) dishes or wheat (refined) preparations deep fried or prepared with large amounts of ghee, butter, and hydrogenated fats (vanaspati) containing *trans* fatty acids.	Use brown rice and whole grain wheat. Boil or bake instead of frying. Fry with canola, olive, or corn oil or *trans*-free margarine instead of solid or hydrogenated fat. Limit to 1/4 cup oil.
Whole milk/cheese/cream/yogurt used to prepare rice dishes, vegetables, desserts, and shakes. Yogurt cheese (panir) prepared with whole milk.	Substitute low-fat or non-fat milk, milk powder, cheese, cream, yogurt, buttermilk, or soymilk instead.
Omelettes and desserts prepared with egg yolks.	Substitute egg whites for yolks.
Snacks such as fried legumes "bhel".	Snack on fruits, rice cakes, and puddings made with low-fat milk instead. Use oat and whole wheat cereal to prepare savory snacks.
Salt used to enhance flavor.	Use herbs (e.g. cilantro, mint), spices (e.g. cumin, black pepper, cardamom, cinnamon), or flax seed powder to enhance flavor.

Source: Karmally W. Multicultural Nutrition Strategies: Asian Indians. In *Cardiovascular Nutrition: Disease Management and Prevention*. American Dietetic Association, Chicago, IL. 2004.

Stress The death of his father and stress at work has placed much pressure on MG, which causes him to eat more, exercise less, and avoid focusing on his own health. Discuss meditation, yoga, and massage therapy, all of which may fit into his cultural belief systems.

Preparation of family meals Now that MG's mother is living with his family on a full-time basis, she is taking care of their child and cooking all their meals. As a result, he states that he has gained 15 pounds in the past few years. His BMI of 29, combined with an increased WC to 39 inches, significantly increases his risk of CHD. To help improve adherence, include his mother as part of the conversation with the registered dietitian to ensure that she can still prepare and enjoy a healthier Indian cuisine.

Chapter and Case References

Adrogué HJ, Madias NE. Sodium and potassium in the pathogenesis of hypertension. *N Engl J Med.* 2007;356(19):1966–78.

American Dietetic Association. ADA Evidence Analysis Library. Heart Failure. Available at www.adaevidencelibrary.com.

American Dietetic Association. ADA Evidence Analysis Library. Disorders of lipid metabolism. Available at www.adaevidencelibrary.com.

Appel LJ, Brands MW, Daniels SR, et al. Dietary approaches to prevent and treat hypertension. *Hypertension.* 2006;47:296–308.

Appel LJ, Champagne CM, Harsha DW, et al. Effects of comprehensive lifestyle modification on blood pressure control: main results of the PREMIER clinical trial. *JAMA.* 2003;289:2083–2093.

Appel LJ, Moore TJ, Obarzanek E, et al. A clinical trial of the effects of dietary patterns on blood pressure. DASH Collaborative Research Group. *N Engl J Med.* 1997;336:1117–1124.

Balk EM, Lichtenstein AH, Chung M, Kupelnick B, Chew P, Lau J. Effects of omega-3 fatty acids on coronary restenosis, intima-media thickness, and exercise tolerance: a systematic review. *Atherosclerosis.* 2006;184:237–246.

Beyer FR, Dickinson HO, Nicolson DJ, Ford GA, Mason J. Combined calcium, magnesium, and potassium supplementation for the management of primary hypertension in adults. *Cochrane Database of Systematic Reviews.* 2006, Issue 3. Art No.:CD004805. DOI:10.1002/14651858.CD004805.pub2.

Bosworth HB, Olsen MK, Neary A, et al. Take Control of Your Blood pressure (TCYB) study: A multifactorial tailored behavioral and educational intervention for achieving blood pressure control. *Patient Educ Couns.* 2008;70(3):338–347.

Carson JAS, Grundy SM, Van Horn L, et al. Medical nutrition therapy in the prevention and management of coronary heart disease. In Carson JAS, Burke FM, Hark LA. *Cardiovascular Nutrition: Disease Management and Prevention.* Chicago, IL: American Dietetic Association, 2004.

Carson JAS. Cardiovascular Section. American Dietetic Association Nutrition Care Manual, 2007. Available from www.nutritioncaremanual.org.

Carson JS, Burke FM, Hark LA (editors). Multicultural Nutrition Strategies. In Cardiovascular Nutrition. Disease Management and Prevention. American Dietetic Association, Chicago, IL. 2004.

Chobanian AV. Prehypertension revisited. *Hypertension.* 2006;48:812–814.

Chobanian AV, Bakris GL, Black HR, Cushman WC, Green LA, Izzo JL Jr., Jones DW, Materson BJ, Oparil S, Wright JT Jr, Roccella EJ, for The National High Blood Pressure Education Program Coordinating Committee. The seventh report of the Joint National Committee on Prevention, Detection, Evaluation, and Treatment of High Blood Pressure: the JNC 7 report. *JAMA.* 2003;289:2560–2572.

Collier SR, Kanaley JA, Carhart R Jr, et al. Effect of 4 weeks of aerobic or resistance exercise training on arterial stiffness, blood flow and blood pressure in pre- and stage-1 hypertensives. *J Hum Hypertens.* 2008;22(10):678–686.

Dickinson BD, Havas S; Council on Science and Public Health, American Medical Association. Reducing the population burden of cardiovascular disease by reducing sodium intake: a report of the Council on Science and Public Health. *Arch Intern Med.* 2007;167(14):1460–8.

Dickinson BD, Havas S. Reducing the population burden of cardiovascular disease by reducing sodium intake. *Arch Intern Med.* 2007;167(14):1460–1468.

Eckel RH, Grundy SM, Zimmet PZ. The metabolic syndrome. *Lancet.* 2005;365:1415–1428.

Elmer PJ, Obarzanek E, Vollmer WM, Simons-Morton D, Sevens VJ, Young DR, et al. for PREMIER Collaborative Research Group. Effects of comprehensive lifestyle modification on diet, weight, physical fitness and blood pressure control: 18-month results of a randomized trial. *Ann Intern Med.* 2006;144:485–495.

Enas EA, Chacko V, Pazhoor SG, Chennikkara H, Devarapalli HP. Dyslipidemia in South Asian patients. *Curr Atheroscler Rep.* 2007;9(5):367–374.

Expert Panel on Detection, Evaluation, and Treatment of High Blood Cholesterol in Adults. Executive summary of the third report of the national cholesterol education program (NCEP) expert panel on detection, evaluation, and treatment of high blood cholesterol in adults (Adult Treatment Panel III). *JAMA.* 2001;285:2486–2497.

Finckenor MA, Byrd-Bredbenner C. Nutrition intervention group program based on preaction stage–oriented change processes of the Transtheoretical Model promotes long-term reduction in dietary fat intake. *J Am Diet Assoc.* 2000;100:335–342.

Grundy SM, Cleeman JI, Merz CN, et al. Implications of recent clinical trials for the National Cholesterol Education Program Adult Treatment Panel III guidelines. *Circulation.* 2004;110:227–239.

Grundy SM. *Contemporary Diagnosis and Management of the Metabolic Syndrome.* Newtown, PA: Handbooks in Health Care Co., 2005.

Gupta R, Joshi P, Mohan V, Reddy KS, Yusuf S. Epidemiology and causation of coronary heart disease and stroke in India. *Heart.* 2008;94:16–26.

Hanninen SA, Darling PB, Sole MJ, Barr A, Keith ME. The prevalence of thiamin deficiency in hospitalized patients with congestive heart failure. *J Am Coll Cardiol.* 2006;47:354–361.

Havas S, Dickinson BD, Wilson M. The urgent need to reduce sodium consumption. *JAMA.* 2007;298(12):1439–41.

Hoogeveen RC, Gambhir JK, Gambhir DS, et al. Evaluation of Lp(a) and other independent risk factors for CHD in Asian Indians and their USA counterparts. *J Lipid Res.* 2001;42:631–638.

Hunt SA, Abraham WT, Chin MH, et al. ACC/AHA guideline update for the diagnosis and management of chronic heart failure in the adult: summary article. *Circulation.* 2005;112:1825–1852.

Institute of Medicine. *Dietary Reference Intakes for Energy, Carbohydrates, Fiber, Fat, Protein and Amino Acids (Macronutrients).* Washington, DC: National Academy Press, 2002.

International Diabetes Federation. Ethnic and gender waist circumference criteria for central obesity. Available at www.idf.org.

Jen KL, Brogan K, Washington OG, et al. Poor nutrient intake and high obese rate in an urban African American population with hypertension. *J Am Coll Nutr.* 2007;26(1):57–65

Joshi P, Islam S, Pais P, et al. Risk factors for early myocardial infarction in South Asians compared with individuals in other countries. *JAMA.* 2007;297:286–294.

Koelling TM, Johnson ML, Cody RJ, Aaronson KD. Discharge education improves clinical outcomes in patients with chronic heart failure. *Circulation.* 2005;111:179–185.

Kollipara UK, Mo V, Toto KH, et al. High sodium food choices by southern, urban African-Americans with heart failure. *J Card Fail* 2006;12:144–148.

Kotchen TA. Hypertension control: trends, approaches, and goals. *Hypertension.* 2007;49(1):19–20.

Kris-Etherton PM, Lichtenstein AH, Howard BV, Steinberg D, Witztum JL. Antioxidant vitamin supplements and cardiovascular disease. *Circulation.* 2004;110:637–641.

Kshirsagar AV, Carpenter M, Bang H, Wyatt SB, Colindres RE. Blood pressure usually considered normal is associated with an elevated risk of cardiovascular disease. *Am J Med.* 2006;119:133–141.

Lichtenstein AH, Appel LJ, Brands M, et al. Diet and Lifestyle Recommendations Revision 2006. A Scientific Statement from the American Heart Association Nutrition Committee. *Circulation.* 2006;114:82–96.

Lin PH, Appel LJ, Fun K, et al. The PREMIER intervention helps participants follow the dietary approaches to stop hypertension dietary pattern and the current dietary reference intake recommendations. *J Am Diet Assoc.* 2007;107:1541–1551.

Liszka HA, Mainous AG, King DE, Everett CJ, Egan BM. Prehypertension and cardiovascular morbidity. *Ann Fam Med.* 2005;3294–299.

Mellen PB, Gao SK, Vitolins MZ, Goff DC Jr. Deteriorating dietary habits among adults with hypertension: DASH dietary accordance, NHANES 1988–1994 and 1999–2004. *Arch Intern Med.* 2008;168(3):308–14.

Mitka M. DASH dietary plan could benefit many, but few hypertensive patients follow it. *JAMA.* 2007;298:164–165

Misra A, Vikram NK. Insulin resistance syndrome (metabolic syndrome) and obesity in Asian Indians: evidence and implications. *Nutrition. 2004*;20:482–491.

Morton SP, Hardy M. Effect of Supplemental Antioxidants Vitamin C, Vitamin E, and Coenzyme Q10 for the Prevention and Treatment of Cardiovascular Disease. Evidence Report/Technology Assessment No. 83 (Prepared by Southern California-RAND Evidence-based Practice Center). AHRQ Publication No. 03-E043. Rockville, MD: Agency for Healthcare Research and Quality. July 2003.

Mozaffarian D, Katan MB, Ascherio A, et al. Trans fatty acids and cardiovascular disease. *NEJM.* 2006;354:1601–1613.

Myers VH, Champagne CM. Nutritional effects on blood pressure. *Curr Opin Lipidol.* 2007;18:20–24.

National Heart, Lung, and Blood Institute. *Facts about DASH Diet.* Available at http://www.nhlbi.nih.gov.,

Ong KL, Cheung BM, Man YB, Lau CP, Lam KS. Prevalence, awareness, treatment, and control of hypertension among United States Adults 1999–2004. *Hypertension.* 2007;49:69–75.

Rajeshwari R, Nicklas TA, Pownall HJ, Berenson GS. Cardiovascular diseases – a major health risk in Asian Indians. *Nutrition Research.* 2005;25:515–533.

Sacks FM, Lichtenstein A, van Horn L, Harris W, Kris-Etherton P, Winston M for the American Heart Association Nutrition Committee. Soy protein, isoflavones, and cardiovascular health. *Circulation.* 2006;113:1034–1044.

Sacks FM, Svetkey LP, Vollmer WM, et al. Effects on blood pressure of reduced dietary sodium and the Dietary Approaches to Stop Hypertension (DASH) diet. DASH-Sodium Collaborative Research Group. *N Engl J Med.* 2001;344:3–10.

Sipahi I, Tuzcu EM, Schoenhagen P, Wolski KE, Nicholls SJ, Balog C, Crowe TD, Nissen SE. Effects of normal, pre-hypertensive, and hypertensive blood pressure levels on progression of coronary atherosclerosis. *J Am Coll Cardiol.* 2006;48:833–838.

The Seventh Report of the Joint National Committee on Prevention, Detection, Evaluation, and Treatment of High Blood Pressure. *JAMA.* 2003;289:2083–2093.

van Horn L, McCoin M, Kris-Etherton PM, et al. Evidence base for dietary prevention and treatment of cardiovascular disease: a 21st century perspective. *J Am Diet Assoc.* 2008;108:287–331.

von Eckardstein A, Schulte H, Cullen P, et al. Lipoprotein(a) further increases the risk of coronary events in men with high global cardiovascular risk. *J Am Coll Cardiol* 2001;37:434–439.

Wang C, Harris WS, Chung M, et al. N-3 fatty acids from fish or fish-oil supplements, but not alpha-linolenic acid, benefit cardiovascular disease outcomes in primary- and secondary-prevention studies: a systematic review. *Am J Clin Nutr.* 2006;85:5–17.

Welty FK, Nasca MM, Lew NS, Gregoire S, Ruan Y. Effect of onsite dietitian counseling on weight loss and lipid levels in an outpatient physician office. *Am J Cardiol* 2007;100:73–75.

Williams MA, Haskell WL, Ades PA, et al. American Heart Association Council on Clinical Cardiology; American Heart Association Council on Nutrition, Physical Activity, and Metabolism. Resistance exercise in individuals with and without cardiovascular disease: 2007 update: a scientific statement from the American Heart Association Council on Clinical Cardiology and Council on Nutrition, Physical Activity, and Metabolism. *Circulation.* 2007;116(5):572–84.

7 Gastrointestinal Disease

Gary R. Lichtenstein[1], Emily Gelsomin[2], and Julie Vanderpool[3]

[1] University of Pennsylvania Health System, Philadelphia, PA
[2] Massachusetts General Hospital, Boston, MA
[3] Brigham and Women's Hospital, Boston, MA

OBJECTIVES

- To incorporate nutrition into the medical history, review of systems, and physical examination of patients with gastrointestinal diseases.

- To identify the causes of malnutrition in inflammatory bowel disease, liver diseases, and malabsorption syndrome.

- To describe why sodium and fluid restriction may be necessary for patients with liver disease.

- To explain the association between diet and lower esophageal sphincter pressure in patients with gastroesophageal reflux disease.

*Source: Objectives for chapter and cases adapted from the NIH Nutrition Curriculum Guide for Training Physicians. (www.nhlbi.nih.gov/funding/training/naa)

Peptic Ulcer Disease

The goals of nutritional intervention in the treatment of peptic ulcer disease (PUD) are to reduce and neutralize the secretion of gastric acid and to maintain the resistance of the gastrointestinal epithelial tissue in order to combat the effect of gastric acid. Historically, prior to the introduction of our current medical armamentarium to treat individuals with peptic ulcer disease, patients were prescribed special bland diets that restricted their intake of foods and beverages thought to irritate the gastric mucosa or promote excessive gastric acid secretion. In the past, dietary therapy for PUD included small, frequent feedings with mechanically soft foods such as milk and eggs. Frequent feedings were thought to provide constant buffering, and small feedings were thought to limit the amount of gastric distention and thus gastric acid secretion. However, this dietary treatment has not been sufficiently supported by scientific evidence.

Randomized, controlled clinical trials have shown no differences between unrestricted and therapeutic diets when assessing the endpoint of healing of the ulcer or remission of symptoms. In addition, foods with high protein content, such as milk, were found to be the most powerful stimuli of gastric acid secretion, an outcome

---

Medical Nutrition and Disease: A Case-Based Approach, 4th edition. Edited by Lisa Hark.
© 2009 Wiley-Blackwell Publishing, ISBN: 978-1-4051-8615-5.

Table 7-1 Medical Nutrition Therapy for Peptic Ulcer Disease

- Limit caffeine intake by reducing consumption of coffee, tea, cola, chocolate, and other foods and beverages that contain caffeine.
- Limit alcohol intake and avoid drinking on an empty stomach.
- Avoid cigarette smoking, which may increase gastric acid secretion and delay the healing process. Cigarette smoking also affects the gastric mucous layer, and is also associated with an increased frequency of duodenal ulcers. The gastric mucous layer acts as a lubricant, and as a discrete layer, it helps to establish a gradient between the acidity of the gastric lumen and the neutral pH at the apical surface of the gastric cells.
- Eat three meals daily, avoid skipping meals, and limit intake of spicy, fatty, or otherwise bothersome foods.
- Avoid bedtime snacks to prevent acid secretion if symptoms often occur in the middle of the night.

Source: Gary Lichtenstein, MD. Used with permission.

counterproductive to the goals of dietary therapy in these patients. Therefore, current nutritional therapy is based on the individual's tolerance to foods and beverages that may cause abdominal discomfort. Nutritional advice is thus offered as an adjunct to conventional medical and pharmacologic therapy in this cohort; the primary focus of pharmacologic therapy has been to reduce gastric acid secretion.

Nutrition Therapy for Peptic Ulcer Disease

The acid-secreting parietal cells are primarily located in the fundus of the stomach. The sight or smell of food and distention of the stomach trigger neurally mediated reflexes, which initiate gastric acid secretion by stimulating the parietal cells. Caffeine and other alkaloids in coffee, polypeptides, and amino acids (products of protein digestion), and alcohol stimulate the release of the hormone gastrin, thereby triggering gastric acid secretion. Although alcohol and caffeine consumption have not been directly implicated in the development of PUD, excessive intake of these substances may cause abdominal discomfort. It has been well recognized that ethanol is a direct irritant to the stomach. Individuals who abuse alcohol (ethanol) appear to have an increased risk of developing PUD. Medical nutrition therapy for patients with PUD is shown in Table 7-1.

Gastroesophageal Reflux Disease

Gastroesophageal reflux (GER) is the regurgitation of gastric contents into the esophagus typically as a consequence of transient, increased abdominal pressure or transient relaxation of the lower esophageal sphincter (LES). When the gastric acid, bile, and pepsin in the stomach are in frequent and prolonged contact with the esophagus, gastroesophageal reflux disease (GERD) may develop, and the patient typically becomes symptomatic.

Heartburn, described as a burning epigastric or substernal pain, is a major symptom of GERD. Findings that have been known to be associated with GERD include decreased esophageal clearance, weak or incompetent LES, delayed gastric emptying, and irritation of the esophageal mucosa. The role of the LES tone in preventing

GERD is known to be important. If the pressure exerted by the LES to prevent the refluxate from entering the esophagus is not greater than the pressure exerted by the stomach, which promotes propulsion of the contents of the stomach back up into the esophagus, then GERD does occur.

The goals of nutrition therapy for patients with GERD include:

- avoiding decreases in LES pressure,
- decreasing the frequency and volume of the refluxate,
- reducing irritation of sensitive or inflamed esophageal tissue,
- improving esophageal clearing ability.

Because the severity of symptoms varies greatly among individuals with GERD, nutrition therapy is based on the individual's tolerance of foods and beverages that may cause discomfort.

Nutrition Therapy for GERD

Maintaining Lower Esophageal Sphincter Pressure

A major goal in the treatment of GERD is to avoid decreasing lower esophageal sphincter pressure. From a nutritional standpoint, the following measures have proven to be helpful in patients with this disorder:

- *Limiting dietary fat intake:* High-fat meals tend to decrease LES pressure and delay gastric emptying time. As a consequence, the time that the esophagus is exposed to irritants increases, as does the gastric volume available for reflux.
- *Losing weight:* Obesity promotes GERD by increasing abdominal pressure and thus the likelihood of reflux.
- *Limiting alcohol, chocolate, and coffee:* These substances decrease LES pressure. Alcohol is also a powerful stimulus of gastric acid secretion.

Decreasing Reflux Frequency and Volume

The following steps have proven useful to decrease the frequency and volume of gastroesophageal reflux:

- eating small meals and eating more frequently if necessary,
- losing weight if overweight,
- drinking most fluids between meals rather than with meals,
- consuming adequate fiber to avoid constipation because straining increases intraabdominal pressure.

Decreasing Esophageal "Irritation"

To decrease "irritation" of the esophagus, patients with GERD should be counseled to monitor their dietary intake in the following ways:

- Limit intake of citrus fruits (oranges, grapefruit, and lemons), tomato products, spicy foods, and carbonated beverages. Although most of these foods do not irritate the esophagus, they can cause heartburn and other GERD symptoms in individuals with a sensitized esophagus.
- Avoid any other foods that regularly cause heartburn.

Improving Esophageal Clearing Time

To improve the clearance of food from the esophagus, patients should take the following precautions:

- Do not recline after eating. Sit upright or take a walk.
- Avoid eating for at least 2 to 3 hours before bedtime (or prior to assuming a supine position).
- Elevate the head of the bed.

Malabsorption

Malabsorption involves defective digestion and absorption of carbohydrates, proteins, fats, vitamins, and minerals, either jointly or independently. From a clinical standpoint malabsorption should be differentiated from maldigestion. A thorough history and a careful physical examination are essential to help detect the signs and symptoms of malabsorption. Successful management of malabsorption hinges on identifying the underlying defect and implementing specific therapy to correct it. Malabsorption can be treated, and the treatment invariably improves the patient's quality of life.

Defect Associated with Malabsorption

Four categories of defects have been identified as the major causes of malabsorption:

- impairment of mechanical digestion,
- impairment of chemical digestion,
- impairment of solubilization,
- pathologic impairment of absorption.

Malabsorption of Specific Nutrients

Carbohydrate Malabsorption Malabsorption of carbohydrates causes osmotic diarrhea. The most commonly seen carbohydrate malabsorption is lactose intolerance. Lactose is a disaccharide found in milk and dairy products. Normally, lactose is hydrolyzed to its constituent moieties, glucose and galactose, by an enzyme indigenous to the small bowel called lactase. Lactose intolerance occurs when lactase is not present in adequate quantities to digest lactose. The development of clinical symptoms of lactose intolerance – bloating, abdominal cramps, and diarrhea – depends on whether the level of lactase activity is adequate to fully hydrolyze the lactose load delivered to the intestine. Typically, these symptoms will occur between 30 minutes and 2 hours after the lactose-containing food has been ingested. About 15 percent of Caucasians, up to 80 percent of African-Americans, and more than 90 percent of Asian Americans are lactase deficient.

Nutrition therapy for lactose intolerance or lactase deficiency involves the following measures, individually or in combination, according to the severity of the patient's intolerance:

- reducing or avoiding lactose intake (milk and dairy products),
- pretreating milk with lactase derived from bacteria,
- ingesting only lactase-treated dairy products (such as Lactaid milk).

Individuals who avoid all products containing lactose may not meet their daily calcium requirements from dairy products alone. In this case, calcium supplementation and encouragement to consume non-dairy sources of calcium is advised. Non-dairy sources of calcium include almonds, fortified soy milk, sardines, salmon with edible bones, broccoli, kale, and calcium set tofu. It should be noted that some leafy greens, such as Swiss chard and spinach, do contain calcium; however, they also contain oxalate, which binds to calcium and prevents it from being significantly absorbed. There are also certain dairy sources of calcium that can be well tolerated in some patients with lactose intolerance. Yogurts and hard cheeses, such as cheddar and Swiss, can be suggested depending on the patient's individual tolerance. Yogurt contains bacteria that aid in the digestion of lactose. The bacteria produce the enzyme lactase thus enhancing the individual patient's ability to digest some of the lactose. Additionally, patients are advised to eat hard cheeses rather than soft cheeses since hard cheeses usually contain only small amounts of lactose.

For severely lactose intolerant individuals, they may need to avoid sources of lactose in unlikely places: baked goods, energy bars, instant mixes, candies, and processed meats can all be sources of lactose. It should be emphasized that lactose is occasionally used as a binder for pills of various types. Product ingredients such as whey, curds, dry milk, and milk solids indicate that the product may contain enough lactose to cause discomfort in individuals severely sensitive to lactose. Pregnant and lactating women and the elderly require higher calcium levels, depending on their intake of non-dairy calcium sources, but most healthy adults need between 1000 to 1200 mg per day. Calcium supplements should also contain vitamin D to aid in absorption.

Fat Malabsorption

Lipids are a group of compounds with drastically different chemical and physical properties: triglycerides, diglycerides, monoglycerides, fatty acids, phospholipids, cholesterol, cholesterol esters, and bile acids. Lipids (primarily triglycerides), a major source of calories, require the most complicated sequence of digestive and absorptive processes. A typical Western diet contains at least 70 grams of fat per day, accounting for approximately one-third of total dietary calories. The absorption coefficient of triglycerides (the amount absorbed as a percentage of what is ingested) in normal individuals is greater than 99 percent. Due to the complexity of the digestive and absorptive processes involved in the body's utilization of fats, a number of problems can arise in individuals whose intake of these substances exceeds their capacity to break them down.

Clinical Manifestations of Fat Malabsorption

Malabsorption of fat can present with a unique clinical manifestation of excessive fat loss in the stool called steatorrhea, the result of impairment of either the digestive or the absorptive process. Clinical manifestations of fat malabsorption include the

following general signs and symptoms:
- weight loss, muscle wasting;
- failure to thrive, growth retardation, and fatigue, especially in infants, children, and adolescents;
- tetany, osteomalacia, bone pain, compression fracture of vertebral bodies due to hypocalcemia secondary to calcium malabsorption;
- infertility, dysmenorrhea, amenorrhea.

In addition, fat malabsorption is often responsible for a number of fat-soluble vitamin deficiencies. Clinical signs vary as follows according to the vitamin deficiency involved:

Vitamin A: night blindness, hyperkeratosis, skin changes

Vitamin D: hypocalcemia, osteomalacia, rickets, hypophosphatemia

Vitamin K: prolongation of prothrombin time, easy bruisability

Vitamin E: neuropathy, hemolytic anemia.

Renal Stone Manifestation with Fat Malabsorption

Oxalate kidney stones can be caused by bile salt malabsorption resulting from a pathologic disease process in the luminal digestive tract. Most dietary oxalic acid is normally precipitated in the lumen after it binds with free calcium as calcium oxalate and is excreted in the feces without being absorbed. However, in the presence of certain pathologic processes, such as extensive ileal resection in Crohn's disease, the damaged portion of the small intestine is unable to absorb bile salts completely. The resulting excess bile salt loss in the stool eventually leads to bile salt pool depletion, despite the liver's attempts to compensate by increasing the amount of bile salts it produces.

In individuals with extensive ileal disease, an excess of fatty acids in the lumen depletes calcium by binding with it to form a calcium soap. Consequently, dietary oxalic acid in these patients bonds with sodium (as opposed to calcium, as it would usually do) to form sodium oxalate, which is more soluble than the calcium salt. Oxalic acid thus becomes available for absorption, which occurs primarily in the colon. In the presence of bile acid malabsorption, bile acids alter colonic permeability, and as a result, the colon absorbs the sodium oxalate produced in the lumen. The kidney excretes this oxalate, which contributes secondarily to the formation of oxalate stores. In addition, these patients with fat malabsorption tend to be volume depleted secondary to diarrhea, with low urine output, another factor contributing to increased oxalate stone formation. To avoid the formation of stones, patients with bile salt malabsorption should avoid foods high in oxalate such as spinach, rhubarb, cocoa, chocolate, tea, green beans, collards, kale, peanut butter, and beer. They should also drink adequate volumes of liquid to help "flush" the fluids through. (Oxalate kidney stones are discussed in detail in Chapter 10).

Liver Disease

The liver is involved in many of the body's metabolic processes, including regulation of protein, fat and carbohydrate metabolism, vitamin storage and activation, and detoxification and excretion of waste products. Thus, impaired liver function can lead to nutrient deficiencies, and eventually, protein-energy malnutrition. Conversely, malnutrition can further impair liver function by affecting the liver's structural integrity.

There exists a large spectrum of liver abnormalities that range from fatty liver (steatosis), to fatty liver with inflammation (steatohepatitis), to permanent destruction of normal liver tissue (cirrhosis). Chronic alcoholism is the most common cause of cirrhosis in the United States. According to the American Liver Foundation, about 40 percent of people who die from cirrhosis each year have a strong history of alcohol abuse. Hepatitis C and Hepatitis B infections are the second leading cause of cirrhosis. Nonalcoholic Steatohepatitis (NASH) can also lead to cirrhosis and has been linked to obesity, diabetes, coronary artery disease, and severe malnutrition. Regardless of the cause, patients with end-stage liver disease usually develop malnutrition. It is estimated that 65 to 90 percent of patients with advanced liver disease have some degree of protein–calorie malnutrition. Higher rates of complications associated with liver disease such as hepatic encephalopathy, infection, variceal bleeding, and ascites are found in malnourished patients.

Causes of Malnutrition

The major causes of malnutrition in patients with liver disease are:
- poor dietary intake,
- maldigestion and malabsorption,
- abnormalities in the metabolism and storage of macro- and micronutrients.

The goals of nutritional management in patients with liver disease are to correct preexisting malnutrition and supply adequate calories as well as protein to encourage hepatic regeneration without precipitating hepatic encephalopathy.

Poor Dietary Intake

Poor oral intake resulting in malnutrition stems from multiple factors. In patients with alcohol-related liver disease, dietary assessment should include an evaluation of the pattern, quantity, and duration of alcohol intake, usual dietary intake, and various socioeconomic factors affecting eating habits. Alcohol provides 7 kcal/g that can be fully utilized and metabolized, but it contains no vitamins or minerals. Individuals who substitute alcohol for other sources of carbohydrate and fat calories find that their appetite decreases proportionally to the amount of alcohol they ingest, largely because their need for calories is satisfied.

Patients with chronic liver disease frequently present with a poor dietary intake resulting from nausea, vomiting, diarrhea, abdominal pain, and early satiety. Early satiety is felt in part related to mechanical compression from ascites and also from the liver externally compressing the stomach (if hepatomegaly is present) thus not enabling it to fill to its capacity. Some studies have also shown elevated levels of serum leptin in patients with liver disease, which can lead to both anorexia and early satiety. Deficiencies in vitamin A and zinc have been associated with altered sense of taste and decreased oral intake in these patients. Dietary restrictions in sodium and fluid, often imposed on patients with ascites, can also discourage adequate oral intake. In addition, encephalopathy, weakness, and fatigue contribute to poor dietary intake in patients with advanced liver disease.

Maldigestion and Malabsorption (Chapter 7: Case 7.2)

Individuals with chronic liver disease frequently present with both maldigestion and malabsorption of fat. High concentrations of alcohol can disrupt the gastric and duodenal mucosa, causing diarrhea and malabsorption of thiamin, folate, and vitamin B_{12}. Steatorrhea, the most common manifestation of malabsorption, occurs in approximately 50 percent of patients with cirrhosis. Cholestasis, which is associated with decreased bile salt secretion and pancreatic insufficiency, may contribute to fat malabsorption. These patients may have deficiencies of the fat-soluble vitamins A, D, E, and K. Clinical manifestations include night blindness caused by vitamin A deficiency, osteomalacia caused by vitamin D deficiency, neuropathy caused by vitamin E deficiency, and easy bruisability or bleeding caused by vitamin K deficiency. An additional factor that may contribute to malabsorption is the administration of medications such as neomycin and lactulose, which are used to treat encephalopathy, and can cause excessive loose stool and diarrhea.

Abnormal Metabolism and Storage of Nutrients

Liver disease causes many metabolic problems and can reduce the body's ability to utilize ingested nutrients appropriately, therefore contributing to malnutrition.

Protein In patients with liver disease, there is reduced hepatic synthesis of transport proteins, which can result in low levels of serum albumin and transferrin. Hepatic synthesis of clotting factors is also reduced, interfering with blood coagulation, as evidenced by an abnormal prothrombin time (PT) and partial thromboplastin time (PTT).

Blood urea nitrogen (BUN) levels are reduced and plasma ammonium levels may be increased in liver disease subsequent to decreased hepatic urea synthesis. The failure to detoxify ammonia and the abnormal amino acid profile (increased aromatic amino acids and decreased branched chain amino acids) that is seen in patients with cirrhosis may augment their risk for the development of hepatic encephalopathy.

Carbohydrate Liver disease can also lead to disturbances in glucose metabolism, resulting in either hypoglycemia or hyperglycemia. The hypoglycemia sometimes seen in acute liver disease may be due to impaired glycogenesis, glycogenolysis, or gluconeogenesis. Hyperglycemia, often observed in cirrhosis and chronic hepatitis, may be associated with increased glucagon levels and insulin resistance.

Fat Disturbances in fat metabolism can be associated with the development of decreased lipid clearance and increased serum triglyceride and cholesterol levels. Excessive alcohol consumption is associated with increased accumulation of triglycerides in the liver and the development of fatty liver. Poor utilization of fat increases dependence on gluconeogenesis as an energy source.

Vitamins and Minerals Poor absorption and reduced storage of vitamins and minerals occur commonly in patients with chronic liver disease. Chronic liver disease also contributes to frequent deficiencies of thiamin, folate, pyridoxine, and vitamin D by decreasing the conversion of these vitamins to their active forms.

Nutritional Assessment for Malabsorption

Since malnutrition contributes to the development of complications that may be commonly encountered in patients with end-stage liver disease, a thorough nutrition assessment is of paramount importance when developing a plan of care for the patient. As discussed above, liver disease commonly causes many metabolic problems. These problems may affect assessment parameters commonly used to evaluate a patient's nutritional status.

Reduced hepatic synthesis of transport proteins may result in low serum albumin, prealbumin, and transferrin values in these patients. In turn, low levels of serum proteins, particularly albumin, result in decreased serum oncotic pressure, which is the most probable cause of ascites and edema. The presence of ascites and edema affects measured body weight. The presence of extra fluid may also further dilute serum protein levels. Therefore, measurement of patient's albumin, prealbumin, and weight is not a reliable indicator of malnutrition in this population.

Studies have investigated the use of anthropometric measurements to assess these patients; however, limitations were found including poor interobserver reproducibility and overestimation because of third spacing. The Subjective Global Assessment is a tool that aids in classifying malnutrition based upon features of a patient's medical history and physical examination. The components include weight loss during the previous six months, changes in dietary intake, gastrointestinal symptoms, functional capacity, metabolic demands, signs of muscle wasting, and presence of edema. This method has been shown to have an acceptable interobserver reproducibility rate, and may be more useful in assessing patients with end-stage liver disease than other traditional methods.

Nutrition Therapy for Liver Disease

The goals of nutrition therapy for patients with liver disease are to provide adequate protein and calories to maintain nitrogen balance and support hepatic regeneration, while preventing such complications as encephalopathy. Abstinence from alcohol is an essential part of managing alcohol-related liver disease.

Calories

Estimating energy requirements for patients with cirrhosis is controversial. Studies have been mixed with some showing no significant increase in metabolism in patients with liver disease, and others suggesting hypermetabolism in up to one-third of patients with stable cirrhosis. In 1997, the European Society for Parenteral and Enteral Nutrition created guidelines for meeting nutritional goals in patients with liver disease. These guidelines were updated in 2006 to include recommendations for nutrition support. They recommend that patients who have compensated cirrhosis should strive to achieve intakes of 25 to 35 kcal/kg/day. For those with complicated cirrhosis and associated malnutrition, they suggest 35 to 40 kcal/kg/day. Adjustments must be made in individuals who have infection, trauma, surgery, or loss of nutrients due to disorders such as steatorrhea, because additional calories are needed to minimize endogenous protein catabolism. In patients with ascites, all calculations must be based on estimated "dry" weight (total weight minus the weight of the ascites fluid). One liter of fluid is equivalent to approximately 1 kg of body weight. When fluid is seen only in the abdominal cavity, the amount is estimated at least 5 liters, or at least 5 kg of body weight. If fluid is present in both the abdominal cavity and the extremities, the amount is estimated at least 10 liters, or at least 10 kg of body weight.

For patients who are unable to meet their needs, enteral nutrition by means of oral nutrition supplementation or tube feeding may be utilized. Tube feeding in patients with liver disease is often avoided due to fears of bleeding with tube placement if esophageal or gastric varices, or coagulopathy, are present. Recent evidence suggests tube feeding can be safely considered in some of these patients, although the risks versus the benefits must be appropriately assessed. For most patients, supplementation with a standard enteral formula is effective. There are conflicting data about the benefit of enteral formulas supplemented with branched chain amino acids; however these are widely available and sometimes utilized in malnourished patients with hepatic encephalopathy. Parenteral nutrition should be reserved only for patients in whom enteral feeding is not an option.

Fat

Fat intake amounting to 20 to 40 percent of daily caloric requirements should be encouraged as tolerated in the absence of steatorrhea, because fat contributes to the non-protein caloric intake and additionally contributes to the increased palatability of the diet. Providing fat calories in the form of oil composed solely of medium-chain triglycerides (MCTs) may be necessary in the presence of fat malabsorption. MCTs are more efficiently absorbed than long-chain triglycerides (LCTs) because they are absorbed directly into the portal vein and subsequently are transported to the liver.

Protein

Achieving positive nitrogen balance in patients with cirrhosis involves individualizing protein prescriptions. ESPEN guidelines suggest 1.0 to 1.2 gm/kg/day for patients with stable cirrhosis, and up to 1.5 gm/kg/day for patients with complicated cirrhosis and underlying malnutrition. After the diagnosis of hepatic encephalopathy is established, it is important that precipitating factors such as infection, electrolyte imbalance, and GI bleeding be identified and treated. Recent evidence suggests protein restriction should not be instituted during periods of episodic encephalopathy; however, dietary intervention may be considered if hepatic encephalopathy persists. Dietary protein may be restricted to lower plasma ammonium levels because ammonia, a by-product of protein metabolism, can contribute to the development of hepatic encephalopathy. Drastic, long-term protein restriction is not indicated because many of these patients are protein depleted already when they present for treatment of their hepatic encephalopathy. Additional protein deprivation may promote catabolism of lean body tissue and contribute to malnutrition, and reduce host defenses to infection.

Sodium

In the severely sodium-retentive patient who has liver disease with ascites, sodium and fluid restrictions are necessary. The extent to which sodium needs to be restricted is controversial. Moderate sodium restriction (2 to 3 g/day), coupled with the use of effective diuretics, can make the diet more palatable and nutritious, while minimizing biochemical complications such as hyponatremia and the hypokalemia associated with potassium-wasting diuretics. However, cirrhotic patients have limited ability to excrete sodium, and those who are severely sodium retentive should be restricted initially to less than 500 mg of sodium per day. Once the patient shows rapid diuresis, the diet can be liberalized.

Fluid

By consensus, patients with hyponatremia (serum sodium under 130 mEq/L) require a fluid restriction of 1000 to 1500 cc/day. Massive fluid shifts result from edema, ascites, and diuretic therapy in these patients. Malnutrition is associated with a fluid shift from the intravascular space to the extravascular space and a concurrent decrease in lean body mass.

Vitamins and Minerals

Patients with chronic liver disease are at an increased risk for developing vitamin and mineral deficiencies secondary to poor intake, malabsorption, impaired metabolism, and decreased storage. The physical examination therefore should include evaluation of the physical signs and symptoms associated with the presence of vitamin and mineral deficiencies. A combined multivitamin and mineral preparation should be routinely provided for patients with chronic liver disease. If the patient is still consuming alcohol, thiamin and folate supplements should be prescribed to prevent Wernicke's encephalopathy and macrocytic anemia, respectively. Patients with advanced chronic liver disease may have problems with vitamin storage, metabolism, and transport, and thus may require subcutaneous injections of vitamins. In particular, these patients have been found to have fat-soluble vitamin deficiencies. Calcium deficiency and osteoporosis can result from decreased intestinal absorption and vitamin D deficiency, and should be monitored. Serum potassium, magnesium, and zinc levels should be monitored closely when diuretics are prescribed for these patients.

Inflammatory Bowel Disease

Inflammatory bowel disease (IBD) refers to idiopathic, chronic, inflammatory conditions affecting the gastrointestinal tract, primarily Crohn's disease and Ulcerative Colitis. Because of the chronic involvement of the GI tract, most patients with IBD have some form of nutritional deficiency. Therefore, careful attention to diet can prevent nutritional deficiencies and help in the medical and surgical management of these diseases.

Protein–energy malnutrition is prevalent among patients with IBD. Nutritional assessment is essential because of the consequences of malnutrition, which include growth retardation in children, impaired healing of the inflamed bowel, and enhanced susceptibility to infection in children and adults. In addition, a malnourished patient with IBD may present with defects in GI function that further limit the absorption and utilization of nutrients.

Causes of Malnutrition

Malnutrition occurs in patients suffering from IBD as a consequence of:
- decreased dietary intake,
- increased nutrient losses,
- increased nutrient requirements.

Decreased Dietary Intake The most important factor contributing to the poor nutritional status seen in patients with IBD is inadequate dietary intake. Gastrointestinal symptoms such as nausea, diarrhea, and recurrent abdominal pain at mealtimes often decrease patient's appetite and food intake. Also, eating certain foods may increase the likelihood of particular complications of IBD. For example, in Crohn's disease, where the lumen of the small bowel is narrower, impaction of bulky food in an inflamed area may precipitate an obstruction.

Increased Nutrient Losses In Crohn's disease, small and large bowel inflammation, bacterial overgrowth, and multiple bowel resections can decrease the absorptive surface area of both the small and large intestine and cause malabsorption of essential nutrients. Resections of the ileum can cause bile salt deficiency, resulting in steatorrhea or fat malabsorption and subsequent deficiency of the fat-soluble vitamins A, D, E, and K. Vitamin B_{12} is coupled with intrinsic factor secreted by the parietal cells of the stomach. Because the vitamin B_{12}-intrinsic factor complex is absorbed in the ileum, complete ileal resection produces a vitamin B_{12} deficiency that requires treatment with parenteral repletion (intramuscular injections of this vitamin, use of vitamin B_{12} nasal spray, or use of sublingual vitamin B_{12}).

IBD also can result in protein-losing enteropathy, or excessive intestinal secretion of protein-rich fluids through the inflamed bowel wall. Severe diarrhea causes depletion of electrolytes, minerals, and trace elements such as zinc. Gastrointestinal bleeding can contribute to iron-deficiency anemia.

Increased Nutrient Requirements The inflammatory process of IBD may increase resting energy expenditure, thereby contributing to weight loss and depletion of fat stores that occur when patients do not consume adequate calories and protein. Patients with fever or sepsis and those undergoing surgery also have greater requirements for protein, calories, and other nutrients than do patients who are less severely ill. Increased intestinal cell turnover can also raise nutrient requirements in patients with IBD.

Medical Nutrition Therapy for IBD

The goals of nutrition therapy for patients with IBD are to prevent symptoms associated with malabsorption such as diarrhea; to correct and prevent nutritional deficiencies; to promote healing of the intestinal mucosa; to minimize stress on inflamed and often narrowed segments of the bowel (Crohn's disease); and, in children, to promote normal growth and development. Oral nutritional repletion may be difficult to achieve during symptomatic, active IBD, since most patients' symptoms worsen both during and following meals. To decrease both the symptoms associated with eating and bowel activity during the healing process, patients hospitalized for IBD are sometimes placed on bowel rest. However, prolonged bowel rest without nutrition support can lead to nutritional depletion. An oral diet may be tolerated when active IBD is less severe. To control diarrhea and malabsorption, a low-fat, low-fiber, low-lactose diet is often prescribed. Small, frequent feedings may help to limit gastrointestinal secretions as well as reduce the volume of food that the damaged bowel must handle at any one time. During a flare, the diet should be individualized according to the patient's clinical condition and food tolerances.

Many patients with inflammatory bowel disease believe that diet plays a role in the development of a flare. While certain foods have been associated with causing increased GI pain, they are not believed to cause disease relapses. Unnecessary restriction of diet when individuals do not have active IBD is not encouraged because it can further limit nutrient intake (unless there are fixed narrowings in the GI tract). Patients should be advised to eat foods per their tolerance; however there are certain foods that can be discouraged because they offer few redeeming nutritional qualities and have been associated with intestinal distress. Of note, this can also allow patients to feel as though they have some control over their disease. Alcohol and caffeine can trigger diarrhea because they stimulate the GI tract: many times this can occur within 30 minutes following consumption. Similarly, diet foods and beverages containing sugar alcohols, such as sorbitol, xylitol, and mannitol, can also cause intestinal discomfort and diarrhea, and patients should be encouraged to look for these items on ingredient labels. Though controversial, heavily spiced foods, fried foods, and concentrated sweets have also been associated with inducing diarrhea. Individuals who experience intense GI pain after eating may benefit from keeping a food log to determine if any specific foods or beverages they are consuming may be acting as a GI irritant.

Calories

In adults, ingested calories should be provided in amounts sufficient to maintain or restore body weight. In children, the amount of ingested calories should be adequate to support growth and development, as is measured on the pediatric growth charts.

Complications, such as sepsis and fistulas, may increase caloric requirements in adults to as high as 35 to 45 kcal/kg per day, or approximately 1.5 to 1.7 times the basal energy expenditure according to the Harris–Benedict equation. If a patient is severely malnourished and his or her calorie intake is significantly low, usually 20 to 25 kcal/kg/day is initially prescribed to help avoid complications of refeeding syndrome; the patient should be assessed by a Registered Dietitian to help determine the most appropriate feeding plan. Supplemental calories can be given in the form of glucose polymers or medium chain triglyceride (MCT) oil.

Protein
Protein needs are often increased in IBD due to intestinal inflammation and infections such as abscesses (in Crohn's disease patients). The majority of IBD patients have daily protein needs of 1 to 1.5 g/kg body weight, if free of complications, such as chronic renal failure, that would otherwise limit protein requirements.

Vitamins and Minerals
IBD patients are at higher risk for vitamin, mineral, and trace element deficiencies. Higher doses of specific nutrients are indicated if clinical or laboratory evidence identifies a deficiency due to possible poor absorption or increased requirements. Patients with Crohn's disease who have extensive damage and/or have undergone resection of the terminal ileum are likely to suffer from defective vitamin B_{12} absorption and thus require supplementation with parenteral sources of this vitamin. IBD patients with persistent, watery diarrhea may have difficulty maintaining adequate zinc and magnesium levels and require supplementation.

Chronic blood loss and altered iron absorption, frequently observed in patients with IBD, can cause iron deficiency anemia. However, iron supplements in full therapeutic doses may exacerbate "GI distress." In particular, oral iron may cause symptoms of nausea, constipation, and abdominal cramping. Slower iron supplementation along with ascorbic acid may be more effective, because ascorbic acid enhances the absorption of iron by converting the ferric ions to the ferrous form, which is absorbed primarily in the duodenum. Only 25 to 50 mg of ascorbic acid is needed daily to enhance the absorption of iron.

Long-term treatment with corticosteroids requires calcium and vitamin D supplementation because corticosteroids decrease calcium absorption and increase calcium excretion. Patients treated with sulfasalazine (Azulfidine) should receive folate supplements because this medication inhibits uptake of folate by competitive inhibition of the enzyme folate conjugase in the jejunum. Mexthotrexate also requires folate supplementation because it is a folate antagonist (it inhibits the enzyme dihydrofolate reductase). If a patient is taking cholestyramine, fat soluble vitamins A, D, E, K can bind with the medication; folate and magnesium absorption can also be impaired by cholestyramine.

Fiber
A low-fiber diet is often prescribed for patients with narrowed sections of bowel to decrease the possibility of intestinal obstruction, minimize physical irritation to

the inflamed bowel, reduce stool weight and stool frequency, and slow the rate of intestinal transit. The diet consists of white bread and refined cereals and avoidance of high-fiber fresh fruits and vegetables, nuts, skins, and seeds. Controversy exists over the benefits of a low-fiber diet because its efficacy in managing symptoms or affecting the course of IBD remains unclear. Diets should be recommended depending on a patient's individual tolerance and intolerance; intake of fiber-rich nutrient-dense foods can generally be encouraged if the patient does not have GI discomfort after eating these items, pending there are no bowel strictures. A fiber-rich diet is not encouraged with strictures as this could potentially contribute to a small bowel obstruction.

Lactose
Patients with IBD may malabsorb lactose because of decreased brush border epithelial cell lactase activity and rapid intestinal transit. The enzyme lactase is most prevalent in the jejunum. Given that Crohn's disease is most prevalent in the ileocecal region it is not unexpected that the incidence of lactose intolerance among those suffering from IBD is similar to that of the general population.

Fat
Decreased fat intake may help control the symptoms of steatorrhea, especially in patients with Crohn's disease involving the small bowel. MCT oil is more easily absorbed than other fats; MCT oil can be added to other foods, but this may change the palatability of the food. Doses should be given in less than 15 gram amounts.

Omega-3 Fatty Acids
It has been demonstrated that gene mutations that affect the immune system, causing inflammation, are associated with IBD; consequently, it has been hypothesized that the ratio of polyunsaturated fats in the diet may play a role in helping to control inflammation. Current intake of omega-6 fats, are being consumed in much larger amounts compared with omega-3 fats. An increase in consumption of omega-3 fats and a decrease in omega-6 fats decreases arachidonic acid in the body: arachidonic acid is involved in the production of pro-inflammatory cytokines. It is hypothesized that when there is a reduction of omega-6 fat sources and an increase in omega 3-fatty acids there may be a reduction of inflammation in the body. While research has not been able to demonstrate that supplementation with omega-3 pills is beneficial in helping to sustain remission, the food sources of omega-3 fats pose little harm to IBD patients and should be encouraged, if tolerated. Dietary sources of omega-3 fats include fatty fish, walnuts, soy, flaxseed, canola oil, and in small amounts in certain leafy greens.

Oxalate
Calcium oxalate kidney stones following ileal resection are a common complication in patients with Crohn's disease. Limiting fat intake and foods with a high oxalate content is recommended to help reduce the formation of these stones (Chapter 10).

Prebiotics and Probiotics

Gene mutations that affect bacterial recognition, leading to an excessive immune response, are also thought to be associated with IBD: if the ratio of pathogenic bacteria in the gut is too high, significant inflammation in the gut may occur. Probiotics – microorganisms thought to have a beneficial effect on gut health – have been hypothesized to be beneficial to IBD patients. There are currently too few conclusive studies to be certain of the effect of probiotics in IBD, specifically with regards to probiotic supplementation. However, dietary sources of probiotics, such as yogurt and kefir, can be advised as they contain probiotics and are also sources of protein and calcium. Patients should look for food labels of such sources to say "contains live and active cultures," indicating that the bacteria are viable. Caution should be taken in giving probiotics to patients who are immunocompromised; have short bowel of less than 150 cm; or are otherwise critically ill, as a few complications have been associated with probiotics in these populations. Prebiotics are non-digestable ingredients that may stimulate the growth of healthy bacteria found in the gut and may improve gut health. Dietary sources of prebiotics include bananas, chicory root, Jerusalem artichoke, onions, asparagus, garlic, and barley. More studies need to be done to support prebiotic supplementation in IBD patients.

Nutrition Support

Enteral nutrition support should be the primary source of nutrition if it is safe to provide and oral nutrition consumption is not an option. The liquid formula used to provide enteral nutrition support in patients with IBD should be low in fat, low residue, and lactose-free. Elemental formulas (formulas that contain protein in the form of amino acids) for enteral tube feeding have been used successfully in this population. Because these formulas are completely absorbed in the upper small intestine and seem to be effective in reducing residue in the bowel, they are particularly appropriate for patients with Crohn's disease. Elemental formulas are also well tolerated because of their low fat content. Parenteral nutrition support is indicated only in severe cases of IBD when bowel rest is considered necessary and enteral nutrition support is not an option, as in such cases of bowel obstruction or severe strictures; distal fistulas that prohibit feeding; or a length of less than 150 cm of functional small intestine (short bowel) remaining (Chapter 12).

Case 1 **Alcohol and Vitamin Deficiencies**

Gail Morrison and Lisa D. Unger

University of Pennsylvania School of Medicine, Philadelphia, PA

OBJECTIVES

- Explain how excessive alcohol consumption contributes to nutritional deficiencies.
- Describe the biochemical and pathophysiologic abnormalities that occur with excessive alcohol intake.
- Recognize the importance of assessing a patient's alcohol intake during a routine social history.
- Describe the nutritional recommendations for patients who consume alcohol.

CT, a 52-year-old car salesman, presents to his family physician for his yearly physical examination reporting fatigue, burning in his feet, decreased memory, and heartburn. He has also noticed a recent weight gain and increased waist circumference and complains of increase in abdominal girth in association with weight gain and decreased endurance when exercising. He denies blurred vision, headaches, night sweats, or hearing loss.

Past Medical History

CT has no prior history of heart disease, stroke, or peripheral vascular disease. He has been told in the past that his liver is "damaged," but he has never received specific treatment for this. He is not taking any medications and has no known drug or food allergies.

Social History

CT states that he usually consumes three "healthy" meals every day, but his appetite has been poor for the past week. He has smoked one pack of cigarettes per day for 30 years (30-pack year history).

Family History

CT's family history is negative for the presence of heart disease, stroke, cholesterol, and lipid disorders, or neurologic diseases.

Review of Systems

General: The patient reports lethargy, decreased appetite, and recent bloating; he relates that his pants are tighter in the waist than usual.
GI/abdomen: No vomiting or diarrhea.

Medical Nutrition and Disease: A Case-Based Approach, 4th edition. Edited by Lisa Hark.
© 2009 Wiley-Blackwell Publishing, ISBN: 978-1-4051-8615-5.

Neurologic: No history of seizures, no tinnitus, no syncope. He has reported some memory loss.

Physical Examination
Vital Signs
Temperature: 98.2 °F (36.8 °C)
Heart rate: 104 BPM
Respiratory rate: 16 BPM
Blood pressure: 120/90 mm Hg
Height: 5'8" (173 cm)
Current weight: 160 lb (73 kg)
Usual weight (1 month ago): 150 lb (68 kg)
BMI: 24 kg/m^2

Exam
General: Well-dressed male who appears to be in mild distress.
Skin: Jaundiced; spider angiomas on the upper chest (central blood vessels feeding small, dilated vessels, characteristic of chronic liver disease).
Eyes: Pale conjunctiva, sclera icteric; no ophthalmoplegia or nystagmus.
Cardiac: Resting tachycardia; heart sounds are normal; no murmurs are present.
Chest/Pulmonary: Lungs clear to auscultation and percussion bilaterally; mild gynecomastia (excessive development of male mammary glands).
Abdomen: Distended abdomen; presence of an abdominal fluid wave and shifting dullness, consistent with ascites (physical finding of fluid accumulation in the peritoneal cavity that can be associated with severe liver disease); enlarged liver size (14 cm span) with a firm, non-tender edge; no splenomegaly.
Extremities: slight (1+) bilateral lower extremity edema.
Neurologic: decreased vibratory sensation in the lower legs; bilaterally decreased knee reflexes; no asterixis; normal sensation and position sense in upper and lower extremities; cranial nerves II through XII grossly intact.
Mental status: alert; oriented to time, place, and person.

CT's Laboratory Data

Measure	Patient's Values	Normal Values
Red blood cells (RBC):	3.8 million/mm^3	4.3–5.9 million/mm^3
Hemoglobin:	10 g/dL	13.5–17.5 g/dL
Hematocrit:	35%	41–53%
Mean corpuscular volume (MCV):	104 fL	80–100 fL
Albumin:	2.8 g/dL	3.5–5.8 g/dL
Prothrombin time:	15 seconds	11.0–13.2 seconds
International Normalized Ratio (INR):	1.3	1.0
Total bilirubin:	5 mg/dL	0.1–1.0 mg/dL
Aspartate aminotransferase (AST):	140 IU/L	8–20 U/L
Alanine aminotransferase (ALT):	80 IU/L	8–20 U/L
Sodium:	135 mmol/L	133–143 mmol/L

Case Questions:

1. What additional information is important to obtain from a patient who presents with these symptoms?
2. What are the biochemical consequences of excessive alcohol consumption?
3. What is the prevalence of alcoholism in the United States and what are the associated medical consequences?
4. What are the nutritional consequences of excessive alcohol consumption?
5. What evidence from CT's history, physical examination, and laboratory data suggests complications of alcoholism and nutritional deficiencies?
6. What does CT's serum albumin level indicate?
7. What additional laboratory tests would you request before giving CT a folate supplement?

Answers to Questions: Case 1

1. What additional information is important to obtain from a patient who presents with these symptoms?

Assessment of a patient's alcohol intake should always be included in the social history because many people who actively drink alcohol may not voluntarily admit to having a drinking problem. In addition, particular attention must be paid to those signs, symptoms, and lab tests that are likely to be abnormal in the alcoholic patient. Neurologic signs, combined with fatigue, gynecomastia, ascites, enlarged liver, possible gastroesophageal reflux, and abnormal liver function tests all alert the clinician to probe for chronic alcohol ingestion. Once the patient admits to drinking, specific information regarding quantity, type, frequency, and duration of consumption should be obtained.

CT has been drinking heavily for 10 years. His daily routine consists of two cocktails before dinner, a few glasses of wine with dinner, and two cocktails after dinner, totaling six drinks per day. Considering that CT is a heavy drinker, as evidenced by his consumption of 42 drinks per week, he is a candidate for the CAGE test. The CAGE test was developed as a diagnostic tool for alcoholism. CT is asked the following questions, which are assigned a value of one point if answered "yes."

Have you ever felt you should **C**ut down on your drinking? ___(Yes)
Have people **A**nnoyed you by criticizing your drinking? ___(No)
Have you ever felt bad or **G**uilty about your drinking? ___(Yes)
Have you ever had a drink the first thing in the morning (**E**ye opener) to steady your nerves or to get rid of a hangover? ___(No)

When interpreting the CAGE test, take into account the patient's answers to the preliminary questions about alcohol use. A key question is "When was the last time you had a drink?" Because CT reports drinking within the past 30 days and scored two on the CAGE test, he is very likely to have a current alcohol problem.

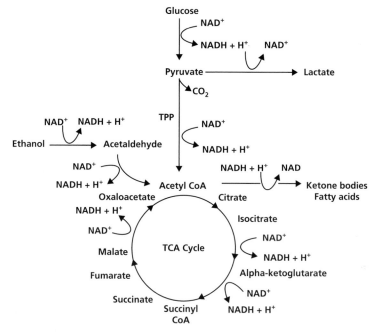

Figure 7-1 Alcohol Metabolism and the Altered Redox State.
Source: Adapted from Berg JM, Tymoczko JL, Stryer L. *Biochemistry*. Paperback Edition, WH Freeman: New York. 2008.

2. What are the biochemical consequences of excessive alcohol consumption?

Excessive alcohol consumption can cause metabolic acidosis by interfering with the oxidation of acetyl CoA in the TCA cycle. Ethanol is oxidized to acetaldehyde by the enzyme alcohol dehydrogenase, which also simultaneously reduces NAD^+ to NADH $+ H^+$. Next, the enzyme acetylaldehyde dehydrogenase oxidizes acetaldehyde to acetyl CoA and reduces another NAD^+ to NADH $+ H^+$. This enzyme requires NAD^+ to accept the hydrogen ions.

The increased ratio of NADH to NAD^+ in the presence of excess alcohol, called an altered redox state, drives pyruvate to lactate instead of to acetyl CoA. High levels of lactate generated from pyruvate suggest an abnormality in the recycling of NADH to NAD^+ caused by excessive alcohol ingestion. In addition, instead of entering the TCA cycle, where more NADH is produced, acetyl CoA is converted to ketone bodies and fatty acids. As a result, a ketoacidotic state develops and fatty acids are converted to triglycerides. In turn, a significant rise in triglyceride levels can lead to fatty liver (Figure 7-1).

3. What is the prevalence of alcoholism in the United States and what are the associated medical consequences?

Alcoholism is a major problem in the United States. Each year, about 100,000 deaths in the United States are related to alcohol consumption. According to the 2000 National Household Survey on Drug Abuse, almost half of Americans (46.6 percent) aged 12 and older reported being consumers of alcohol in some form or another. This translates into an estimated 103 million people. In addition, nearly 5.6 percent of people aged between 25 and 44 were heavy drinkers (five or more drinks per day). The harm associated with the intake of large amounts of alcohol has been well documented.

Alcohol intake over 30 grams per day (more than 2 drinks) has been associated with increased mortality due to hypertension, pancreatitis, gastrointestinal malignancies, stroke, cardiomyopathy, cirrhosis, motor vehicle accidents, and breast cancer. Alcoholics can also experience marital/family difficulties and also may lose their jobs as a result of work absenteeism. In addition, alcohol can interact with many different medications affecting their potency.

4. What are the nutritional consequences of excessive alcohol consumption?

Alcohol provides 7 kcal/gram, which can be utilized and metabolized when substituted for calories from food, but provides no protein, vitamins, or minerals. Drinking causes a decrease in appetite that generally is proportional to the amount of ingested calories from alcohol and can significantly affect the nutritional adequacy of a patient's diet. High concentrations of alcohol can also disrupt the gastric and duodenal mucosa, affect the digestive and absorptive processes, and as a consequence, reduce significantly the absorption of vitamins.

One of the most important vitamin supplements routinely given to alcoholics is thiamin, since alcohol interferes with thiamin absorption, even in healthy individuals. Thiamin is important in carbohydrate metabolism. Its predominant form, thiamin pyrophosphate (TPP), functions as a coenzyme for pyruvate dehydrogenase, which converts pyruvate to acetyl CoA. Inadequate thiamin intake forces pyruvate to be converted to lactate, further contributing to the development of lactic acidosis (Figure 7-1). Thiamin deficiency manifests as anorexia, irritability, fatigue, and decreased memory. Later stages present with peripheral neuropathy, confusion, and tachycardia.

Chronic alcohol consumption has also been associated with folate deficiency; however, the etiology is unclear. Alcohol may affect folate levels by decreasing dietary intake, impairing absorption and metabolism, increasing urinary excretion of folate, and may also be directly toxic to bone marrow and other cells. Tetrahydrofolate (THF), the coenzyme derived from this vitamin, is involved in one-carbon-unit transfers including amino acid interconversions and purine and pyrimidine biosynthesis. The interconversion of homocysteine to methionine requires methyl tetrahydrofolate as the coenzyme for methionine synthase. Vitamin B_{12} also acts as a cofactor in the methylation of homocysteine to methionine, in which methyl tetrahydrofolate is converted to THF. As a result, in vitamin B_{12} deficiency, the demethylation of methyl THF is prevented, blocking folate metabolism, or trapping folate.

Folate is also required for normal purine and pyrimidine biosynthesis. The methylation of deoxyuridine monophosphate (dUMP) to thymidine monophosphate (dTMP,) catalyzed by thymidylate synthase, requires 5,10-methylene THF, which is synthesized from THF.

Folate deficiency alters red blood cell production, resulting in enlarged, oval erythrocytes, manifested as megaloblastic anemia. It often cannot be distinguished from the anemia associated with a vitamin B_{12} deficiency. However, the neurologic abnormalities that occur with a vitamin B_{12} deficiency are rarely seen in folate deficiency.

5. What evidence from CT's history, physical examination, and laboratory data suggests complications of alcoholism and nutritional deficiencies?

Decreased lower extremity reflexes, decreased lower extremity vibratory sensation, and paresthesias are all neurologic signs and symptoms associated with thiamin deficiency due to prolonged alcohol abuse. The diagnosis of thiamin deficiency is highly likely because this patient has been drinking heavily for 10 years. This condition is considered a medical emergency because, if left untreated, it can progress quickly and cause irreversible damage.

This patient's hematology lab data reveal that anemia is present, which may explain his fatigue. An elevated mean corpuscular volume (MCV) indicates the presence of large red blood cells, a characteristic finding in megaloblastic anemia. Megaloblastic anemia can be caused by either vitamin B_{12} or folate deficiency; however, alcoholics are not usually vitamin B_{12} deficient.

6. What does CT's serum albumin level indicate?

CT's serum albumin value may reflect moderately depleted protein status and overall nutritional status. Decreased albumin, however, may not accurately reflect protein status in patients with severe liver disease because albumin is synthesized in the liver and is also influenced by hydration status. Usually, the liver retains its capacity to produce albumin until end-stage liver disease. The liver also synthesizes the vitamin K-dependent clotting factors, which explains CT's prolonged prothrombin time, since the liver's ability to produce factors II, VII, IX, and X can be affected early in liver disease.

7. What additional laboratory tests would you request before giving CT a folate supplement?

Serum and RBC folate and serum vitamin B_{12} levels should be checked. Serum folate levels are greatly affected by current diet intake; however, RBC folate levels are a better measure of tissue folate status. Although alcoholics are not usually vitamin B_{12} deficient, it is important to check CT for vitamin B_{12} deficiency because if CT's megaloblastic anemia is due to vitamin B_{12} deficiency, prescribing folate without vitamin B_{12} will improve the anemia but mask the vitamin B_{12} deficiency and its progression with the associated neurologic damage. It is important to remember that neurologic impairments due to vitamin B_{12} deficiency do not respond to folate supplementation alone and are not reversible; however, hematologic abnormalities do respond both to folate and to vitamin B_{12}.

CT's results from the recommended tests support the diagnosis of folate deficiency.

CT's Values	Normal Values
Vitamin B$_{12}$: 520 pg/mL	220–960 pg/mL
Serum folate: 2 ng/mL	3.0–17 ng/mL
RBC folate: 90 ng/mL	280–903 ng/mL

Based on his clinical presentation and laboratory data, CT should receive thiamin, folate, and multivitamin supplements, especially if he continues to drink alcohol. CT should be advised to eliminate drinking alcohol and enroll in an appropriate outpatient therapy program.

Case 2 **Malabsorption**

Gary R. Lichtenstein[1] and Barbara Hopkins[2]

[1] University of Pennsylvania Health System, Philadelphia, PA
[2] Georgia State University, Atlanta, GA

OBJECTIVES

- Evaluate the clinical, anthropometric, and laboratory data of a patient with malabsorption.
- Explain how dietary factors affect a patient with malabsorption.
- Identify nutrient deficiencies associated with malabsorption and develop a nutritional care plan to treat these problems.

JR, a 27-year-old graduate student, is referred to the GI clinic by his primary care physician because of persistent complaints of loose bowel movements. JR's history is significant for a gunshot wound to his abdomen 5 years ago, requiring intestinal resection of approximately 75 percent of his small intestine (the ileum and most of the jejunum) with anastomosis (surgical re-attachment) of the proximal jejunum to the cecum. Post-operatively he noted about five liquid bowel movements daily, described as oily and foul smelling, which have persisted until the present time. After surgery he did not seek medical follow-up. JR takes no medications.

Social History

After surgery he was instructed to eat 5 to 6 small meals per day, to follow a high-calorie, high-protein diet with 5 to 10 grams of soluble fiber and a limited intake of oxalates, and to take a daily multivitamin and mineral supplement. JR chose to discontinue the vitamin and mineral supplement 1 year ago. JR does not smoke cigarettes, but he reports drinking two beers per week and three cups of coffee daily. He states that he does not have the energy to exercise.

Diet History

JR reports the following recall as his "typical" intake.

Medical Nutrition and Disease: A Case-Based Approach, 4th edition. Edited by Lisa Hark.
© 2009 Wiley-Blackwell Publishing, ISBN: 978-1-4051-8615-5.

JR's 24-Hour Dietary Recall:

Breakfast (Diner)

Fried eggs	2 large
Margarine	1 Tbsp.
Bacon	3 slices
White toast	2 slices (enriched)
Butter	2 Tbsp.
Cranberry juice	12 ounces
Coffee	1 6-ounce cup
Sugar	4 packets

Snack (Food truck)

Coffee	1 6-ounce cup
Sugar	4 packets
Jelly doughnut	1 regular

Lunch (Fast-food)

Double cheeseburger	1 large
French fries	1 large order
Chocolate milkshake	12 ounces (360 mL)

Dinner (Home)

Baked ham	8 ounces (227 g)
Baked potato	1 medium
Butter	2 Tbsp.
White bread	2 slices (enriched)
Butter	2 Tbsp.
Apple pie	1/6 of 9 inch pie
Coffee	1 cup
Sugar	2 packets

Snack (Home)

Corn chips	3 ounces bag (85 g)
Beer	12 ounces (360 mL)

Total Calories: 4462 kcal
Protein: 143 g (13% of calories)
Fat: 204 g (43% of calories)
Saturated fat: 85 g (17% of total calories)
Monounsaturated fat: 31 g (6% of total calories)
Polyunsaturated fat: 6 g (1.5% of total calories)
Cholesterol: 852 mg
Carbohydrate: 488 g (44% of calories)
Dietary fiber: 25 g
Sodium: 6902 mg
Calcium: 544 mg

Review of Systems

General: 27-year-old male who appears very thin and wears loose-fitting clothes; weight loss (10 pounds or 4.5 kg) over the past year, fatigue, and weakness. Appetite good, but patient reports that he must eat "twice as much food" as he did prior to his operation and that he still continues to lose weight.

Skin: Dry and scaly.

Eyes: Difficulty driving at night due to poor night vision.

GI: Five liquid bowel movements daily, described as oily and foul-smelling.

Physical Examination

Vital Signs

Temperature: 98.0 °F (37 °C)

Heart rate: 80 BPM

Respiration: 16 BPM

Blood pressure: 94/60 mm Hg

Height: 5′10″ (178 cm)

Current weight: 125 lb (57 kg)

Usual body weight: 165 lb (75 kg); has lost 40 pounds (18 kg) since surgery 5 years ago

BMI = 18 kg/m^2

Exam

General: Thin, underweight man in mild distress

Skin: Flaky dermatitis, ecchymoses

Head: Bilateral temporal muscle wasting

Mouth: Glossitis, cheilosis

GI/abdomen: Protuberant abdomen, bowel sounds with no activity, no hepatosplenomegaly

Extremities: Skeletal pain, interosseous muscle wasting, subcutaneous fat wasting, skeletal muscle wasting

Laboratory Data

Patient's Lab Values	Normal Values
Albumin: 2.5 g/dL	3.5–5.8 g/dL
Cholesterol: 120 mg/dL	desirable <200 mg/dL
Calcium: 5.5 mg/dL	9–11 mg/dL
Vitamin B$_{12}$: 100 pg/mL	220–960 pg/mL
Vitamin A: 13 mg/dL	28–94 mg/dL
25(OH)D: 5 ng/mL	20–30 ng/mL
Vitamin E	
Alpha tocopherol: 3 mg/L	4.6–14.5 mg/L
Beta/gamma tocopherol: 0.6 mg/L	1.4–4.8 mg/L
Prothrombin time: 16 seconds	<11–15 seconds
Parathyroid hormone: 50 pg/mL	10–55 pg/mL
Serum folate: 2.5 ng/mL	>3–17 ng/mL

Zinc: 300 mg/dL   550–1400 mg/dL

Magnesium: 1.2 mg/dL   1.8–2.9 mg/dL

Fecal fat (72 hours): 28 g   <6 g daily

Case Questions:

1. Explain why JR continues to lose weight even though he eats a large volume of food.
2. What is the cause of JR's steatorrhea?
3. What are the causes and associated clinical signs or symptoms of each laboratory abnormality with which JR presents?
4. Using JR's actual body weight, calculate the percentage change from his usual weight and interpret these results.
5. What conclusions can you draw regarding the fat, calorie, vitamin, and mineral content of JR's diet?
6. How does JR's current caloric intake compare with his requirements?
7. JR notes that his symptoms worsen when he eats fried or fatty foods. What should be done to correct these symptoms and his laboratory abnormalities?

Answers to Questions: Case 2
Part 1: Diagnosis

1. Explain why JR continues to lose weight even though he eats so much food.

Weight loss may be a result of fat malabsorption (steatorrhea). Moreover, while luminal digestion of starch into oligosaccharides and proteins into oligopeptides should be unaffected, decreased small bowel surface area interferes with brush border and cytoplasmic digestion, as well as transport across enterocytes. Transit time through the small intestine is decreased in patients who have undergone partial resection. Therefore, reduced exposure of nutrients to the intestinal mucosa also interferes with optimal absorption.

2. What is the cause of JR's steatorrhea?

JR does not have an ileum and thus is unable to reabsorb bile salts. Bile salts are essential for the absorption of fats and fat-soluble vitamins. Normally, bile salts are reabsorbed through the ileum, transported to the liver via the enterohepatic circulation, and recycled back to the intestinal lumen to meet the need for bile salts. Following ileal resection, bile salt loss through the stool increases because these salts are no longer being absorbed. The liver increases bile salt production in an attempt to compensate for the losses, but often fails to adequately accommodate them. As a result, absorption of fat, fat-soluble vitamins (A, D, E, and K), calcium, and magnesium decreases as the bile salt pool becomes depleted. In spite of greatly increased hepatic synthesis of bile salts, a deficiency of conjugated bile salts may result.

The inability to reabsorb bile salts results in an increased rate of conversion of cholesterol to bile acids by the liver. Depletion of intracellular free cholesterol upregulates the low-density lipoprotein receptors in these cells, resulting in an elevated rate of removal of cholesterol from the blood. This could explain the relatively low serum cholesterol level in the face of a high cholesterol intake. However, the rate of conversion of cholesterol to bile acids is inadequate in this patient to prevent symptoms of steatorrhea.

Bile salt deficiency leads to impairment in the body's ability to incorporate ingested dietary lipids (primarily long-chain triglycerides) into the micellar phase. This inability leads to decreased mucosal absorption of ingested lipids and fat-soluble vitamins resulting in subsequent steatorrhea, a condition called cholerrheic enteropathy. The deficiency of bile acids/salts diminishes the emulsification needed for efficient digestion of triacylglycerols to fatty acids by pancreatic lipase, due to the small surface area for enzyme attachment.

When treating patients who have undergone ileal resection, it is important to remember that although bile salt absorption occurs passively through the upper small intestine, active sodium-coupled uptake of bile salts in the ileum normally is responsible for retrieval of over 95 percent of the intraluminal bile salts.

Part 2: Laboratory Evaluation

Several laboratory abnormalities were observed in this patient. JR's nutritional problems reflect his decreased small bowel absorptive area, which renders him less able to absorb fat, protein, carbohydrate, vitamins, and minerals

3. What are the causes and associated clinical signs or symptoms of each laboratory abnormality with which JR presents?

Albumin JR's value: 2.5 g/dL   Normal value: 3.5–5.8 g/dL

A serum albumin level of 2.1 to 2.7 g/dL is an indication of a moderate degree of visceral protein depletion caused by decreased protein absorption. Muscle wasting and weakness are signs of skeletal protein depletion.

Calcium JR's value: 5.5 mg/dL   Normal value: 9–11 mg/dL

Because calcium is bound to albumin, it is always important to determine the serum calcium corrected for the patient's albumin level to account for the ionized calcium in serum, which is determined by an equilibrium between free calcium and calcium bound to serum protein. We use the following equation to determine the corrected calcium:

(Normal albumin − Serum albumin) × (Correction factor) + Serum calcium
Correction factor = 0.8 Normal albumin = 4.0 g/dL
Therefore, in JR's case
Corrected calcium = (4.0 − 2.5)(0.8) + 5.5 = 6.7 mg/dL

This calcium value of 6.7 mg/dL, corrected for JR's albumin level, still is not in the normal range of 9 to 11 mg/dL.

Most calcium absorption occurs in the duodenum, but all small intestinal segments absorb calcium. When adjustments are made for transit time and the relative lengths of the different intestinal segments, both the jejunum and ileum contribute substantially to overall calcium absorption. JR's resection has reduced the available absorptive surface area of the small intestine and this accounts in part for his low serum calcium value.

A second cause for the low serum calcium seen in this patient is the reduction in the size of the bile salt pool with impairment of micellar solubilization. This condition leads to decreased calcium absorption due to intraluminal binding of dietary calcium to unabsorbed fatty acids (soap formation). Third, vitamin D malabsorption and deficiency also lead to calcium malabsorption.

JR suffers from hypocalcemia, a low serum calcium level. Evaluation of ionized calcium would help in assessing the severity of calcium depletion. Clinical manifestations of calcium deficiency include skeletal pain, tetany, paresthesia, osteoporosis, and stunted growth in children. (See Appendices G and H for dietary sources of calcium.)

Vitamin B_{12} JR's value: 100 pg/mL   Normal value: >220–960 pg/mL

After vitamin B_{12} complexes with the binding protein, intrinsic factor (which is produced in the stomach), it is absorbed in the terminal ileum. Patients who have undergone removal of the terminal ileum thus cannot absorb vitamin B_{12} and require intramuscular injections of this nutrient to prevent long-term deficiency and associated peripheral neuropathy, which generally first becomes apparent after 5 to 10 years. An intranasal form of vitamin B_{12} has gained favor as a supplement. Clinical manifestations of vitamin B_{12} deficiency include megaloblastic anemia, peripheral neuropathy, glossitis, and cheilosis. The only dietary sources of vitamin B_{12} are foods of animal origin such as meat, chicken, fish, eggs, dairy products, and fortified soymilk. Some breakfast cereals are also fortified with vitamin B_{12}. Since JR has no ileum, dietary sources are unimportant since absorption is not feasible.

Vitamin A JR's value: 13 mg/dL   Normal value: 28–94 mg/dL

Vitamin A, in the form of dietary retinyl ester, is a fat-soluble vitamin that is hydrolyzed to retinol by pancreatic and intestinal brush border esterases prior to uptake from the gut lumen. Absorption occurs in the proximal small intestine and is aided by the presence of bile salts. Another source of retinol is the vitamin precursor beta-carotene. After uptake and transport, vitamin A is stored in the liver cells called stellate cells. Clinical manifestations of vitamin A deficiency include xerophthalmia (with clinical findings ranging from night blindness to corneal ulceration and irreversible blindness), poor wound healing, and loss of epithelial integrity (in the skin, GI tract, and urinary and respiratory systems). Dietary sources of vitamin A and beta-carotene are listed in Appendix A. These nutrients also are found in meats, wheat and rice germ, nuts, and legumes. Vitamin A absorption is also limited by fat malabsorption.

Vitamin D JR's value: 5 ng/mL   Normal value: 20–30 ng/mL

Vitamin D is a fat-soluble vitamin, naturally occurring in two forms, vitamin D_2 and vitamin D_3. Fat malabsorption conditions adversely affect vitamin D absorption. Once absorbed and transported to the liver as a component of the chylomicrons or bound to a serum carrier protein, DBP (vitamin D binding protein), vitamin D undergoes hydroxylation to 25-hydroxy vitamin D 25(OH)D with further conversion to its physiologically active form, 1,25-dihydroxy-vitamin D 1,25(OH)$_2$D, in the kidneys. The synthesis and metabolism of vitamin D is closely coupled to calcium homeostasis; therefore when calcium levels in the blood are low, the body releases parathyroid hormone (PTH), which stimulates the kidney to convert calcidiol to calcitriol, its active form. Elevations in 1,25(OH)$_2$D stimulate the gastrointestinal tract to increase calcium absorption from about 10 to 30 percent and phosphorous absorption from about 60 to 80 percent.

Vitamin D deficiency due to fat malabsorptive disorders can result in rickets in infants and children and osteomalacia (softening of the bones) in adults. Osteomalacia may lead to pain in the legs, ribs, hips, and muscles, and easily broken bones. (See Appendix B for dietary sources of vitamin D.)

Parathyroid hormone (PTH) and vitamin D: It is important to consider PTH levels in patients who have low vitamin D levels because it is likely that the upper limit of normal for the PTH range – especially in elderly subjects – is set too high. Low vitamin D levels – by reducing calcium absorption – will tend to raise PTH secretion and may affect the PTH reference range. PTH tends to increase as vitamin D levels fall below 10 to 15 ng/mL. Severe vitamin D deficiency is likely to raise PTH to levels above the reference range ("secondary hyperparathyroidism"), irrespective of the plasma calcium or phosphate level. However not all patients with hypovitaminosis D will necessarily show "hyperparathyroidism".

Vitamin E   JR's alpha tocopherol value: 3.0 mg/L
                            Normal value: 4.6–14.5 mg/L
                            JR's beta gamma tocopherol value: 0.6 mg/L
                            Normal value: 1.4–4.8 mg/L

Vitamin E is absorbed passively in the proximal small intestine. Bile salts serve as an important factor in normal vitamin E absorption. Like other fat-soluble vitamins, vitamin E is packaged into chylomicrons and delivered into the mesenteric lymphatics. It is stored primarily in the liver and in the adipose tissue. Clinical manifestations of vitamin E deficiency include neurologic dysfunction in the form of cerebellar ataxia, loss of deep tendon reflexes, and diminished vibratory and position sense. Hemolytic anemia may also result from vitamin E deficiency. (See Appendix C for dietary sources of vitamin E.)

Vitamin K   JR's PT: 16 seconds   Normal PT: <11–15 seconds

Vitamin K is obtained from dietary sources and also produced by colonic flora. Absorption of vitamin K occurs primarily in the proximal small bowel and requires bile salts. Following intestinal absorption, vitamin K is taken up largely by the liver and accumulated in the microsomal fraction. In the liver, vitamin K is a required cofactor for the enzymatic gamma-carboxylation of glutamic acid on vitamin K–dependent coagulation proenzymes (factors II [prothrombin], VII, IX, and X) and other proteins involved in coagulation and fibrinolysis (proteins C, S, M, and Z).

Clinical manifestations of vitamin K deficiency include prolonged clotting time resulting in bleeding problems (oral, genitourinary, gastrointestinal, and skin). Long-term use of antibiotics may eliminate bacterial production of vitamin K for patients, rendering them prone to clinical deficiency if they do not receive exogenous sources of vitamin K. (See Appendix D for dietary sources of vitamin K.)

Folate JR's value: 2.5 ng/mL   Normal value: >3–17 ng/mL

The jejunum absorbs folate for subsequent delivery into the portal circulation. Following intestinal resection, the remaining portions of the small intestine may increase their uptake of folate to compensate for poor absorption; however, JR's folate intake is low due to poor intake of fruits and vegetables. Serum folate levels reflect very recent dietary ingestion rather than total body folate stores. Therefore, a normal serum folate test does not exclude folate deficiency. A better reflection of total body folate stores would be an erythrocyte folate level. Clinical manifestations of folate deficiency include megaloblastic anemia and glossitis. (See Appendix F for dietary sources of folate.) Folate is easily destroyed in cooking or processing.

Zinc JR's value: 300 mg/dL   Normal value: 550–1400 mg/dL

Zinc absorption occurs throughout the small intestine, but its rate of absorption is greater in the jejunum than in the ileum or duodenum. In patients who have undergone intestinal resection, transit time and surface area for absorption decrease, especially for zinc absorption. Intestinal reabsorption of zinc is impaired further in these patients because the jejunum and ileum have been removed. Clinical manifestations of zinc deficiency include anorexia, hypogeusia, alopecia, delayed onset of puberty, dermatitis, and poor wound healing. Oysters, meats, nuts, and legumes are all excellent dietary sources of zinc.

Magnesium JR's value: 1.2 mg/dL   Normal value: 1.8–2.9 mg/dL

Magnesium is absorbed primarily in the jejunum and ileum by a passive mechanism. In patients with steatorrhea, unabsorbed fatty acids inhibit Mg absorption by forming insoluble complexes in a reaction called chelation. Magnesium absorption is reduced in patients who have undergone small intestinal resections because of the decreased available surface area. Clinical manifestations of magnesium deficiency may include neuromuscular weakness, confusion, fatigue, tetany, and paresthesias. (See Appendix K for dietary sources of magnesium.)

Fecal Fat 28 grams over 72 hours   Normal <6 grams per day.

Normal fat excretion on a diet of 80 to 100 grams of fat is up to 6 grams of fat per day. A larger amount of fat excretion is associated with a disorder of fat digestion and/or fat malabsorption.

Part 3: Clinical Assessment

4. Using JR's current body weight, calculate the percentage change from his usual weight and interpret these results.

$$\% \text{ Weight change} = \frac{\text{Usual weight} - \text{Current weight}}{\text{Usual weight}} \times 100$$

$$\% \text{ Weight change} = \frac{165 \text{ lb} - 125 \text{ lb}}{165 \text{ lb}} \times 100 = 24\%$$

A value of this magnitude (24% weight change) indicates a clinically significant and severe weight loss.

5. What conclusions can you draw regarding the fat, calorie, vitamin, and mineral content of JR's diet?

According to JR's 24-hour dietary recall analysis, his diet is high in fatty and salty foods and sweets. He is consuming more than 200 grams of fat per day. JR's diet lacks foods from three major food groups: fruits, vegetables, and dairy products. The fact that he rarely selects foods from these food groups places him at high risk for vitamin and mineral deficiencies compounded by malabsorption of fat and several vitamins and minerals.

6. How does JR's current caloric intake compare with his requirements?

According to the Harris–Benedict equation or 35 kcal/kg estimate, JR should consume 2700 to 2800 kcal/day to achieve a weight of 166 pounds (75 kg). However, according to JR's actual intake, he is consuming 4462 kcal/day. Normally, fat weight gain can be expected even when excess intake amounts only to a few hundred calories, but JR's significant malabsorption problem has resulted in weight loss instead.

Part 4: Treatment

7. JR notes that his symptoms worsen when he eats fried or fatty foods. What should be done to correct these symptoms and his laboratory abnormalities?

JR is experiencing fat malabsorption secondary to his surgery. Because his ileum was resected, JR cannot reabsorb the bile acids required for fat digestion. Thus his dietary fat intake, at 43 percent of total calories, far exceeds his ability to digest and absorb fat properly. Referral to a registered dietitian for individualized counseling and reinforcement of the following suggestions is highly recommended in JR's case.

Low-fat foods should be substituted for fried and fast foods. However, because JR may find gaining weight difficult if his diet is too low in fat, monitoring his weight carefully is important. JR should be encouraged to eat small frequent meals. Not all patients with malabsorption require a low-fat diet. JR should consume a wide variety of foods and increase his intake of soluble fiber (e.g. legumes, fruits, oats). Because many patients with malabsorption due to intestinal resection tend to be lactose-intolerant as a consequence of their reduced levels of lactase enzyme, a lactose-free diet may be beneficial.

Vitamin and mineral supplementation is indicated, since his surgery has significantly increased his intestinal motility and decreased transit time and the available absorptive area for the vitamins and minerals described previously. In addition, as a result of bile salt depletion, his absorption of fat and fat-soluble vitamins A, D, E, and K also has decreased. Other food factors that are troublesome in patients with resected small intestines include insoluble fiber (whole-wheat products), oxalates (chocolate, cocoa, coffee, most berries (especially strawberries and cranberries)), most nuts (especially peanuts), beans, beets, bell peppers, black pepper, parsley, rhubarb, spinach, Swiss chard, summer squash, sweet potatoes, and tea) and concentrated sweets.

Case 3 **AIDS with Opportunistic Infection**

Cade Fields-Gardner

The Cutting Edge, Cary, IL

OBJECTIVES

- Assess the nutritional status of a patient with advanced HIV disease.
- Explain the nutritional consequences of weight loss, diarrhea, and malabsorption in patients with HIV disease.
- Develop appropriate medical nutrition therapy goals for patients with HIV disease.
- Describe the role of medications in supporting nutritional status in HIV disease.

MD is a 38-year-old Hispanic man who presented to the outpatient clinic with weight loss. He was in his usual state of health until 3 years ago, when he presented to an AIDS Service organization (ASO) for an HIV test, shortly after his brother died of AIDS. When the results came back positive, he was provided with a list of physicians and clinics for follow-up care. However, he stated that he felt well at that time and remained without complaints until 6 months prior to this presentation.

MD works in the construction industry as a finish carpenter. His daily activities were becoming increasingly limited by the several bouts of watery diarrhea, which was associated with nausea. MD compensated by reducing his food intake. After several days of decreased intake, his diarrhea would decrease, but he became weak and ultimately lost his appetite. His job was threatened by frequent absenteeism because of weakness and diarrhea. He noted additional weight loss and loose-fitting clothes. MD denied fever, chills, night sweats, or muscle or joint pain.

Usual Dietary Intake

Food intake: Primarily crackers, rehydrating sports drinks, and juices, approximately 500 calories per day over the past two weeks.
Alcohol intake: None recently
Tobacco: None
IV drug use: None

Medical Nutrition and Disease: A Case-Based Approach, 4th edition. Edited by Lisa Hark.
© 2009 Wiley-Blackwell Publishing, ISBN: 978-1-4051-8615-5.

Physical Examination
Vital Signs
Temperature: 97.0 °F (36.1 °C)
Heart rate: 100 BPM
Respiration: 15 BPM
Blood pressure: 100/60 mm Hg
Height: 5′6″ (173 cm)
Current weight: 117 lb (53 kg)
Usual weight (6 weeks ago): 145 lb (66 kg)
Percent weight change: 19% (145–117/145)
BMI: 18.9 kg/m^2

MD's Body Composition Data

Parameter	Patient's Value	Normal Value
Fat free mass (kg)	105.7	>102.3
Body cell mass (kg)	48.1	>55.4
Extracellular tissue (kg)	57.6	47–53
Fat (kg)	11.3	12–24
Mid-upper arm circumference (percentile)	27.5 cm (<5th percentile)	30.5–34.2 cm (25th–75th percentile)
Triceps fatfold (percentile)	4 mm (<5th percentile)	8–16 mm (25th–75th percentile)

Exam
General: Thin, cachectic male in no apparent distress
Skin: Cold, dry
Head/neck: Bilateral temporal wasting and nasolabial fat loss, thin hair
Mouth: Gums red around tooth edges
Cardiac: Normal
Abdomen: Bowel sounds present, scaphoid, soft, non-tender, no organomegaly.
Extremities: Interosseous muscle wasting bilaterally
Neurologic: Non-focal grossly

Laboratory Data

Patient's Lab Values	Normal Values
HIV viral load: >500,000 copies/mL	0 copies/mL
CD4 count: 50 cell/mm^3	600–1800 cells/mm^3
Albumin: 2.5 g/dL	3.5–5.8 g/dL
Hemoglobin: 10.0 g/dL	13.5–17.5 g/dL
Hematocrit: 31%	41–53 %
ALT: 22 IU/L	0–35 IU/L
AST: 22 IU/L	0–35 IU/L
Alkaline phosphatase (ALP): 160 IU/L	53–128 IU/L
Total cholesterol: 85 mg/dL	<200 mg/dL
LDL-C: 60 mg/dL	<160 mg/dL

HDL-C: 20 mg/dL	>40 mg/dL
Triglycerides: 300 mg/dL	<150 mg/dL
Glucose: 120 mg/dL	70–99 mg/dL
Testosterone (total): 300 ng/dL	500–1000 ng/dL

Case Questions

1. Compare MD's weight and body composition to appropriate goal levels. What do the results suggest for his level of wasting and medical problems?
2. What factors have contributed to MD's wasting?
3. What is your overall impression of MD's nutritional status and what intervention strategies should be initiated?
4. Based on MD's nutritional evaluation, what medical nutrition therapy is appropriate at this time?
5. What medical therapies may be necessary to improve MD's nutritional status?
6. Once MD is being treated with antiviral medications, what follow-up recommendations would be appropriate?

Answers to Questions: Case 3
Part I. Nutrition Assessment

1. Compare MD's weight and body composition to goal levels. What do the results suggest for his level of wasting and medical problems?

The Centers for Disease Control and Prevention (CDC) case reporting definition of AIDS includes a loss of weight of greater than 10 percent with diarrhea or fever for more than 30 days. MD qualifies for that definition, but of even more concern, his body composition suggests that he also qualifies for a more evidence-based definition of wasting that is associated with a significant decline in health and functional capacity as shown in Table 7-2.

MD has lost 28 pounds (12.7 kg) or nearly 20 percent of his usual body weight. While the fat-free mass level is adequate, the body cell mass compartment (muscle and organ tissues) has been depleted by more than 16 pounds (7.3 kg), or nearly 15 percent from ideal. The other portion of the fat free mass, extracellular tissues (representing bone, collagen, and fluids outside of body cell mass), is slightly

Table 7-2 Definition of Wasting

- Greater than 10% loss of weight over a 12-month period
- Greater than 7.5% loss of weight over a 6-month period
- BMI <20 kg/m²
- 5% loss of body cell mass over a 6-month period
- Body cell mass <35% of weight in men (if BMI <27 kg/m²)
- Body cell mass <23% of weight in women (if BMI <27 kg/m²)

Source: Polsky B, Kotler D, Steinhart C. HIV-associated wasting in the HAART era: guidelines for assessment, diagnosis, and treatment. *AIDS Patient Care*. 2001;15:411–423.

elevated. These values are calculated using Kotler's equations for body mass composition that were validated for use in chronic HIV infection.

We would expect that with poor appetite and decreased food intake, along with diarrhea, MD would present with a picture of starvation where all body compartments decline. In MD's case, even though there has been significant diarrhea, extracellular fluids are elevated, which is a common finding in the state of infection or injury. It may be suspected that in the absence of injury, the lack of fever with fluid shifts may indicate the presence of an underlying infection with severe body cell mass depletion and the inability to mount an adequate inflammatory response.

2. What factors have contributed to MD's wasting?

A combination of several factors contributed to wasting in MD's case. High HIV viral load and low CD4 counts increase his risk for an opportunistic infection, which can initiate weight loss and body cell mass wasting. Opportunistic infections are commonly complicated by the development of anorexia. Diarrhea can increase fluid and nutrient losses leading to wasting. While serum testosterone levels are commonly low in HIV infection, a large weight loss can also lead to reduced testosterone synthesis, compromising the maintenance of body cell mass. In addition to total testosterone, free testosterone levels should be documented because globulin levels in HIV are frequently elevated, leading to an artificially normal testosterone.

3. What is your overall impression of MD's nutritional status and what strategies should be initiated?

MD's nutritional status is quite poor based on his weight, BMI, and body composition. While his triglycerides are high, as would be expected during non-specific inflammation or stress, the low albumin and low cholesterol levels combined with anemia are findings consistent with the presence of advanced HIV disease. Intervention to improve nutritional status and reduce mortality includes both medical and nutritional management. MD's high viral load and very low CD4 count require treatment to limit the effects of HIV infection, immune suppression, and opportunistic infection on his poor nutritional status.

Simultaneously, expediting nutritional status restoration will be important to support both survival and adequate tissue stores to process and support the efficacy of anti-HIV and other medications. Additional support for the restoration of weight and body composition will be essential to improving MD's health status. These interventions may include adequate oral intake or enteral or parenteral nutrition support, additional medications, and social support strategies.

Part 2: Medical Nutrition Therapy and Treatment

4. Based on MD's nutritional evaluation, what medical nutrition therapy is appropriate at this time?

Establishing a goal weight of 140 to 145 pounds (64 to 66 kg) and restoration of body composition levels will help MD and his health care team to formulate appropriate goals. These include adherence to anti-HIV therapies, treatment of opportunistic infections that may be present, diet adequacy, and increased physical activity. Dietary intervention should include both a personalized plan of action and education. Personalized exercise recommendations can be based on an evaluation by a physical therapist to evaluate capabilities and limitations or risks.

In this case, nutritional repletion strategies should be approached with caution since the risks associated with refeeding include restoration of a capacity for mounting a difficult-to-control inflammatory response. Combined with the reconstitution of immunity after initiation of anti-HIV therapy, the ensuing inflammatory response can be substantial.

Malabsorption may be an issue and in severe cases, parenteral nutrition and fluid resuscitation can be considered. Some form of oral intake should be maintained, as it will be important to maintain gut integrity, particularly with HIV infection. Oral feeding strategies may include a low-residue diet in small, frequent meals to improve digestibility and possibly lactose-free if he is lactose intolerant.

Because MD is significantly underweight, it may be counterproductive to rely on an extremely restrictive diet (such as the "BRAT" diet: bananas, rice, apples, and toast) to help in controlling diarrhea. If such a diet is used, it should be used for just a few days and replaced as quickly as possible with more calorically dense foods.

5. What medical therapies may be necessary to improve MD's nutritional status?

Highly active antiretroviral therapy (HAART) should be introduced and may reduce the influence of HIV infection and immune suppression on nutritional status. There is a significant incidence of transient and intermittent side effects with the introduction of antiretrovirals that can compromise nutritional status and therefore should be carefully monitored and treated as needed. Diarrhea should be worked up, and any appropriate treatments should be initiated for infection or other medical problems that contribute to diarrhea. In the case of general or fat malabsorption, diet strategies may include the use of lactase and pancreatic enzyme supplements to limit malabsorption. In select cases, antidiarrheal medications can be used to overcome short-term diarrhea problems, particularly if no pathogen is found, and the abdominal examination is benign.

Because nearly 20 percent of baseline weight was lost and body cell mass is at a critically low level, one would expect a lower level of testosterone. Physiologic testosterone replacement strategies may include use of topical gel, patches, or injections of testosterone and/or its analogs. Levels of total and free testosterone should be monitored occasionally to assure maintenance of appropriate levels to improve well-being and restore normal muscle mass. Additional therapies that may be employed as required include antinausea and appetite stimulation medications, growth

Table 7-3 Examples of Commonly Used Therapies to Restore Nutritional Status

Categories of Interventions	
Nutrition	Diet therapy, supplements, enteral nutrition, parenteral nutrition
Exercise	Aerobic exercise, progressive resistance exercise
Appetite stimulants	Dronabinol (Marinol)
	Megestrol acetate (Megace)
Hormonal therapy	Replacement testosterone:
	Injection: testosterone cypionate
	Patch: Testoderm, Androderm
	Gel: Androgel
	Anabolic steroid: oxandrolone (Oxandrin), oxymetholone
	(Anadrol) Growth hormone: Serostim
Others	Insulin sensitizers: metformin (Glucophage), rosiglitazone
	(Avandia)
	Anticytokines: thalidomide (Thalidomid) [not commonly used]

Source: Cade Fields-Gardner. Used with permission.

hormone, anabolic steroids, and other symptom management and anabolic agents (Table 7-3).

6. Once MD is being treated with antiviral medications, what follow-up recommendations would be appropriate?

MD initiated combination antiretroviral (anti-HIV) therapy and is monitored closely for symptom management. He continues to gain weight and body cell mass and has returned to a normal diet. MD is back on his construction job and doing well at this time.

MD's immune and nutritional recovery will require close monitoring to make sure he responds appropriately. For instance, while it is normal to replenish some fat tissues during the initial phases of nutrition intervention, body cell mass should return toward normal as body weight is increased. In addition, restored function of tissues should be monitored. MD should be encouraged to self-monitor weight and other body measures as well as to maintain an adequate nutrient intake in spite of bouts of diarrhea, should they continue. The normalization of testosterone levels and any need for additional anabolic therapies should be carefully monitored every few months. To enhance the efficacy of both nutrient and testosterone or other therapies, exercise should be encouraged.

Antiretroviral medications in all classes have been required by the FDA to carry in their labeling that use of the drugs may lead to altered fat metabolism and deposition, known as lipodystrophy. These complications are still a poorly understood disorder that entails the deposition or loss of fat in a number of body sites. Such alterations can have profound implications for patient's health maintenance and well-being. These and other complications of long-term survival with a chronic inflammatory disease, such as HIV infection, should be routinely monitored and appropriate medical nutrition therapy applied.

Chapter and Case References

Alvares-Da-Silva MR, Reverbel-da-Silveira T. Comparison between handgrip strength, subjective global assessment, and prognostic nutritional index in assessing malnutrition and predicting clinical outcome in cirrhotic outpatients. *Nutrition.* 2005;21(2):113–117.

Cave M, Deaciuc I, Mendez C, et al. Nonalcoholic fatty liver disease: predisposing factors and role of nutrition. *J Nutr Biochem.* 2007;18(3):184–195.

Chang E, Sekhar R, Patel S, Balasubramanyam A. Dysregulated energy expenditure in HIV-infected patients: a mechanistic review. *Clin Infect Dis.* 2007;44(11):1509–1517.

Cordoba J, López-Helln J, Planas M et al. Normal protein diet for episodic hepatic encephalopathy: results of a randomized study. *J Hepatology.* 2004;41:38–43.

Crippin JS. Is tube feeding an option in patients with liver disease? *Nutr Clin Pract.* 2006;21:296–298.

Eiden KA. Nutritional considerations in inflammatory bowel disease. *Pract Gastroenterol.* 2003:33–54.

Ferguson LR, Shelling AN, Browning BL, Huebner C, Petermann I. Genes, diet and inflammatory bowel disease. *Mutat Res.* 2007;622:70–83.

Henkel AS, Buchman AL. Nutrition support in patients with chronic liver disease. *Nat Clin Pract Gastroenterol Hepatol.* 2006;3(4):202–209.

Khanna S, Gopolan S. Role of branched chain amino acids in liver disease: the evidence for and against. *Curr Opin Clin Nutr and Metab Care.* 2007;10(3):297–303.

Kotler DP, Burastero S, Wang J, Pierson RN Jr. Prediction of body cell mass, fat-free mass, and total body water with bioelectrical impedance analysis: effects of rase, sex, and disease. *Am J Clin Nutr.* 1996; 64(3 Suppl):489S–497S.

Kultstad R, Schoeller DA. The energetics of wasting diseases. *Curr Opin Clin Nutr Metab Care.* 2007;10(4):488–493.

Macdermott, R. Treatment of irritable bowel syndrome in outpatients with inflammatory bowel disease using a food and beverage intolerance and food and beverage avoidance diet. *Inflamm Bowel Dis.* 2007;13(1):91–96.

MacDonald, A. Omega-3 fatty acids as adjunctive therapy in Crohns disease. *Gastroenterol Nurs.* 2006;29(4):295–301.

Mahan K, Escott-Stump S. *Krause's Food Nutrition and Diet Therapy* (11th ed.). 2004:314, 711.

Mangili A, Murman DH, Zampini AM, Wanke CA. Nutrition and HIV infection: review of weight loss and wasting in the era of highly active antiretroviral therapy from the nutrition for healthy living cohort. *Clin Infect Dis.* 2006;42(6):836–842.

Mayo Foundation for Medical Education and Research. Lactose intolerance. 2008. Available from http://www.mayoclinic.com/health/lactoseintolerance/DS00530/DSECTION=7

Montano M, Flanagan JN, Jiang L, Sebastiani P, Rarick M, LeBrasseur NK, Morris CA, Jasuja R, Bhasin S. Transcriptional profiling of testosterone-regulated genes in the skeletal muscle of human immunodeficiency virus-infected men experiencing weight loss. *J Clin Endocrinol Metab.* 2007;92(7):2793–2802.

Morley JE, Thomas DR, Wilson MM. Cachexia: pathophysiology and clinical relevance. *Am J Clin Nutr.* 2006;83(4):735–743.

National Digestive Diseases Information Clearinghouse, A Service of the National Institute of Diabetes and Digestive and Kidney Diseases, NIH. Lactose intolerance. 2006. Available from http://digestive.niddk.nih.gov/ddiseases/pubs/lactoseintolerance/index.htm

Office of Dietary Supplements, NIH. Dietary fact sheet: calcium. 2005. Available from http://dietary-supplements.info.nih.gov/factsheets/calcium.asp# h8

Park GH, Kim JW, et al. A case of percutaneous endoscopic gastrostomy in a patient with liver cirrhosis accompanied by both esophageal and gastric varices. *Korean J Gastroenterol.* 2006;48(1):51–54.

Plauth M, Merli M, et al. ESPEN guidelines for nutrition in liver disease and transplantation. *Clin Nutr.* 1997;16:43–55.

Testa R, Franceschini R, et al. Serum leptin levels in patients with viral chronic hepatitis or liver cirrhosis. *J Hepatology.* 2000;33:33–37.

Thomas AM, Mkandawire SC. The impact of nutrition on physiologic changes in persons who have HIV. *Nurs Clin North Am.* 2006;41(3):455–468.

8   Endocrine Disease: Diabetes Mellitus

Marion J. Franz

Nutrition Concepts by Franz, Inc. Minneapolis, MN

OBJECTIVES[*]

- Describe the most common macrovascular and microvascular complications associated with diabetes mellitus and describe the role of glycemic control, nutrition therapy, and physical activity in reducing these complications.

- Summarize the current nutrition recommendations and interventions for diabetes, and compare and contrast the nutrition strategies for persons with type 1 vs. type 2 diabetes.

- Complete a thorough food and nutrition history of a person with diabetes, including an assessment of the (a) family history of diabetes, (b) onset and duration of diabetes symptoms, (c) evidence of complications, (d) weight history, (e) usual food intake, (f) frequency, intensity, and duration of physical activity, (g) use of medications, and (h) alcohol consumption. Identify any problem areas.

- Recognize the central importance of medical nutrition therapy and physical activity in the maintenance of health, and demonstrate a commitment to support patient adherence to nutrition interventions proven to be effective.

*Source: Objectives for chapter and cases adapted from the *NIH Nutrition Curriculum Guide for Training Physicians.* (www.nhlbi.nih.gov/funding/training/naa)

Introduction

Diabetes mellitus is manifested in three primary forms: type 1 diabetes, type 2 diabetes, and gestational diabetes. Diabetes is group of diseases characterized by hyperglycemia resulting from defects in insulin secretion, insulin action, or both. Pathogenic processes involved in the development of diabetes range from autoimmune destruction of the beta cells of the pancreas with resultant insulin deficiency – type 1 diabetes – to abnormalities that result in resistance to insulin action and an inadequate compensatory insulin secretory response – type 2 diabetes.

Without sufficient insulin, hyperglycemia occurs, resulting in short-term and long-term microvascular and macrovascular complications. Acute, life-threatening consequences of uncontrolled hyperglycemia are ketoacidosis and nonketotic hyperosmolar syndrome. Long-term complications include retinopathy, nephropathy, and peripheral and autonomic neuropathy. Patients with diabetes are also at high risk for atherosclerotic, cardiovascular, peripheral arterial, and cerebrovascular

---

Medical Nutrition and Disease: A Case-Based Approach, 4th edition. Edited by Lisa Hark.
© 2009 Wiley-Blackwell Publishing, ISBN: 978-1-4051-8615-5.

disease. Hypertension and lipoprotein abnormalities are other common problems. It is, therefore, essential that effective therapy to achieve as normal glycemia as possible be initiated early to prevent the deleterious effects of hyperglycemia.

In the United States, 20.8 million people of all ages are reported to have diabetes. Of these 14.6 million are diagnosed, and 6.2 million are undiagnosed. Diabetes prevalence increases with increasing age, affecting 18.4 percent of those 65 years of age or older and is particularly prevalent in high-risk ethnic populations, such as African-American, Latino, Native American, Asian American, and Pacific Islander. Among children with newly diagnosed diabetes, the prevalence of type 2 diabetes increased from less than 4 percent prior to 1990 to as high as 45 percent in certain racial/ethnic groups in recent years.

At high risk for type 2 diabetes are the greater than 41 million people estimated to have pre-diabetes and the 47 million with metabolic syndrome. Not only are these individuals at high risk for type 2 diabetes, but they are also at high risk for cardiovascular disease, if lifestyle prevention strategies are not implemented. (Chapter 1: Case 1.1; Chapter 9: Case 9.2.)

Diagnosis of Diabetes Mellitus or Pre-Diabetes

Three ways to diagnose diabetes are available, and each must be confirmed on a subsequent day unless unequivocal symptoms of hyperglycemia are present. Any of the following glucose values are diagnostic of diabetes:

- Fasting plasma glucose (FPG) $\geq$126 mg/dL (7.0 mmol/L);
- Casual plasma glucose $\geq$200 mg/dL (11.1 mmol/L) plus the classic symptoms of polyuria, polydipsia, and unexplained weight loss; or
- 2-hr plasma glucose (PG) $\geq$200 mg/dL (11.1 mmol/L) during an oral glucose tolerance test (OGTT) using a glucose load containing the equivalent of 75 grams of anhydrous glucose dissolved in water.

Fasting plasma glucose is the preferred test to diagnosis diabetes in children and non-pregnant adults because of ease of use, acceptability to patients, and lower cost.

Hyperglycemia that does not meet diagnostic criteria for diabetes is categorized as either impaired fasting glucose (IFG) or impaired glucose tolerance (IGT). Both IFG and IGT are officially termed pre-diabetes and are risk factors for future diabetes and cardiovascular disease:

- IFG = FPG 100 mg/dL (5.6 mmol/L) to 125 mg/dL (6.9 mmol/L).
- IGT = 2-h plasma glucose 140 mg/dL (7.8 mmol/L) to 199 mg/dL (11.0 mmol/L).

Testing for Pre-Diabetes and Diabetes

Testing to detect pre-diabetes and type 2 diabetes in asymptomatic adults should be considered in adults who are overweight or obese (BMI $\geq$25 kg/m^2) and who have one or more additional risk factors for diabetes listed in Table 8-1. In those without risk factors, testing should begin at age 45. If tests are normal, repeat testing should done at 3-year intervals.

Consistent with screening recommendations for adults, children, and youth at age 10 years or onset of puberty, at increased risk for type 2 diabetes should be tested

Table 8-1 Risk Factors for Development of Diabetes

- Physical inactivity
- First-degree relative with diabetes
- Member of a high-risk ethnic population (e.g. African-American, Latino, Native American, Asian American, or Pacific Islander)
- Women who delivered a baby weight >9 lbs (4 kg) or were diagnosed with gestational diabetes mellitus (GDM)
- Hypertension (blood pressure ≥140/90 mm Hg)
- High-density lipoprotein cholesterol (HDL-C) level ≤35 mg/dL (0.90 mmol/L) and/or triglyceride level ≥250 mg/dL (2.82 mmol/L)
- Women with polycystic ovarian syndrome (PCOS)
- IGT or IFG on previous testing
- Other clinical conditions associated with insulin resistance (e.g. severe obesity and acanthosis nigricans)

Source: Adapted from American Diabetes Association. Standards of medical care in diabetes – 2008 (Position Statement). *Diabetes Care* 2008;31 (Suppl1):S12–S54.

if risk factors listed below are present. If test are normal, testing should be repeated every 3 years:

- Overweight (BMI >85 percentile for age and sex, weight for height >85th percentile, or weight >120 percent of ideal for height).
- Plus any two of the following risk factors: family history of type 2 diabetes in first- or second-degree relative, member of high-risk ethnic populations, signs of insulin resistance (e.g. acanthosis nigricans (gray-brown skin, pigmentations) hypertension, dyslipidemia, or PCOS), maternal history of gestational diabetes mellitus (GDM).

Pathophysiology of Diabetes
Type 1 Diabetes
Type 1 diabetes accounts for 5 to 10 percent of all diagnosed cases of diabetes. The primary defect is pancreatic beta-cell destruction leading to absolute insulin deficiency (insulinopenia), and resulting in hyperglycemia, polyuria, polydipsia, weight loss, dehydration, electrolyte disturbance, and ketoacidosis. The capacity of a healthy pancreas to secrete insulin is far in excess of what is needed normally; therefore, the clinical onset of diabetes may be preceded by an extensive asymptomatic period (months to years), during which beta cells are undergoing gradual destruction. Persons with type 1 diabetes are dependent on exogenous insulin to prevent ketoacidosis and death. Although it can occur at any age, most cases are diagnosed in people younger than 30 years of age, with peak incidence between 10 to 12 years in girls and 12 to 14 years in boys.

Type 1 diabetes is a result of a genetic predisposition combined with autoimmune destruction of the islet beta cells. At diagnosis, 85 percent to 90 percent of persons with type 1 diabetes have one or more circulating autoantibodies. Antibodies identified as contributing to the destruction of beta cells are (1) islet cell autoantibodies

(ICAs); (2) insulin autoantibodies (IAAs), which may occur in persons who have never received insulin therapy; (3) autoantibodies to glutamic acid decarboxylase (GAD$_{65}$), a protein on the surface of beta cells (GAD autoantibodies appear to provoke an attack by the T cells [killer T lymphocytes], which may be what destroys the beta cells in diabetes); and (4) autoantibodies to the tyrosine phosphatases IA-2 and IA-2β.

Frequently, after diagnosis and the correction of hyperglycemia, metabolic acidosis, and ketoacidosis, endogenous insulin secretion recovers. During this "honeymoon phase," exogenous insulin requirements decrease dramatically. However, the need for exogenous insulin is inevitable, and within 8 to 10 years after clinical onset, beta-cell loss is complete and insulin deficiency is absolute.

Type 2 Diabetes

Type 2 diabetes accounts for 90 to 95 percent of all diagnosed cases of diabetes and is a progressive disease that is often present long before it is diagnosed. Although approximately 50 percent of men and 70 percent of women are obese at the time of diagnosis, type 2 diabetes also occurs in non-obese individuals, especially in elderly individuals. An affected individual may or may not experience the classic symptoms of uncontrolled diabetes, and they are not prone to develop ketoacidosis. Insulin resistance begins and progresses for many years before the development of diabetes, but impaired beta cell insulin secretory function must be present before hyperglycemia is present. By the time diabetes is diagnosed, the individual has lost as much as 50 percent of beta cell function.

In type 2 diabetes, the normal biphasic insulin response to glucose is altered, resulting in postprandial hyperglycemia. The inadequate first-phase insulin response is also unable to suppress pancreatic alpha cell glucagon secretion, resulting in increased glucagon hypersecretion, which leads to an increase in hepatic glucose production and fasting hyperglycemia. The second major metabolic abnormality is a decrease in the ability of insulin to act on target tissues: muscles, liver, and fat cells. Compounding the problem is the deleterious effect of hyperglycemia itself – glucotoxicity – on both insulin sensitivity and insulin secretion; hence, the importance of achieving near-euglycemia in persons with type 2 diabetes.

Insulin resistance is also demonstrated in adipocytes, leading to lipolysis and an elevation in circulating free fatty acids. Increased free fatty acids cause a further decrease in insulin sensitivity at the cellular level, impair insulin secretion, and augment hepatic glucose production (lipotoxicity). All the defects (cellular, hepatic, and beta-cell) contribute to the development and progression of type 2 diabetes.

As type 2 diabetes progresses, insulin production progressively declines. Therefore, patients with diabetes usually require more medication(s) over time; eventually exogenous insulin will be required. This is not a "diet" or medication failure, but rather a failure of beta cell function.

Treatment of Diabetes

Optimal control of diabetes requires the restoration of normal carbohydrate, protein, and fat metabolism. Insulin is both anticatabolic and anabolic and facilitates cellular transport. In general, the counterregulatory hormones – glucagon, growth hormone, cortisol, epinephrine, and norepinephrine – have the opposite effect of insulin.

Diabetes is a chronic disease that requires lifetime changes in lifestyle. The management of diabetes includes appropriate medical nutrition therapy, regular physical activity, self-management education, and medications. An important goal is to provide the individual with the necessary tools to achieve the best possible control of glycemia, lipids, and blood pressure to prevent, delay, or arrest the microvascular and macrovascular complications of diabetes while minimizing hypoglycemia and excess weight gain.

Two large, long-term studies demonstrated the clear link between glycemic control and the development of microvascular complications in persons with type 1 and type 2 diabetes. They also provided strong evidence for the role of medical nutrition therapy in the management of diabetes. The Diabetes Control and Complications Trial (DCCT) was a long-term, randomized, controlled, multi-center trial that studied approximately 800 young adults (aged 13 to 39 years) with type 1 diabetes who were treated with either intensive therapy (multiple injections of insulin or use of insulin pumps guided by blood glucose monitoring data) or conventional therapy (1 or 2 insulin injections per day). Both groups received nutrition therapy counseling. The DCCT clearly showed that even small improvements reduced the rate of microvascular complications. Patients in the intensive treatment group showed a 50 percent to 75 percent reduction in the risk of progression to retinopathy, nephropathy, and neuropathy. Subjects in the intensive therapy arm who reported following their meal plan greater than 90 percent of the time had A1C levels one percent lower than those who reported following their meal plan only 40 percent of the time.

In a mean 17-year follow-up study of DCCT patients, intensive treatment during the trial reduced the risk of any cardiovascular event by 42 percent and the risk of non-fatal myocardial infarction, stroke, or death from cardiovascular disease (CVD) by 57 percent compared to the conventional therapy group. Thus, the importance of early intensive therapy for reducing risk of diabetes complications is essential.

The United Kingdom Prospective Diabetes Study (UKPDS) demonstrated that reduction of elevated blood glucose levels reduced microvascular complications in type 2 diabetes just as in type 1 diabetes. The UKPDS followed 5102 newly diagnosed individuals with type 2 diabetes for an average of 10 to 11 years who were randomized into a group treated conventionally and an intensively treated group. The intensively treated group experienced a 25 percent reduction in the rate of retinopathy and nephropathy. Additionally, for every percentage point decrease in hemoglobin A1c (A1C), there was a 25 percent reduction in diabetes-related deaths, a 7 percent reduction in all-cause mortality, and an 18 percent reduction in combined fatal and non-fatal myocardial infarction. Improved blood pressure control resulted in a 34 percent reduction in all macrovascular endpoints and a 37 percent reduction in all microvascular endpoints.

The UKPDS also illustrated the progressive nature of type 2 diabetes. At diagnosis and before randomization into intensive or conventional treatment, subjects received individualized intensive nutrition therapy for 3 months. During this period A1C levels decreased by approximately 2 percent from 9 to 7 percent and patients lost an average of 3.5 kg (8 lb). Researchers concluded that a reduction of energy intake was at least as important, if not more important, than the actual weight lost in determining glucose improvements. However, as the study progressed nutrition therapy alone was not enough to keep the majority of the patient's A1C levels at 7 percent. Medication(s) and for many, insulin, needed to be combined with nutrition therapy. It was not the "diet" failing, but instead was as stated above the pancreas failing to secrete enough insulin to maintain adequate glucose control.

Monitoring of Metabolic Outcomes

Individuals can assess day-to-day glycemic control by self-monitoring of blood glucose (SMBG). Persons with diabetes can use SMBG to determine the impact that food choices and physical activity have on blood glucose levels and to make adjustments in lifestyle and medications required to achieve glycemic goals. SMBG should be done three to more times daily by patients using multiple insulin injections or insulin pump therapy. For persons on non-insulin therapy SMBG should be done sufficiently to facilitate reaching glucose goals. To achieve postprandial glucose goals, postprandial SMBG is helpful. The accuracy of SMBG is instrument and user dependent and monitoring techniques must be evaluated on a regular basis. Patients also should be taught how to use the data to adjust food intake, exercise, or medications to achieve glycemic goals.

Continuous glucose monitoring (CGM) measures interstitial fluid glucose (which correlates with blood glucose) in a continuous and minimally invasive manner. Continuous glucose sensors have alarms for hypo- and hyperglycemia and small studies have shown use of CGM to decrease the average time patients spend in hypo- and hyperglycemic ranges. Currently, its use is recommended as a supplement to SMBG for selected patients with type 1 diabetes.

Complementing day-to-day testing are measurements of glycosylated hemoglobin (simplified as A1C) reflecting a weighted average of plasma glucose over the preceding six to eight weeks, and long-term glycemic control. When hemoglobin and other proteins are exposed to glucose, the glucose becomes attached to the protein in a slow, non-enzymatic, and concentration-dependent manner. In non-diabetic persons, A1C values are 4.0 percent to 6.0 percent, which correspond to mean plasma glucose levels of approximately 90 mg/dL (5.0 mmol/L). Measurements approximately every three months determine whether a patient's glycemic goals have been reached and maintained. Lowering A1C to an average of approximately 7 percent has clearly been shown to reduce complications of diabetes; however, some epidemiologic studies have reported benefit to lowering A1C into the normal range.

Lipid levels and blood pressure should also be monitored. Lipids should be measured annually and blood pressure at every visit. The American Diabetes Association (ADA) glycemic, lipid, and blood pressure goals are listed in Table 8-2.

Medical Nutrition Therapy

The primary goal of medical nutrition therapy (MNT) for diabetes mellitus is to assist in attaining and maintaining optimal metabolic outcomes,

Table 8-2 Clinical Goals for Diabetes Therapy

Recommendations for Adults with Diabetes	Goal
Glycemic	
A1C	<7.0 percent*
Preprandial capillary plasma glucose	70–130 mg/dL(3.9–7.2 mmol/L)
Peak postprandial capillary plasma glucose†	<180 mg/dL (<10.0 mmol/L)
Lipids	
LDL-C (without overt CVD)	<100 mg/dL (<2.6 mmol/L)
LDL-C (with overt CVD)	<70 mg/dL (<1.8 mmol/L
Triglycerides	<150 mg/dL (<1.7 mmol/L)
HDL-C	>40 mg/dL (>1.0 mmol/L) in men and
	>50 mg/dL (>1.3mmol/L in women)
Blood Pressure	
Blood pressure	<130/80 mm Hg

*Referenced to a nondiabetic range of 4.0–6.0 percent using a DCCT-based assay
† Postprandial glucose measurements should be made 1–2 h after the beginning of the meal
Source: Adapted from American Diabetes Association. Standards of medical care in diabetes – 2008
(Position Statement). *Diabetes Care* 2008;31 (Suppl 1):S12–S54.

including:

- Blood glucose levels in the normal range to the greatest extent possible to prevent the microvascular complications of diabetes;
- A lipid and lipoprotein profile that reduces the risk for cardiovascular diseases; and
- A blood pressure level that reduces the risk for vascular diseases.

Clinical trials and outcome studies support medical nutrition therapy as an effective therapy in reaching diabetes treatment goals. The American Dietetic Association Evidence-Based Nutrition Practice Guidelines (EBNPG) for diabetes documented decreases in A1C of 1 to 2 percent (range: −0.5 percent to −2.6 percent) depending on the type and duration of diabetes. These outcomes are similar to those from glucose-lowering medications. Many different types of nutrition interventions were effective. Central to these interventions are multiple encounters to provide education and counseling initially and on a continued basis. These outcomes highlight the importance of the registered dietitian (RD) determining the most effective nutrition intervention for each individual and coordinating care with an interdisciplinary team.

Reducing saturated fat to less than 7 percent of daily energy intake and dietary cholesterol to 200 mg/day lowers LDL-C on average by 16 percent (~25 mg/dL). In hypertensive patients who consume excessive sodium, reducing intake to approximately 2400 mg/day can lower systolic blood pressure by 6 mm Hg and diastolic blood pressure by 2 mm Hg.

The outcomes of nutrition interventions on glycemia, lipids, and blood pressure are usually evident by 6 weeks to 3 months. At this point, it needs to be determined if medications need to be added (or adjusted) with MNT to achieve target goals.

Prior to 1994, the ADA nutrition recommendations attempted to define "ideal" macronutrient percentages for a diabetes nutrition prescription. Then by determining an individual's energy needs based on theoretical calorie requirements and using the ideal percentages of carbohydrate, protein, and fat, a nutrition prescription was ordered. This approach limited individualization. In 1994, the ADA recommended a different approach. Instead of rigid percentages, the nutrition prescription is to be based on an assessment of lifestyle changes required to assist the individual with diabetes in achieving and maintaining therapeutic goals, implementing changes the patient is able and willing to make.

This transition to a more flexible and realistic approach to MNT continues in the 2002 and 2008 ADA diabetes nutrition recommendations. To achieve nutrition-related objectives requires a coordinated team effort that includes registered dietitians, diabetes educators, physicians, and the person with diabetes who must be involved in problem solving. A system of care that provides ongoing support and education is essential.

Prioritizing Nutrition Strategies for Diabetes

Historically, nutrition advice has been given to patients with diabetes, such as "don't eat foods with sugar" or "go home and lose weight." This advice has often been accompanied by a calorie-level "diet sheet" or a pamphlet or brochure with general guidelines. Patients often find such information difficult to understand and implement. To achieve positive outcomes, appropriate priorities should be set for each patient.

Type 1 Diabetes The first priority for persons requiring insulin therapy is to integrate an insulin regimen into the patient's lifestyle. After an initial food/meal plan is determined (with the patient's input), it should be reviewed with the health professional planning the insulin regimen. With the many insulin options now available, an insulin regimen can usually be developed that will conform to the patient's preferred meal times and food choices. Flexible insulin regimens using basal (background) insulin and bolus (mealtime) insulin or insulin pumps give the patient freedom in timing and composition of meals and are the preferred mode of therapy to maximize blood glucose control and minimize complications.

The total amount of carbohydrate in the meal (and snacks, if desired) is the major determinant of the bolus rapid-acting insulin dose and postprandial glucose response. After determining the amount of insulin required to cover the patient's usual meal carbohydrate, patients can be taught how to adjust bolus insulin doses based on the amount of carbohydrate they are planning to eat (insulin-to-carbohydrate ratio). For persons receiving fixed insulin regimens and not adjusting mealtime insulin doses, consistency of day-to-day carbohydrate amounts at meals is important.

Type 2 Diabetes Previously, nutrition advice focused on losing weight and avoiding sugars. Today, the focus of medical nutrition therapy for type 2 diabetes is to implement lifestyle strategies that will assist in improving glycemia, dyslipidemia, and blood pressure. Since many persons with type 2 diabetes are insulin resistant and overweight, MNT often begins with lifestyle strategies that reduce energy intake and increase energy expenditure through physical activity. However, many individuals have already tried unsuccessfully to lose weight and it is important to note that other lifestyle strategies, even without weight loss, can improve glycemia. Teaching individuals how to make appropriate food choices, often through the use of carbohydrate counting, encouraging physical activity, and using data from blood glucose monitoring to evaluate effectiveness will improve success for individuals with type 2 diabetes. These strategies should be implemented as soon as the diagnosis of diabetes is made.

Some studies, but not all, demonstrate that modest amounts of weight loss improve metabolic abnormalities in some individuals. Weight loss, especially of intra-abdominal fat, reduces insulin resistance and helps correct dyslipidemias in the short-term. However, as individuals move from being primarily insulin resistant to insulin deficiency, therapeutic strategies change. At later stages of the disease when medications, including insulin, need to be combined with MNT, prevention of weight gain often becomes an issue, although glycemic control must take precedence over concern about weight. Thus far, no study has reported weight loss/maintenance for a long enough time period to know whether there are long-term benefits of weight loss on prevention of diabetes complications. The Look AHEAD (Action for Health in Diabetes) trial is a 12-year multicenter trial examining the effects of weight loss achieved through an intensive lifestyle program in overweight and obese individuals with diabetes. The goal is for individuals to lose 7 to 10 percent of their body weight and maintain the weight loss for the duration of the study. The study will examine the effects of weight loss on CVD, diabetes control, myocardial infarction, and stroke.

In weight loss studies in subjects with type 2 diabetes, weight loss appears to plateau at 6 months, and it appears that weight loss is more difficult in people with diabetes. Furthermore, in the evidence review for the American Dietetic Evidence-Based Nutrition Practice Guidelines for diabetes in 11 studies with weight loss arms, six weight loss arms reported no improvement in A1C, whereas five reported improvement in A1C with fairly similar weight losses (range: 0.8 to 5.1 kg). Therefore, it was recommended that if weight loss is a goal for persons with diabetes who are overweight or obese, the RD should advise that glycemic control is the primary focus. While decreasing energy intake may improve glycemic control, it is unclear whether weight loss alone will improve glycemic control, as sustained weight loss interventions lasting one year or longer reported inconsistent effects on A1C.

Regular physical activity improves blood glucose control and insulin sensitivity independent of weight loss. In addition, physical activity reduces CVD risk factors, improves well-being, and is important for long-term weight maintenance.

Macronutrient Recommendations

Carbohydrate Because carbohydrate and adequacy of insulin determine postprandial glucose response, it is addressed first. With the continued popularity of low-carbohydrate diets, it should be remembered that foods containing carbohydrates – fruits, vegetables, whole grains, legumes, and low fat-milk – are important components of a healthy diet and should be included in a food/meal plan for persons with diabetes.

Areas of controversy involve how much carbohydrate to recommend in a food/meal plan and the value of the glycemic index (GI). Evidence can be found to support either a low or high-carbohydrate diet for persons with diabetes. Both the American Diabetes Association and the American Dietetic Association recommend using the Dietary Reference Intakes (DRI) as a guideline. Some, but not all, short-term studies had reported modest benefits from low GI diets compared to high GI diets in persons with diabetes. However, the Canadian Trial of Carbohydrate in Diabetes, a one-year study comparing low or high GI diets, reported no significant difference in A1C or lipids by altering the GI or the amount of carbohydrate.

All patients can, however, benefit from basic information about carbohydrates: what foods contain carbohydrate (starches, fruit, starchy vegetables, milk, sweets, and desserts; one average serving is equivalent to 15 grams) and how many servings to select for meals (and snacks if desired). The following are other recommendations for food carbohydrates:

- In persons on MNT alone, glucose-lowering medications, or fixed insulin doses, meal (and snack) carbohydrate should be kept consistent on a day-to-day basis, as consistency in carbohydrate intake has been shown to result in improved glycemic control. In persons with type 1 or type 2 diabetes who adjust their mealtime insulin or who are on insulin pump therapy, insulin doses should be adjusted to match carbohydrate intake.
- The concept of the GI may be best used for fine-tuning postprandial responses after first focusing on total carbohydrate. Because of the large intravariability and intervariability of the glucose response to equal amounts of carbohydrate, testing of blood glucose before and after eating a particular food or meal may be the best way to determine an individual's glycemic response, and the concept of a personal GI can be used to fine-tune food choices.
- Recommendations for fiber intake are similar to recommendations for the general public (DRI: 14 g/1000 kcal per day). Diets containing 44 to 50 grams of fiber per day are reported to improve glycemic control; however, more usual fiber intakes (up to 24 g/day) have not shown beneficial effects on glycemia. It is unknown if free-living individuals can daily consume the amount of fiber needed to improve glycemia. However, diets high in total and soluble fiber, as part of cardioprotective nutrition therapy, have been shown to reduce total cholesterol by 2 to 3 percent and LDL-C up to 7 percent.
- If persons with diabetes choose to eat foods containing sucrose, the sucrose-containing foods should be substituted for other carbohydrate foods. Sucrose intakes of 10 to 35 percent of total energy intake do not have a negative effect on glycemic or lipid responses when substituted for isocaloric amounts of starch.
- Non-nutritive sweeteners and sugar alcohols are safe when consumed within the accepted daily intake levels established by the Food and Drug Administration. However, some of these products may contain energy and carbohydrate from other sources.
- Eating a minimum of 5 servings of fruits and vegetables daily is recommended for both prevention and treatment of high blood pressure.

Protein Aside from sugars, protein is probably the most misunderstood nutrient with inaccurate advice frequently given to persons with diabetes. Although non-essential amino acids serve as substrates for gluconeogenesis, in subjects with controlled diabetes, this glucose does not enter the general circulation. Protein also does not slow the absorption of carbohydrate, but can increase acute insulin responses without increasing glucose concentrations. Therefore, protein should not be used to treat acute or prevent nighttime hypoglycemia.

There is no evidence to suggest that usual intake of protein (15 percent to 20 percent of energy intake) be changed in persons who do not have renal disease.

There is some evidence that lowering protein intake to 0.8 to 1.0 g/kg per day in patients with diabetes and earlier stages of chronic kidney disease (CKD) and to 0.8 g/kg per day in the later stages of CKD may improve renal function and is recommended. In persons with diabetic nephropathy, diets with less than 1.0 g/kg per day have been shown to improve albuminuria, but they have not been shown to have significant effects on glomerular filtration rates. For persons in CKD Stages 3 to 5, hypoalbuminemia (an indicator of malnutrition) and energy intake must be monitored and changes in protein and energy intake made to correct deficits. Protein intakes of ~ 0.7 g/kg per day have been associated with hypoalbuminemia, whereas protein intakes of ~ 0.9 g/kg per day have not.

Dietary Fat Limiting intake of saturated fatty acids to less than 7 percent of total energy, minimal *trans* fatty acids, and dietary cholesterol less than 200 mg/day are recommended. Reducing saturated fatty acids may reduce HDL-C, but importantly, the ratio of LDL-C to HDL-C is not adversely affected. Polyunsaturated fatty acids have effects similar to monounsaturated fatty acids and either type can replace saturated or *trans* fatty acids.

The ADA also recommends two or more servings of fish per week (with the exception of commercially fried fish filets). Plant sterol and stanols esters have also been shown to lower total and LDL-C in persons with type 2 diabetes and can be substituted for other fats in the diet, such as margarine or cream cheese.

Micronutrient Recommendations

Vitamins and Minerals There is no evidence of benefit from vitamin or mineral supplementation in persons with diabetes who do not have underlying deficiencies. Routine supplementation of the diet with antioxidants is not recommended because they have not proven beneficial and concerns have been raised related to long-term safety. Benefits from chromium supplementation in individuals with diabetes or obesity have not been clearly demonstrated and therefore can not be recommended.

Sodium For both normotensive and hypertensive individuals, a reduction in sodium intake lowers blood pressure. The goal should be to reduce sodium intake to 2300 mg or less per day and a diet high in fruits, vegetables, and low-fat dairy products is recommended.

Alcohol Recommendations for alcohol intake are similar to those for the general public. If individuals choose to drink, alcoholic beverage consumption should be limited to no more than 2 drinks per day for men and no more than 1 drink per day for women. One drink is defined a 12 ounces beer, 5 ounces wine, or 1.5 ounces of distilled spirits, each of which contains approximately 15 g of alcohol. For individuals using insulin or insulin secretagogues, alcohol should be consumed with food to reduce the risk of hypoglycemia. Occasional use of alcoholic beverages should be considered an addition to the regular meal plan, and no food should be omitted.

Moderate amounts of alcohol, when ingested with food, have minimal acute effects on glucose and insulin concentrations and light to moderate alcohol intake (one to two drinks per day) are associated with a decreased risk of CVD. The type of alcohol-containing beverage does not make a difference. On the other hand, excessive amounts of alcohol (three or more drinks per day), on a consistent basis, contribute to hyperglycemia, hypertension and other medical conditions.

Physical Activity

Physical activity should be an integral part of the treatment plan for persons with diabetes. Exercise helps improve insulin sensitivity, reduce cardiovascular risk factors, control weight, and improve well-being. People with diabetes can exercise safely. The exercise plan will vary depending on age, general health, and level of physical fitness. A minimum of 150 min/week of moderate intensity aerobic physical activity (50 to 70 percent of heart rate) is advised. In the absence of contraindications, resistance training three times per week is encouraged. Persons taking insulin or insulin secretagogues should monitor their blood glucose and take appropriate precautions to avoid hypoglycemia; carbohydrate should be eaten if pre-exercise glucose levels are less than 100 mg/dL (5.6 mmol/L).

Medications

Glucose-Lowering Medications If metabolic goals are not being met in persons with type 2 diabetes, there are now six classes of oral medications as well as injectable medications, including insulin, that can be combined with nutrition therapy. This provides numerous options for achieving euglycemia in persons with type 2 diabetes. Many people benefit from taking two or more of the medications because each addresses a different problem. Such combination therapy is so common that a number of combination pills are also available. However, because of the progressive nature of type 2 diabetes, many individuals will also require two or more daily insulin injections to achieve glycemic control.

The six classes of oral medications are:

- *Alpha-glucosidase inhibitors* (acarbose, miglitol), which work in the small intestine to inhibit enzymes that digest carbohydrates, thereby delaying carbohydrate absorption and lowering postprandial glycemia;
- *Biguanides* (metformin), which suppress hepatic glucose production, lower insulin resistance, but do not stimulate insulin secretion;

- *DPP-4 inhibitors* (sitagliptin), which inhibit dipeptidyl peptidase-4 (DDP-4) enzyme that degrades glucose dependent insulinotropic polypeptide (GIP) and glucose-like polypeptide (GLP), whose actions are to increase insulin secretion in the presence of elevated plasma glucose and to reduce postmeal glucagon secretion;
- *Meglitinides* (nateglinide and repaglinide), which acutely promote insulin secretion and are taken at the start of a meal;
- *Sulfonylureas* (first-and second-generation), whose actions are to promote insulin secretion by the beta cells of the pancreas over longer periods of time;
- *Thiazolidinediones* (pioglitazone, rosiglitazone), which decrease insulin resistance in peripheral tissues and thus enhance the ability of muscle and adipose cells to take up glucose.

There are a number of combination medications. Metformin is combined with sulfonylureas and thiazolidinediones and thiazolidinediones are combined with sulfonylureas.

The injectable drugs approved for use in persons with type 2 diabetes are Byetta (exenatide) and Symlin (pramlintide acetate). Byetta enhances insulin secretion in the presence of hyperglycemia, decreases postmeal glucagon production, delays gastric emptying, and may suppress appetite. Pramlintide is used by persons with type 2 or type 1 diabetes taking mealtime insulin. It lowers glucose levels after meals by decreasing postmeal glucagon production and delaying gastric emptying.

Insulin All persons with type 1 diabetes and many persons with type 2 diabetes who no longer produce adequate endogenous insulin need replacement of insulin that mimics normal insulin action. After eating, plasma glucose and insulin concentrations increase rapidly, peak in 30 to 60 minutes and return to basal concentrations within 2 to 3 hours in non-diabetics. To mimic this, rapid-acting insulin, such as lispro, aspart, or glulisine, is given at mealtime; doses are adjusted based on the amount of carbohydrate in the meal.

Basal or background insulin, such as determir, glargine, or NPH, is required in the post-absorptive state to restrain endogenous glucose output primarily from the liver and to limit lipolysis and excess flux of free fatty acids to the liver. Glargine and detemir are insulin analogs of 24-hour duration with no peak action time. They can be injected any time during the day, as long as they are taken around the same time each day, and can not be mixed with other insulins. NPH is also occasionally used as background insulin but usually has to be given twice a day. The type and timing of insulin regimens should be individualized based on eating and exercise habits and blood glucose concentrations.

There are also premixed insulins that are usually used in persons with type 2 diabetes, often when insulin is initiated. A listing of insulins, their onset of action, peak action time, and usual effective duration is shown in Table 8-3.

Many patients find insulin pens to be a convenient way to inject their insulin doses. Insulin pens are available containing regular, NPH, lispro, aspart, glulisine, or 70/30 or 7/25 premixed insulin.

Table 8-3 Action Times of Human Insulin Preparations

Type of insulin	Onset of action	Peak action	Effective duration
Rapid-acting			
Lispro (Humalog)	<15 min	1–2 hr	2–4 hr
Aspart (Novolog)	<15 min	1–3 hr	3–5 hr
Glulisine (Apidra)	<15 min	0.5–1 hr	3 hr
Short-acting			
Regular	0.5–1 hr	2–4 hr	3–5 hr
Intermediate-acting			
NPH	2–4 hr	4–10 hr	10–16 hr
Long-acting			
Glargine (Lantus)	4–6 hr	None	24 hr
Detemir (Levemir)	3–4 hr		5.7–24 hr
Mixtures			
Humalog Mix (75/25)	< 15 min	Dual	
Novolog Mix (70/30)	<15 min		10–16 hr
Humalog Mix (50/50)	<15 min		
Humulin (70/30)	0.5–1 hr		10–16 hr
Novolin (70/30)	0.5–1 hr		10–16 hr

Source: Adapted from American Diabetes Association. Insulin. *Diabetes Forecast 2008 Resource Guide.* 2008;RG11–RG14.

Insulin pump therapy delivers insulin in two ways: in a steady, measured, and continuous dose (the basal insulin), and as a surge (bolus) dose at mealtime. Insulin pumps can also deliver precise insulin doses for different times of day, which may be necessary to correct for situations such as the dawn phenomenon (increase in blood glucose level that occurs in the hours before and after waking). Pump therapy requires a committed and motivated person who is willing to do a minimum of four blood glucose tests per day, keep blood glucose and food records, and learn the technical features of pump usage.

Treatment of Hypoglycemia

Any available carbohydrate-containing food will raise glucose levels, including glucose tablets, sucrose, juice, regular soda, and syrup. Glucose is the preferred treatment, and commercially available glucose tablets have the advantage of being pre-measured to help prevent over-treatment. Treatment begins with 15 to 20 gram of glucose and an initial response should be seen in approximately 10 to 20 minutes. Blood glucose should be evaluated again in approximately 60 minutes as additional treatment may be necessary. Adding protein has no benefit in treatment or in the prevention of subsequent hypoglycemia. Severe hypoglycemia (the individual is unable to ingest oral carbohydrate) requires administration of glucagon. For insulin users, prevention of hypoglycemia is a critical component of diabetes management.

Self-Management Education

For metabolic goals to be achieved there must be open communication and self-management education. With chronic illnesses such as diabetes, the role of health care providers shifts from providing direct medical care to facilitating self-management by individuals with diabetes and their families. Many health care providers choose to use a team approach with registered dietitians (as well as other team members) in their medical center or clinic or delegate the educational and skill-building components by referring to a registered dietitian and/or a diabetes education center.

It is reported that individuals who hold two important beliefs are more likely to engage in effectively self-management behaviors than are those who do not hold these beliefs: (1) consider diabetes to be serious and (2) believe that their own actions make a difference. An individual's self-efficacy and self-confidence in making and maintaining a change are significant predictors of later adherence. A simple, but effective role that all health care providers can provide is to endorse and support lifestyle changes and to express confidence in the patient's ability to make change.

Nutrition Recommendations for the Prevention of Diabetes

The increase in diabetes worldwide has made prevention of type 2 diabetes a high priority. Individuals with pre-diabetes are at high risk for the development of diabetes and cardiovascular disease. The Finnish Diabetes Prevention Study and the Diabetes Prevention Program investigated the effects of lifestyle interventions on the prevention of diabetes in those at high risk (impaired glucose tolerance). In both studies, the incidence of diabetes was reduced by 58 percent in the intensive lifestyle intervention group. In a 7-year follow-up of participants in the Finnish Diabetes Study, participants still undiagnosed with diabetes after the first four years of an active lifestyle intervention reported continuing lifestyle changes and experienced a 43 percent lower diabetes risk.

Several trials have tested how efficacious drugs (i.e., metformin, acarbose, orlistat, rosiglitazone) would be in the prevention of diabetes. Each decreased incident diabetes to various degrees. Based on cost and side effects the ADA recommends that only metformin use, in combination with lifestyle counseling, be considered in those who are at very high risk (combined IFG and IGT plus other risk factors) and who are obese and under 60 years of age.

Based on the evidence the following are nutrition recommendations for prevention of diabetes:

- Structured programs that emphasize lifestyle changes including education, reduced fat and energy intake, regular physical activity, and regular participant contact can produce a long-term weight loss of 5 to 7 percent of starting weight and reduce the risk of developing diabetes and are therefore recommended.
- All individuals, especially family members of individuals with type 2 diabetes, should be encouraged to engage in regular physical activity (150 min/week) to decrease risk of developing type 2 diabetes.
- A dietary fiber intake of 14 g fiber/1000 kcal per day and consuming foods containing whole grains (one-half of grain intake) are encouraged.

Case 1 **Type 1 Diabetes Mellitus**

Judith Wylie-Rosett[1] and Brian W. Tobin[2]

[1] Texas Tech University Health Sciences Center Paul L. Foster School of Medicine, El Paso, TX
[2] Albert Einstein College of Medicine, Bronx, NY

OBJECTIVES

- Describe the role of exogenous insulin and medical nutrition therapy in the management of type 1 diabetes and in the prevention and/or treatment of acute and long-term diabetic complications.

- Take an appropriate medical and lifestyle history of a person with type 1 diabetes.

- Recognize the importance of individualizing rapid-acting insulin algorithm based on carbohydrate intake, physical activity, and blood glucose monitoring.

- Evaluate and identify potential metabolic complications of diabetes mellitus based on nutritional and physical activity history, use of medications, and alcohol consumption.

MN is a 33-year-old Hispanic woman with type 1 diabetes, whose HbA1c is 7.8 percent. She reports feeling lightheaded in the late afternoon and notes that she feels better after eating. MN also reports difficult sleeping. Her blood glucose monitor log indicated from before breakfast to before dinner blood glucose. Tests range from 70 mg/dL and 150 mg/dL. MN is 5'4" (163 cm) tall and currently weighs 132 pounds (60 kg). Recent assessment of her kidney function and an eye examination were normal.

Past Medical History

MN was diagnosed with type 1 diabetes three years ago after being brought to the emergency room by her mother in ketoacidosis. At the time of her diagnosis, MN recalls losing 9 pounds (4.1 kg) in two days after coming down with a cold and suffered from dizziness, fatigue, and frequent urination and experienced excess thirst and hunger.

Family History

MN's mother developed type 1 diabetes in her late 30s and had poorly controlled diabetes until a hospitalization for a myocardial infarction six months ago. Her mother also has hypertension and microalbuminuria. Her paternal grandfather developed diabetes in his late 60s and was treated with oral medication.

Medical Nutrition and Disease: A Case-Based Approach, 4th edition. Edited by Lisa Hark.
© 2009 Wiley-Blackwell Publishing, ISBN: 978-1-4051-8615-5.

Social History

MN has a hectic schedule during the week. She works long hours at a law firm and attends classes two nights a week. MN tries to go to the gym before work, but is often too tired. MN does not smoke and drinks alcohol only socially on occasional weekends when she goes dancing with friends. She may have two or three frozen margaritas when she goes out dancing, but feels weak shortly after drinking and reports that she "is just too tired to dance the way she used to."

MN's usual schedule and food intake consist of the following:

1. Biosynthetic human insulin (Humulin) given subcutaneously as 16 units NPH and 6 units regular before breakfast and 5 units NPH and 5 units regular before dinner. She takes no other medications.
2. A 2000 calorie food plan distributed among 3 meals and 3 snacks, which she received from the nutritionist at the hospital when she was first diagnosed 3 years ago. It consists of 50 percent carbohydrate, 20 percent protein, and 30 percent fat. MN has noted that "sticking to her diet" is one of the most difficult aspects of her diabetes self-care.
3. Monitoring and recording capillary glucose by means of a glucose monitor before breakfast and dinner. Her goal is to maintain her fasting capillary glucose level between 80 and 150 mg/dL, but it is above 150 mg/dL about 50 percent of the time. Her morning readings are usually elevated. Her glucose self-monitoring results are rarely below 60 mg/dL.

MN's Usual Intake
Breakfast (office 7:30 a.m.)

Instant oatmeal (flavored, apple-cinnamon)	1 package
Coffee	12 ounces (360 mL)
Whole milk	2 Tbsp.
Sugar	2 packets
Orange juice	12 ounces (360 mL)

Lunch (fast food restaurant 1:00 p.m.)

Hamburger	4 ounces (113 g)
Roll	1 each
Lettuce	1 leaf
Tomato	2 slices
Apple juice	12 ounces (360 mL)

Snack (vending machine 5:00 p.m.)

Pretzels	1 ounces (28 g)
Cola	20 ounces (600 mL)

Dinner (home 8:00 p.m.)

Chicken breast (baked)	6 ounces (170 g)
Rice	1 cup

Spicy black beans	1 cup
Olive oil	1 Tbsp.
Mixed salad	1 cup
French dressing	2 Tbsp.
Iced tea (sweetened)	16 ounces (480 mL)

Snack (home 11:00 p.m.)

| Chocolate chip cookies | 3 small |
| Whole milk | 8 ounces (240 mL) |

Total calories: 2863 kcal

Protein: 124 g (17% of total calories)

Total fat: 87 g (27% of total calories)

 Saturated fat 27 g (8% of total calories)

 Monounsaturated fat: 35 g (11% of total calories)

Cholesterol: 287 mg

Carbohydrate: 403 g (56% of total calories)

Dietary fiber: 25 g

Sodium: 2386 mg

Physical Examination
Vital signs

Temperature: 101.3 °F (38.5 °C)

Heart rate: 120 BPM

Respiratory rate: 28 BPM

Blood pressure: 120/60 mm Hg

Height: 5′4″ (163 cm)

Weight: 132 lbs (60 kg)

BMI: 22.7 kg/m2

Exam

General appearance: Sick-looking woman with rapid respirations. Acetone was noted on her breath. By examination she was assessed to have lost at least 10 percent of her body weight.

Eyes: Dry conjunctivae. Normal fundoscopy.

Throat: Erythematous, but tonsils were neither large nor pustular. Her buccal mucous membranes were dry.

Neck: No thyromegaly.

Heart: Normal S_1 and S_2, no murmurs, rubs, or gallops.

Lungs: Clear to oscultation.

Abdomen: Soft but diffusely tender. No hepatosplenomegaly.

Extremities: Cool and mottled in the periphery with weak but equal pulses.

Neurological: Lethargic but easily aroused. Once aroused, she is able to provide a coherent history. She responded to verbal orders and was oriented to person, place, and time.

The rest of her examination was normal.

ML's laboratory test during her previous hospitalization

Measure:	Patient's Lab Values	Normal Values
White blood cells:	20,800/mm³	4500–11000/mm³
		2.5–7.5 (10³/L)
Segmented neutophils:	7.2 10³/L	2.5–7.5 (10³/L)
Hematocrit:	47%	36–46%
Glucose:	720 mg/dL	70–99 mg/dL
Sodium (Na):	128 mEq/L	133–143 mEq/L
Potassium (K):	4.5 mEq/L	3.5–5.3 mEq/L
Chloride (Cl):	95 mEq/L	98–108 mEq/L
Bicarbonate:	7 mEq/L	22–28 mEq/L
BUN:	35 mg/dL	7–18 mg/dL
Creatinine:	2.0 mg/dL	0.6–1.2 mg/dL
Calcium (Ca):	9.2 mg/dL	9.0–11.0 mg/dL
Phosphate (PO_4):	2.4 mg/dL	2.5–4.6 mg/dL
Acetone:	4+	Negative
Venous pH:	7.10	7.35–7.45
Triglyceride:	300 mg/dL	desirable <150 mg/dL
Cholesterol:	220 mg/dL	desirable <200 mg/dL
Hemoglobin A1c:	8.5%	4–6%
	Urinary Lab Values	**Normal Values**
Specific gravity:	1.031	1.002–1.030
pH:	4.5	5–6
Glucose (Chem strip):	4+	negative
Ketone bodies (Chem strip):	4+	negative
Protein (Chem strip):	negative	negative

Treatment and Course
New Insulin Regimen
To reduce her risk of hypoglycemia and to help improve her HbA1c, MN's inter-mediate acting (NPH) insulin was changed to 24 units of long-acting glargine to provide basal insulin. Depending on her carbohydrate intake, NM takes between 5 and 10 units of rapid-acting lispro before meals to give her more flexibility in her lifestyle. The glargine insulin provides basal insulin without peaks and is proven to decrease the incidence of both hypoglycemia and prebreakfast hyperglycemia caused by the Somogyi effect.

Case Questions
1. Explain how MN's symptoms and laboratory tests at the time of her diagnosis were related to a deficiency of insulin.
2. How are acute and long-term chronic (microvascular and macrovascular) complications associated with diabetes controlled?
3. Why is medical nutrition therapy a vital component of managing patients with type 1 diabetes?
4. What are the goals of medical nutrition therapy in patients with type 1 diabetes?
5. How should insulin be adjusted to carbohydrate intake?

6. What adjustments to her MNT are needed for exercise?
7. How can acute complications (ketoacidosis and hypoglycemia) be prevented in this patient?

Answers to Questions: Case 1
Part 1: Diagnosis and Pathophysiology

1. Explain how MN's symptoms and laboratory tests are related to the absence of insulin at the time of her diagnosis.

Insulin-dependent tissues require insulin for glucose uptake and normal energy metabolism. Type 1 diabetes develops after approximately 80 to 90 percent of the beta cells of the pancreas have been destroyed (usually as the result of an autoimmune inflammatory reaction involving primary insulitis, cytotoxic T-lymphocytes, and secretion of interleukins and tumor necrosis factor alpha). The insulin secretory capacity of the pancreas normally exceeds the body's need. The decline of the islet cell mass, therefore, remains non-symptomatic for a long time, unless the body's insulin requirements increase, such as during infection or stress. When insulin secretory capacity becomes insufficient to regulate hepatic glucose output and glucose uptake by peripheral tissues, hyperglycemia occurs.

MN begins to excrete glucose in her urine when her plasma glucose has exceeded the reabsorption capacity of her kidneys. The kidney threshold for glucose is about 180 to 220 mg/dL. Above this plasma glucose level, osmotic diuresis begins. As her kidneys begin to filter more glucose, urinary volume and water loss increase. Hyperglycemia results in polyuria (increased urinary volume and frequency) that in turn leads to hypovolemia (decreased volume of circulating plasma) and secondary polydipsia (increased thirst prompting fluid intake). Polyphagia (increased appetite) presents concurrently because insulin-dependent cells are in a "starved state," despite hyperglycemia.

In the absence of insulin, the body releases fatty acids from adipose tissue due to increased adenylate cyclase activation and decreased inhibition of hormone sensitive lipase. The liver produces ketone bodies (beta-hydroxybutyrate, acetoacetate, acetone) from the increased levels of acetyl CoA formed from the oxidation of free fatty acids. Ketone bodies accumulate in the blood (ketonemia) and are excreted in the urine (ketonuria). Ketonemia is a normal response to starvation; in starvation-induced ketonemia blood glucose is low-normal.

In diabetic ketoacidosis (DKA), blood glucose levels are elevated. The primary source of blood glucose in DKA is hepatic gluconeogenesis. Gluconeogenesis is a process whereby certain amino acids, pyruvate, lactate, and intermediates of the TCA (tricarboxylic acid) cycle are converted to glucose. Gluconeogenesis is directly stimulated by stress-induced hormones (cortisol, adrenaline, glucagon). These hormones, in antagonism with insulin, increase lipolysis in adipose tissue and raise free fatty acid levels in plasma. The increased levels of free fatty acids provide energy (ATP, NADH) and reducing equivalents for gluconeogenesis. Insulin primarily inhibits hepatic gluconeogenesis by its antilipolytic action in adipose tissue.

Ketone bodies are relatively weak acids that generate large numbers of hydrogen ions by dissociation, causing metabolic acidosis. The serum bicarbonate level – an indicator of the partial pressure of CO_2 – decreases as hyperventilation decreases CO_2 in alveolar air and in arterial blood, and as the excess hydrogen ions are buffered by bicarbonate and eliminated with urine. Acidosis means the accumulation of protons. These protons in the extracellular fluid are exchanged with intracellular potassium. The potassium and other electrolytes are lost in the urine. A patient in DKA may display hypokalemia, hyperkalemia, or normokalemia depending on the stage of the condition and fluxes of potassium. Regardless of plasma potassium concentration, total body potassium stores are significantly decreased.

With insulin deficiency, weight loss can occur as body fat and protein stores are reduced because of increased rates of lipolysis and proteolysis. MN's rapid weight loss (9 pounds in two days) is likely to occur in severe insulinopenia and hyperglycemia despite an increase in appetite and caloric intake. This weight loss is due to fluid loss and not from loss of muscle mass and adipose tissue.

2. How are acute (hyperglycemia and hypoglycemia) and chronic (macrovascular and microvacular) complications associated with diabetes controlled?

The acute complications of type 1 diabetes include hypoglycemia and hyperglycemia often resulting in ketoacidosis Factors associated with increased risk of hypoglycemia include intensive therapy, better glycemic control, irregular schedule, and alcohol consumption (especially if combined with exercise or decreased carbohydrate intake). Counterregulatory hormones responded to the stress of her illness resulting in a release of glucose from her liver. MN's pancreatic beta cells were unable to respond by producing insulin to facilitate tissue uptake of the excess glucose.

Chronic microvascular complications that affect smaller blood vessels in the eyes and kidneys and neurological functioning are closely related to elevation of blood glucose. The Diabetes Control and Complications Trial (DCCT) demonstrated that intensive treatment of patients with type 1 diabetes dramatically reduces the risk of progression to retinopathy, nephropathy, and neuropathy by 50 to 75 percent. The DCCT intensified diabetes management included self-monitoring blood glucose at least 4 times a day and the use of multiple insulin injections or the use of a continuous insulin infusion pump to reduce hemoglobin A1C from approximately 9 to 7 percent. The DCCT intensive treatment was, however, associated with an increased risk of hypoglycemia and weight gain. Use of nutritional strategies, such as more regular meal times, use of snacks, and adjustments to match insulin dosage to carbohydrate intake were stressed as an essential component of behavior modification. Because weight gain will adversely affect glycemia, lipid levels, blood pressure, and general health, prevention of weight gain should be advised.

The duration of diabetes is an important component in the development of diabetic complications. The risk of complications increases with longer duration of diabetes and poorer metabolic control. Microvascular complications are related to the direct impact of high glucose levels, but elevated blood pressure contributes to excretion of protein and renal complications. Macrovascular complications are associated with an abnormal plasma lipoprotein profile as well as with atherosclerosis, ischemic heart disease, and stroke. Diabetes, especially when accompanied by insulin resistance, is associated with increased triglycerides and cholesterol (VLDL and LDL). The DCCT showed 25 percent less hypercholesterolemia with tight control.

Control of blood pressure and lipid levels is essential to prevent or ameliorate the macrovascular complications of diabetes. The improvement of glycemic control resulted in a borderline significant reduction in macrovascular complications during the 7 to 10 years of follow-up in the DCCT. This result is most likely due to the fact that the cohort was below the age of 40 years on study entry and too young. Microalbuminuria is an indication of increased risk for both atherosclerosis and diabetic nephropathy, and the American Diabetes Association recommends the use of angiotensin-converting enzyme (ACE) inhibitors as a means to slow down the progression of nephropathy.

Part 2: Medical Nutrition Therapy

3. Why is medical nutrition therapy a vital component of managing patients with type 1 diabetes?

Medical nutrition therapy (MNT) is vital to achieving more stable glycemic control. The goals of MNT are to match insulin regimens to the patient's usual schedule of meals, carbohydrate intake, physical activity, and energy needs. The timing and dosage of insulin therapy need to "mimic" how the beta cells of the pancreas normally secrete insulin in response to food intake. The Dose Adjustment for Normal Eating (DAFNE) trial determined that patients with type 1 diabetes experienced a better quality of life by adjusting insulin for their normal eating pattern despite needing more injections.

Insulin needs to be provided for basal needs (long-acting such as insulin glargine Lantus or insulin determir Levemir). Long-acting insulin has a relatively flat action curve, resulting in a lower risk of hypoglycemia than with the intermediate acting insulin, and has a peak action that occurs between 4 to 8 hours after the insulin is injected. Preferred meal-time bolus insulins are rapid-acting insulins such as insulin lispro (Humalog), insulin aspart (Novolog), or insulin glulisine (Apidra). Regular insulins (Humulin R and Novolin R) are also available, but because of their peak times of action often require snacks to prevent hypoglycemia. Insulin pumps can also be programmed to provide basal and bolus insulin.

The amount of rapid-acting insulin is based on the carbohydrate content of meals. If the patient prefers snacks with more than 15 grams of carbohydrate, rapid-acting insulin may also be needed before the snack. If the patient prefers snacks on a daily basis, regular insulin before meals may work better than a rapid-acting insulin, since this would cover those carbohydrates. Patients who have a fixed insulin dose and schedule must be consistent with both the amount of carbohydrate eaten and the timing of meals and snacks. However, patients on flexible insulin regimens can adjust their bolus insulin and accommodate changes in the times and amounts of carbohydrate eaten. Adjustments in insulin and/or carbohydrate intake are also important for planning physical activity and in managing sick days. For planned physical activity, it may be necessary to decrease bolus insulin doses or to consume additional carbohydrates.

To reduce her long-term risk for cardiovascular disease, MN's diabetes goals include an LDL-cholesterol of less than 100 mg/dL, and a blood pressure goal of less than 130/85 mm Hg. To achieve this goal, cholesterol synthesis inhibitor drugs ("statins") and hypertensive medications are often needed in addition to increased physical activity and a diet low in saturated fat, cholesterol, and sodium.

4. What are the goals of medical nutrition therapy in patients with type 1 diabetes?

The process of intensifying type 1 diabetes management to improve glycemic control involves several stages and individualization. At the time of diagnosis, the insulin dose can be calculated based on current body weight with approximately 0.5 to 0.6 units of insulin/kg per day with approximately half for basal needs and half as boluses for meals and snacks. During this initial stage, which usually includes three to four visits, diabetes management and MNT will focus on basic skills. Nutrition counseling should emphasize tailoring insulin therapy to carbohydrate intake and eating times. Blood glucose monitoring data can be used to refine the dosage of basal insulin and meal-related insulin boluses. Patients need to master a basic understanding of the relationship between insulin action and lifestyle before moving on to more complex planning to achieve better glycemic control and a more flexible lifestyle.

Guidelines for Coordinating Insulin Therapy and Food Carbohydrate

A) Make adjustments to reduce elevated glucose based on self-monitoring blood glucose. Obtain self-monitoring blood glucose at 2 a.m. if patient encounters difficulty sleeping or evidence of hypoglycemia overnight (especially for intermediate acting insulin at dinner time).

B) Individualize adjustment of insulin for changes in carbohydrate.

Self-monitoring blood glucose four or more times per day provides useful information to help intensify therapy and improve glycemic control. Estimate bolus of insulin needed for usual meal intake while keeping carbohydrate intake as consistent as possible to determine the ratio between carbohydrate intake and amount of insulin that is needed.

Adjustments are made for individual needs based on a diary indicating the number of grams of carbohydrate consumed at each meal and measuring blood glucose before eating and 2 hour after the meal. If blood glucose levels are elevated (>140 mg/dL), more insulin is needed (e.g., 1 unit of rapid-acting insulin for every 12 g of carbohydrate). Fine-tune the ratio as needed. If hypoglycemia develops within 3 hours after the meal, the ratio of carbohydrate to insulin needs to be adjusted in the other direction (e.g., 1 unit of rapid-acting insulin for every 18 g of carbohydrate).

C) Try to evaluate the effects of one change for three days before making another change in carbohydrates or insulin therapy.

Patients learn to adjust insulin and/or carbohydrate intake based on blood glucose levels. This estimate can be based on the number of carbohydrate exchanges or servings from the food groups that contain approximately 15 grams of carbohydrate per carbohydrate serving (milk and yogurt (1 cup); starches: rice (1/3 cup cooked), potatoes, pasta, starchy vegetables (1/2 cup); breads (1 slice or 1 ounce); cereals (3/4 cup dry), and fruit and fruit juices (1/2 cup or 1 small)). A more precise estimate can be made from a detailed listing of the carbohydrate content of foods.

Time	Food Intake	Carbohydrate Serving	Carbohydrate (grams)
Breakfast	12 ounces orange juice	3	45
	Instant oatmeal	2	30
	Coffee, milk and 2 packets sugars	1	15
Breakfast Total			(90)
Lunch	Hamburger with roll	2	30
	Lettuce and tomato		
	12 ounces Apple juice	3	45
Lunch Total			(75)
Snack 5pm	Pretzels, 1 ounces	1.5	22
	Cola 20 ounces (regular)	5	45
Snack Total			(67)
Dinner	Chicken		
	Rice 1 cup	3	45
	Spicy black beans 1 cup	2	30
	Green Salad		
	16 ounces bottle of ice tea (sweetened)	3	45
Dinner Total			(120)
Snack	Cookies 2 small	1	15
	Milk 8 ounces	1	15
Snack Total			(30)

Source: Judith Wylie-Rosett, PhD, RD. Used with permission.

MN eats approximately 90 grams of carbohydrate at breakfast, 75 grams at lunch, and 120 grams at dinner. Her afternoon snack contains 67 grams of carbohydrate and her night snack contains 30 grams of carbohydrate. Trying to match her bolus insulin dose to cover the amount of the carbohydrate at meals and snacks may increase risk of hypoglycemia. Reducing her carbohydrate intake from beverages (fruit juices and sugar-containing beverages) may help in synchronizing carbohydrate and insulin intake. If nutritional needs are met, sugar can be incorporated into a diabetic meal plan substituting for other carbohydrates on a gram for gram basis.

5. How should insulin be adjusted to carbohydrate intake?

Most patients need 1 unit of insulin for between 8 grams and 16 grams of carbo-hydrate, although some children may need 1 unit for 20 grams of carbohydrate, and some obese patients may need 1 unit for every 5 grams of carbohydrate. When information is limited, start by trying 1 unit of rapid-acting insulin for 15 grams of carbohydrate for an average-size adult.

6. What adjustments to her MNT are needed for exercise?

Patients with type 1 diabetes need to develop an algorithm for adjusting insulin dose to accommodate frequent or typical activity considering the intensity and duration of the activity. Testing blood glucose before the exercise session, immediately after exercise, and again 45 minutes later can help estimate the blood glucose decrease for the specified activity. For example, half an hour of brisk walking (2 to 3 miles per hour) may reduce blood glucose by about 40 mg/dL Patients can use past experience to estimate the amount of carbohydrate that should be eaten to raise blood glucose by 40 mg/dL. If the blood glucose level is elevated right before exercising (e.g. 170 mg/dL), exercise can be used to help reduce the blood glucose level to the normal range within an hour after the exercise session.

Patients with type 1 diabetes should be advised to monitor their blood glucose prior to and after exercise in order to detect and prevent hypoglycemia. Insulin dosage may need to be reduced when exercise is planned to prevent hypoglycemia. Additional carbohydrates may be needed for unplanned exercise depending on the glucose levels. If blood glucose is less than 100 mg/dL, about 15 grams of carbohydrate is needed for 30 minutes of walking or other low-to-moderate intensity activities; about 30 to 60 grams of carbohydrate is needed for 1 hour of moderate to strenuous activity (monitor glucose accordingly).

If blood glucose is 100 to 200 mg/dL, no additional carbohydrate is usually needed for 30 minutes of walking or low-intensity activity; about 15 grams of carbohydrate is needed for 1 hour of moderate activity. If glucose is 200 to 300 mg/dL, about 15 grams of additional carbohydrate is needed for strenuous activity. If glucose is greater than 300 mg/dL, physical activity should wait until blood glucose is lower.

7. How can acute complications (ketoacidosis and hypoglycemia) be prevented in this patient?

Strategies to reduce the risk of hypoglycemic episodes include frequent blood glucose monitoring especially when eating and activity patterns change. Caution is needed with regard to consuming alcoholic beverages. Individuals with type 1 diabetes should follow the guidelines for the general public with regard to the amount of alcohol they consume (a daily limit of no more than one 1 drink for women and 2 drinks for men). Food containing carbohydrate should be consumed with the alcoholic beverage.

An effective diabetes education program includes counseling on sick day management, which includes the use of short-acting insulin, monitoring of blood glucose and urinary ketones, and consumption of fluids containing sugar and salt (i.e. sports drinks that contain glucose and electrolytes). Patients should be taught to continue taking their insulin and to contact their physician early in their illness. Guidelines should be provided as to when to seek medical treatment including a weight loss of 5 percent or more of body weight, a persistent elevation in blood glucose concentration, respiration rate of greater than 35 BPM, or uncontrolled fever, nausea, or vomiting.

Case 2 **Type 2 Diabetes Mellitus**

Samuel N. Grief[1] and Frances Burke[2]

[1] University of Illinois at Chicago, Chicago, IL
[2] University of Pennsylvania School of Medicine, Philadelphia, PA

OBJECTIVES

- Describe the differences between pre-diabetes and type 2 diabetes.
- Identify the components of a healthy lifestyle for the prevention of type 2 diabetes.
- Take an appropriate medical history, including family, social, food and nutrition, physical activity, and weight histories, of a person with type 2 diabetes.
- Provide effective medical nutrition therapy for patients with both pre-diabetes and type 2 diabetes.

MA, a 55-year-old Hispanic female, presents to her family physician with a 6-month history of fatigue and lethargy, mostly noticeable after meals and in the evening. She also periodically experiences transient hot flashes. She denies any recent change in weight or appetite, shortness of breath, skin or hair changes, change in urinary frequency, bowel irregularity, or memory impairment. She has noticed some increased irritability, both at home and at work, which she attributes to her fatigue.

Past Medical History

MA denies any personal history of diabetes, high blood pressure, high cholesterol, or heart disease. She has no history of previous hospitalizations or other illnesses.

Family History

MA has one sibling, a 49 year-old brother, who has no known medical problems. Both her parents have high blood pressure and are overweight.

Social History

MA is married with two children. She leads a very sedentary lifestyle. She is a nursing supervisor who spends the majority of her workday in meetings. On the advice of a co-worker, MA has recently begun taking black cohosh for her hot flashes. She is taking no other medications or over-the-counter vitamins and/or supplements. MA rarely eats breakfast and buys sandwiches at work for lunch. Her dinner consists of store-bought frozen dinners, which are often accompanied by a dessert. She has never smoked cigarettes or other tobacco products and drinks alcohol on social occasions; on average about two glasses of wine twice per month. Her sex life is less active lately, which she attributes to her fatigue.

Medical Nutrition and Disease: A Case-Based Approach, 4th edition. Edited by Lisa Hark.
© 2009 Wiley-Blackwell Publishing, ISBN: 978-1-4051-8615-5.

Review of Systems

General: Fatigue, lethargy for past 6 months.

Endocrine: Negative for polyuria, polydipsia, or changes in appetite or weight.

Genito-Urinary: Last remembered menstrual period was 1 year ago. She has no pain with intercourse.

Neurological: Negative for headache, change in vision, numbness, or tingling in extremities.

Physical Examination

Examination

General: Obese female in no acute distress.

Head, ears, eyes, nose, throat (HEENT): Normal, visual acuity 20/20 bilaterally, normal funduscopic examination

Neck: No carotid bruits, thyromegaly, or lymphadenopathy

Lungs: Clear

Heart: Regular rate and rhythm, no murmurs

Abdomen: Obese, non-tender without organomegaly; no femoral bruits

Pelvic: Normal sized uterus, no adnexal masses or tenderness

Genitourinary: Normal introitus and labia, no lesions noted

Vital Signs (Initial Visit)

Temperature: 98.8 °F (37.1 °C)

Heart rate: 92 beats per minute (BPM)

Respiration: 16 BPM

Blood pressure: 145/90 mm Hg

Height: 5′4″ (163 cm)

Current weight: 187 lbs (85 kg)

BMI: 32 kg/m^2

Waist circumference: 37 inches (94 cm)

Weight history: MA describes a gradual weight gain since giving birth to her children, now ages 24 and 20.

Laboratory Data

Random capillary glucose: 210 mg/dL (normal: 70 to 99 mg/dL)

MA returned the following day for fasting blood work and was told to come back the following week to review and discuss the test results with her family physician:

MA's Laboratory Values	(Second Visit)	Normal Values
Plasma glucose:	135 mg/dL	70–99 mg/dL
Hemoglobin A1C:	8.5%	4–6 %
Cholesterol:	220 mg/dL	desirable <200 mg/dL
HDL-C:	48 mg/dL	desirable >50 mg/dL
LDL-C:	122 mg/dL	desirable <100 mg/dL
Triglycerides:	250 mg/dL	desirable <150 mg/dL
TSH	2.5	0.4–4.0 (μIU/mL)
Hemoglobin	12.5 mg/dL	12.0–16.0 mg/dL

Based on her history and laboratory data, MA's problem list includes:
1. Type 2 diabetes mellitus
2. Class I obesity
3. Stage 1 hypertension
4. Dyslipidemia
5. Peri-menopausal hot flashes

MA was counseled to lose weight, begin a regular exercise program, and was given a prescription for metformin 500 mg to take twice daily with meals. She was referred to a registered dietitian who is also a certified diabetes educator for nutrition and diabetes counseling, which included instruction on how to use a glucose-monitoring device. MA was also referred to a gynecologist to discuss the pros and cons of beginning hormone replacement therapy.

Three months later, MA returned to her family physician. She reported that her fatigue and hot flashes had improved and she lost 10 pounds. Her blood pressure was 135/85 mm Hg and the rest of her physical examination was unchanged. Fasting lab data obtained one week prior to this visit was as follows:

MA's Laboratory Values	(Three Months Later)	Normal Values
Plasma glucose:	115 mg/dL	70–99 mg/dL
Hemoglobin A1C:	7.7%	4–6 %
Cholesterol:	180 mg/dL	desirable <200 mg/dL
HDL-C:	51 mg/dL	desirable >50 mg/dL
LDL-C:	102 mg/dL	desirable <100 mg/dL
Triglycerides:	135 mg/dL	desirable <150 mg/dL

MA was started on the following medications:
Atorvastatin: 10 mg once daily
Enalapril: 2.5 mg once daily
Enteric coated aspirin: 325 mg once daily

Her metformin dose was maintained and combined with sitagliptin 50 mg twice daily to improve her glycemic control. On the advice of her gynecologist, MA had also started taking a combination pill of conjugated estrogen and medroxyproges-terone acetate (doses of 0.3 mg and 1.5 mg, respectively) two months ago to offset her menopausal hot flashes.

Case Questions
1. What medical conditions and risks do MA's symptoms and laboratory values represent?
2. Describe insulin resistance as it pertains to both pre-diabetes and type 2 diabetes mellitus.
3. What specific evidenced-based nutrition recommendations would you offer MA given her current diagnosis?
4. What is the role of exercise in patients with pre-diabetes and type 2 diabetes?
5. What evidence exists regarding the prevention of type 2 diabetes for patients with pre-diabetes?

Answers to Questions: Case 2
Part 1: Assessment

1. What medical conditions and risks do MA's symptoms and laboratory values represent?

MA came to her family physician complaining of fatigue and lethargy and periodic hot flashes. This may represent many conditions. Physical and psychological causes should initially be considered. Taking a careful history and performing a pertinent physical examination and obtaining laboratory tests should reveal the underlying cause of MA's symptoms.

Acute changes in blood glucose levels have been associated with feelings of fatigue. Additionally, focus groups of patients with diabetes mention fatigue as a common symptom. MA's initial laboratory values indicate that her glycemic control is poor. The recommended hemoglobin A1c (A1C) goal for patients with diabetes is less than 6.5 percent. MA's A1C is 8.5 percent, indicating her average blood glucose during the previous three-month period was in the range of 210 to 220 mg/dL. The United Kingdom Prospective Diabetes Study (UKPDS) demonstrated that a 0.9 percent reduction in A1C resulted in a 25 percent reduction in microvascular complications.

Periodic hot flashes are likely to indicate the onset of menopause. Observationally, hormone replacement therapy had been shown to reduce the risk for cardiovascular disease in women during and after menopause. As determined by the Women's Health Initiative study, hormone replacement therapy in post-menopausal women should be undertaken with caution and only with the guidance of an experienced health professional.

Dyslipidemia often accompanies diabetes. MA presents with abdominal obesity as indicated by a waist circumference of 37 inches (94 cm). She is physically inactive. These three conditions – dyslipidemia, abdominal obesity, and physical inactivity – increase MA's risk for cardiovascular disease per the National Heart, Lung and Blood Institute's 10-year risk calculator.

Diabetes confers a risk of disease and death from cardiovascular disease similar to someone with known cardiovascular disease. A major focus of the National Cholesterol Education Program ATP III Guidelines is the identification and treatment of patients with metabolic syndrome. MA's initial laboratory values and physical examination show that she meets all five ATP III criteria for diagnosis of metabolic syndrome: hypertension (BP greater than 130/85 mm Hg), high triglycerides (greater than 150 mg/dL), low HDL-C (less than 50 mg/dL in women), diabetes (or insulin resistance and glucose intolerance in pre-diabetes), and abdominal obesity (indicated by a waist circumference greater than 35 inches or 89 cm for women). MA's stage 1 hypertension, according to the *JNC VII*, mandates immediate therapeutic lifestyle changes and pharmacotherapy as the standard of care.

2. Describe insulin resistance as it pertains to both pre-diabetes and type 2 diabetes mellitus.

Insulin resistance can be defined as the diminished sensitivity of cells to the action of insulin. Insulin resistance is associated with type 2 diabetes, hypertension, dyslipidemia, central abdominal obesity, hyperinsulinemia, and other abnormalities.

Insulin resistance is present in most individuals who develop diabetes many years before the development of diabetes and often heralds the onset of pre-diabetes. However, impaired beta-cell function must be present before hyperglycemia develops. As long as the pancreas produces adequate insulin, blood glucose levels remain normal. However, it is reported that by the time diabetes develops, the individual has lost as much as 50 percent of beta-cell function. Treating insulin-resistant individuals may help to possibly reverse pre-diabetes and delay or prevent the onset of type 2 diabetes mellitus.

The reasons for the development of insulin resistance are becoming better defined, and it is now apparent that genetics, diet, and level of physical activity all play a vital role. Those at increased risk of developing insulin resistance are those with a personal history of impaired glucose tolerance, a first-degree relative with type 2 diabetes, and in women, a history of gestational diabetes or polycystic ovarian syndrome (PCOS). The condition is also associated with obesity, especially abdominal or central obesity.

Pre-diabetes and type 2 diabetes are characterized by both a progressive decrease in insulin production by the pancreas and the development of insulin resistance in skeletal muscle, adipose cells, and the liver. The effects of insulin resistance in muscle tissue are postprandial hyperglycemia and impaired glucose tolerance.

Medical nutrition therapy and regular physical activity can be very effective and may be sufficient treatment when insulin resistance is moderate or in the pre-diabetic stage when the pancreatic beta cells are still producing insulin. However, as the disease progresses, nutrition and pharmacological therapy may need to be combined to achieve the desired glucose and lipid outcomes, and to treat other co-morbidities such as hypertension and obesity.

As mentioned above, MA was successful at losing 10 pounds in the three months between medical visits, which helped to improve her lipid, glycemic, and blood pressure control. Not all patients are as likely to succeed at weight loss. If and when failure to lose weight occurs, it is worthwhile to spend time assessing a patient's readiness for change. Clinicians often find when patients focus on "what they can eat" rather than "what they cannot eat" they are more likely to lose weight. Motivational interviewing should be used to identify what a patient wants to learn, what he/she feels are areas of difficulty, and to help identify problem-solving strategies to successfully implement lifestyle changes. Involving a patient's spouse or partner in these discussions would also be helpful (see Chapter 1).

Part 2: Medical Nutrition Therapy

3. What specific evidenced-based food/nutrition recommendations would you offer MA given her current diagnosis?

Randomized controlled trials have documented the effectiveness of medical nutrition therapy (MNT) for diabetes provided by registered dietitians. Continual, multiple encounters improve glycemic and other metabolic outcomes. Depending on the type and duration of the disease, MNT has been shown to decrease A1C by approximately 1 to 2 percent. The American Dietetic Association has developed evidenced-based nutrition practice guidelines for the treatment of diabetes, which are similar to the American Diabetes Association recommendations.

MA presents with type 2 diabetes, dyslipidemia, hypertension, and obesity. Her A1C goal is less than 6.5 percent and her LDL-C goal is less than 100 mg/dL. Recent scientific evidence supports an LDL-C goal in diabetic patients at very high risk for cardiovascular disease (CVD) of 70 mg/dL or lower. MNT goals for patients with diabetes are to achieve and maintain normal or near normal glucose, blood pressure, and lipid levels to prevent or reduce the complications of diabetes and risk for CVD, and to address individual nutrition preferences and willingness to change. An analysis of a three-day food record can be undertaken to assess ways to modify or improve MA's eating habits. Since MA is considered obese with a BMI of 32 kg/m^2, reducing her total calorie intake and increasing her activity level are important goals. Because her LDL-C is elevated, MA should be advised to reduce her saturated and *trans*-fat intake, to less than 7 percent of her total calorie intake per the American Heart Association (AHA) and ATP III guidelines. Substituting foods containing phytosterols, at a maximum dose of 2 grams per day, for other foods in her diet may be beneficial in reducing her LDL-C an additional 10 percent. The AHA, ATP III, and the American Dietetic Associations' MNT Evidence-Based Guidelines provide recommendations for the nutritional management of dyslipidemia (see Chapter 6).

For individuals with diabetes, both the amount and source of carbohydrate contained in foods influence postprandial glucose levels as well as overall glycemic control. The total amount of carbohydrate depends on individual preference, weight management goals, and diabetes medication therapy. A common and effective strategy used for meal planning in patients with diabetes is carbohydrate counting. One carbohydrate serving is equal to the amount of food providing 15 grams of carbohydrate. Foods containing carbohydrate include, for example, fruit and fruit juice, milk and yogurt, starches and baked desserts. A carbohydrate counting meal plan provides guidance and consistency by tracking either the number of grams of carbohydrate or carbohydrate servings per meal and snack. Choosing carbohydrate foods according to their glycemic index is another strategy for meal planning. The glycemic index classifies carbohydrate foods according to their effect on post-prandial glucose levels. Foods rich in fiber, such as apples, whole grain breads, beans, legumes, oats, and barley tend to have a low glycemic index. Ebbeling, et. al recently published data supporting low-glycemic index diets' ability to enhance weight loss among obese young adults. Additionally, Jenkins and his colleagues from the University of Toronto reported in the Journal of the American Medical Association that a low-glycemic index diet outperformed a high-cereal fiber diet in lowering hemoglobin A1c in a type 2 diabetic population.

The recommendation for dietary fiber is no different for individuals with diabetes than for the general population. An adequate fiber intake for women is 25 g/day and 38 g/day for men, which can be met with diets rich in fruits, vegetables, and whole grain products. Clinical studies have suggested but not confirmed that increasing dietary fiber intakes above recommended levels ($\sim$ 50 g/day) would influence glycemic outcomes. The possible gastrointestinal side effects, limited food choices, and palatability may make this an impractical recommendation to follow.

MA should be encouraged to consume three meals and 1 or 2 snacks per day. Her prior dietary routine of skipping breakfast discouraged blood glucose stability and thwarted any efforts to increase her metabolism. Weight loss cannot occur or be maintained unless portion-controlled meals are consumed. The addition of a small, low-calorie snack may help to prevent overeating at mealtime. Based on this sample recommended diet, MA should continue to lose 1 to 2 pounds per week. The percent of total and saturated fat calories is within the ATP III guidelines. Increasing consumption of foods rich in calcium such as low-fat milk, yogurt, beans, and green leafy vegetables will help MA reach her daily calcium requirement. Post-menopausal women need 1,200 mg of calcium daily, according to recommendations of the National Osteoporosis Foundation. Consideration can be given to offering MA a calcium plus vitamin D supplement of 500 IU once daily in the morning to boost her calcium intake above 1200 mg per day. To be consistent with the Dietary Approaches to Stop Hypertension (DASH) recommendations, MA should avoid using the saltshaker at meals, watch her intake of soups, processed foods, salty snacks, and condiments, and increase her fruit and vegetable intake. MA can be allowed to use non-nutritive sweeteners (aspartame, sucralose) in her diet. Reduced calorie sweeteners include sugar alcohols (sorbitol, mannitol, and xylitol) and provide 2 calories per gram. Both are approved by the Food and Drug Administration; however, sugar alcohols may cause diarrhea if consumed in large quantities. Note that the dietary recommendations to assist MA in controlling her diabetes, blood pressure, and reducing her cardiovascular risk are all consistent.

Below is a sample menu for MA:

MA's Recommended Sample Diet
Breakfast (home)
Banana	1 medium
Oatmeal, cooked	1 cup (234 g)
Non-fat milk	4 ounces (120 mL)
Tea, brewed	8 ounces (240 mL)

Snack (work)
Fruit-flavored, non-fat yogurt (sweetened with sucralose)	4.4 ounces (125 g)
Tea, brewed	8 ounces (240 mL)

Lunch (home-made)
Turkey breast meat	3 ounces (85 g)
Low-fat Swiss cheese	1 ounces (28 g)
Tossed green salad	2.5 cups
Low-calorie Italian salad dressing	3 Tbsp. (42 g)
Water	12 ounces (360 mL)

Dinner (Mexican Restaurant)

Chicken fajita (chicken breast, pepper, onions, salsa) (no cheese or sour cream)	1 each
Black bean soup	1 cup (240 mL)
Diet carbonated beverage	12 ounces (360 mL)

Snack (home)

Dry roasted mixed nuts, unsalted	1.5 ounces (42 g)
Fresh apple	1 medium

Total calories: 1482 kcal
Protein: 76 g (20 % of total calories)
Total fat: 46 g (28% of total calories)
Saturated fat: 8 g (5% of total calories)
Monounsaturated fat: 21 g (13% of total calories)
Trans fat: 0.5 g
Cholesterol: 87 g
Carbohydrate: 194 g (52% of total calories)
Dietary fiber: 34 g
Calcium: 824 mg
Sodium: 2300 mg

4. What is the role of exercise in patients with pre-diabetes and type 2 diabetes?

A lifestyle that includes physical activity plays an important role in the prevention and management of patients with both pre-diabetes and type 2 diabetes. The American College of Sports Medicine (ASCM), The Centers for Disease Control and Prevention (CDC) and the Surgeon General recommend 30 minutes per day of moderate intensity aerobic exercise. The definition of moderate intensity physical activity is 50 to 70 percent of one's maximal heart rate for age. However, before starting an exercise program the patient should consult with his/her physician.

A meta-analysis done by Boule demonstrated that structured exercise programs greater than 8 weeks duration reduced A1C levels independent of any effect on body weight. Exercise reduces insulin resistance and lowers post-prandial glucose levels by increasing peripheral insulin uptake and increasing insulin sensitivity. Exercise may not contribute to a greater short-term weight reduction than diet alone, but it has been shown to be the single best predictor of long-term weight loss in overweight or obese people.

Additional benefits of exercise include decreasing the risk of CVD, improving one's lipoprotein profile, and increased cardiovascular fitness. It is likely that the beneficial effects of exercise on the prevention of CVD are associated with improvements in the metabolic syndrome. In hypertensive patients with hyperinsulinemia, regular exercise has consistently produced reductions in blood pressure. Regular exercise has also been shown to reduce levels of triglyceride-rich VLDL particles. However, its effects on HDL-C levels have not been as favorable, probably due to the lack of intensive activity used in most studies. Physical activity performed regularly can also reduce stress and anxiety and promote feelings of well-being.

Since MA does not engage in a regular exercise program, asking her to walk at least 3 non-consecutive days a week to start (increasing up to 5 to 7 days) for 30 minutes a day is a reasonable initial exercise program. Ideally, MA would eventually incorporate some physical activity into each day. MA might start out with just 10 minutes every day during lunch, after work, or in the evening and work up to this optimum level gradually. Tailoring exercise to each patient's needs is very important to maximize adherence. Motivating patients to maintain a physically active lifestyle is not a simple task, but it is a worthwhile endeavor.

Given its many health benefits, all patients with diabetes or pre-diabetes should be physically active and encouraged to begin a regular exercise program if they are sedentary.

5. What evidence exists regarding the prevention of type 2 diabetes for patients with pre-diabetes?

There is strong evidence to show that type 2 diabetes can be prevented or delayed. Therefore, individuals at high risk of developing diabetes (those individuals who are overweight or obese or who have a family history of diabetes) need to be aware of the benefits of modest weight loss and participation in regular physical activity.

For people with pre-diabetes, the benefits of therapeutic lifestyle modification have been demonstrated in scientific studies. In the Finnish Diabetes Study, one of four different interventions was used to assist patients with pre-diabetes in preventing the progression to diabetes: weight reduction (5 percent or more), reduction of total and saturated fat (less than 30 percent of energy and less than 10 percent of energy, respectively), increased fiber (25 to 35 grams per day), and increased physical activity (greater than 4 hours per week). After 4 years, the overall risk of diabetes was reduced by 58 percent in those patients who participated in any one of the above lifestyle interventions.

In the Diabetes Prevention Program (DPP), 3234 subjects with impaired glucose tolerance and a mean BMI of 34 kg/m^2 were randomly assigned to one of three intervention groups, which included intensive lifestyle modification or one of the medicine treatment groups (metformin vs. placebo). After an average follow-up of 2.8 years, the lifestyle group reduced the onset of diabetes by 58 percent and the metformin group reduced the onset of diabetes by 31 percent compared to placebo. The goals of the lifestyle intervention were at least a 7 percent weight reduction and a total of 150 minutes per week of physical activity. On average, 50 percent of the lifestyle group achieved this weight reduction goal and 74 percent maintained the required amount of physical activity.

In the DPP, the lifestyle group lost about 12 pounds after 2 years, and 9 pounds after 3 years. Additional research confirms the potential for moderate weight loss (5 to 10 percent) in reducing the risk of developing diabetes. An active lifestyle has also been shown to prevent or delay the development of type 2 diabetes, since both moderate and vigorous exercise decrease the risk of pre-diabetes and type 2 diabetes.

Chapter and Case References

American Diabetes Association. Diagnosis and classification of diabetes mellitus (Position Statement). *Diabetes Care.* 2008;31 (Suppl 1):S55–S60.

American Diabetes Association. Insulin. *Diabetes Forecast 2008 Resource Guide.* 2008; January:RG11–RG14.

American Diabetes Association. Standards of medical care in diabetes – 2008 (Position Statement). *Diabetes Care.* 2008;31 (Suppl 1):S12–S54.

American Dietetic Association. Evidence Analysis Library. Available from http://www.adaevidencelibrary.com.

American Heart Association Scientific Statement. Managing Abnormal Blood Lipids – A Collaborative Approach. Circulation. 2005;112:3184–3209.

Bantle JP, Wylie-Rosett J, Albright AL, et al. Nutrition recommendations and interventions for diabetes. A position statement of the American Diabetes Association. *Diabetes Care.* 2008;31 (Suppl 1):S61–S78.

Barnard ND, Cohen J, Jenkins DJA, et al. Talpers S. A low-fat vegan diet improves glycemic control and cardiovascular risk factors in a randomized clinical trial in individuals with type 2 diabetes. *Diabetes Care.* 2006;29;1777–1783.

Briscoe VJ, Tate DB, Davis SN. Type 1 diabetes: exercise and hypoglycemia. *Appl Physiol Nutr Metab.* 2007;32:576–582.

Centers for Disease Control and Prevention. *National Diabetes Fact Sheet: General Information and Nations Estimates of Diabetes in the United States, 2005.* Department of Health and Human Services, Centers for Disease Control and Prevention; Atlanta, GA: 2005.

Cox DJ, Gonder-Fredrick L, Ritterband L, et al. Prediction of severe hypoglycemia. *Diabetes Care.* 2007;30:1370–1373.

Diabetes Control and Trial (DCCT). Available from http://diabetes.niddk.nih.gov/dm/pubs/dcct_st.

Ebbeling CB, et.al. Effects of a Low-Glycemic Load vs Low-Fat Diet in Obese Young Adults. *J Amer Med Assn.* 2007;297(19): 2092–2102.

Franz MJ, Boucher JL, Green-Pastors J, Powers MA. Evidence-based nutrition practice guidelines for diabetes and scope and standards of practice. *J Am Diet Assoc.* 2008;108 (Suppl 1):S52–S58.

Franz MJ. Lifestyle interventions across the continuum of type 2 diabetes: reducing the risks of diabetes. *Am J Lifestyle Med.* 2007;1:327–334.

Franz MJ. The dilemma of weight loss in diabetes. *Diabetes Spectrum.* 2007;20:133–136.

Hayes C, Kriska A. Role of Physical Activity in diabetes management and prevention. *J Am Diet Assoc.* 2008;108 (Suppl 1):S19–S23.

Jenkins DJA, et.al. Effect of a low-glycemic index or a high-cereal fiber diet on type 2 diabetes. *J Amer Med Assn.* 2008;300(23): 2742–2753.

Kirk JK, Graves DE, Craven TE, Lipkin EW, Austin M, Margolis KL. Restricted-carbohydrate diets in patients with type 2 diabetes: a meta-analysis. *J Am Diet Assoc.* 2008;108:91–100.

Lindström J, Ilanne-Parikka P, Peltonen M, et al., on behalf of the Finnish Diabetes Prevention Study Group. Sustained reduction in the incidence of type 2 diabetes by lifestyle intervention: follow-up of the Finnish Diabetes Prevention Study. *Lancet.* 2006;368:1673–1679.

Look AHEAD Research Group, Bray G, Gregg E, Haffner S, Pi et al. Baseline characteristics of the randomized cohort study from the Look AHEAD (Action for Health in Diabetes) study. *Diab Vas Dis Res.* 2006;3:202–215.

Look AHEAD Research Group. Reduction in weight and cardiovascular disease risk factors in individuals with type 2 diabetes. *Diabetes Care.* 2007;30:1374–1383.

Nathan DM, Davidson MB, DeFronzo RA, et al. Impaired fasting glucose and impaired glucose tolerance: implications for care. *Diabetes Care.* 2007;30:753–759.

Palerm CC, Zisser H, Bevier WC, et al. Prandial insulin dosing using run-to-run control: application of clinical data and medical expertise to define a suitable performance metric. *Diabetes Care.* 2007;30:1131–1136.

Samman A, Muhlhauser I, Bender R, Kloos C, Müller UA. Glycaemic control and severe hypoglycaemia following training in flexible, intensive insulin therapy to enable dietary freedom in people with type 1 diabetes: a prospective implementation study. *Diabetologia.* 2005;48:1965–1970.

Sigal RJ, Kenny GP, Wasserman DH, et al. Physical activity/exercise and type 2 diabetes. *Diabetes Care.* 2006;29:1433–1438.

The Diabetes Control and Complications Trial/Epidemiology of Diabetes Interventions and Complications (DCCT/EDIC) Study Research Group. Intensive diabetes treatment and cardiovascular disease in patients with type 1 diabetes. *N Engl J Med.* 2005;353:2643–2653.

Vega-Lópe, Ausman LM, Griffith JL, Lichtenstein AH. Interindividual variability and intraindividual reproducibility of glycemic index values for commercial white bread. *Diabetes Care.* 2007;30:1412–1417.

Wenzel J, Utz SW, Steeves R, et al. "Plenty of sickness" descriptions by African Americans living in rural areas with type 2 diabetes. *Diabetes Educ.* 2005;31:98–107.

Wheeler ML, Pi-Sunyer X. Carbohydrate issues: type and amount. *J Am Diet Assoc.* 2008;108 (Suppl 1):S34–S39.

Wolever TMS, Gibbs AL, Mehling C, et al. The Canadian Trial of Carbohydrates in Diabetes (CCD), a 1-y controlled trial of low-glycemic-index dietary carbohydrate in type 2 diabetes: no effect on glycated hemoglobin but reduction in C-reactive protein. *Am J Clin Nutr.* 2008;87:114–125.

Your Guide to Lowering Your Blood Pressure with DASH. US Department of Health and Human Services, National Institutes of Health, and the National Heart, Lung, and Blood Institute. NIH Publication No. 06-4082. Originally printed 1998, revised April 2006.

Zisser H, Jovanovic L, Doyle F, Ospina P, Owens C. Run-to-run control of meal-related insulin dosing. *Diabetes Technol Ther.* 2005;7:48–57.

9 Pulmonary Disease

Jessica Dine[1], Jennifer Williams[1], and Horace M. DeLisser[2]

[1] Hospital of the University of Pennsylvania, Philadelphia, PA
[2] University of Pennsylvania School of Medicine, Philadelphia, PA

OBJECTIVES [*]

- Define the nutritional deficits, requirements, and medical nutrition therapy in patients with chronic obstructive pulmonary disease and cystic fibrosis.

- Examine available feeding options and their indications for mechanically ventilated patients and the risk associated with nutritional support.

- Identify the association between obstructive sleep apnea syndrome and obesity, and outline the nutritional recommendations for these patients.

- Recognize the importance of incorporating nutrition into the history, review of systems, and physical examinations of patients with pulmonary diseases.

[*]Source: Objectives for the chapter and cases adapted from the *NIH Nutrition Curriculum Guide for Training Physicians*. (www.nhlbi.nih.gov/funding/training/naa)

Chronic Obstructive Pulmonary Disease (Case 9.1)

Between 25 and 40 percent of patients with advanced chronic obstructive pulmonary disease (COPD) have some degree of nutritional depletion. Weight loss, with reductions in fat reserves and muscle mass, occurs in 30 percent of patients with COPD. Those patients that lose 15 percent or more of their weight within a year are at risk for undernutrition, which is associated with a higher mortality even after adjusting for age, smoking habits, baseline BMI, and lung function. Mean survival of COPD patients with a low BMI is considerably shorter than those who are not underweight.

However, even patients at normal body weight may be undernourished. The prevalence of undernutrition may be underestimated when BMI alone is used for assessment. Fat-free mass (FFM) index is a better marker of lean body mass compared to BMI because it is associated with prognostic indeces such as six-minute walk distance, dyspnea, percentage of predicted FEV_1 and FEV_1/FVC ratio, airway obstruction, lung hyperinflation, and total lung capacity. Depletion of FFM with preservation of body weight occurs in 11 to 25 percent of COPD patients and is associated with impaired peripheral muscle strength. More severe COPD

Medical Nutrition and Disease: A Case-Based Approach, 4th edition. Edited by Lisa Hark.
© 2009 Wiley-Blackwell Publishing, ISBN: 978-1-4051-8615-5.

is associated with an increased risk of undernutrition, as weight loss leads to a reduction in the mass of the respiratory muscles and the diaphragm.

Patients with COPD benefit from nutritional assessment because the consequences of undernutrition include adverse effects on respiratory muscle mass and function that result in decreased respiratory muscle strength and exercise capacity. Furthermore, because undernutrition is also associated with decreased cell-mediated immunity, altered immunoglobulin production, and impaired cellular resistance of the tracheobronchial mucosa to bacterial infection, these patients are at increased risk for respiratory infections, especially pneumonia and bronchitis. Patients with advanced COPD are also at risk for osteoporosis. Low BMI and decreased weight-bearing exercise capacity are independent predictors of osteoporosis.

Interestingly, an imbalance in oxidative status in the setting of undernutrition and low body weight may play a vital role in the pathogenesis and severity of COPD. The imbalances between the formation of reactive oxygen species and antioxidant capacity can cause cell damage, mucous hypersecretion, antiprotease inactivation, and increased pulmonary inflammation. Dietary intake of antioxidant nutrients, including vitamin C, vitamin E, β-carotene, and selenium, has been positively associated with lung function. In fact, studies suggest that foods high in antioxidants, including tea, fruits and vegetables, as well as whole grains and alcohol, may have protective or ameliorative effects on the development of COPD.

Mechanisms of Weight Loss in Patients with COPD

The causes of weight loss in patients with advanced COPD are multiple and still not fully understood. However, they can be separated into processes or conditions that result in poor nutritional intake, altered protein metabolism and a hypermetabolic state. Mechanisms of weight loss in patients with chronic obstructive pulmonary disease are shown in Figure 9-1.

Poor Nutritional Intake

Factors that may cause poor dietary intake in patients with COPD include:

- Appetite is reduced by 45 percent in cachectic patients.
- Chronic sputum production and frequent coughing may alter the desire for and taste of food and may interfere with swallowing (deglutition).
- Severe dyspnea and fatigue may result in an inability to prepare adequate meals.
- Depression from the illness may result in anorexia.
- Hyperinflation of the lungs, causing flattening of the diaphragm and pressure on the abdominal cavity during eating, leading to early satiety and problems with swallowing.
- Oxyhemoglobin desaturation during eating results in increased dyspnea.
- Side effects of medications such as nausea, vomiting, diarrhea, dysgeusia, dry mouth, and gastric irritation may limit dietary intake. Medications may also increase the need for protein, calcium, vitamin A, and folic acid or result in altered serum levels of potassium, magnesium, vitamins, or cholesterol.

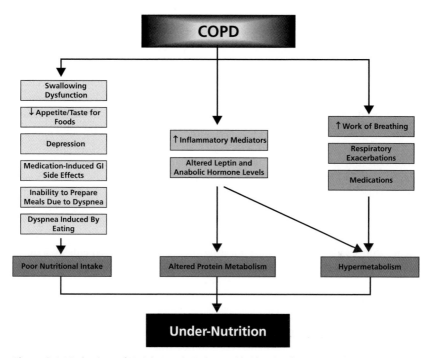

Figure 9-1 Mechanisms of Weight Loss in Patients with Chronic Obstructive Pulmonary Disease. Source: Horace M. DeLisser, MD. University of Pennsylvania School of Medicine. Used with permission.

Hypermetabolism

Several causes of hypermetabolism result in increased energy requirements in patients with COPD. These include:

Increased Work of Breathing In patients with normal lung function, breathing expends 36 to 72 calories per day. Patients with COPD may have up to a tenfold increase in their daily energy expenditure from breathing. Both the increased resistive load and the reduced respiratory muscle efficiency experienced by these patients contribute to this increased daily energy expenditure from breathing. This increased work of breathing results in an increased daily energy requirement. Patients will lose weight if they do not ingest additional calories to meet these increased needs. Alternatively, patients may reduce their activity in an effort to conserve energy.

Frequent, Recurrent Respiratory Infections Depending on the severity of the illness, respiratory infections may increase metabolic rate and, therefore, contribute to weight loss.

Miscellaneous Processes Other potential causes for hypermetabolism include disease-induced inflammatory mediators and the use of corticosteroids, $\beta 2$-agonists, and/or theophylline.

Altered Protein Metabolism Recent studies suggest that elevated levels of the cytokines, especially TNF-alpha, contribute to weight loss, skeletal muscle loss, and increased resting energy requirement in patients with COPD. Low levels of serum leptin and testosterone have been found in patients with COPD, which is believed to cause increased protein catabolism. Increased levels of growth hormone in cachectic COPD patients indicate growth hormone resistance. Reductions in phosphocreatine decrease lactate anaerobic metabolism, resulting in early onset lactic acidosis and exercise intolerance. Several studies suggest that the metabolism of the amino acid leucine is abnormal in patient with severe COPD. In summary, the rate of protein degradation may increase when the effects of inflammatory mediators and stress hormones overpower processes that tend to decrease protein turnover, such as decreased protein-energy intake, leucine levels, tissue oxygen delivery, and physical activity.

Medical Nutrition Therapy for COPD

Patients with COPD have difficulty meeting their caloric requirements and frequently lose weight. Based on survival statistics, the goal for underweight patients is weight gain and the goal for overweight patients is weight maintenance. It is safe to assume that patients who are not ingesting their caloric requirements and present with weight loss may also suffer from vitamin and mineral deficiencies. Certain electrolytes (calcium, magnesium, potassium and phosphorus) are especially important because depletion may contribute to the impairment of respiratory muscle function. When severely undernourished COPD patients are rapidly re-fed with glucose infusions, careful attention must be paid to these electrolytes to avoid refeeding syndrome (Chapter 4: Case 2).

The goals of medical nutrition therapy for COPD patients are shown in Table 9-1.

Table 9-1 Medical Nutrition Therapy for COPD

- Supply adequate calories, protein, vitamins and minerals to maintain desirable body weight (BMI 20 to 24 kg/m^2), energy level, and nutritional status.
- Provide small, frequent meals with nutrient-dense foods, such as peanut butter and jelly sandwiches, and soft-textured, easily consumed foods such as omelets, yogurt, cottage cheese, and casseroles.
- Add high-calorie, high-protein, liquid, or pudding nutritional supplements or milk shakes to the diet. Patients should sip these throughout the day instead of adding them to meals to avoid post-prandial dyspnea.
- Recommend foods that require little preparation, such as frozen dinners heated in a microwave oven.
- Follow *My Pyramid* recommendations.
- Limit consumption of cured and red meat, high-fat daily products, and refined carbohydrates.
- Limit alcohol consumption to no more than two drinks (30 grams alcohol) per day for men and one drink (15 grams alcohol) per day for women.
- Time the main meal when the patient's energy level is the highest.
- Rest before mealtime to conserve energy.
- Prescribe a daily multivitamin and mineral supplement.

Source: Jennifer Williams, MS, RD, CNSD. Used with permission.

Emerging areas of research include the use of anabolic steroids, growth hormones, and appetite stimulants for anabolism. The peptide grehlin, stimulates growth hormone secretion, food intake, and weight gain. Though appetite stimulants often result in an increase in adiposity, grehlin improves body composition by decreasing muscle wasting via inhibition of production of anorectice proinflammatory cytokines. Appetite stimulants may cause hyperglycemia, which may be exacerbated by steroid medication.

Mechanical Ventilation
Rationale for Nutrition Support
Patients with respiratory failure requiring mechanical ventilation cannot ingest food through the mouth because the endotracheal or nasotracheal tube (unless the patient has a tracheostomy). Because many patients require mechanical ventilation for prolonged periods, nutrition support is necessary to prevent undernutrition.

Undernutrition associated with critical illness impairs cell-mediated immunity, alters immunoglobulin production, and impairs cellular resistance to infection. Therefore, patients who have not been fed for seven to ten days are at increased risk of infection. In addition, undernutrition causes difficulty in weaning a patient from the ventilator, presumably due to respiratory muscle weakness. Conversely, ventilated patients with pre-existing undernutrition who are fed have improved respiratory muscle strength and function, which may improve weaning from the ventilator.

Immune-Modulating Enteral Feeding Formulas
Investigations have demonstrated that early enteral nutrition has led to decreased infections, reduced hospital length-of-stay, and even a reduction in mortality. This has led to an interest in the use of immune modulating formulas – enteral formulas containing glutamine, arginine, omega-3 fish oils and anti-oxidants. Omega-3 fish oils, in particular, have been found to improve outcomes in patients with acute lung injury (ALI) or acute respiratory distress syndrome (ARDS). A high content of omega-6 polyunsaturated fatty acids (PUFAs) has been considered unfavorable because of their potential to induce a pro-inflammatory state. This led to the development of emulsions in which part of the omega-6 fatty acid component is replaced by less bioactive fatty acids, such as omega-3 derived from fish oils. Intravenous fish oil has been shown to blunt the physiological response to endotoxin in healthy subjects. More clinical studies are needed to determine the effects of fish oils in the critically ill patient, although early, small, clinical studies suggest an improved outcome in patients with ALI.

Similar interest in enteral nutrition support, enriched with glutamine, has also arisen. Glutamine enhances the immunological barrier in the GI tract via its trophism of enterocytes and colonocytes and serves as a substrate for glutathione, which is an antioxidant. Studies have shown patients had a reduction in days spent in the intensive care unit (ICU) and in the hospital when they received enteral nutrition support containing glutamine compared to those patients fed an enteral diet without glutamine.

Feeding Options

Most patients who require mechanical ventilation for more than several days should receive enteral nutrition via a naso-enteral feeding tube as long as the GI tract is functioning (Chapter 12). Parenteral nutrition should be reserved for patients who are severely undernourished and/or do not have a functioning gut such as those with a bowel obstruction or an ileus (Chapter 13).

Minimizing Effects of Nutrition Support on CO_2 Production

The caloric and nutrient composition of the diet has a profound effect on gas exchange, especially CO_2 production. The respiratory quotient (RQ) is expressed as the ratio of CO_2 produced to oxygen consumed.

$$RQ = \frac{CO_2 \text{ produced}}{O_2 \text{ consumed}}$$

The RQ of carbohydrate is 1.0, while the RQ of fat is 0.7 and of a mixed meal is 0.83. Thus, CO_2 production is greater during carbohydrate metabolism than during fat metabolism. A diet high in carbohydrate therefore requires increased ventilation to eliminate the excess CO_2 and may complicate weaning from the ventilator. Consequently, high-fat, low-carbohydrate enteral feeding products have been formulated and recommended for feeding mechanically ventilated patients with severe COPD. These have not been proven effective, however, probably because excess CO_2 production associated with mixed or high-carbohydrate diets is not clinically relevant unless caloric requirements are exceeded. Thus, it is essential to avoid overfeeding these patients because this can result in excessive CO_2 production, increased RQ, and difficulty in weaning from the ventilator. If indirect calorimetry is available to determine caloric expenditure, this should be recommended; otherwise 100 to 120 percent of predicted caloric expenditure should be used.

Cystic Fibrosis (Chapter 9 Case 9:3)

Cystic fibrosis (CF), a life-threatening genetic disorder usually seen in children and young adults, which presents with profuse, abnormally thick exocrine gland secretions. These excessive secretions may obstruct pancreatic and bile ducts, intestines, and bronchi, resulting in a variety of clinical problems. Chronic lung disease and pancreatic insufficiency are the two most common problems seen in patients with CF. There is a definite association between worsening lung disease and undernutrition, and the degree of undernutrition seen in these patients varies considerably. Nutritional deficiencies of specific micronutrients may be sub-clinical initially, and may progress to clinically evident symptoms and signs if not recognized and treated. Deficiencies of calories, protein, essential fatty acids, fat-soluble vitamins (A, K, E, and D), beta-carotene, zinc, iron, and sodium have been described. Bone disease, such as osteoporosis, is also being increasingly recognized.

Causes of Weight Loss and Undernutrition

The causes of weight loss and undernutrition in patients with CF are multifactorial. These include maldigestion and/or malabsorption (due to pancreatic insufficiency), inadequate oral caloric intake, increased caloric and nutrient needs, and the development of CF-related organ system disease, particularly pulmonary disease, liver disease, intestinal resection, and CF-related diabetes mellitus (CFRD).

Maldigestion and Malabsorption Most patients with CF (80 to 85 percent) have pancreatic insufficiency and consequent malabsorption of fats, proteins, carbohydrates, vitamins, and minerals, which, if untreated, leads to serious nutritional problems. Pancreatic enzyme supplements are administered with meals and snacks to assist with the absorption of nutrients. The amount and type of enzyme supplements depend on the degree of malabsorption and the fat content of the diet. Steatorrhea is considered a clinical indicator of fat malabsorption (Chapter 7: Case 2).

Increased Nutritional Needs Despite pancreatic enzyme supplementation, the energy and protein needs of CF patients are significantly increased. This is due to loss of nutrients secondary to malabsorption and by higher than normal protein catabolism and energy expenditure due to frequent infections.

Increased Work of Breathing Patients with CF commonly suffer from chronic bronchitis, airway obstruction, and recurrent infections, which increase the work of breathing and result in higher energy expenditure. The effects of muscle wasting and undernutrition on respiratory muscles contribute as well.

Other Factors Gastro-esophageal reflux, abdominal pain, and psychosocial stresses may also contribute to low caloric intake. Liver disease with decreased bile salt excretion also worsens malabsorption. CF-related diabetes mellitus with glucosuria also results in increased energy loss. Finally, patients who undergo significant intestinal resection may have decreased intestinal surface area for nutrient absorption.

Medical Nutrition Therapy for Cystic Fibrosis

Patients with CF are typically unable to meet their caloric and protein requirements or maintain their weight due to increased nutrient needs and losses and inadequate caloric intake. CF is usually diagnosed in infancy or early childhood, and monitoring growth and development in these patients is particularly important. Not uncommonly, CF patients remain at or fall below the fifth percentile in both weight-for-age and height-for-age on pediatric growth charts. The goals of nutrition therapy for CF patients:

- Routine nutrition assessment, which includes height, weight, BMI, percent weight change, pediatric growth parameters, dietary history, physical examination, and evaluation of laboratory values.
- Dietary counseling to provide adequate intake of calories, protein, vitamins, and minerals. This will include education about high-calorie, balanced meals

with added salt, nutrient-dense snacks two to three times daily, and nutritional supplements.

• Adequate pancreatic enzyme replacement therapy adjusted to avoid malabsorption.

• Adequate vitamin and mineral supplements according to the *CF Foundation Guidelines.*

If patients continue to experience weight loss and fall below 85 percent of their ideal body weight, witness a significant reduction in their BMI, or have difficulty maintaining their weight, additional nutrition support may be necessary. Both enteral (using nasogastric or gastrostomy tubes) and parenteral feedings may be recommended, as clinically indicated.

Obstructive Sleep Apnea (Chapter 9 Case 9:2)

Obstructive sleep apnea (OSA) is defined as recurrent episodes of apnea during sleep caused by occlusion of the upper airway. A primary risk factor for OSA is obesity. Up to two-thirds of all patients who present with OSA are obese. OSA may be caused by an increased amount of fat surrounding the structures of the upper airway. Although not all obese patients have OSA, and occasional non-obese patients may have it, it is clear that weight loss in obese patients with OSA improves signs and symptoms. Symptoms of sleep apnea, such as snoring and excessive daytime sleepiness, should always be ascertained as part of the medical history in obese patients.

Two groups of inflammatory proteins are produced and released by adipose tissue: cytokines, such as TNF-alpha, and adipokines, such as leptin. These cytokines may play a role in the development of insulin resistance and increased oxidative stress in obese patients.

Studies have suggested a role for the fat cell protein, leptin, in the pathogenesis of respiratory dysfunction in OSA. In fact, mutation in the leptin or leptin receptor gene has been found in some obese human subjects. Other investigations suggest that patients with OSA also have lower plasma levels of orexin. Orexin is a neuropeptide produced in the lateral hypothalamus, which increases appetite and alertness. Researchers hypothesize that lower levels of orexin may result in decreased levels of alertness and may play a role in the pathogenesis of OSA.

In addition to weight loss, patients with OSA are most commonly treated with continuous positive airway pressure therapy (CPAP). A CPAP machine is approximately the size of a toaster, and is connected to tubing that ends with a mask that must be worn snugly over the face. The machine blows air into the throat and splints the airway open during sleep. CPAP eliminates apneas and snoring.

Causes of Weight Gain and Obesity

Fatigue due to chronic sleep disruption, a common symptom of patients with OSA, may influence patients' eating behaviors. Often too tired and lacking in motivation to exercise, they tend to lead sedentary lifestyles. In addition, many patients with OSA report falling asleep often after eating, which further decreases their energy expenditure. Certain overweight patients with OSA may also be prone to binge eating as a result of depression about their illness and/or body image. Whatever the exact causes, a combination of decreased physical activity and increased caloric consumption contributes to weight gain in these patients.

Medical Nutrition Therapy for Obstructive Sleep Apnea

Weight Loss Because obesity contributes to the pathogenesis of OSA, weight loss is of primary importance in obese patients with OSA. Weight loss, even as small as 5 to 10 percent body weight, can dramatically improve breathing and sleep patterns. Patients would benefit from a referral to a registered dietitian for either individual or group nutritional counseling.

Increasing Activity Once patients begin to feel better and have more energy, they should be encouraged to begin a low-intensity exercise program, such as walking 15 minutes once or twice a day.

Lung Transplantation

Lung transplantation has become a viable alternative for some patients with severe pulmonary disease, including COPD, cystic fibrosis, and pulmonary hypertension. The nutritional implications for lung transplantation patients vary depending on whether they are awaiting or have received a transplant, and whether they are breathing spontaneously or mechanically ventilated following surgery. The following recommendations are listed accordingly.

Nutrition Assessment Prior to Lung Transplantation

Routine nutrition assessment prior to lung transplantation entails the following steps:

- Assess nutritional status using BMI and the patient's weight history, and body composition measurement if equipment is available.
- Assess albumin as a predictor of mortality. If protein status is depleted, supplement the diet with high-protein milkshakes and snacks.
- Assess serum lipid levels.
- Monitor the patient's satiety level and gastrointestinal symptoms, such as bloating and gas, which could interfere with adequate dietary intake.
- Assess bone density with a DEXA scan pre- and post-lung transplantation.

Medical Nutrition Therapy Post-Lung Transplantation

Several of the drugs used for immunosuppression after lung transplantation have an impact on nutrition. Cyclosporine can cause hyperkalemia, and may also elevate serum cholesterol and triglyceride levels. These changes may require reducing dietary potassium, saturated fat, and cholesterol intake. Tacrolimus, often substituted for cyclosporine, causes hyperglycemia. The antimetabolite azathioprine causes nausea, vomiting, and diarrhea. The similarly acting mycophenolate mofetil may produce diarrhea and dyspepsia. These problems may interfere with the provision of adequate intake and must be addressed.

Corticosteroids (e.g. prednisone) cause hyperglycemia and increased appetite, which often leads to weight gain and potentially obesity. Patients taking corticosteroids may also experience fluid retention and osteoporosis.

Medical nutrition therapy immediately following lung transplantation is shown in Table 9-2.

Table 9-2 Medical Nutrition Therapy Following Lung Transplant

- Adjust calorie intake to achieve desirable body weight.
- Increase protein to promote repletion as clinically indicated and to assist with wound healing during the catabolic state following surgery.
- Low-sodium and low-fat diet for prevention of fluid retention and hyperlipidemia association with steroid use.
- Carbohydrate-controlled diet for those with steroid induced diabetes.
- Daily multivitamin and mineral supplement.
- Calcium and vitamin D supplementation for prevention of osteoporosis.

Source: Jennifer Williams, MS, RD, CNSD. Used with permission.

Case 1 **Chronic Obstructive Pulmonary Disease**

Jessica Dine[1] and Jennifer M. Williams[2]

[1] Hospital of the University of Pennsylvania, Philadelphia, PA
[2] University of Pennsylvania Health System, Philadelphia, PA

OBJECTIVES

- Review those factors in the history and physical examination important to the nutritional assessment of a patient with COPD.
- Assess the relevance of routine nutritional assessment parameters in a patient with pulmonary disease.
- Explain the causes of weight loss in patients with COPD.
- Outline the appropriate dietary interventions for a COPD patient with weight loss.

PD is a 53-year-old Caucasian woman diagnosed with chronic obstructive pulmonary disease (COPD) 8 years ago, who visits her physician complaining of shortness of breath (dyspnea). This has worsened progressively over the last 3 days since she caught a cold from her grandchildren. She explains that her customary dyspnea worsens when she is sick or under increased stress, when the humidity is high, when the temperature is extremely cold, or when she eats a large meal. Currently, PD has two-pillow orthopnea and bilateral lower extremity edema. She reports an unintentional weight loss of 18 pounds (8.2 kg) within the last year. Pulmonary function tests from last year confirmed severe COPD with a forced expiratory volume (FEV1) of 36 percent predicted, a forced vital capacity (FVC) of 44 percent predicted, and a ratio of FEV to FVC of 39 percent. A recent chest X-ray revealed hyperinflation of lung fields, with diminished lung markings in the upper lung fields.

Past Medical History

PD has been treated for hypertension for 12 years and for hypercholesterolemia for the past 2 years. She has no previous history of diabetes mellitus, thyroid disease, or liver disease.

Medications

PD is currently taking verapamil, furosemide, potassium chloride, atorvastatin, prednisone, tiotropium, alendronate, and albuterol. She does not take any vitamin/mineral or herbal supplements. PD has no known food allergies.

Family History

PD's mother died at age 70 of a heart attack. Her father also died of a heart attack at age 73.

Medical Nutrition and Disease: A Case-Based Approach, 4th edition. Edited by Lisa Hark.
© 2009 Wiley-Blackwell Publishing, ISBN: 978-1-4051-8615-5.

Social History

PD lives with her husband in a two-storey home. They have four children and fourteen grandchildren. PD worked in a local department store as a salesperson until last year, when she retired because of her illness. She formerly attended church regularly with her husband, but lately has been too tired. Her husband has also recently taken over the food shopping. PD usually follows a low-salt, low-fat, low-cholesterol diet at home. She reports the following substance use:

Alcohol intake: None

Tobacco: 45 pack-year smoking history (1 $\frac{1}{2}$ packs per day for 30 years); quit 5 years ago.

Caffeine: One cup of coffee/day

Diet History

PD is on a low-fat, low-cholesterol, low-salt diet for elevated cholesterol and hypertension. PD provided the following 24-hour dietary recall that reflects her typical daily intake. She does not add salt to her food or use salt in cooking.

PD's 24-Hour Dietary Recall

Breakfast (home)

Cream of wheat	1.5 cup
White toast	1 slice
Jelly	2 Tbsp.
Coffee	1 cup
1% milk	4 ounces (120 mL)

Lunch (home)

Low-fat yogurt	1 cup
Apple juice	6 ounces (180 mL)

Dinner (home)

Chicken breast	4 ounces (114 g)
Baked potato	1 medium
Cooked carrots	1/2 cup
Diet margarine	1 Tbsp.
Water	1 glass

Snack (home)

Banana	1 medium

Total calories: 1262 kcal
Protein: 63 g (20% of calories)
Fat: 21 g (15% of calories)
Saturated fat: 7.0 g (5% of calories)
Monounsaturated Fat: 5.0 g (4% of calories)
Cholesterol: 112 mg
Carbohydrate: 209 g (66% of calories)
Fiber: 11 g
Sodium: 1036 mg

Review of Systems
General: Weakness, fatigue, and weight loss
Mouth: Wears dentures (top and bottom; loose fitting)
GI: Poor appetite; no nausea, vomiting, or diarrhea
Extremities: No joint pain; has difficulty walking without a walker

Physical Examination
Vitals Signs
Temperature: 97 °F (36 °C)
Heart rate: 94 BPM
Respiration: 20 BPM
Blood pressure: 150/80 mm Hg

Anthropometric Data
Height: 5'6" (168 cm)
Current weight: 169 lb (77 kg)
Estimated dry weight: 147 lb (67 kg)
[Dry weight is estimated by subtracting the weight of the fluid from the current weight. Fluid weight is estimated at 22 pounds (10 kg) since she has 2+ pitting edema on both ankles. Eleven pounds (5 kg) can be used to estimate fluid in patients with ascites and no peripheral edema]
Usual weight: 187 lb (85 kg)
BMI using estimated dry weight: 24 kg/m^2
Percent weight change using estimated dry weight (over 1 year): 21% decrease [(85–67)/85]

Exam
General: Frail woman in no acute distress
Skin: Ecchymoses
HEENT: Normal non-palpable thyroid
Mouth: Loose-fitting dentures; no sores; symmetrical soft palate and uvula
Cardiac: Regular rate and rhythm; normal first and second heart sounds; jugular venous distention and hepatojugular reflux noted
Lung: Increased A-P diameter, decreased breath sounds throughout; diffuse mild expiratory wheezing with a prolonged expiratory phase

Abdomen: Non-distended, non-tender; no hepatosplenomegaly; normal bowel sounds

Extremities: 2+ pitting edema on both ankles

Rectal: Soft, heme-negative brown stool in vault

Neurologic: Alert; appropriate reactions; good memory; no evidence of sensory loss

Laboratory Data

Patient's Values	Normal Values
Albumin: 4.3 g/dL	3.5–5.8 g/dL
Hemoglobin: 10.8 g/dL	12.0–16.0 g/dL
Hematocrit: 35%	36–46%
Mean corpuscular volume:78 fL	80–100 fL
Cholesterol: 265 mg/dL	desirable <200 mg/dL
LDL-C: 173 mg/dL	desirable <130 mg/dL
HDL-C: 42 mg/dL	desirable >40 mg/dL
Triglycerides: 150 mg/dL	desirable <150 mg/dL
Arterial blood gases (ABG):	
pH: 7.37	7.35–7.45
pCO_2: 63 mm Hg	33–45 mmHg
pO_2: 60 mm Hg	80–100 mm Hg
HCO_3: 35	24–28 mEq/L
SaO_2: 90%	95–100%

Case Questions

1. Does PD's percent weight change indicate a significant weight loss?
2. Estimate PD's caloric needs using the Harris–Benedict equation including a stress factor for COPD.
3. What factors have contributed to PD's weight loss?
4. Based on PD's history, what may account for her severe fatigue?
5. How does poor nutritional status compromise pulmonary function?
6. Discuss the impact of current medications on nutritional status.
7. What is the appropriate medical nutrition therapy for PD, including specific recommendations to improve her nutritional and fluid status?

Answers to Questions: Case 1

Part 1: Nutrition Assessment

1. Does PD's percent weight change indicate a significant weight loss?

Progressive, unintentional weight change of greater than 5 percent in one month or greater than 15 percent of body weight within a 1-year period is considered a severe weight loss, and represents a significant risk for undernutrition. PD had an unintentional weight change of 21 percent over the past year and her current BMI is less than 18.5 kg/m², both considered a risk for undernutrition.

2. Estimate PD's calorie needs using the Harris–Benedict equation including a stress factor for COPD.

The Harris–Benedict equation for women:
Resting energy expenditure (REE)

$$= [655 + (9.7 \times wt^* in\ kg) + (1.8 \times ht\ in\ cm) - (4.7 \times age)] = 1358\ kcal$$

* Use estimated dry weight in this patient with bilateral pitting edema.

Total Energy Expenditure**(TEE) = (REE) × 1.3 (sedentary) or

(pulmonary disease)

TEE = (1358 × 1.3) = 1765 kcal/day

**When defining TEE by Harris–Benedict for activity and stress factors use only one correction (the highest appropriate). In this case both are 1.3.

When the TEE is compared to her current intake, which totals 1262, her calorie needs are about 500 greater than her actual intake. This could explain her continued weight loss.

3. What factors have contributed to PD's weight loss?
Because of reduced lung function, PD requires more energy to breathe. The normal daily intake of calories required to maintain her body weight is insufficient to meet the excessive demands of breathing for COPD patients. Elevated cytokines (e.g. TNF-alpha) and decreased levels of cell-derived protein (e.g. leptin and testosterone) exacerbated by frequent recurrent respiratory infections increase resting energy requirements and promote loss of weight and lean body mass.

PD's diet history reveals that her calorie intake meets only 2/3 of her nutritional requirements. Her low calorie intake is due in part to the low-fat, low-cholesterol diet originally prescribed to manage her hypertension and hypercholesterolemia. Patients with pulmonary disease may ingest even fewer calories because they are too tired to prepare food or to eat a meal. Such patients report dyspnea while chewing and swallowing food, preventing them from breathing adequately and, thereby, increasing the amount of desaturation.

PD is currently retaining fluid, so her actual "dry" weight is 22 pounds (10 kg) lower than her reported weight. PD should be asked about recent lifestyle changes and possible depression, which could be contributing to her reduced appetite and unintentional weight loss. Also, her weight loss likely contributed to her ill-fitting dentures, which decreases her ability to chew meats and other foods.

4. Based on PD's history, what may account for her severe fatigue?
COPD can cause arterial hypercapnia, which limits exercise tolerance, which further contributes to loss of lean body mass. Similarly, arterial hypoxemia reduces the amount of oxygen available to the tissues and other organs. PD has fluid overload, probably due to cor pulmonale (right ventricular failure). Patients with COPD typically have elevated hemoglobin and hematocrit levels due to chronic hypoxia.

PD's hemoglobin and hematocrit are low, further reducing her body's ability to transport oxygen. Her low mean corpuscular volume (MCV) may reflect an iron deficiency or inadequate heme synthesis due to protein-calorie undernutrition. Again, recent lifestyle changes and possible depression may also contribute to her fatigue. PD's current calorie intake is inadequate, adding to her fatigue. Liberalizing the monounsaturated and polyunsaturated fat content in PD's diet will provide additional calories without the potential to increase her lipids.

Part 2: Drug–Nutrient Interactions

5. How does poor nutritional status compromise pulmonary function?

Poor nutritional status can compromise a patient with COPD by impeding pulmonary defense mechanisms and altering respiratory muscle structure and function. Limitations of pulmonary defense mechanisms include decreased surfactant production, decreased immunoglobulin levels, and impaired cellular resistance of the tracheobronchial mucosa to bacterial infection. Poor protein status, mineral deficiencies (calcium, magnesium, and phosphorus), and electrolyte (potassium) wasting can decrease the diaphragmatic muscle mass or function, reduce diaphragmatic strength and contractility, diminish the vital capacity, and depress ventilatory responses even to minimal exertion such as walking.

6. Discuss the impact of current medications on nutritional status and the need for medical nutrition therapy.

Interactions between medications and dietary intake can be complex. Patients with protein-calorie undernutrition have impaired drug metabolism. In this case, a patient with COPD who has lost a significant amount of weight and who is consuming an inadequate diet can be expected to have significant alterations in her drug metabolism which increases the possibility of drug toxicity. The blood pressure lowering effects of verapamil have been shown not to be dependent upon dietary sodium intake but verapamil absorption is lower with increased sodium intake. Corticosteroids increase hepatic glycogen storage to protect glucose sensitive tissues (heart and brain) resulting in gluconeogenesis and increased protein turnover. Prednisone can increase the hypokalemia produced by furosemide and thus the dose of potassium replacement should be monitored closely. With this in mind, the following considerations apply to the specific medications being used by this patient and should be kept in mind if problems arise.

Verapamil-SR

- Slow-release forms need to be swallowed whole with food or milk. Other formulations can be ingested without regard to food.
- Verapamil may cause constipation, dizziness, elevated liver enzymes, bradycardia, and hypotension.
- Patients are advised to avoid alcohol. A diet low in sodium with limited caffeine may also be recommended.

Furosemide

- It is recommended to be taken on an empty stomach but may be taken with food or milk to reduce abdominal distress.
- Furosemide can produce anorexia, increased thirst, or nausea and should be administered with caution to diabetic patients. Furosemide lowers serum potassium, magnesium, sodium, chloride, and calcium and raises glucose, blood urea nitrogen, and may transiently elevate cholesterol levels.
- High intake of dietary sodium will make furosemide less effective. Supplement of potassium, magnesium, and calcium may be recommended.

K-Lyte/Cl

- K-Lyte should be taken with meals and 8 ounces of liquid.
- Possible side effects include gastric irritation, nausea, and iatrogenic elevations in serum potassium and chloride levels.

Lipitor

- Patients should avoid grapefruit juice and limit alcohol consumption.
- Side effects include nausea, dyspepsia, abdominal pain, constipation, flatulence, rhabdomyolysis, and increased liver function tests.
- HMG CoA reductase inhibitors decrease coenzyme Q_{10} synthesis, which may cause fatigue in some patients. This may respond to CoQ_{10} supplements (50–100 mg/day).

Prednisone

- Prednisone should be taken with meals to avoid gastrointestinal intolerance.
- Side effects include esophagitis, nausea, dyspepsia, increased appetite, weight gain, negative nitrogen balance, osteoporosis, fluid retention, hypertension, bruising, and slow wound healing. Hypercholesterolemia and reductions in serum zinc, vitamin A, and vitamin C levels can result from prednisone therapy. Prednisone may reduce absorption of calcium and phosphorous, and antagonizes the action of insulin, often resulting in hyperglycemia.
- Avoid alcohol.
- Supplement with potassium, calcium, phosphorus, folate, and vitamins A, C, and D.

Tiotropium

- This inhaler may cause dry mouth, dyspepsia, abdominal pain, or constipation. Other side effects include possible glaucoma, angioedema, and benign prosthetic hypertrophy.

Alendronate

- Alendronate should be taken before meals with lots of water. Because of the risk of esophagitis, patients should avoid lying down for 30 minutes after taking their medication.

Albuterol (nebulized or inhaled)

- Limit caffeine intake and take with food if gastrointestinal upset occurs.
- Side effects include anorexia, peculiar taste, sore/dry throat, nausea, tremor, headache, dizziness, and increased blood glucose levels.

Part 3: Medical Nutrition Therapy

7. What is the appropriate medical nutrition therapy for PD, including specific recommendations to improve her nutrition and fluid status?

Providing adequate calories and protein for weight and skeletal muscle maintenance is a major goal of medical nutrition therapy. By liberalizing her monounsaturated fat intake, she will increase her calories (see PD's recommended sample diet). The acute risks of weight loss and undernutrition at this time exceed the long-term risks associated with hypercholesterolemia, which can be pharmacologically managed if needed by increasing her dose of Lipitor or waiting until prednisone can be discontinued and rechecking her cholesterol level. Fluid balance is also an important consideration to prevent dehydration or hyponatremia. Consider referring both PD and her husband to a dietitian since he will be shopping and cooking and would benefit from nutritional guidance. Medical nutrition therapy should be aimed at maintaining her BMI between 20 to 25 kg/m^2 and an albumin level of 3.5 to 5.8 g/dL. Since she has microcytic anemia, she should be evaluated for iron deficiency. Medical nutrition therapy should also include the following:

- Rest before mealtime.
- Eat foods that are easy to chew, such as soft meats and casseroles.
- Avoid eating in bed; sit upright when eating.
- Drink Carnation Instant Breakfast, Boost, or Ensure at least one can per day for additional calories, protein, vitamins, and minerals.
- Include milk, which does not usually contribute to mucus/sputum production.
- Use a microwave oven to prepare convenience foods and decrease cooking time.
- Consume small, frequent meals consisting of nutrient-dense foods, such as peanut butter and jelly sandwiches.
- Use additional margarine (tub or liquid) on bread, potatoes, and vegetables as a calorie supplement.
- Consume the main meal at a time of the day when her energy level is highest.
- Avoid foods that cause gas or bloating, which makes breathing more difficult. Examples include cauliflower, broccoli, cabbage, Brussels sprouts, onions, beans, and melons.
- Gradually increase intake of fiber-rich foods to enhance GI motility.
- Limit fluid intake during meals. Instead, drink fluids between meals.
- Avoid salty foods such as canned, smoked, or cured products to minimize fluid retention and bloating.
- Take a multivitamin/mineral supplement and 500 mg/day calcium.
- Patients on home oxygen should be advised to use oxygen when preparing and eating meals, and to avoid cooking on a gas stove. The microwave oven is a safer option.

Recommended Revised Diet for PD
Breakfast (home)
Coffee	1 cup
Instant oatmeal	1 packet
2% milk	6 ounces (180 mL)
Raisins	1/4 cup
Regular margarine	1 Tbsp.

Snack (home)
Apple	1 medium

Lunch (home)
Tuna salad	3 ounces (85 g)
Whole wheat bread	1 slice

Snack (home)
2% milk	1/2 cup
Saltines (low sodium)	6 each
Peanut butter	1 Tbsp.
Jelly	2 Tbsp.

Dinner (home)
Lean ground beef patty	4 ounces
Brown rice	1/2 cup
Tossed salad	1 cup
Olive oil	2 Tbsp.
Balsamic vinegar	1 Tbsp.

Snack (home)
Low-fat yogurt	4 ounces
Orange	1 medium

Total calories: 1919 kcal
Protein: 76 g (16% of calories)
Fat: 89 g (42% of calories)
Saturated fat: 22 g (10% of calories)
Monounsaturated fat: 45 g (21% of calories)
Cholesterol: 143 mg
Carbohydrate: 213 g (44% of calories)
Fiber: 21 g
Sodium: 1346 mg

Case 2 **Obstructive Sleep Apnea and Metabolic Syndrome**

Lisa Hark[1], Indira Gurubhagavatula[2], and Sharon Drozdowsky[3]

[1] Jefferson Medical College, Philadelphia, PA
[2] Philadelphia VA Medical Center, Philadelphia, PA
[3] Washington State Department of Labor and Industries, Tumwater, WA

OBJECTIVES

- Understand how to effectively use a medical interpreter.
- Recognize the importance of eliciting the patients' explanatory model.
- Examine how socio-cultural factors may influence the healthcare decisions of patients.

CC is a 34-year-old Mexican immigrant who works as a truck driver. He presents to his primary care physician complaining of daytime sleepiness, loud snoring, and fatigue. He is referred to the pulmonary clinic for an expedited sleep study, which confirms a diagnosis of severe sleep apnea. He is prescribed continuous positive airway pressure (CPAP) therapy and instructed to use the CPAP machine during all periods of sleep in order to minimize his risk of falling asleep while driving. He is told that his usage of the CPAP will be monitored through a small electronic chip in the CPAP machine. He is further informed that if he does not comply, and if he is still sleepy while driving, the physician is obligated under state law to report him to the Department of Transportation for possible suspension of his commercial driver's license. He is advised to make sure he sleeps for 7.5 to 8 hours each night with the CPAP machine on, to lose weight, limit alcohol, and is educated about safe driving habits. CC returns to the clinic one month later and his symptoms are minimally improved. The CPAP usage is checked and indicates that he used the device only 20 percent of the time and less than four hours per night.

Past Medical History

CC has no history of cardiovascular disease. He takes no medications, vitamins, or herbal supplements. He admits to loud snoring at night and occasionally falling asleep during the day when he visits truck stops.

Family History

CC's family history is positive for overweight. His two brothers and one sister are overweight. His father has hypertension and had a myocardial infarction at the age of 63. His mother is obese, hypertensive, and has type 2 diabetes.

Medical Nutrition and Disease: A Case-Based Approach, 4th edition. Edited by Lisa Hark.
© 2009 Wiley-Blackwell Publishing, ISBN: 978-1-4051-8615-5.

Social History
CC is single and has never been married. He does not smoke. He averages two to three bottles of beer daily. He eats three meals per day, mostly on the road, and admits to snacking during the day while driving. He states that he has no opportunity to exercise since he is driving a truck 6 days a week and frequently traveling.

Review of Systems
Skin: No history of rashes
HEENT: No visual complaints
Neurological: No headaches, tremors, seizures, or depression
Endocrine: Denies abnormal heat or cold intolerances
GI: Constipation
Cardiovascular: Normal rate and rhythm. No orthopnea or dyspnea
Joints: No swelling, heat, or redness

Physical Examination
Vital signs
Temperature: 98.4 °F (36.9 °C)
Heart rate: 88 BPM
Blood pressure: 135/88 mm Hg
Height: 5′9″ (176 cm)
Current weight: 215 lbs (98 kg)
BMI: 32 kg/m^2
Waist circumference: 43 inches (109.2 cm)

General: Obese man in no acute distress; no Cushingoid features.
Exam: Non-palpable thyroid. Acanthosis nigricans. Negative hirsutism or striae; no dorsal, cervical, or supraclavicular fat. His limbs are not edematous.

Laboratory Data

Patient's Fasting Values	Normal Values
Glucose: 116 mg/dL	70–99 mg/dL
Potassium: 3.8 mEq/L	3.5–5.0 mEq/L
Cholesterol: 216 mg/dL	desirable <200 mg/dL
Triglycerides: 275 mg/dL	desirable <150 mg/dL
HDL-C: 32 mg/dL	desirable for male ≥40 mg/dL
Calculated LDL-C: 129 mg/dL	desirable <130 mg/dL

When asked about his usual intake, he reports the following:
Breakfast (truck stop or motel)

Coffee	24 ounces (720 mL)
Half and half cream	3 ounce (90 mL)
Sugar	4 packets
Conchas (Mexican Sweet Bread)	2 pieces
Orange juice	8 ounces (240 mL)

Lunch (fast food)

Deluxe beef burrito	1 whole
Nachos with cheese	large
Cola soda	24 ounce large (720 mL)

Snack (truck stop)

Oreo cookie snack-pack	6 cookies
Cola Soda	12 ounce (360 mL)

Dinner (home)

Beef Enchiladas with cheese	2
Mexican rice	1 cup
Cheesecake	1 slice
Beer	12 ounces (360 mL)

Snack (home)

Beer	12 ounces (360 mL)
Corn chips	6 ounces

Total calories: 4539 kcal
Protein: 88 g (8% of calories)
Fat: 164 g (32% of calories)
Saturated fat: 59 g (12% of calories)
Monounsaturated fat: 31 g (6% of calories)
Cholesterol: 393 mg
Carbohydrate: 632 g (55% of calories)
Fiber: 27 g
Sodium: 7436 mg

Case Questions

1. How was CC diagnosed with sleep apnea and what are the risk factors and appropriate treatment recommendations?
2. In addition to OSA, what other medical conditions does CC present with?
3. How does CC's occupation as a truck driver impact his medical condition?
4. How should the clinician go about determining whether CC understands his diagnosis of sleep apnea and its treatment?
5. How can communication be improved between CC and the health care team?
6. How should CC's low CPAP adherence be addressed?
7. Now that communication issues have been discussed, what specific dietary recommendations would be appropriate and realistic for CC to implement?
8. How can CC increase his physical activity level?

Answers to Questions: Case 2
Part 1: Diagnosis and Treatment

1. How was CC diagnosed with sleep apnea and what are the risk factors and appropriate treatment recommendations?

Obstructive sleep apnea (OSA) is a characterized by intermittent airway closure during sleep, leading to arousals, sleep fragmentation, and daytime sleepiness. Sleep apnea carries a significant morbidity; risk factors include male gender, middle-age, and obesity.

The diagnostic gold standard for sleep apnea is an in-laboratory polysomnography (PSG) or an overnight "sleep study." PSG provides an estimate of OSA severity by reporting the apnea-hypopnea index (AHI), a value that expresses the hourly number of breathing disturbances during sleep. PSG is relatively costly, requires technical expertise to perform. and is difficult to access.

A large prospective study found that persons with apnea experience increased risk of future development of hypertension. Prospective data also link sleep apnea to increased incidence of myocardial infarction, stroke, coronary artery bypass grafting, coronary angioplasty, and to death from cardiovascular events. Cross-sectional data link sleep apnea with myocardial infarction, stroke, and insulin resistance.

The first-line treatment for sleep apnea is not a medication, but a device, which is worn during sleep, called continuous positive airway pressure (CPAP). A CPAP machine is approximately the size of a toaster, and is connected to tubing that ends with a mask that must be worn snugly over the face. The machine blows air into the throat and splints the airway open during sleep. CPAP eliminates apneas and snoring.

Randomized, controlled trials show that CPAP therapy reduces blood pressure and insulin resistance and improves neuro-cognitive function. These data hold true even after controlling for important confounding variables such as obesity. CPAP may also reduce highway crash risk, as assessed by performance in driving simulators.

The major problem with CPAP therapy is adherence; up to 50 percent of patients offered CPAP refuse it at the outset, and close to 25 percent abandon this treatment within 3 years. Improving adherence to therapy so that its benefits may be realized by all affected patients remains an active area of investigation, and an elusive goal for many sleep medicine specialists.

2. In addition to OSA, what other medical conditions does CC present with?

According to CC's physical examination and laboratory data, he also presents with metabolic syndrome. Laboratory tests reveal elevated triglycerides and blood sugar and low HDL-C, and physical examination shows an abnormally high waist circumference (43 inches). He therefore meets four of the five criteria for the diagnosis of metabolic syndrome. Metabolic syndrome has been identified as an independent risk factor for CVD by ATP III and increases the risk of developing type 2 diabetes (Chapter 1: Case 1.1).

The diagnosis of metabolic syndrome can serve as a starting point for discussing lifestyle modification. Metabolic syndrome represents a cluster of metabolic abnormalities associated with abdominal obesity. Obesity frequently leads to insulin resistance, which in turn may lead to elevated BP, atherogenic dyslipidemia, and impaired fasting glucose levels. Clinicians should add waist circumference measurement to their clinical examination or assign clinical support staff to obtain this along with the patient's blood pressure prior to the clinician's evaluation. Waist circumference is an important marker of visceral fat, which is more prognostic of metabolic syndrome than body mass index (BMI). Waist circumferences should always be measured, since self-reported pant size will almost always be smaller than the patient's true girth. To get the correct waist measurement, wrap a tape measure around the smallest area below the rib cage and above the umbilicus. Accuracy is important, especially for patients at risk, because abdominal obesity is a crucial pathophysiologic link to other features of metabolic syndrome, particularly insulin resistance. A waist circumference of greater than 40 inches for men and greater than 35 inches for women defines significant abdominal obesity. The International Federation of Diabetes has developed lower cut-off measurements for waist circumference specific to ethnicity (Chapter 6: Case 6.3).

3. How does CC's occupation as a truck driver impact his medical condition?

The association between sleep apnea and sleepiness should be highlighted in the population of commercial drivers. This is because sleepiness among commercial drivers impairs task performance and accounts for 31 to 41 percent of major crashes of commercial vehicles. Overall, large trucks are involved in nearly half-million traffic accidents each year. These accidents injure 130,000 victims each year, and incur huge costs. While we know little about the role of OSA in crashes in commercial vehicles, we do know that drivers of passenger cars who have OSA experience increased crash risk. A recent meta-analysis quantified a 2.5-fold increase in crash risk among sleep apnea sufferers.

Given the increased prevalence of risk factors in truck drivers, it is not surprising that OSA occurs more commonly in this occupational group compared to the general population. As many as 60 percent of commercial drivers may have sleep-disordered breathing, with 16 percent having OSA – the combination of sleep-disordered breathing plus daytime sleepiness. These figures contrast starkly with the prevalence among the general group of all middle-aged employed adults affecting 4 percent of men and 2 percent of women.

Part 2: Enhancing Patient Communication

4. How should the clinician go about determining whether CC understands his diagnosis of sleep apnea and its treatment?

Ensuring that a patient understands his/her diagnosis is critical to promoting adherence (compliance) to recommended or prescribed treatments. Patients enters the clinician's office with their own beliefs, concerns, and expectations about their illness

Table 9-3 Questions to Elicit a Patient's Explanatory Model

- What do you think has caused your problem?
- Why do you think it started when it did?
- What do you think your sickness does to you? How does it work?
- How severe is your sickness? Will it have a short or long course?
- What kind of treatment do you think you should receive?
- What are the most important results you hope to receive from this treatment?
- What are the chief problems your sickness has caused for you?
- What do you fear most about your sickness?

Source: Adapted from Kleinman A, Eisenberg L, Good B. Culture, illness, and care: clinical lessons from anthropologic and cross-cultural research. *Ann Intern Med.* 1978. 88:251–8

and the medical encounter. This conceptualization of the illness experience can be described as the patient's explanatory model. This is the patient's understanding of the cause, severity, and prognosis of an illness; the expected treatment; and how the illness affects his or her life. In essence, it is the meaning of the illness for the patient. Patients' explanatory models of illness are to a large extent culturally determined.

Kleinman and associates, in their seminal paper referenced below, further discuss the importance of the explanatory model: "Eliciting the patient's (explanatory) model gives the clinician knowledge of the beliefs the patient holds about his/her illness, the personal and social meaning he/she attaches to their disorder, their expectations about what will happen to them and what the health care professional will do, and their own therapeutic goals."

Comparison of the patient's model with the clinician's model enables the clinician to identify major discrepancies that may cause problems for clinical management. Such comparisons also help the clinician know which aspects of the explanatory model need clearer exposition to patients (and families), and what sort of patient education is most appropriate. And they clarify conflicts not related to different levels of knowledge but different values and interests. Part of the clinical process involves negotiations between these explanatory models, once they have been made explicit.

Eliciting the patient's explanatory model of illness through a set of targeted questions (shown in Table 9.3) is an important tool for facilitating cross-cultural communication, ensuring patient understanding, and identifying areas of conflict that will need to be negotiated. The wording and number of questions used will vary depending on the characteristics of the patient, the problem, and the setting.

5. How can communication be improved between CC and the health care team?

To improve communication between a Mexican immigrant, who may not speak English as a first language, and any member of the health care team, it would be helpful to invite a bilingual staff member, if available, to join the conversation. CC could also be asked if there is someone else who is more proficient in English to

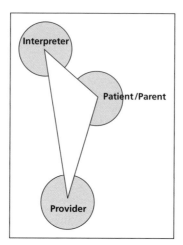

Figure 9-2 Proper Positioning for a Medical Interpreter
Source: Horace M. DeLisser, MD. University of Pennsylvania School of Medicine. Used with permission.

join him either on the phone or at the next visit. By saying: "*CC, I am not sure I explained everything well enough for you to understand,*" the clinician is able to address any concerns without causing embarrassment for the patient or making him defensive.

Subsequently, the office staff needs to be informed so that they can prepare for CC's visit by ensuring that interpreter services will be available. Depending on available resources, this may involve the patient bringing someone or ensuring that bilingual staff is available for the visit, or arranging for a trained interpreter, either live or via telephone.

The following should be done to effectively use an interpreter, particularly when someone other than a trained medical interpreter is used:

- Have a pre-interview discussion with the interpreter. (Tell the interpreter what you hope to accomplish with this interview and give a brief description of how the patient came to the current situation.)
- Position the interpreter to the side and slightly behind the patient (see Figure 9.2).
- Look at the patient and not at the interpreter. (Experienced interpreters actually avoid eye contact with everyone in order to promote optimal interaction between the clinician and the parent and/or patient).
- Speak in short sentences and avoid jargon and phrases that may not translate well from English into another language, such as "the ball is your court." (It is important to note that "interpretation" refers to the spoken word, while "translation" is about the written word.)

6. How should CC's low CPAP adherence be addressed?

Most patients with severe sleep apnea, and particularly those who are very sleepy, who use the CPAP device as recommended, feel significantly better. They notice significant improvements in daytime sleepiness and as a result, tend to use the CPAP more consistently. It is therefore worrisome, given the severity of CC's apnea, that he is still not using the CPAP device. This strongly suggests there are other factors that may be compromising his adherence.

It would be important to begin by ensuring that CC understands his disease and its treatment. Assuming he understands how to use the CPAP machine, the next step would be to ascertain the barriers he encountered when using this device. Given that his low adherence may potentially involve embarrassing, sensitive, and/or personal issues, it is important to continue this conversation with non-judgmental, open-ended questions.

To this end, it is essential to separate patient-related factors (social stigma of CPAP, stigma of diagnosis, health and cultural belief system that promotes or dissuades compliance) from machine-related factors (the CPAP machine is too noisy, the mask is leaking, the mask irritates the skin, the pressure is uncomfortable). Patients may worry about how the CPAP device will impact their social functioning, including their sexual behavior. Since 80 percent of patients with sleep apnea are obese, their self-esteem may also be low, which could affect their motivation to adhere to the treatment. For this patient, since he is a truck driver, barriers that may have influenced his adherence include sleeping in his truck on a regular basis and being on the road most of the time.

Part 3: Medical Nutrition Therapy

7. Now that communication issues have been discussed, what specific dietary recommendations would be appropriate and realistic for CC to implement?

CC's labs and physical examination revealed elevated triglycerides and blood sugar, low HDL-C, borderline hypertension, and an abnormally high waist circumference. He therefore meets all five of the criteria for the diagnosis of metabolic syndrome. He is also at risk for diabetes and hypertension. CC's current diet is high in total fat, saturated fat, cholesterol, sodium, and sugar. He is also obese, with a BMI of 32 kg/m2 and a waist circumference of 43 inches. At present, there is no single dietary recommended for all individuals with metabolic syndrome, therefore it is best to focus on the specific patient's metabolic alterations when offering nutrition counseling.

His current job is very stressful, he is on the road all the time, and says that he does not have time to exercise and has limited choices for healthy foods. These are all challenges for CC to improve his health. Because of his strong family history of obesity, diabetes, and hypertension, he is at risk of also developing these medical problems. It is important to help him understand that his current diet may make it more likely that he will develop those conditions. His goals should therefore include reducing this total calories, fat, saturated fat, sodium, sugar, cholesterol, and alcohol intake. As shown in his diet analysis, his current total caloric intake

Table 9-4 Tips for Truck Drivers While Eating on the Road

- It's all about choice as well as portions.
  - Ask for nutritional information at the places you like to eat.
  - Ask "What do I like?" and "What do I need?" rather than "What do I want?"
- Have a plan:
  - Walk in knowing what you will choose based on what you need.
  - Stick to your plan.
- Request that food is prepared the way you want it . . . no gravy, broiled rather than fried, dressing on the side for you to control.
- Look for steamed, baked, broiled, braised, poached, or grilled and skip the sautéed, pan-fried, or deep-fried items.
- Look for health-focused entrees.
- A box of crayons. Keep in mind that a colorful plate containing more veggies than meat should be a goal!
- Forget the "clean plate" notion. At restaurants ask for a doggie bag and then refrigerate it for your next meal.
- Avoid asking for *super-size* or *value size* items.

Source: Sharon Drozdowsky, MES. Used with permission.

is 4539 kcal/day and his saturated fat intake represents 12 percent of his daily intake.

Nutritional goals could encourage CC to refuel his body just as he refuels his truck. Healthy eating practices will allow his body to perform at its best, provide extra energy, and increase his alertness for long hours on the road. Tips for eating on the road are shown in Table 9.4.

For sedentary patients with hypertriglyceridemia and insulin resistance (particularly those who are obese or have elevated waist circumference) a lower carbohydrate diet that limits sodas, juice drinks, refined grains such as sweetened cereals, baked goods, and desserts may be beneficial. The long-term effects of low-carbohydrate diets have not been adequately studied but short-term research shows that these diets lower triglycerides, raise HDL-C, and reduce body weight.

In addition, alcohol intake should always be quantified. Although alcohol has been shown to be cardioprotective in certain patients, it contributes a significant amount of calories and can raise triglyceride levels. For example, 6 ounces of red wine has approximately 120 calories, and 12 ounces of beer has 150 calories, equivalent to a 12-ounces can of regular soda. In addition, excessive alcohol consumption may cause hypertension, atrial arrhythmias, stroke, cirrhosis, pancreatitis, breast cancer, and accidents. Finally, alcohol also weakens the patient's resolve not to overeat and can thus contribute to many collateral calories. Limit alcohol in patients with metabolic syndrome to 1 drink per day or a maximum of 7 drinks per week.

If CC follows the recommended diet as shown below, he will have a reduction in calories, total fat, saturated fat, cholesterol, alcohol, sodium, and simple sugars. He will meet the recommendations for saturated fat of less than 7 percent, cholesterol of

Table 9-5 Healthy Snacks for the Road

Bananas	Low sodium tomato juice	Cherries
100% Juice	Baby carrots	Apples
Raisins	Celery	Oranges
Pretzels	Snap peas	Pears
Fig cookies	Grape or cherry tomatoes	Plums
Graham crackers	Grapes	Broccoli
Whole grain crackers	Other fresh produce	

Source: Sharon Drozdowsky, MES. Used with permission.

less than 200 mg per day, and fiber of 20 to 30 grams per day. He will also increase his fruit and vegetable consumption as recommended by the DASH diet (Table 6-6). Fish and nuts were included to increase MUFAs. Fruits and vegetables are ideal carbohydrate-rich foods, high in fiber and containing important phytonutrients such as antioxidant vitamins and flavonoids. This approach will also improve his constipation.

Two percent milk was suggested as a way to help CC reduce his consumption of half and half. After he becomes accustomed to the 2 percent, he can be encouraged to switch to 1 percent milk. Decaffeinated beverages were interspersed with caffeinated beverages to help lower his caffeine tolerance, prevent dehydration, and reduce truck stops. By lowering his caffeine tolerance, he will ensure that caffeine will be more effective when he does need it to stay awake.

A fast food meal was included because drivers avoid regular restaurants due to parking options and time constraints. Truck stops and fast food restaurants do offer healthy options. He can improve his diet and "limited choices" by purchasing one of the electric coolers now available for trucks. This will enable him to pack healthy foods and maintain their freshness. Examples of healthy snacks for the road and tips for buffet style truck stops are shown in Tables 9.5 and 9.6.

Table 9-6 Tips for Buffet-Style Truck Stops

- First take a look at everything that's on the buffet.
- Avoid the temptation to choose a little bit of everything.
- Use medium-sized plates use the serving utensils at a serving line to dictate the amount to take.
- Concentrate on fresh vegetables at the salad bar and avoid pre-dressed salads.
- Keep in mind that a colorful plate containing more vegetables than meat should be a goal.
- For an entree, select small portions of one or two main dishes and round out the meal with cooked vegetables.
- Buffets often have a great selection of fresh fruits – try these for dessert.
- Try a serving fresh fruit and top it off with a little bit of soft-serve ice cream.
- Drink water or tea without sugar.

Source: Sharon Drozdowsky, MES. Used with permission.

Recommended Revised Diet for CC:

Breakfast (truck stop or motel)

Coffee	16 ounces (480 mL)
2 percent milk	8 ounces (240 mL)
Sweetener	4 packets
Oatmeal	1 cup (with milk)
Banana	1 medium

Snack (on-board cooler)

Apple	1 medium
Peanut butter	2 tablespoons
Decaf iced tea (unsweetened)	12 ounces (360 mL)

Lunch (fast food and on-board cooler)

Grilled steak soft taco	1 whole
Orange	1 medium
Iced tea (unsweetened)	24 ounces (720 mL)

Snack (on-board cooler)

Fresh baby carrots	1 cup
Almonds	11
Decaf iced tea (unsweetened)	12 ounces (360 mL)

Dinner (home)

Grilled salmon tacos	2
Onions and peppers	1 cup
Diced tomatoes	$\frac{1}{2}$ cup
Mexican rice	1 cup
Pinto beans	$\frac{1}{2}$ cup
Beer	12 ounces (360 mL)

Snack (home)

Decaf iced tea (unsweetened)	12 ounces (360 mL)
Air pop popcorn	2 cups

Total calories: 2219 kcal
Protein: 92 g (17% of calories)
Fat: 55 g (22% of calories)
Saturated fat: 12 g (5% of calories)
Cholesterol: 92 mg
Carbohydrate: 339 g (61% of calories)
Dietary fiber: 40 g
Sodium: 1909 mg

Table 9-7 Tips for Exercising on the Road

- Walk at rest stops and truck stops (around facility or on walking path nearby).
- Walk around truck or bus several times at each stop.
- Walk when truck is being loaded/unloaded at the delivery site.
- Park far from the building.
- Take exercise equipment on the truck.
- Ride a stationary bike at a truck stop fitness center.
- Jump rope in the rest stop parking lot.
- Pack low-weight dumbbells or cans to do arm curls.
- Use resistant elastic bands for 5–10 minutes at rest stops.
- Do crunches or push-ups in your cab (build up to this).
- Tighten stomach muscles while driving, hold for 30 seconds, then release.

Source: Sharon Drozdowsky, MES. Used with permission.

8. How can CC increase his physical activity level?

Skeletal muscle is the most-insulin sensitive tissue in the body and therefore a primary target for impacting insulin resistance (IR). Physical training has been shown to reduce skeletal muscle lipid levels and IR regardless of BMI. Exercise has been shown to lower systolic blood pressure by an average of 4 to 9 mm Hg in patients with elevated blood pressure. The impact of exercise on insulin sensitivity is evident for 24 to 48 hours and disappears within 3 to 5 days. Thus, regular physical activity should be a part of any effort to reverse the effects of IR. In a meta-analysis of studies published on the impact of exercise in patients with type 2 diabtetes, Boule and colleagues concluded that exercise should be considered a desirable end-point and not just a means to achieve weight loss.

Exercise Prescription

A recent Institute of Medicine report recommends 1 hour of physical activity daily for health maintenance. The American Heart Association calls on health professionals to prescribe 30 minutes or more of brisk walking on most or all days of the week. The greatest health benefits occur when sedentary individuals incorporate moderate-intensity exercise as part of their lifestyle. Low-intensity exercise can have a significant impact and may be easier for patients to comply with these regimens, since compliance declines as frequency increases. Encourage patients to find their own comfort level when it comes to physical activity. Help each patient find a level of activity that he or she can accomplish over the long-term. A combination of resistance and aerobic exercise is advisable, but any activity is better than none and patients who have been sedentary need to start with walking and increase duration and intensity gradually.

CC should exercise 30 to 60 minutes per day, on most days. Explain to him that exercise will make him healthier, reduce stress, help with sound sleep, help him look better and move easier. Exercise will help muscles and joints become stronger and a strong body is less susceptible to strains, sprains, and other injuries. Ways to exercise on the road are listed in Table 9.7.

Case 3 **Cystic Fibrosis**

Andrea J. Nepa and Maria R. Mascarenhas

The Children's Hospital of Philadelphia, Philadelphia, PA

OBJECTIVES

- Explain the nutritional abnormalities commonly observed in patients with cystic fibrosis.
- Conduct a nutritional assessment of patients with cystic fibrosis.
- Develop an appropriate nutritional care plan for patients with cystic fibrosis.
- Recognize the importance of medical nutrition therapy in the long-term survival and well-being of patients with cystic fibrosis.

JF, a 21-year-old Caucasian female with cystic fibrosis (CF), presents to the pulmonary clinic with a 1-week history of increased cough, shortness of breath, and a 3-pound weight loss. She reports increased mucus production with a change in color from yellow to green. She has also been passing three or four foul-smelling, floating stools daily for the past several months.

Past Medical History

JF was diagnosed with CF at 5 years of age based upon recurrent upper respiratory tract infections, bulky, foul-smelling stools, and hepatomegaly. In addition, JF has scoliosis, diagnosed 2 years ago, and hearing loss due to frequent intravenous antibiotic therapy. She has been hospitalized two times over the past year for acute exacerbations of CF. JF has no known food or drug allergies.

Medications

JF's current medication regimen includes pancrealipase (Pancrease MT 10) (six capsules per meal, three capsules with snacks), Azithromycin, albuterol, and acetyl-cysteine solutions via nebulizer, cromolyn sodium (Intal metered dose inhalers), triamcinolone acetonide (metered dose inhaler), rhDNase (Pulmozyme via inhalation), and ranitidine. She also receives frequent chest percussion therapy.

Diet History/Vitamin and Mineral Supplements

JF follows a high-calorie, high-protein, high-fat, extra-salt diet that includes three meals and three snacks daily. She also drinks two servings per day of a high-calorie, high-protein powder supplement that is mixed with whole milk, but recently ran out of supply at home. JF's current vitamin/mineral therapy includes a standard adult multivitamin with iron twice a day, vitamin E (400 IU) once a day, and vitamin

---

Medical Nutrition and Disease: A Case-Based Approach, 4th edition. Edited by Lisa Hark.
© 2009 Wiley-Blackwell Publishing, ISBN: 978-1-4051-8615-5.

K (5 mg 3 times per week). JF prepares her breakfast and lunch, and her mother prepares dinner.

Social History
JF is a junior in college and lives at home with her parents. She denies smoking, alcohol, drug use, and sexual activity.

Review of Systems
Remainder of the review of systems was unremarkable except for poor appetite, shortness of breath, and increased frequency of bulky, foul-smelling stools.

Physical Examination
Vital Signs
Temperature: 101.4 °F (40 °C)
Heart rate: 110 BPM (tachycardia)
Respiration: 24 PM (tachypnea)
Blood pressure: 134/74 mm Hg
Height: 5′2″ (158 cm)
Current weight: 88 lb (40 kg)
Usual weight: 91 lb (41 kg)
BMI: 16 kg/m2
Triceps skinfold (TSF): 13 mm (<25th percentile)
Mid-arm muscle circumference (MAMC): 200 mm (20 cm) (<25th percentile)

Exam
The patient's physical examination is normal except for the following observations:
General: Thin, ill-appearing female
Skin: Warm to the touch
HEENT: Right nasal polyp
Chest: New rales and rhonchi in right upper lung zone, no wheezing or dullness to percussion
Cardiac: Elevated rate, normal rhythm, no murmurs

Laboratory Data

Patient's Values	Normal Values
Albumin: 4.2 g/L	3.5–5.8 g/L
Hemoglobin: 13.4 g/dL	12.0–16.0 g/dL
Prothrombin time: 14 seconds	<15 seconds
Random glucose: 220 mg/dL	70–99 mg/dL
25(OH)D: 18 ng/dL	20–30 ng/dL

Treatment
Because of her worsening symptoms, abnormal physical examination, and decreasing pulmonary function, JF is diagnosed with an acute exacerbation of CF and admitted to the hospital. During her 1-week hospital admission, she received

intravenous antibiotics, respiratory treatments, and vigorous chest percussion to help mobilize her secretions. A DEXA scan was ordered to obtain additional body composition data and to determine her bone mineral density.

In addition, random blood glucose levels were consistently elevated suggesting CF-related diabetes. After consultation with endocrinology, an insulin regimen was initiated using short-acting insulin matched to the carbohydrate content of her meals. Despite these therapies, JF's appetite has remained poor, and she has lost an additional 4 pounds (1.8 kg). Three-day calorie counts reveal that JF consumes approximately 1500 calories and 40 grams of protein per day. A high-calorie, high-protein oral supplement was ordered to help her meet her calorie goals.

Follow-up
JF was discharged to home when her weight reached 91 pounds (41 kg). She was advised to continue monitoring her blood glucose levels until her post-hospitalization office visit.

Case Questions
1. What factors are most likely contributing to JF's weight loss?
2. What nutritional problems are patients with CF at risk for developing?
3. Is albumin a valid indicator of JF's nutritional status?
4. What is the significance of an elevated blood glucose level?
5. Are JF's current nutrition and vitamin therapy appropriate?
6. Is JF's current enzyme therapy appropriate?
7. What dietary recommendations would you give JF upon discharge?
8. What parameters should be used to monitor changes in JF's nutritional status after she is discharged from the hospital?

Answers to Questions: Case 3
Part 1: Nutrition Assessment

1. What factors are most likely contributing to JF's weight loss?
A negative calorie balance accounts for JF's weight loss, compounded by ongoing malabsorption and by increased energy needs due to fever and infections. JF's poor appetite may be due to her current lung infection and to her antibiotic therapy. Decreased appetite in CF patients may also be due to esophagitis, cholelithiasis, salt depletion, and vitamin and mineral deficiencies leading to altered taste (dysgeusia). Psychosocial factors also commonly contribute to anorexia. JF's bulky, foul-smelling stools suggest fat malabsorption. In addition, JF has protein losses due to maldigestion caused by pancreatic enzyme insufficiency. Finally, JF has elevated serum glucose levels. Hyperglycemia is frequently seen with CF exacerbations and can contribute to weight loss via glucosuria.

2. What nutritional problems are patients with CF at risk for developing?
The importance of uncompromised nutritional status in the long-term survival and well-being of patients with CF is well documented. Pancreatic insufficiency occurs in about 85 percent of CF patients. Analysis of pancreatic secretions reveals

a marked decrease in the amounts of water, electrolytes, and enzymes (lipase, protease, and amylase). This results in inadequate digestion of food, producing malabsorption and undernutrition with growth retardation and weight loss. Protein-energy undernutrition impairs immune responses, increases the risk for pulmonary infections, and leads to muscle wasting. Declining respiratory muscle strength may adversely affect survival. Protein deficiency can lead to hypoalbuminemia, which may result in edema.

Patients with CF are at risk for developing multiple vitamin deficiencies with their associated clinical manifestations. Vitamin K deficiency results in coagulopathy, a commonly encountered deficiency. Vitamin E deficiency can lead to hemolytic anemia in infants; and to neuropathy, ophthalmoplegia, ataxia, and diminished vibration sense and proprioception in older children and adults. Vitamin D deficiency causes rickets in young children and osteomalacia in adults and contributes to reduced bone mineral density. Vitamin A deficiency leads to night blindness, conjunctival xerosis, and epithelial keratinization.

Deficiencies of water-soluble vitamins are less common; however, vitamin B_{12} deficiency produces macrocytic anemia and neuropathy. Pancreatic insufficiency, which occurs when CF patients are not receiving (or are not complying with) enzyme therapy, impairs the digestion of the glycoproteins known as R binders, which are necessary for the transfer of vitamin B_{12} to intrinsic factor (IF). Salt depletion leads to lethargy, weakness, dehydration, and metabolic alkalosis. Essential fatty acid deficiency results in desquamation, thrombocytopenia, and poor wound healing.

Osteopenia is also commonly seen in CF patients, which may be due to malabsorption, decreased calcium intake, vitamin D deficiency, delayed puberty, reduced physical activity, and medications (e.g. corticosteroids) and high circulating levels of inflammatory cytokins related to lung infections. A DEXA scan is recommended for all adults and children 8 years old and up who are at nutritional risk.

JF's DEXA scan indicates very low bone density. According to her 24-hour diet recall, JF's calcium intake was only 800 mg of elemental calcium. JF's estimated calcium needs were 2000 mg of elemental calcium per day. Therefore, JF was started on an oral calcium supplement to provide 400 mg, three times a day. Her serum 25(OH)D level was only 18 units. Currently, the goal is to achieve levels greater than 30. JF was started on vitamin D_2 (ergocalciferol – 50,000 units once a week for 8 weeks). There is evidence that vitamin D3(cholecalciferol) may be more effective at increasing low serum vitamin D levels than vitamin D2 (ergocalciferol) (See Chapter 2 and 7: Case 7.2).

3. Is albumin a valid indicator of JF's nutritional status?

Serum albumin indicates visceral protein status. JF's albumin was normal, indicating good protein stores. Hypoalbuminemia reflects poor protein intake and/or increased protein losses, and suggests acute visceral protein depletion. Protein deficiency may develop in as little as two weeks. Most commonly, patients with CF are undernourished at the time of diagnosis and throughout their lives, but their albumin levels are normal until the end stages of their disease because the body preserves visceral protein in chronically ill patients. Therefore, the clinical diagnosis of undernutrition should be based on physical examination findings, such as temporal and interosseus muscle wasting, and information gathered in the medical and diet history. Similarly, anthropometric results, such as BMI, percent weight change, and diminished triceps skinfold thickness (TSF) and mid-arm muscle circumference (MAMC), reflect fat and muscle wasting due to chronically inadequate protein and energy intake (See Chapter 1).

Part 2: Medical Nutrition Therapy

4. What is the significance of an elevated blood glucose level?

Hyperglycemia is frequently seen during CF exacerbations and can lead to increased morbidity and mortality in this population. Studies have shown that weight loss and declining pulmonary function can occur several years prior to the diagnosis of CF-related diabetes (CFRD). Glucose intolerance and CFRD often develops around 18 to 21 years of age in patients with CF. CFRD can be diagnosed by the following criteria: fasting glucose levels of greater than or equal to 126 mg/dL two or more times; fasting glucose level greater than or equal to 126 mg/dL plus a random glucose level of greater than 200 mg/dl; or elevated random glucose levels greater than 200 mg/dL on two or more occasions with symptoms. It is important to aggressively treat hyperglycemia and to closely monitor fasting glucose levels for resolution of glucose intolerance as acute infections resolve. Increased glucose levels may occur temporarily during pulmonary exacerbations and with steroid use.

5. Are JF's current nutrition and vitamin therapy appropriate?

Medical nutrition therapy   A high-calorie, high-protein, high-fat (greater than 30 percent of total calories), balanced diet is indicated for patients with CF because of their significantly increased work of breathing and potential for malabsorption and maldigestion. A BMI of at least the 50th percentile is ideal for children andado-lescents from 2 to 20 years of age. For adults older than 20 years of age, women should have a BMI of at least 22 and men should have a BMI of at least 23 according to the current CF Foundation recommendations. Despite hyperglycemia, calories should not be restricted. Extra salt is needed to replace the large amounts of sodium lost in perspiration. Six small meals per day are better tolerated than fewer, larger meals by patients with high caloric requirements. According to the *Cystic Fibrosis Consensus Report*, a patient whose weight is less than 85 percent of ideal body weight should receive enteral supplementation via a nasogastric tube (NG) tube or enterostomy. With the addition of oral high-calorie supplements JF was able to meet her caloric needs. Two Scandishakes (a high-calorie powder supplement to mix with milk) were added daily between meals, which provided JF with an additional 1200 calories per day.

Vitamin therapy   Even with appropriate pancreatic enzyme therapy, fat malabsorption and associated fat-soluble vitamin deficiencies may still persist in CF patients. A daily multivitamin supplement, enriched in fat-soluble vitamins that are in a water-miscible form to improve absorption, is indicated. Typically-CF patients are instructed to consume two times the RDA for vitamins and minerals to prevent the associated deficiencies. CF patients are encouraged to supplement their diets with 200 to 400 IU of vitamin E per day to ensure adequate absorption of this vitamin. Vitamin K is produced by gut micro-organisms. Antibiotic therapy significantly decreases gut bacteria and, as a result, diminishes vitamin K production. Therefore, vitamin K supplements should be given to all patients, especially those receiving chronic antibiotic therapy (at least 2.5 to 5 mg per week). CF patients should receive 400 to 800 IU of vitamin D and 10,000 units of vitamin A daily.

6. Is JF's current enzyme therapy appropriate?
Malabsorption should be suspected in any patient with CF who reports an increased incidence of foul-smelling, floating stools. Such patients require higher enzyme dosages to help them digest and absorb fat. Currently, JF is taking six capsules per meal and three capsules per snack of Pancrease MT 10 (10,000 units of lipase per capsule), which provides 1500 lipase units per kilogram per meal. Instead of increasing the number of MT 10s, changing the prescription to MT 20s (2,000 units of lipase per capsule) and altering the dosage to four capsules per meal and two capsules per snack will increase the total units of lipase the patient receives to 20,000 lipase units per kilogram per meal. This will also minimize the number of capsules the patient must ingest with each meal and snack. The usual recommended dose is 500 to 2500 units of lipase/kg per meal. The use of gastric acid blocking medications can optimize duodenal pH, which enhances enzyme activity. If symptoms of malabsorption persist despite optimizing enzyme dose, then other causes of malabsorption should be explored.

7. What dietary recommendations would you give JF upon discharge?
Because patients with CF have such high caloric and protein needs (up to two times the RDA to prevent undernutrition), it is very important *not* to limit calories to control hyperglycemia. Instead, insulin therapy should be adjusted to optimize glucose control by matching the carbohydrate content of meals and snacks. If patients consume concentrated sweets, these should accompany a meal to reduce the glycemic response.

Upon discharge, JF should be instructed to increase her caloric intake with small, frequent nutrient-dense meals and Scandishakes (a high-calorie powder supplement to mix with milk) to promote weight gain. Her insulin regimen may need to be adjusted based on her blood glucose levels, which she should continue to monitor at least once a day. Her blood glucose log will be brought to her office visit to assess improvement in glycemic control with the resolution of her acute infection.

8. What parameters should be used to monitor changes in JF's nutritional status after she is discharged from the hospital?
Weight change Weight should be monitored three times a week during an inpatient admission and then re-checked at each outpatient appointment. Due to her worsening symptoms and poor appetite, JF's weight was 88 pounds (40 kg) when admitted to the hospital. Her BMI of 16 kg/m^2 suggests that she is undernourished. A BMI of less than 18.5 kg/m^2 is considered significant malnutrition in adults. She lost an additional 4 pounds (1.8 kg) reflecting an 8 percent weight change from her usual body weight, which is indicative of significant weight loss. Arm anthropometrics

(TSF and MAMC) are also useful in screening and following a patient's body fatness and lean body mass. Patients with CF are often hypermetabolic because of their increased work of breathing, inflammatory responses, and infections. They need at least 20 to 50 percent more calories than a person without CF.

Dietary intake/appetite JF's energy requirements are approximately 2525 calories per day for weight gain. This is based on her basal metabolic rate of 1084 calories per day with an activity factor of 1.5 plus 0.2 for moderate lung disease, times 1.1 for malabsorption, and 500 added for weight gain. Her daily intake in the hospital was approximately 1500 calories – a 1000 calorie per day deficit – which can lead to continued weight loss. Calorie intake should be increased to prevent further weight loss and promote weight gain. JF's intake should be assessed periodically to ensure that her calorie intake is adequate. Protein needs are 1.5 to 2.0 grams/kg/day.

Laboratory data Relevant laboratory tests to be monitored are prothrombin time (to assess adequate vitamin K stores), fat-soluble vitamin levels (vitamins A, D, and E levels should be checked annually), and iron stores. Albumin and pre-albumin levels can be affected by acute infection and therefore may not reliably detect a change in nutritional status.

Chapter and Case References

Aranguri C, Davidson B, Ramirez R. Patterns of communication through interpreters: a detailed sociolinguistic analysis. *J Gen Intern Med.* 2006;21:623–629.

Becker HF, Jerrentrup A, Ploch T, et al. Effect of nasal continuous positive airway pressure treatment on blood pressure in patients with obstructive sleep apnea. *Circulation.* 2003;107(1):68–73.

Boulé NG, Kenny GP, Haddad E, et al. Meta-analysis of the effect of structured exercise training on cardiorespiratory fitness in type 2 diabetes mellitus. *Diabetologia.* 2003;46(8):1071–81.

Consensus Statement: Guide to bone health and disease in cystic fibrosis. *J Clin Endoc Metab.* 2005;90:1888–1896.

Dysart-Gale D. Communication, models, professionalism, and the work of medical interpreters. *Health Commun.* 2005;17:91–103.

Flores G. The impact of medical interpreter services on the quality of health care: a systematic review. *Med Care Res Rev.* 2005;62:255–299.

Goodpaster BH, He J, Watkins S, et al. Skeletal muscle lipid content and insulin resistance: evidence for a paradox in endurance-trained athletes. *J Clin Endocrinol Metab.* 2001;86:5755–5761.

Harsch IA, Schahin SP, Radespiel-Tröger M, et al. Continuous positive airway pressure treatment rapidly improves insulin sensitivity in patients with obstructive sleep apnea syndrome. *Am J Respir Crit Care Med.* 2004;169(2):156–162.

Hayek K. Medical nutrition therapy for cystic fibrosis: beyond pancreatic enzyme replacement therapy. *J Amer Dietet Assoc.* 2006;106 (8):1186–1188.

Howard ME, Desai AV, Grunstein RR, et al. Sleepiness, sleep disordered breathing and accident risk factors in commercial vehicle drivers. *Am J Respir Crit Care Med.* 2004;170:1014.

Hsieh E. Conflicts in how interpreters manage their roles in provider–patient interactions. *Soc Sci Med.* 2006;62:721–730.

Hsieh E. Understanding medical interpreters: reconceptualizing bilingual health communication. *Health Commun.* 2006;20:177–186.

Institute of Medicine. *Dietary reference intakes for energy, carbohydrates, fiber, fat, protein, and amino acids (macronutrients).* National Academy Press; Washington, DC. 2002.

Ip MS, Lam B, Ng MM, et al. Obstructive sleep apnea is independently associated with insulin resistance. *Am J Respir Crit Care Med.* 2002;165(5):670–676.

Kalnins D, Durie P, Pencharz P. Nutritional management of cystic fibrosis patients. *Curr Opin Clin Nutr Metab Care.* 2007;10:348–354.

Keller C, Trevino RP. Effects of two frequencies of walking on cardiovascular risk factor reduction in Mexican American women. *Res Nurs Health.* 2001;24:390–401.

Kleinman A, Eisenberg L, Good B. Culture, illness, and care: clinical lessons from anthropologic and cross-cultural research. *Ann Intern Med.* 1978;88:251–8.

Lui S, Manson JE. Dietary carbohydrates, physical inactivity, obesity, and the 'metabolic syndrome' as predictors of coronary heart disease. *Curr Opin Lipidol.* 2001;12:395–404.

Maqbool A, Stallings V. Update on fat-soluble vitamins in cystic fibrosis *Curr Opin Pulm Med.* 2008;14:574–581.

Marin JM, Carrizo SJ, Vicente E, et al. Long-term cardiovascular outcomes in men with obstructive sleep apnoea–hypopnoea with or without treatment with continuous positive airway pressure: an observational study. *Lancet.* 2005;365(9464):1046–1053.

Misra M, Pacaud D, Petryk A, et al. Vitamin D deficiency in children and its management: review of current knowledge and recommendations. *Pediatrics* 2008;122;398–417.

Peppard PE, Young T, Palta M, et al. Prospective study of the association between sleep-disordered breathing and hypertension. *NEJM.* 2000;342(19):1378–1384.

Pepperell JC, Ramdassingh-Dow S, Crosthwaite N, et al. JR, Davies RJ. Ambulatory blood pressure after therapeutic and subtherapeutic nasal continuous positive airway pressure for obstructive sleep apnoea: a randomised parallel trial. *Lancet.* 2002;359(9302):204–210.

Pratt M. Benefits of lifestyle activity vs. structured exercise. *JAMA.* 2001;281(4):375–376.

Punjabi NM, Sorkin JD, Katzel LI, et al. Sleep-disordered breathing and insulin resistance in middle-aged and overweight men. *Am J Respir Crit Care Med.* 2002;165(5):677–682.

Sassani A, Findley LJ, Kryger M, et al. Reducing motor-vehicle collisions, costs, and fatalities by treating obstructive sleep apnea syndrome. *Sleep.* 2004;27(3):453–458.

Shahar E et al. Sleep-disordered breathing and cardiovascular disease: cross-sectional results of the Sleep Heart Health Study. *Am J Respir Crit Care Med.* 2001;163(1):19–25.

Stallings VA, Stark LJ, Robinson KA, Feranchak AP, Quinton H; Clinical Practice Guidelines on Growth and Nutrition Subcommittee; Ad Hoc Working Group. Evidence-based practice recommendations for nutrition-related management of children and adults with cystic fibrosis and pancreatic insufficiency: results of a systemic review. *J Am Diet Assoc.* 2008;108:832–839.

Stoohs RA, Bingham LA, Itoi A, et al. Sleep and sleep-disordered breathing in commercial long-haul truck drivers. *Chest.* 1995;107(5):1275–1282.

The Seventh Report of the Joint National Committee on Prevention, Detection, Evaluation, and Treatment of High Blood Pressure JNCVII. *JAMA.* 2003;289:2560–2572.

Thompson PD, Buchmer D, Pina IL, et al. Exercise and physical activity in the prevention and treatment of atherosclerotic cardiovascular disease. *Circulation.* 2003;107:3109–3116.

Update on Enteral Nutrition Support for Cystic Fibrosis. *Nutr Clin Pract.* 2007;22:223–232.

Yankaskas et al. Cystic fibrosis adult care consensus conference report. *Chest.* 2004;125:1S–39S.

Young T et al. Sleep-disordered breathing and motor vehicle accidents in a population-based sample of employed adults. *Sleep.* 1997;20:608–613.

10 Renal Disease

Jean Stover[1] and Gail Morrison[2]

[1] DaVita Dialysis, Philadelphia, PA
[2] University of Pennsylvania School of Medicine, Philadelphia, PA

OBJECTIVES*

- Describe the specific medical nutrition therapy for acute renal failure, chronic kidney disease, nephrotic syndrome, and nephrolithiasis.
- Describe the goals of medical nutrition therapy for patients on hemodialysis and peritoneal dialysis.
- Identify the impact of various forms of renal replacement therapy and renal transplant on a patient's nutritional status.
- Explain the importance of regulating the intake of protein, calories, sodium, potassium, phosphorus, fluid, vitamins, and other minerals in patients with renal disease.

*Source: Objectives for chapter and cases adapted from the *NIH Nutrition Curriculum Guide for Training Physicians*. (www.nhlbi.nih.gov/funding/training/naa)

Acute Renal Failure

Acute renal failure (ARF) is characterized by a sudden decline in the glomerular filtration rate (GFR) of the kidney due to insults such as infection, exogenous nephrotoxins, trauma, dehydration, and shock resulting in ischemia. Patients with ARF are at high risk for malnutrition because of underlying illnesses, recent surgical procedures, or trauma, all of which place them in a catabolic, pro-oxidative, and proinflammatory state. In ARF precipitated by major trauma, critical illness, or sepsis, patients frequently undergo metabolic changes that accelerate degradation of protein and amino acids and result in the loss of lean body mass. The dramatic effects of this catabolic state include poor wound healing, increased infection, and higher mortality rates.

Medical Nutrition Therapy for Acute Renal Failure

Since malnutrition is so often seen in patients with ARF and is known to be an independent risk factor contributing to increased mortality, implementation of medical nutrition therapy is very important. Decisions on when to implement and how aggressive medical nutrition therapy should be depend on the patient's nutritional status and catabolic rate, the phase of ARF, the amount of urine output, and clinical indications such as uremia or volume overload requiring dialysis or

---

continuous renal replacement therapy (CRRT). Thus, medical nutrition therapy for the patient with ARF must be highly individualized. Goals are to preserve protein stores and prevent nutritional deficiencies until renal function returns, while maintaining fluid, electrolyte, and acid-base homeostasis.

Protein

Restricting protein intake to 0.8 g/kg per day is indicated only for patients with ARF whose GFR falls to less than 10 mL/min and who are not catabolic or on any form of dialysis or Continuous Renal Replacement Therapy (CRRT). All forms of dialysis and CRRT contribute to protein losses. The protein intake of patients who are receiving hemodialysis should be at least 1.2 g/kg per day and patients receiving peritoneal dialysis (although infrequently used with ARF) are encouraged to ingest 1.2 to 1.3 g/kg of protein each day. Severely catabolic patients with ARF may have even higher protein needs and require CRRT or aggressive dialytic therapy to allow for sufficient protein intake.

Calories

Caloric requirements for patients with ARF vary depending on their degree of hypermetabolism. Usual recommendations are 35 kcal/kg per day, however, needs may actually be closer to only 20 to 30 kcal/kg per day. The most accurate determination of caloric requirements is by indirect calorimetry. Complications from slightly underfeeding are not as harmful as overfeeding. Calories from the dextrose utilized in dialysate with PD, as well as in replacement fluids with CRRT, must be considered.

Patients who have adequate gastrointestinal (GI) tract function but cannot tolerate food by mouth because of mechanical ventilation, altered mental status, anorexia, nausea, or poor compliance, should receive nourishment by enteral tube feeding (Chapter 12). Those with a dysfunctional GI tract require parenteral nutrition (Chapter 13). Peripheral insulin resistance may cause hyperglycemia in catabolic patients with ARF, therefore blood glucose levels should be closely monitored. Insulin may be required, especially with the use of parenteral nutrition. Also, there may be alterations in lipid metabolism in patients with ARF. Lipids are not precluded in parenteral feedings, but triglyceride levels must also be monitored closely.

Vitamins and Minerals

Vitamin and mineral requirements for patients with ARF vary depending on their nutritional status and whether they are receiving dialysis or CRRT. Serum electrolytes must be closely monitored in all patients with ARF. Initially, serum potassium and phosphate are likely to be elevated and serum sodium lowered in nondialyzed patients who are oliguric (urine output less than 400 mL/day). Patients with acute intrinsic renal failure (usually defined as acute tubular necrosis – the major cause of ARF) may experience salt and water overload during the oliguric phase and salt and water depletion during the diuretic or recovery phase of the disease (when urine output can exceed 2 to 3 liters per day). In the recovery phase, sodium, potassium, and fluid may need to be replaced to offset urinary losses. Oliguric or anuric patients receiving hemodialysis usually require a sodium restriction of 2 to 3 g/day and a potassium restriction of 2 to 3 g/day. Those undergoing peritoneal dialysis, frequent hemodialysis (more than three times per week), and some forms of CRRT generally have more liberal sodium and potassium requirements. Patients with ARF undergoing any form of dialysis or CRRT should receive supplemental water-soluble vitamins above the Recommended Dietary Allowances (RDA) to compensate for losses with these treatments.

Fluid

Daily fluid intake for oliguric patients should equal urine output plus approximately 500 mL to replace insensible losses; fluid needs increase if the patient has a fever. Most anuric patients can tolerate approximately 1000 mL/day with hemodialysis three times per week. These restrictions may be liberalized in patients receiving continuous or daily peritoneal dialysis CRRT, or hemodialysis more frequently than three times per week.

Continuous Renal Replacement Therapy

Continuous arteriovenous hemofiltration (CAVH) utilizes catheters that are placed into a large artery and vein (often the femoral artery and vein). The arterial blood flows through a small filtering device with a large porous membrane where plasma is filtered of water, minerals, and uremic toxins, and albumin and blood products return to the vascular space through the vein. This form of therapy removes large volumes of essentially albumin-free plasmanate, leaving water and electrolytes in a concentration equal to normal serum levels. Parenteral nutrition can be combined with CAVH to provide intravenous nutrition while controlling salt and water balance and removing small amounts of metabolic waste products that accumulate in renal failure.

Continuous arteriovenous hemodiafiltration (CAVHD) combines hemodialysis and hemofiltration simultaneously and removes larger amounts of solutes as well as large volumes of fluid. CAVH and CAVHD use systemic arterial blood flows; other forms of CRRT including continuous venovenous hemofiltration (CVVH) and continuous venovenous hemodiafiltration (CVVHD) use a pumping machine that may result in less erratic blood flows and ultrafiltration rates.

Chronic Kidney Disease (Predialysis)

In 2002, the National Kidney Foundation (NKF) published clinical care guidelines for those with chronic kidney disease (CKD). These guidelines help determine the stage of kidney disease based on kidney damage and/or level of glomerular filtration rate (GFR) as shown in Table 10-1. Stage 1 includes kidney damage (e.g. proteinuria) with normal GFR or a GFR of 90 or above. Stage 2 includes mild kidney damage and a GFR of 60 to 89. Stage 3 includes a moderate decrease in GFR to 30 to 59. In Stage 4 the GFR is 15 to 29 and in Stage 5 the GFR is less than 15. Medical nutrition

Table 10-1 Clinical Care Guidelines for Chronic Kidney Disease

Stage	GFR (mL/min)
Stage 1 – Proteinuria	≥90
Stage 2 – Mild kidney damage	60–89
Stage 3 – Moderate decrease	30–59
Stage 4	15–29
Stage 5	≤15

Source: National Kidney Foundation. Used with permission.

therapy goals for patients with CKD Stages 1 to 4 prior to dialysis or renal transplantation are to retard the progression of CKD while providing adequate calories to maintain or achieve ideal body weight, and to prevent or alleviate the symptoms of uremia and restore biochemical, calcium/phosphorus, vitamin, and iron balance.

Medical Nutrition Therapy for CKD
Protein

In CKD, as the GFR and excretion of nitrogenous wastes decline, it is necessary to control the level of protein intake while continuing to maintain a positive nitrogen balance. Protein restriction can minimize the symptoms of uremic toxicity by reducing the production of nitrogenous wastes in the blood. Evidence also suggests that protein restriction early in the course of CKD due to glomerular damage may slow the progression of the disease and delay the need to initiate dialysis therapy. The generally accepted level of protein restriction for patients with CKD stages 1 to 3 is 0.75 g/kg per day, which is approximately what the DRIs recommend for normal, healthy adults. This is actually a restriction for most individuals, as the American diet is generally much greater in protein content. For stages 4 and 5 (GFR <25 mL/minute), 0.6 g/kg per day (using an adjusted body weight if the patient is obese) is suggested.

Approximately 50 percent of high biological value protein is usually encouraged to ensure that essential amino acid requirements are met. The biological value of a dietary protein is determined by its constituent amino acids, with the highest value given to proteins that contain all essential amino acids, such as eggs, meats, and other animal proteins. It has also been shown, however, that with diabetic nephropathy, carefully planned low-protein vegetarian diets containing soy and plant-based protein may reduce proteinuria, improve serum protein levels, and retard the progression of CKD. Nutritional status must be monitored closely in patients prescribed protein-restricted diets, especially when they are ingesting protein at 0.6 g/kg per day or less.

When patients exhibit proteinuria, as in diabetic nephropathy, the daily urinary protein losses may be added to the daily allowance. Additional increased protein needs due to catabolism from use of glucocorticoid (steroid) therapy or recent surgery may contraindicate limiting dietary protein.

Calories

The recommendations for adequate energy intake for individuals with CKD not yet on dialysis are generally 35 kcal/kg per day to maintain body weight and allow for effective protein utilization. It has been recommended that 30 kcal/kg per day be used for those greater than sixty years of age due to a more sedentary lifestyle. Calories from complex and simple carbohydrates must be included in the diet to provide adequate energy to prevent weight loss.

Lipids

Additional fat, in the form of monounsaturated and polyunsaturated fats, may also be recommended to provide adequate calories for patients with CKD. Since dyslipidemia is prevalent in patients with CKD, lipid levels should be monitored, and an effort made to keep total cholesterol, LDL-C, HDL-C, and triglyceride levels within normal limits (Chapter 6). Pharmacologic therapy may need to be considered to manage lipid levels, as some studies utilizing statins have shown cardiovascular risk reduction for patients with CKD stages 2 to 3.

Sodium

As renal failure progresses to a GFR of about 10 percent of normal, renal sodium excretion subsequently falls. Sodium intake may have to be limited to prevent sodium retention, generalized edema, hypertension, and/or congestive heart failure, especially in the advanced stages of CKD when excretion diminishes. *The NKF/KDOQI Clinical Practice Guidelines on Hypertension and Antihypertensives* recommend a sodium intake of less than 2.4 grams per day unless a sodium wasting disease is present or medications causing sodium loss are prescribed.

Measuring urinary sodium in a 24-hour urine collection may be helpful in determining how much sodium is being excreted. Urinary sodium is reported in milliequivalents (mEq), making it necessary to convert from milligrams to milliequivalents to determine how many milliequivalents of sodium are associated with any given diet. To convert milligrams of sodium to milliequivalents, divide the number of milligrams by the molecular weight of sodium (23 mg Na = 1 mEq Na). For example, assuming that a low-sodium diet is limited to 2000 mg/day, it contains 87 mEq of sodium (Table 10-2).

Potassium

The kidney usually handles potassium efficiently until the GFR is significantly reduced (less than 10 mL/min). Thus, a dietary potassium restriction may be necessary only during the latter stages of CKD. Exceptions include renal diseases such as diabetic nephropathy, in which aldosterone deficiency develops and potassium excretion declines. Use of an angiotensin-converting enzyme (ACE) inhibitor to control blood pressure in some individuals may also require a mild-to-moderate potassium restriction, even with good urine output. ACE inhibitors suppress the renin-angiotensin system, resulting in decreased aldosterone levels and subsequent elevations in serum potassium levels. Angiotensin receptor antagonists used to control hypertension can also cause hyperkalemia, though the likelihood is probably

Table 10-2 Foods With High Sodium Content

Bacon	Ham	Smoked meats or fish
Barbecue sauce	Hotdogs	Soy sauce
Bouillon cubes*	Meat tenderizers	Steak sauce
Canned seafood*	Nuts, salted*	Soups, canned* & dried mixes
Cheeses, processed	Olives	Tomato juice*
Chinese food	Packaged or prepared	Tomato sauce
Cold cuts	casserole dishes	Vegetable juice*
Corned Beef	Popcorn	Worcestershire sauce
Corn chips	Pickles	
Crackers*	Potato chips, Pretzels*	
Dried beef	Relish	
"Fast Foods"	Salt pork	
Frozen dinners (unless of a	Sauerkraut	
healthy variety). Gravy, canned	Sausages	
or packaged	Scrapple	

Generally, any labeled food with a sodium content greater than 400 mg per serving is considered high in sodium; some of the above foods may be acceptable if allowed in small servings.
*These items may be purchased "salt-free" or "low sodium" in many grocery stores.
Source: Lisa Hark, PhD, RD. Used with permission.

lower than with ACE inhibitors. When serum potassium levels are consistently greater than 5.0 mEq/L, a potassium-restricted diet of 2 to 3 g/day (51 to 77 mEq/day) should be initiated (Table 10-3).

Calcium and Phosphorus

Renal osteodystrophy refers to the complex lesions of bone present in the majority of patients with CKD, including osteitis fibrosa and osteomalacia. Restriction of dietary phosphorus has been shown to prevent the development of secondary hyperparathyroidism, which is frequently seen in patients with CKD. Also, in the past decade increased vascular and soft tissue calcifications have been seen in this population, believed to be related to calcium/phosphorus metabolism and treatment to maintain proper balance of these minerals. As a result, the *NKF/KDOQI Clinical Practice Guidelines for Bone Metabolism and Disease* recommend a phosphorus restriction of 800 to 1000 mg/day for individuals with CKD stages 3 and 4 when the serum phosphorus level is greater than 4.6 mg/dL (Table 10-4). With a protein-restricted diet, this is usually feasible, as animal protein-based foods are also high in phosphorus content. If dairy products are avoided in a vegetable-based low-protein diet utilizing soy products, this level of phosphorus restriction is also feasible.

Generally, calcium acetate is also prescribed with meals as a "phosphate binder," which interferes with the absorption of phosphate in the small intestine to keep the serum phosphate levels within normal range. Sevelamer hydrochloride or sevelamer carbonate, non-absorbed phosphate-binding polymers without calcium or aluminum and lanthanum carbonate have also been utilized (Table 10-5). These medications are used "off-label" for CKD patients not yet on hemodialysis; sometimes, a

Table 10-3 Foods With High and Low-To-Medium Potassium Content

High-potassium vegetables	High-potassium fruits and juices
Artichokes	Apricots
Beans (navy, lentil, kidney, pinto)	Avocados
Broccoli	Bananas
Brussels sprouts	Cantaloupes
Carrots, raw	Dates
French fries,	Figs
Greens	Honeydew melons
Lima beans	Mangos
Parsnips	Nectarines
Potato, baked	Oranges, orange juice
Pumpkin	Papayas
Spinach	Prunes
Sweet potato	Raisins
Tomato	Rhubarb
Winter squash (butternut, acorn)	Watermelon
Tomato juice	Apricot nectar
Vegetable juices	Prune juice

Other high-potassium foods	
Milk (more than 4 to 8 ounces/day)	Salt substitutes (containing KCL)
Chocolate	Molasses
Nuts	Potato chips
Bran Cereal	

Low-to-medium potassium vegetables*	**Low-to-medium potassium fruits and juices***
Asparagus	Apples, apple juice
Beets	Applesauce
Cabbage	Blueberries
Carrots, cooked	Cherries
Cauliflower	Cranberries, cranberry juice
Celery	Fruit cocktail
Corn	Grapefruits, grapefruit juice (only 4 ounces/day)
Cucumber	Grapes, grape juice
Eggplant	Lemons
Green beans	Limes
Green peppers	Peaches, fresh (small)
Kale	Pears, fresh (small), pear nectar
Lettuce	Pineapples, pineapple juice (only 4 ounces/day)
Okra	Plums
Onions	Raspberries (1 cup)
Peas	Strawberries (1 cup)
Potato (only when presoaked)	Tangerines
Radishes	
Wax beans	
Zucchini	

*Please note that even low-to-medium potassium foods must be consumed in limted amounts daily
Source: Lisa Hark, PhD, RD. Used with permission.

Table 10-4 Phosphorus Content of Selected Foods.

Foods	Portion size	Phosphorus content (mg)
Dairy		
Cheese, cheddar	1 ounces	145
Cheese, cream	1 Tbs.	15
Frozen yogurt	½ cup	95–100
Half-and-half	½ cup	110
Ice cream	½ cup	70–100
Milk (whole, low-fat, skim)	8 ounces	220–230
Pudding (vanilla/chocolate dry mix regular made with 2% milk)	½ cup	115–135
Pudding (chocolate dry mix instant made with 2% milk)	½ cup	350
Pudding, (vanilla/chocolate/ tapioca/ rice-ready-to-eat)	½ cup	45–75
Yogurt (all kinds)	8 ounces	215–350
Protein foods		
Beef, cooked	3 ounces	150–200
Eggs, whole	1 large	95
Liver, Beef (panfried)	3 ounces	410
Peanut butter	1 Tbs.	55
Sardines, Atlantic, canned in oil	3 ounces	415
Tuna	3 ounces	140–265
Vegetables		
Baked beans and pork and beans	½ cup	95–150
Dried beans	½ cup	130
Chickpeas	½ cup	110–140
Lentils, boiled	½ cup	180
Soybeans, green boiled	½ cup	140
Soybeans, mature boiled	½ cup	210
Bread and cereals		
Barley, pearled cooked	1 cup	85
Bread, white	1 slice	25
Breads whole grain	1 slice	60
Cornbread (from mix)	1 piece	225
Raisin Bran	1 cup	225
Miscellaneous		
Chocolate	1 ounces	70
Nuts, mixed, dry	1 ounces	125
Peanuts, dry roasted	1 ounces	100
Beverages		
Beer	12 ounces	50
Coffee, brewed	6 ounces	5
Colas	12 ounces	60

Source: USDA National Nutrient Database for Standard Reference, Release 20.

Table 10-5 Selected Phosphate-Binding Medications.

Medication	Dose	Ca2+ (mg) (elemental)	Al (mg)	Manufacturer
Calcium carbonate*				
Calcium carbonate, 1250 mg	1 tab	500	0	Roxane Labs
Oscal 500	1 tab	500	0	GlaxoSmithKline
Tums—Regular	1 tab	200	0	GlaxoSmithKline
Extra-strength	1 tab	300	0	GlaxoSmithKline
Ultra	1 tab	400	0	GlaxoSmithKline
500	1 tab	500	0	GlaxoSmithKline
Calcium acetate				
PhosLo	1 tab	169	0	Fresenius Medical Care_
Calphron	1 tab	169	0	Nephro-Tech,
Calcium Acetate	1 tab	169	0	Hillestad Pharmaceuticals
Sevelamer HCL				
Renagel, 800 mg	1 tab	0	0	Genzyme
400 mg	1 tab	0	0	Genzyme
Sevelamer carbonate				
Renvela, 800 mg	1 tab	0	0	Genzyme
Lanthanum carbonate				
Fosrenol, 1000 mg	1 tab	0	0	Shire
750 mg	1 tab	0	0	Shire
500 mg	1 tab	0	0	Shire

*Calcium carbonate is now rarely used for phosphate-binding due to its calcium content relative to current suggested guidelines for calcium intake in CKD
Source: Jean Stover, RD, LDN. Used with permission.

combination of sevelamar and calcium acetate is sometimes used to provide phosphate binding without adding significant calcium. Serum calcium levels may not decrease until the GFR is less than 30 mL/minute, thus initially eliminating any need for specific calcium supplementation until later stages of CKD. Since foods rich in calcium (primarily dairy products) are also high in phosphorus content and must be restricted, calcium carbonate and calcium acetate may be used between meals to increase serum calcium levels. The *K/DOQI Clinical Practice Guidelines for Bone Metabolism and Disease* recommend 1.5 to 2.0 grams of calcium (including dietary and supplemental calcium) for CKD stages 3 and 4 and 1.5 to 1.8 grams for stages 4 and 5 not yet on dialysis. Goals are to keep serum calcium levels within normal range.

Water Balance and Fluid Restriction
Fluid intake for individuals with CKD should be balanced by their ability to eliminate fluid. As long as the urine output essentially equals the daily fluid intake, fluid balance is maintained. If edema becomes apparent, prescribing loop diuretics often increases sodium and water excretion sufficiently to maintain balance. In the latter

stages of CKD, a fluid limit equal to the volume of urine output plus 500 mL/day for insensible fluid losses may be necessary to prevent edema and hyponatremia.

Vitamins and Iron

Protein and mineral restrictions to manage CKD usually result in a diet deficient in vitamins. Supplementation with folic acid (1 mg/day), pyridoxine (5 mg/day), the RDA for other B-complex vitamins, and ascorbic acid (60 to 100 mg/day) is often necessary. Because of the kidney's inadequate conversion of vitamin D from 25-hydroxycholecalciferol [25(OH)D] to its active form, 1,25-dihydroxycholecalciferol [1,25(OH$_2$)D], supplementation of this active form or other analog of vitamin D is often required and individualized to keep serum parathyroid hormone (PTH) levels within goal range for the various stages of CKD. Vitamin A, on the other hand, may accumulate as CKD progresses and should not be supplemented. Vitamin preparations designed specifically for individuals with renal failure are available to meet these needs.

Most individuals with CKD develop anemia primarily because of the kidney's decreased production of the hormone erythropoietin. This hormone stimulates the bone marrow to produce red blood cells. Many individuals with CKD begin treatment with erythropoietin stimulating agents (ESAs) in the form of epoetin alfa or darbepoetin alfa prior to initiating dialysis. To promote red blood cell production, iron supplementation is often necessary for patients receiving erythropoietin therapy, but varies depending on iron status.

Dialysis

The goals of medical nutrition therapy for patients on maintenance hemodialysis (HD), both in-center and home hemodialysis (HHD), and maintenance peritoneal dialysis (PD), both continuous ambulatory peritoneal dialysis (CAPD) and continuous cycling peritoneal dialysis (CCPD), are to maintain:

- protein equilibrium to prevent a negative nitrogen balance while avoiding excessive weight gain;
- serum potassium and sodium concentrations within an acceptable range and maintain total body sodium as close to normal as possible;
- fluid homeostasis by preventing fluid overload or volume depletion;
- serum calcium, phosphorus and parathyroid hormone (PTH) levels within an acceptable range to prevent renal osteodystrophy and metastatic calcification; and
- adequate levels of vitamins and other minerals.

Medical Nutrition Therapy for Dialysis

Protein

Protein intake for patients undergoing maintenance dialysis must at least equal minimum dietary protein requirements but not worsen the uremic syndrome by causing retention of urea, electrolytes, and various minerals. The loss of amino acids, the catabolic stress of dialysis, and the level of protein intake in the pre-dialysis period may all contribute to poor protein status in the chronic dialysis patient. A protein allowance of 1.2 g/kg per day for in-center HD patients and 1.2 to 1.3 g/kg per day for HHD and PD patients will often minimize the accumulation of excessive nitrogenous wastes, maintain a positive nitrogen balance, and replace the amino acids lost during dialysis. During episodes of peritonitis, patients receiving peritoneal dialysis have increased dietary protein needs due to greater losses of protein across an inflamed peritoneum. Many patients on both HD and PD periodically require supplemental commercial or homemade nutritional drinks, bars, or protein powders in order to achieve adequate protein intake.

Calories

The caloric intake for patients undergoing maintenance dialysis should be adequate to maintain or achieve ideal body weight. Unless the diet provides sufficient calories from carbohydrate and fat, endogenous protein is used for energy production, and the patient develops a negative nitrogen balance and loses significant muscle mass. With PD, calories gained from glucose absorbed from the dialysate must be considered when determining total caloric needs to prevent excess weight gain and obesity. Patients on both HD and PD, however, may also require nutritional supplements to meet caloric as well as protein intake goals.

Lipids

As mentioned previously, lipid abnormalities are frequently prevalent in patients with kidney disease. Commonly, patients undergoing HD present with normal or high total cholesterol, LDL-C, and triglyceride levels. Patients on PD frequently have high total cholesterol, LDL-C, and triglyceride levels, and low HDL-C levels. Medical nutrition therapy is aimed at normalizing cholesterol and triglyceride levels without adversely affecting protein and overall caloric intakes in dialysis patients. Pharmacologic therapy for dyslipidemia is often initiated in order to avoid further restrictions to an already complex diet regime.

Sodium and Fluid

Daily sodium recommendations are determined by the patient's blood pressure, weight, and level of kidney function. Excessive ingestion of sodium may promote excessive fluid intake and precipitate edema. The sodium and fluid allowances for maintenance dialysis patients depend largely on their interdialytic weight gains. For patients on HD, sodium intake is generally restricted to 2 to 3 g/day, with a fluid allowance of 1000 mL/day plus the amount of urine output, if any. This will allow an acceptable fluid weight gain of approximately 1 pound per day. Sodium and water may be removed more easily with PD because it is performed daily or continuously, as well as HHD because it is usually done five to six times per week. A more liberal sodium and water intake is therefore possible for PD and HHD patients. It is, however, very important to encourage PD patients to limit sodium and fluid intake more strictly if they need to consistently use more concentrated dextrose solutions to remove excess fluid. The issue is that excessive use of such solutions can cause eventual damage to the peritoneum and thus decrease the ultrafiltration capacity of PD over time.

Potassium

Potassium intake must be individualized to maintain normal serum potassium levels. Patients on maintenance HD usually can maintain serum potassium levels between 3.5 and 5.5 mEq/L with diets containing 2 to 3 g/day (50 to 75 mEq/day). When serum potassium levels are persistently high, despite dietary counseling, the dialysate potassium content may be lowered or a sodium exchange resin added to the medication regime. When serum potassium levels are consistently low (hypokalemia), the dietary intake may be liberalized and/or dialysate potassium content increased. This is especially important for patients receiving digoxin therapy, as hypokalemia can cause arrhythmias. Patients on maintenance PD usually maintain a normal serum potassium level without restricting potassium intake. If serum potassium levels fall below normal, dietary potassium is increased, and if unsuccessful, potassium supplements may be required. For those on HHD, the diet may be more liberal in potassium as well, depending upon frequency of and amount of dialysis performed (Table 10-3).

Calcium and Phosphorus

As renal function diminishes, phosphorus excretion decreases. With a GFR less than 25 mL/min, filtration is inadequate to excrete a normal dietary phosphorus load (1000 to 1800 mg). Dialysis therapy does remove phosphorus, but not efficiently enough to allow an unrestricted diet for those receiving three to four treatments per week. Nocturnal HHD may remove more phosphorus, especially if treatments are four to six times per week. The goal of medical nutrition therapy is to achieve and maintain a serum phosphate level of approximately 3.5 to 5.5 mg/dL, and a calcium × phosphorus product less than 55. Phosphorus is widely distributed in foods, but is found primarily in muscle tissue (meats, poultry, and fish) and dairy products (Table 10-4). Therefore, reducing dietary phosphorus intake often involves a concomitant reduction in total protein intake.

For patients undergoing in-center HD and PD at home, in order to allow adequate protein intake, the usual phosphorus restriction is 1000 to 1200 mg/day. For those at home receiving more frequent HD treatments, the allowance may be greater. It is now also necessary to read labels of many beverages and convenience foods to determine if additives containing phosphate are present. Those foods or beverages that do contain such additives should be avoided as much as possible.

Controlling serum phosphorus by diet alone is usually not possible if the patient is consuming recommended protein levels (1.2 to 1.3 g/kg per day). As a consequence, most dialysis patients are prescribed phosphate binders, such as calcium acetate, sevelamer hydrochloride (Renagel), sevelamer carbonate (Renvela), or lanthanum carbonate (Fosrenol) as mentioned for predialysis patients. All of these medications are prescribed with meals and snacks to promote phosphate-binding in the gut, which decreases phosphorus absorption. Calcium carbonate is not utilized for phosphate binding as frequently now that goals are to keep serum calcium levels lower. Renagel, Renvela, or Fosrenol may be better choices for phosphate-binding medication than calcium-containing binders in efforts to avoid excessive calcium intake and the potential for increased risk of soft tissue and cardiac/vascular calcifications. The *K/DOQI Clinical Practice Guidelines for Bone Metabolism in Disease* recommend keeping serum calcium levels between 8.4 and 9.5 mg/dL. Some practitioners still use calcium acetate, however, and feel that if the product of the serum calcium multiplied by the serum phosphorus product is less than 55, the chance for calcification is diminished. Practical issues including cost and insurance coverage must be considered when prescribing the newer non-calcium binders.

Vitamins and Iron

Patients on both PD and HD generally receive supplementation of folic acid (1 mg/day), pyridoxine (10 mg/day), the RDA for other B-complex vitamins, and ascorbic acid (60 to 100 mg/day) due to probable existing dietary deficiencies of these vitamins and losses occurring during dialysis. Previously, there had been speculation that even higher doses of folic acid may be beneficial for patients with CRF, as this vitamin can reduce serum homocysteine levels, which are two to three times normal in this population. It has now been shown, however, that reducing homocysteine levels with folic acid in patients with ESRD is not associated with decreased rates of cardiovascular events.

As mentioned above and in the pre-dialysis phase of CKD, dialysis patients also may require supplements containing the active form of vitamin D, administered either orally or parenterally. This therapy is highly individualized. Intermittent or daily doses of oral calcitriol, doxercalciferol, or paracalcitol are generally utilized for PD and HHD patients to suppress high levels of parathyroid hormone (PTH). Intravenous doses are generally used for HD patients and administered during the treatment. These may be used in conjunction with the calcimimetic medication, cinicalcet (Sensipar), to suppress elevated PTH levels. Sensipar also controls serum calcium, which helps keep these levels in the ranges now suggested. Intravenous calcitriol is not generally used for suppression of PTH for HD patients any longer due to causing hypercalcemia. It may be utilized for patients who have had parathyroidectomies, however, to maintain normal serum calcium levels.

Iron supplementation for patients receiving either PD or HD is usually necessary if they are receiving erythropoietin stimulating agents for anemia. Periodic – weekly or monthly – doses of intravenous preparations of iron gluconate or iron sucrose are often given to HD patients to maintain a serum transferrin saturation greater than 20 percent and ferritin greater than 200 ng/mL. Iron dextran is rarely used now due to potential adverse reactions being more likely than with the other iron preparations mentioned. Oral iron, because it is poorly absorbed and not always tolerated, is frequently given only to those with intravenous iron allergies. PD and HHD patients often benefit from coming to the dialysis facility periodically for intravenous iron when iron stores are decreased. When transferrin saturation is greater than 50 percent and/or ferritin levels are greater than 800 ng/mL, iron therapy is discontinued until repeat levels are obtained. Recent updates to the *NKF K/DOQI Clinical Practice Guidelines for Anemia* state that there is no sufficient evidence to supplement iron when the ferritin is above 500 ng/mL.

Renal Transplantation

The goal of medical nutrition therapy for patients who have undergone renal transplant surgery is to provide optimal nutrition without exacerbating the metabolic side effects of immunosuppressive drugs and other medical therapy. During acute tubular necrosis (ATN) and/or organ rejection, nutrient modifications may be necessary to prevent hyperkalemia, and to control hypertension and circulating blood volume.

Medical Nutrition Therapy for Renal Transplant

Protein

Protein catabolism may occur in the post-operative period secondary to the stress of surgery and increased catabolic effects of high doses of steroids and other immunosuppressive medications. The recommended protein intake for these patients is 1.3 to 1.5 g/kg per day in efforts to reach net nitrogen balance. This level may be difficult to attain initially after surgery, but is a realistic goal considering the patient may have already been protein depleted prior to this surgery. A long-term protein intake of approximately 1 g/kg per day is suggested with successful transplantation. It has been suggested that regular exercise may also help overcome some of the muscle wasting due to the catabolism of steroids.

Calories

Adequate calories are necessary in the post-operative period in order to utilize the protein ingested to promote wound healing and to withstand rejection, infection, and other complications. The recommended caloric intake for these patients is 30 to 35 kcal/kg per day, based on dry weight or usual body weight (UBW). Because increased appetite is a common side effect of steroid therapy, the long-range goal is weight maintenance with controlled caloric intake, once a reasonable weight is achieved. It has been shown that early intensive nutritional counseling and follow-up are successful in preventing unwanted weight gain in the first year post-transplant. Also, regular exercise should be encouraged to aid in weight maintenance.

Carbohydrate

Hyperglycemia may also occur as a consequence of high-dose steroids and other immunosuppressive drugs such as cyclosporine and tacrolimus. The patient may then require a diet controlled in carbohydrate content and sometimes oral hypoglycemic agents or insulin therapy is prescribed. Need for such medications may subside with time, but a calorie-controlled diet should still be encouraged to prevent unwanted weight gain.

Lipids

Dyslipidemia frequently occurs after renal transplantation primarily due to immunosuppressive therapy as well as obesity. Consequently, total dietary fat may need to be limited, with emphasis on decreasing saturated fat and substituting monounsaturated and polyunsaturated fats in the long-term, chronic post-transplant period. Pharmacologic therapy has also been shown to correct dyslipidemia in this population, but should be used cautiously in conjunction with immunosuppressive medications.

Sodium, Fluid, and Potassium

If steroid therapy results in sodium and fluid retention, reduced sodium intake is encouraged. In the absence of edema and hypertension, a more liberal sodium intake is acceptable. Fluid generally is not restricted unless (ATN) or rejection of the transplanted kidney is present. A higher incidence of hyperkalemia with the use of cyclosporine may indicate periodic potassium restriction, even in patients with a good functioning kidney. Rejection or ATN may also require potassium restriction.

Calcium and Phosphate

Generally, neither dietary phosphate restriction nor phosphate-binding medication is needed when the transplanted kidney is functioning well. In fact, hypophosphatemia due to increased phosphate excretion and bone uptake sometimes develops in the acute post-transplant period and may require a high-phosphorus diet and/or phosphate supplementation. Calcium supplementation may be required in the chronic post-transplant period because steroid therapy interferes with calcium absorption.

Vitamins and Iron

Renal vitamin preparations may be continued temporarily for the post-transplant patient, especially if dietary restrictions are needed to treat ATN or rejection. Iron therapy may also continue if erythropoietin stimulating agents are necessary to treat anemia.

Herbal and Dietary Supplement Use in CKD

In recent years, complimentary or alternative medicine (CAM) has become very popular in industrialized countries. Patients with CKD prior to initiating dialysis, while undergoing dialysis, or after renal transplantation must be very cautious when considering the use of herbal remedies and dietary supplements. These products are not FDA regulated and despite the fact that some of them are already known to be unsafe because they are carcinogenic, hepatotoxic, or nephrotoxic, patients may not be getting what they think they are taking. There have been reported laboratory analyses of products lacking their stated ingredients or being contaminated with pesticides, poisonous plants, heavy metals, or conventional drugs. Also, for patients with CKD, herbal supplements may be especially dangerous due to the unpredictable pharmokinetics of these products. There is potential for drug-supplement interactions, due to the large number of medications required for most dialysis and transplant patients. One example is St. John's Wort, which interferes with the bioavailability of cyclosporine and tacrolimus, and has been reported to cause organ transplant rejection. Also, though fish oils may have many positive effects for patients with CKD, they must be used with caution for patients taking anticoagulant or antiplatelet medications, as they can increase the risk of bleeding (Chapter 2: Case 2.2).

Some bulk-forming laxatives, such as flaxseed, require large amounts of fluid intake, and therefore should be used with caution for CKD patients requiring fluid limitation. Also, Noni juice, a very popular beverage supplement used to cure many ills, should be avoided by CKD patients requiring a potassium-restricted diet due to its high potassium content.

It is therefore very important to ask about the use of herbs and dietary supplements when taking a medication or diet history from all patients, especially those with CKD. Clinicians who care for these patients should be aware of CAM therapies and treatments and appropriately advise patients.

Nephrotic Syndrome

Nephrotic syndrome, a kidney disorder with many etiologies, is characterized by large quantities of protein (greater than 3.0 g/day) in the urine. In all cases, this proteinuria is a consequence of damage to the glomerular basement membrane resulting in its increased permeability to protein. Patients often exhibit poor appetite, muscle wasting, and undernutrition (primarily protein deficiency) secondary to these large protein losses. Nephrotic syndrome is also characterized by edema, when it is associated with a decrease in serum albumin, resulting in decreased plasma oncotic pressure. Dyslipidemia, with elevations either in serum cholesterol and/or triglycerides, also occurs in nephrotic syndrome and correlates with the degree of proteinuria.

Medical Nutrition Therapy for Nephrotic Syndrome

Medical nutrition therapy for patients with nephrotic syndrome should aim to reduce proteinuria, prevent negative nitrogen balance, control dyslipidemia, and minimize edema.

Protein

A high-protein diet may exacerbate albumin excretion through the damaged glomerular membrane. A moderate protein restriction is recommended early in the diagnosis of nephrotic syndrome to reduce the amino acid load to the glomerulus, subsequently diminishing the quantity of albumin crossing the damaged glomerular membrane. The currently recommended protein intake for patients on a moderate restriction is 0.8 to 1.0 g/kg per day. This amount may need to be adjusted based on nutritional status, clinical condition, and degree of proteinuria. Vegetarian diets utilizing soy protein rather than meat-based protein may also be beneficial for patients with nephrotic syndrome.

Calories

Adequate calories from non-protein sources are needed to utilize protein and promote weight maintenance or weight gain in patients with nephrotic syndrome. Small frequent meals may be better tolerated if ascites is present; caloric needs for weight maintenance are estimated to be 35 kcal/kg per day. Because these patients are often edematous, dry weight should be used for this calculation.

Lipids

Dyslipidemia due to reduced lipoprotein clearance from the blood by lipoprotein lipase and a proteinuria-induced alteration in the structure of lipoproteins is common in patients with nephrotic syndrome. Elevated very-low-density lipoprotein (VLDL), intermediate-density lipoprotein, LDL-C, total cholesterol, and triglyceride levels, along with normal or decreased HDL-C levels, may warrant a dietary fat restriction to less than 30 percent of total calories with an equal balance among saturated, monounsaturated, and polyunsaturated fats. Dietary cholesterol should be limited to less than 200 mg/day. Pharmacologic therapy may be necessary if diet has no effect and the nephrotic syndrome is prolonged.

Sodium and Fluid

Controlling edema through sodium restriction and appropriate use of diuretics is essential in the management of nephrotic syndrome. Because edema is commonly associated with nephrotic syndrome, restricting sodium intake to 2 g/day or less may be necessary. The exact level of restriction must be individualized based on the degree of edema. Fluid restriction is not generally recommended unless the patient is hyponatremic.

Potassium

Abnormal potassium levels may occur in patients with nephrotic syndrome depending on the diuretic prescribed to control their edema or if ACE inhibitors are used to control the proteinuria. Monitoring serum potassium levels is essential to determine whether alterations require a low or high potassium diet.

Calcium

Hypocalcemia frequently occurs in individuals with nephrotic syndrome if they are hypoalbuminemic. Serum calcium measurements include both free calcium and calcium bound to serum albumin. When attempting to determine if a calcium deficiency is present, it is therefore essential to use the following equation to correct the patient's serum calcium level to reflect the degree of hypoalbuminemia:

$$[(\text{Normal albumin} - \text{serum albumin})\,(\text{correction factor})] + \text{serum calcium}$$

Correction factor $= 0.8$

Normal albumin $= 4.0$ mg/dL

A concurrent vitamin D deficiency may lead to inadequate calcium absorption from the GI tract in a number of these patients. As a result, if the serum calcium level, corrected for the degree of hypoalbuminemia, still falls below normal levels, a calcium deficiency is likely. Vitamin D supplementation is also recommended for these individuals.

Nephrolithiasis

The goals of medical nutrition therapy for patients with nephrolithiasis (kidney stones) are to eliminate the diet-related risk factors for stone formation and prevent the growth of existing stones. The influence of fluid and specific nutrients such as calcium, oxalate, protein, refined carbohydrates, and sodium on the risk factors for calcium stone formation is discussed in the following section.

Medical Nutrition Therapy for Nephrolithiasis

Fluid

First and most importantly, a high fluid intake is the essential component of diet therapy for patients with nephrolithiasis. An increase in urine volume to 2 liters per day or more is needed to maintain a dilute urine and reduce the concentration of stone-forming substances. Producing this volume of urine requires a fluid intake of approximately 2.5 to 3 liters per day. Observational studies have suggested that coffee, tea, beer, and wine may reduce the risk of stone formation while grapefruit juice and apple juice may increase the risk. It is usually recommended, however, that most fluids be derived from water.

Calcium

Hypercalciuria (usually idiopathic) is one of the common urinary abnormalities seen in patients who form calcium stones. Although much attention is directed toward the effect of dietary calcium on urinary calcium excretion, in reality most cases of calcium urolithiasis are not attributed to high dietary calcium intake. In fact, a very low-calcium diet has been shown to increase the absorption and subsequent excretion of oxalate, which promotes formation of calcium oxalate stones in susceptible individuals. Large studies have also shown that the risk of becoming a stone former is much lower when dietary calcium intake is greater than 1000 mg per day compared to those with dietary calcium intakes less than 600 mg per day. Adequate calcium intake will also prevent long-term negative calcium balance.

Oxalate

Changes in oxalate excretion are more important than calcium excretion in altering the probability of developing calcium oxalate stones. Oxalate has a greater relative effect than calcium on urine supersaturation of calcium oxalate. The role of dietary oxalate in the formation of calcium oxalate stones is not clear, and the proportion of urinary oxalate that comes from the diet is controversial (estimated to range from

Table 10-6 Foods With High-Oxalate Content*

Apricots, dried	Kiwi
Barley, raw (1/2 cup)	Leeks
Beans	Lentil and potato soup
Chili	Miso
Black beans	Nuts, nut butters
White beans	Okra
Great northern beans	Poppy seeds
Navy beans	Potatoes, fried
Pink beans	Raspberries (black)
Beets	Red currants
Bran cereals, shredded wheat, cream of wheat	Rhubarb
Buckwheat flour	Sesame seeds
Carob powder	Soy products
Chocolate/cocoa	Sweet potatoes
Cornmeal, yellow (1/2 cup)	Tumeric, ground
Dark leafy greens	Tomato, canned paste
Spinach	Wheat bran, crude (2T.)
Collards	
Swiss chard	
Mustard	
Figs	
Granola	
Grits (white corn)	

*The oxalate content of foods is variable depending on climate, soil, portion of the plant analyzed, as well as method used for measurement. The above list is based on the "Very High" and "High" lists compiled from the website listed below. This list should only be used as a guide, as some of the "Medium" oxalate-containing foods not listed may become high oxalate foods if eaten in significant amounts.
Source: The Oxalate Content of Food: http://www.ohf.org/docs/Oxalate2008.pdf

10 to 50 percent, but usually closer to 10 percent) (Table 10-6). The remainder of urinary oxalate is a product of endogenous metabolism.

Gastrointestinal disorders that cause malabsorption are the most common cause of enteric hyperoxaluria. Oxalate absorption tends to be excessive when malabsorbed fat forms soaps and binds calcium in the gut. Free oxalate is then easily absorbed in the intraluminal intestine. Small increases in urinary oxalate concentration greatly increase the potential for crystal formation. Hyperoxaluria has now been seen in an increasing number of patients who have undergone Roux-en-Y bariatric surgery for obesity (Chapter 1: Case 1.2). Control of dietary oxalate therefore may benefit those susceptible to oxalate stones, because large fluctuations in urinary oxalate are attributable to variations in diet. Oxalate in the urine can be decreased by reducing oxalate in the diet while maintaining enough calcium to achieve a proper balance between these two elements. Vitamin C supplements should be discouraged since ascorbic acid breaks down to oxalic acid and is excreted in the kidney.

Protein

Most studies have shown that animal proteins cause an unfavorable effect on stone formation because they increase calcium, phosphate, and uric acid excretion, while reducing citrate and urine pH. The increase in urinary phosphate and uric acid is due to the high purine and phosphorus content of animal proteins. The increase in urinary calcium and decrease in citrate and urine PH are due to their high content in sulfurated amino acids. Limiting intake of foods such as meat, fish, poultry, and eggs, to achieve a total protein intake of 60 to 70 grams per day, may be helpful for patients with nephrolithiasis.

Sodium

A high-sodium intake increases calcium excretion by expanding extracellular fluid volume, increasing the GFR, and decreasing renal tubular calcium reabsorption. These alterations result in an increased quantity of calcium-containing crystals in the urine. A moderate reduction of high-sodium foods is recommended (2 to 4 grams per day).

Carbohydrate

Refined carbohydrates are also known to be calciuric, but those high in fiber are anticalciuric. Thus, a diet lower in simple sugars and products made from refined flour, but higher in complex carbohydrates made from whole grains, as well as fresh fruits and vegetables, is recommended.

Case 1 **Chronic Kidney Disease Advancing to Dialysis**

Jean Stover[1] and Gail Morrison[2]

[1] DaVita Dialysis, Philadelphia, PA
[2] University of Pennsylvania School of Medicine, Philadelphia, PA

OBJECTIVES

- Given the medical history, physical examination, and laboratory data identify factors affecting the nutritional status of a patient with chronic kidney disease (CKD).

- Describe the appropriate medical nutrition therapy for a patient with CKD prior to initiation and during continuous ambulatory peritoneal dialysis or hemodialysis.

AB, a 22-year-old Malaysian college student, presented to the emergency room with headaches and shortness of breath. He was admitted to the hospital for evaluation when he was found to have a blood pressure of 200/120 mm Hg and mild congestive heart failure (CHF) by chest X-ray. AB reports that over the past year, his weight has increased about 10 pounds (4.5 kg), although his diet has remained unchanged. He attributed this weight gain to decreased exercise and irregular eating habits due to a busy class schedule.

Past Medical History

AB has had no recent viral illness, sore throat, or upper respiratory infections. He has never had rheumatologic symptoms, and has no knowledge of his family history of renal disease. He grew up in Malaysia and came to the United States when he was 12 years old. He had a history of multiple streptococcal infections of the throat as a child, some of which were treated with antibiotics and some went undiagnosed. He is currently not taking any medications, vitamins, minerals, or herbal supplements and has no known drug or food allergies.

Social History

AB shares a dormitory room with a fellow student who is in good health. He occasionally drinks alcohol, but denies tobacco and intravenous or oral drug use.

Medical Nutrition and Disease: A Case-Based Approach, 4th edition. Edited by Lisa Hark.
© 2009 Wiley-Blackwell Publishing, ISBN: 978-1-4051-8615-5.

AB's 24-Hour Dietary Recall
Breakfast (home)
Coffee	8 ounces (240 mL)
Whole milk	2 Tbsp.

Lunch (fast food)
Hamburger and bun	4 ounces (113 g)
French fries	large
Iced tea	16 ounces (480 mL)

Dinner (home)
2 slices of chicken breast	6 ounces (170 g)
Baked potato	1 medium
Butter	2 tsp.
Broccoli, spinach	1/2 cup each
Chocolate cake	1 slice
Cola soda	16 ounces (480 mL)

Snack (movies)
Salted nuts	small bag
Cola soda	16 ounces (480 mL)

Total calories: 2493 kcal
Protein: 110 g (18% of calories)
Fat: 98 g (35% of calories)
Carbohydrate: 303 g (48% of calories)
Potassium: 3487 mg
Sodium: 1648 mg

Review of Systems
General: Fatigue, weakness, shortness of breath
GI: Anorexia

Physical Examination
Vital Signs
Temperature: 97 °C (36 °C)
Heart rate: 96 BPM
Respiration: 24 BPM
Blood pressure: 200/120 mm Hg
Height: 5'9" (176 cm)
Current weight: 170 lb (77.3 kg)
Usual weight: 155 lb (70.5 kg) 6 months ago (Use for estimated "dry" weight)

Exam
General: Well-developed male
Lungs: Decreased breath sounds with faint crackles at the right base
Cardiac: Regular rate and rhythm, systolic murmur at the apex, S_3 gallop
Abdomen: Soft, non-tender, no hepatomegaly
Extremities: 3+ peripheral edema on both legs, ring tight on finger
Skin: Warm to touch
Neurologic: Intact, mild asterixis

Initial Laboratory Data

Patient's Values	Normal Values
Sodium: 135 mEq/L	133–143 mEq/L
Potassium: 4.4 mEq/L	3.5–5.3 mEq/L
Chloride: 111 mEq/L	98–108 mEq/L
CO2: 15 mEq/L	24–32 mEq/L
Calcium: 7.5 mg/dL	9–11 mg/dL
Adjusted calcium: 8.1 mg/dL	9–11 mg/dL
Phosphorus: 10.2 mg/dL	2.5–4.6 mg/dL
BUN: 108 mg/dL	7–18 mg/dL
Creatinine: 14.0 mg/dL	0.6–1.2 mg/dL
Albumin: 3.2 g/dL	3.5–5.8 g/dL
Hemoglobin: 8.3 g/dL	13.5–17.5 g/dL
Hematocrit: 24.3%	41–53%
Transferrin saturation: 18%	20–50%
Ferritin: 142 ng/mL	20–300 ng/mL
Mean corpuscular volume: 70 fL	80–100 fL
White blood cells (WBC): 8.7 10^9/L	4.5–11 10^9/L
Urinalysis: 3+ heme by dipstick, 1+ protein by dipstick	

Sediment: 15–20 red blood cells (RBC)/HPF, 3–5 WBC/HPF, 2–4 red blood cell casts and broad waxy casts/HPF

Electrocardiogram: Normal sinus rhythm at 100, no ischemic changes
Chest X-ray: Cardiomegaly, CHF

Go to Questions 1-7
Dialysis Treatment Plans
AB received a peritoneal dialysis (PD) catheter during his hospitalization and was discharged from the hospital on a special diet and medications in efforts to delay dialysis until training for Continuous Ambulatory Peritoneal Dialysis (CAPD) could be initiated 2 weeks later. The plan was for him to eventually do additional training for dialyzing on the PD automated cycler machine. At the end of the training period a diet plan was developed. He would now be receiving four 2-liter PD exchanges daily. The following data were available after one week of training:

Laboratory Data #2 (after one week on CAPD):

Patient's Values	Normal Values
Sodium: 136 mEq/L	133-143 mEq/L
Potassium: 4.5 mEq/L	3.5-5.3 mEq/L
Chloride: 102 mEq/L	98-108 mEq/L
CO_2: 18 mEq/L	24-32 mEq/L
Calcium: 8.8 mg/dL	9-11 mg/dL (8.4–9.5)*
Corrected calcium: 9.4 mg/dL	9-11 mg/dL (8.4–9.5)*
Phosphorus: 6.0 mg/dL	2.5-4.6 mg/dL (3.5–5.5)*
BUN: 70 mg/dL	7–18 mg/dL
Creatinine: 9.2 mg/dL	0.6–1.2 mg/dL
Albumin: 3.3 g/dL	3.5-5.8 g/dL
Hemoglobin: 9.8 g/dL	13.5–17.5 g/dL (11–12 g/mL)*
Hematocrit: 27%	41–53% (33–36%)*

* These are guidelines established for patients with Chronic Kidney Disease (CKD) by the National Kidney Foundation Kidney Disease Outcomes Quality Initiatives (NKF K/DOQI) committees.

Go to Questions 8 and 9.
Follow-up

AB did well on CAPD for about three months, until he began missing dialysis exchanges due to class schedules and social activities. He had been encouraged to train on the cycler machine, so that he could more efficiently remove fluid and toxins overnight while he slept, but he kept delaying the training. He was subsequently readmitted to the hospital for nausea, vomiting, and congestive heart failure due to fluid overload. He admitted that he was not performing dialysis exchanges as prescribed. AB was aggressively dialyzed during the hospitalization to remove fluid more rapidly with frequent PD exchanges via the cycler machine. A hemodialysis (HD) catheter and permanent arteriovenous access were then placed during the hospitalization, as AB decided to switch to HD. He no longer wanted responsibility for doing his own treatment, and would take some time off from school and then plan his next term of classes around in-center HD treatments. He then started regular hemodialysis treatments three times per week at a nearby outpatient facility. At that time his urine output had declined to less than 200 mL/24 hours.

Laboratory Data #3 (after 1 week on hemodialysis):

Patient Values	Normal Values
Sodium: 138 mEq/L	133–145 mEq/L
Potassium: 4.8 mEq/L	3.5–5.3 mEq/L
Chloride: 106 mEq/L	98–108 mEq/L
CO_2: 22 mEq/L	24–32 mEq/L
Calcium: 9.2 mg/dL	9–11 mg/dL (8.4–9.5 mg/dL)*
Phosphorus: 8.4 mg/dL	2.5–4.6 mg/dL (3.5–5.5 mg/dL)*
Albumin: 3.5 g/dL	3.5–5.8 g/dL ($\geq$4.0 g/dL)*

Hemoglobin: 9.3 g/dL	13.5–17.5 g/L (11–12 g/dL)*
Hematocrit: 28%	41–53% (33–36%)*
Transferrin saturation: 23%	>20–50%*
Ferritin: 185 ng/dL	>200 ng/dL*

Go to Question 10.
Case Questions

1. Based on AB's history, physical examination, and laboratory data, what is the most likely diagnosis?
2. What additional laboratory tests or studies help confirm this diagnosis?
3. What medications are indicated to manage his clinical condition at this time?
4. Based on AB's physical examination, should his current body weight be used to estimate his caloric and protein needs?
5. How can AB's caloric and protein requirements be estimated?
6. What dietary recommendations are indicated before dialysis based on his initial laboratory data values and what fluid and electrolyte management does AB require?
7. Using AB's lab values to estimate renal function and his vital signs and chest X-ray results to determine his hemodynamic status, what are the immediate and long-term treatment modalities you would recommend?
8. What modifications in phosphate-binding medication should be made once AB's phosphate level improves?
9. What dietary modifications are indicated once AB begins receiving CAPD?
10. When AB's dialysis modality changes to hemodialysis, what dietary modifications are appropriate based on his weight and laboratory data?

Answers to Questions: Case 1
Part 1: Diagnosis and Medications

1. Based on AB's history, physical examination, and laboratory data, what is the most likely diagnosis?

AB has a history of recurrent streptococcal infections in childhood, which most likely increased his risk of developing acute post-streptococcal glomerulonephritis. Approximately 5 to 10 percent of patients with a history of streptococcal infections and acute glomerulonephritis (AGN) develop chronic glomerulonephritis (CGN) 15 to 20 years following the acute infections. CGN results in a markedly decreased GFR, which prevents sodium and water excretion and causes increased sodium and water retention. The result is volume-induced high blood pressure, and with significant sodium and water retention, eventually CHF. This renal disease is irreversible and not amenable to treatment with any form of drug therapy. It seems likely then that CGN is the diagnosis for this patient, and that he will require dialysis therapy.

2. What additional laboratory tests or studies help confirm this diagnosis?
Urinalysis The urinalysis having blood and protein by dipstick indicates renal glomerular damage. Red blood cell casts are highly suggestive of glomerulonephritis and broad waxy casts suggest dilated renal tubules associated with CGN.

24-hour urine collection This procedure reveals the quantity of protein and creatinine excreted over 24 hours. If the amount of urinary creatinine can be measured in a 24-hour urine specimen, a creatinine clearance can be calculated.

Protein excretion 2.2 g/24 hours, normal value 0.1–0.2 g/24 hours.

Creatinine excretion 900 mg/24 hours, normal value 1.0–1.6 g/24 hours.

Creatinine clearance Estimation of creatinine clearance can be calculated using the Cockroff–Gault formula. This may be necessary if urine values are incomplete or not available. The calculation gives an adequate estimation of creatinine clearance as long as the serum creatinine value is stable over time.

Men: $(140 - \text{Age})(\text{Weight in kg})/(72)(\text{serum creatinine in mg/dL}) = \text{c.c.}$

Women: $(140 - \text{Age})(\text{Weight in kg})/[(72)(\text{serum creatinine in mg/dL})] \times 0.85 = \text{c.c.}$

> AB's estimated creatinine clearance $= (140 - 22)(77.3\text{kg})/(72)(14.0 \text{ mg/dL}) = 9121.4/1008 = 9.05 \text{ mL/min}$
>
> (normal creatinine clearance for a male $= 97$–137 mL/min)

Renal ultrasound Renal ultrasound reveals small kidneys bilaterally, which indicates irreversible renal disease (9 and 10 cm, right and left, respectively). Only a renal biopsy could actually confirm the diagnosis of CGN, but it is not done once small kidneys are identified since no treatment can reverse the kidney damage. AB's significantly increased serum phosphate and decreased serum calcium levels suggest that the GFR is less than 30 mL/min, indicating significant renal dysfunction. Tests to eliminate other possible causes of CGN include

Compliment levels CH_5O, C_3, and C_4 within normal limits (which makes the diagnosis of membranoproliferative disease, subacute bacterial endocarditis, and acute post-streptococcal glomerulonephritis highly unlikely).

24-hour protein collection Eliminates the diagnosis of nephrotic syndrome. AB's history and physical examination eliminate other causes of CGN such as Alport's syndrome.

3. What medications are indicated to manage his clinical condition at this time?

AB should be discharged on the following medications:

Diuretic (generally a loop diuretic) To control sodium and water balance (as long as he has urine output).

Phosphate binder Consider the use of a phosphate-binding polymer without calcium and aluminum, since AB's serum phosphorus level is so high. However, due to the risk of worsening the metabolic acidosis (low CO_2 level) with sevelamer hydrochloride, which contains chloride and no "buffer," sevelemer carbonate or lanthanum carbonate could be used instead.

Antihypertensive medication Use as necessary to achieve blood pressure less than 140/90 mm Hg. His hypertensive medication dosage will decrease as excess sodium and water are removed.

Renal multivitamin A supplement to correct dietary deficiencies seen in patients with CKD.

Epoetin alfa Use for anemia.

Iron sucrose Use IV (if feasible) or an oral iron preparation to boost transferrin saturation and support epoetin alfa in red blood cell production.

Part 2: Nutrition Assessment

4. Based on AB's physical examination, should his current body weight be used to estimate his caloric and protein needs?

This patient's total body water is elevated, as evidenced by 3+ peripheral edema of his legs and CHF; his current weight therefore does not reflect his "dry" weight. To estimate "dry" weight, first ascertain the patient's usual weight. AB's usual body weight 6 months ago was 155 pounds (70.5 kg), and this is the value that should be used to estimate his protein and caloric requirements.

5. How can AB's caloric and protein requirements be estimated?

The normal estimated total daily caloric requirement is 35 kcal/kg. In AB's case, this amounts to (35 kcal)(70.5 kg) = 2468 kcal/day.

Daily protein recommendations for CKD stage 5 without dialysis are 0.6 g/day. If proteinuria is present, the urinary protein losses may be added to the daily protein allowance. The 24-hour urine collection indicated a protein loss of 2.2 grams in AB's case. His daily protein intake therefore should be

$$(0.6 \text{ g})(70.5 \text{ kg}) = 42 \text{ g/day} + 2.2 \text{ g} = 44.2 \text{ g/day}$$

Part 3: Medical Nutrition Therapy

6. What dietary recommendations are indicated before dialysis based on his initial laboratory data and what fluid and electrolyte management does AB require?

Protein AB's current meal plan, before any treatment intervention, contained 2493 calories and 110 grams of protein. To achieve a protein restriction of 45 grams per day, the following modifications are recommended:

- Limit milk in coffee to 1 to 2 ounces (30 to 60 mL) per cup.
- Substitute a plain hamburger on a bun, or an equivalent, such as 2 ounces (57 g) of roast beef, turkey, chicken, or rinsed water-packed tuna on two slices bread for a cheeseburger at lunchtime.
- Limit the amount of chicken at dinner to 2 ounces (57 grams).
- Omit all cheese and nuts because they are high in protein, phosphorus, and sodium; and substitute unsalted pretzels or chips as a night snack.
- Replace calories lost from lowering the protein content of the diet by adding sugar to coffee/tea and polyunsaturated fats to potato and vegetables.

Electrolytes AB's total body water and sodium are elevated, as evidenced by 3+ peripheral edema and mild CHF on his chest X-ray. Therefore, a low-sodium diet (2 to 3 g/day) is indicated at this time (which AB is already following). AB's potassium level is within the normal range; thus, no potassium restriction is indicated at this time.

His initial serum calcium and phosphorus levels of 7.5 and 10.2 mg/dL, respectively, are a result of decreased GI calcium absorption and phosphate retention. Lowering serum phosphorus levels by dietary restriction and phosphate-binding medication will improve serum calcium initially without calcium supplementation between meals.

Restricting the daily allowance of dietary phosphorus to 800 to 1000 mg is indicated. An aluminum- and calcium-free phosphate-binding polymer was added in small doses in combination with calcium acetate to AB's medication regimen. The goal was to reduce serum phosphorus levels to less than or equal to 5.5 mg/dL and to normalize serum calcium levels.

Fluid Given that AB's 24-hour urine output was 700 mL in the hospital, a total fluid intake of 1200 mL/day or 40 ounces (700 mL plus 500 mL for insensible fluid losses) should be recommended. To stay within the fluid restriction of 1200 mL/day, limit morning coffee to 8 ounces (240 mL), the lunch beverage to 12 ounces (360 mL), the dinner beverage to 8 ounces (240 mL), and the snack beverage to 8 ounces (240 mL). Allowing for an additional 4 ounces (120 mL) of juice with medications is acceptable.

7. Using AB's lab values to estimate renal function and his vital signs and chest X-ray results to determine his hemodynamic status, what are the immediate and long-term treatment modalities you would recommend?

From these data, AB has a creatinine of 14 mg/dL, blood pressure of 200/120 mm Hg, and CHF. Therefore, AB underwent two acute HD treatments, which effectively removed sodium and water as well as the buildup of uremic products secondary to CGN. He chose PD instead of HD for his long-term treatment. PD allows him to perform dialysis exchanges himself in his dormitory room and have more freedom during the day rather than receiving HD treatments in an out-patient dialysis unit. A catheter (used to instill peritoneal dialysis solution into the peritoneal cavity) was placed during AB's hospitalization. PD is usually started two weeks after a PD catheter is inserted to allow for adequate wound healing. He will initially do continuous ambulatory peritoneal dialysis (CAPD) training, as this modality requires less training time than PD done overnight by the automated cycler machine. This way he can get back to his classes sooner, and then plan to train for continuous cycling peritoneal dialysis (CCPD) when he is on a break from school.

Go to Dialysis Treatment Plans on Page 5

8. What modifications in phosphate-binding medication should be made once AB's phosphate level improves?

At this time, since AB's corrected calcium level is reasonable, no change would be made in phosphate-binding medications unless the sevelamer hydrochloride was not tolerated or feasible for AB due to cost. A change to all-calcium acetate would then be acceptable, but goals are not to exceed 1500 to 1800 mg total calcium intake for CKD stage 5 not yet on dialysis. This recommendation includes the calcium content of both food and medications.

9. What dietary modifications are indicated once AB begins receiving CAPD?

The protein allowance should increase because AB's laboratory values at the start of CAPD exhibit a mildly depleted albumin level at 3.3 g/dL (normal 3.5–5.8 g/dL), and CAPD will remove significant amounts of protein. Since AB has been adherent with his previously prescribed low-protein diet, he will now be able to increase his protein intake. A protein intake of 1.2 to 1.3 g/kg per day (based on usual body weight (UBW) or "dry" weight) is 85 to 92 g/day. To reach that goal, the meat, fish, or poultry portions at lunch and dinner need to be increased to 4 ounces (113 g), and AB should be encouraged to eat a sandwich with at least 2 ounces (57 g) of meat as his nightly snack.

AB remains at least 11 pounds (5 kg) over his previous usual body weight of 155 pounds (70 kg). Current weight is 166 pounds (76 kg): (170 pounds (77 kg) minus the 4 pounds (1.8 kg) of PD fluid indwelling), he remains at least 11 pounds (5 kg) over his previous usual body weight of 155 pounds (70 kg), the same sodium (2 to 3 g/day) and fluid restrictions (1200 mL/day) are indicated until a regular schedule of PD exchanges can be performed. A potassium restriction is still unnecessary because AB's serum potassium level is normal and may drop as a result of continuous removal of potassium with daily PD.

Phosphorus should still be restricted to maintain phosphate levels between 3.5 and 5.5 mg/dL, but the restriction can be liberalized somewhat to allow a greater protein intake (animal protein sources are the foods highest in phosphate). By continuing to limit milk to no more than 4 ounces per day, and limiting cheese to two times per week and eliminating cola and other sodas and beverages containing phosphoric acid, AB can achieve the new daily phosphorus allowance of 1000 to 1200 mg/day. An extra one or two Renagel tablets may be prescribed with the night sandwich as well.

Go to Follow-Up on Page 407

10. When AB's dialysis modality changes to hemodialysis, what dietary modifications are appropriate based on weight and laboratory data?
Pre-dialysis weight: 74 kg (163 lb)
Estimated dry weight: 70.5 kg (155 lb)
AB has the potential to gain fluid weight between HD treatments, because he receives them only three times per week (his predialysis weight is 3.5 kg greater than his dry weight). In addition, AB's urine output is diminished further because of his renal dysfunction. Thus, his fluid intake should be decreased to 1 L/day, and he should be encouraged to maintain a sodium restriction of 2 to 3 g/day. The recommended daily protein allowance is now 1.2 g/kg for a total of 85 grams, which is the lower end of the previous recommendations. Because HD is intermittent, and AB reports that his urine output is minimal, he should be advised to limit his potassium intake to approximately 70 mEq/day. AB can accomplish this goal by eliminating fruits and vegetables high in potassium such as bananas, orange juice, potatoes, and dark-green, leafy vegetables. Phosphorus restrictions for HD are similar to those for PD because no significant change is recommended in the protein content of AB's diet. However, because his phosphorus level is now rising again, AB is advised to avoid dairy products completely except for 4 ounces (120 mL) of milk per day.

Chapter and Case References

Bailie GR, Johnson CA, Mason NA, St. Peter WL, editors. Chronic Kidney Disease 2006: A Guide to Select NKF-KDOQI Guidelines and Recommendations. The National Kidney Foundation, 2006.

Bertolatus, JA. Nutritional requirements of renal transplant patients. In: Mitch WE, Klahr S, editors. *Handbook of Nutrition and the Kidney,* 5th ed. Lippincott Williams & Wilkins: Philadelphia 2005.

Bickford A, Schatz S. Nutrition management in acute renal failure. In: Wiesen K, Byham-Gray L, editors. *Nutrition Care in Kidney Disease.* The American Dietetic Association, Chicago IL. 2004.

Borghi L, Meschi T, Maggiore U, Prati B. Dietary therapy in idiopathic nephrolithiasis. *Nutr Rev.* 2006;64(7):301–312.

Burrowes JD, Van Houten G. Use of alternative medicine by patients with stage 5 chronic kidney disease. *Adv Chronic Kidney Dis.* 2005;12(3):312–325.

Cheung AK. Hemodialysis and hemofiltration. In: Greenberg A, (editor). *Primer on Kidney Diseases,* 4th ed. Elsevier Saunders: Philadelphia 2005.

Colson CE, DeBroe ME. Kidney injury from alterative medicines. *Adv Chronic Kidney Dis.* 2005;12(3):261–275.

Drueke TB, Moe SM, Langman CB. Treatment approaches in CKD. In: Olgard K, editor. *Clinical Guide to Bone and Mineral Metabolism in CKD*. National Kidney Foundation, Inc., 2006.

Druml, W. Nutritional management of acute renal failure. *J Ren Nutr.* 2005;15(1):63–70.

Fedje L, Karalis M. Nutrition management in early stages of chronic kidney disease. In: Wiesen K, Byham-Gray L, editors. *Nutrition Care in Kidney Disease*. The American Dietetic Association, Chicago IL. 2004.

Goldstein-Fuchs J. Nutrition intervention for chronic renal diseases. In: Mitch WE, Klahr S, editors. *Handbook of Nutrition and the Kidney,* 5th ed. Philadelphia: Lippincott Williams & Wilkins, 2005.

Hollander-Rodriguez JC, Calvert JF Jr. Hyperkalemia. *Am Fam Physician.* 2006;73(2):283–90.

Kooienga L. Phosphorus balance with daily dialysis. *Semin Dial.* 2007;20(4):342–345.

Masud T. Trace elements and vitamins in renal disease. In: Mitch WE, Klahr S, editors. *Handbook of Nutrition and the Kidney,* 5th ed. Lippincott Williams & Wilkins: Philadelphia 2005.

McCann L. Nutritional management for the adult peritoneal dialysis patient. In: Wiesen K, Byham-Gray L, editors. *Nutrition Care in Kidney Disease*. The American Dietetic Association, Chicago IL. 2004.

Molitch ME. Management of dyslipidemias in patients with diabetes and chronic kidney disease. *Clin J Am Soc Nephrol.* 2006;1(5):1090–1099.

Moreau K, Chauveau P, Martin S, El-Haggan W, Barthe N, Merville P, Aparicio M. Long-term evolution of body composition after renal transplantation: 5-year survey. *J Ren Nutr.* 2006;16(4):291–299.

Nolan CR, Qunibi WY. Treatment of hyperphosphatemia in patients with chronic kidney disease on maintenance hemodialysis. *Kidney Int.* 2005;67:S13–S20.

Pierratos A, McFarlane P, Chan CT, Kwok S, Nesrallah G. Daily dialysis 2006: state of the art. *Minerva Urol Nefrol.* 2006;58(2):99–115.

Sinha MK, Collazo-Clavell ML, Rule A, et al. Hyperoxaluric nephrolithiasis is a complication of Roux-en-Y gastric bypass surgery. *Kidney Int.* 2007;72(1):100–107.

Smith L. Nutritional management of the chronic kidney disease patient. *Renal Nutrition Forum.* 2006;25(2).

Taylor EN, Curhan GC. Diet and fluid prescription in stone disease. *Kidney Int.* 2006;70:835–839.

Wanner C, Krane V. Management of lipid abnormalities in the patient with renal disease. In: Mitch WE, Klahr S, editors. *Handbook of Nutrition and the Kidney,* 5th ed. Lippincott Williams & Wilkins: Philadelphia 2005.

Yeun JY, Kaysen GA. The nephrotic syndrome: nutritional consequences and dietary management. In Mitch WE, Klahr S, (editors). *Handbook of Nutrition and the Kidney,* 5th ed. Lippincott Williams & Wilkins: Philadelphia 2005.

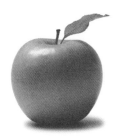

Part IV
Fundamentals of Oncology and Nutrition Support

11 Cancer Prevention and Treatment

Tamara Bockow[1] and Satya S. Jonnalagadda[2]

[1] University of Pennsylvania School of Medicine, Philadelphia, PA
[2] General Mills Bell Institute of Health and Nutrition, Minneapolis, MN

OBJECTIVES

- Discuss the role of dietary and lifestyle factors in the prevention of cancer.
- Evaluate the impact of cancer on nutritional status of individuals with cancer.
- Examine the nutrition-related side effects of cancer therapy.
- Observe the role of Medical Nutrition Therapy in the treatment of cancer.

*Source: Objectives for chapter and cases adapted from the NIH Nutrition Curriculum Guide for Training Physicians. (www.nhlbi.nih.gov/funding/training/naa)

Introduction

Cancer is a major chronic disease that contributes significantly to worldwide morbidity and mortality. Every year ten million people around the world develop cancer, and seven million die as result of the disease (12 percent of the nearly 56 million deaths from all causes worldwide). This year, cancer will impact one out of every three people before the age of 75. In North America alone, 600,000 people will die from cancer.

It is estimated that 50 percent of cancer incidence and 30 to 35 percent of cancer mortality in Americans is related to poor diet and excessive alcohol use. While genetics certainly play a role in predisposing one to cancer, lifestyle factors may have a significant influence on cancer risk as well.

Obesity and Cancer

Obesity is strongly associated with increased risk of colon, kidney, pancreatic, esophageal, endometrial, and postmenopausal breast cancer. The idea that excess weight may be linked to cancer risk is supported by evidence that calorie restriction protects against various types of tumors. The American Institute for Cancer Research (AICR) recently published a new report titled "Food, Nutrition, Physical Activity and the Prevention of Cancer: a Global Perspective." The AICR reviewed over 7000 research studies, and conclusively established the link between obesity and cancer.

Several mechanisms have been proposed to explain how obesity affects cancer, but one important factor is the excess adipose tissue that causes alterations in hormone metabolism. One hypothesis is that high levels of insulin and insulin-related growth

---

Medical Nutrition and Disease: A Case-Based Approach, 4th edition. Edited by Lisa Hark.
© 2009 Wiley-Blackwell Publishing, ISBN: 978-1-4051-8615-5.

factors in obese people may promote tumor development. Insulin and insulin-like growth factor-1 (IGF1) stimulate cell proliferation, inhibit apoptosis, and promote angiogenesis. These cellular mechanisms potentially lead to uncontrolled cell growth and ultimately cancer.

Breast Cancer

Scientists first suggested that there may be a link between excess body weight and breast cancer in the 1970s. Now, studies show that this link depends on the menopausal stage of the woman. There is a strong relationship between obesity and increased breast cancer risk in postmenopausal women, but not in pre-menopausal women. Interestingly, research shows that among pre-menopausal women, a high BMI actually reduces the risk of breast cancer. However, postmenopausal women who gain a considerable amount of excess weight dramatically increase their risk of breast cancer. Cohort studies have shown that postmenopausal women whose BMI is in the top quartile or quintile increase their breast cancer risk by about 40 percent. Additionally, in the Women's Health Study (1999–2004), women with a BMI greater than 40 kg/m^2 had a 60 percent higher risk of dying from cancers of all causes than women with a normal BMI. This increased risk is not impacted by lifestyle factors or physical activity. Researchers hypothesize that this heightened breast cancer risk after menopause may be mediated by the increase in endogenous estrogen production from excess adipose tissue. According to the National Cancer Institute (NCI), weight gain during adulthood is the most consistent and strongest predictor of breast cancer risk.

Endometrial Cancer

There seems to be a positive linear relationship between excess weight gain and risk for endometrial cancer, irrespective of menopausal status. Some studies suggest a linear increase risk of 200 to 400 percent for women with a BMI over 25 kg/m^2. Regardless of menopausal status, obese women are two to four times more likely to develop a uterine cancer than normal weight women.

Colon Cancer

Colon cancer also occurs more frequently in those who are obese compared to those who are of normal weight. Men with high BMI levels consistently show an increase risk of colon cancer; however, the evidence for women is not quite as strong. Weight gain in certain parts of the body may influence this risk. Abdominal fat seems to play a significant role in the risk of colon cancer. Overweight men tend to collect fat in their abdomen, while in some women, fat is more likely to be distributed in the hips, thighs, and buttocks. Thus, it will be important for researchers to define the relationship between colon cancer and waist-to-hip ratio or waist circumference.

Nutrition and Cancer Prevention
Meat and Protein

According to the report issued by the AICR, there is significant evidence that red meat intake from beef, pork, lamb, and processed meats such as bacon, sausage, hot dogs, salami, ham, sandwich meat, and pepperoni significantly increase the risk of colorectal cancer. Researchers recommend eating a maximum of 18 ounces of cooked red meat per week and avoiding processed meat completely. In fact, for every additional ounce of processed meat consumed per day, the risk of colorectal cancer increases dramatically. Processed meats have also been linked to a higher incidence of stomach cancer.

Swedish researchers found a statistically significant increased incidence of stomach cancer in those who consumed high amounts of processed meat in a cohort study of over 60,000 women. Researchers hypothesize that this increase risk may be due to the nitrates and nitrosamines found in these processed meats. Nitrites and nitrates react with amino acids to form cancer-causing nitrosamines. These compounds are used to provide a pink hue to cured meat without which the meat would turn brown during storage.

Other concerns with meat consumption involve cooking methods that use high temperatures such as frying, broiling, or barbequing. When meats such as beef, pork, poultry, and fish cook at high temperatures, the amino acids and creatine may form carcinogenic compounds called heterocyclic amines (HCAs). Researchers at the NCI have found 17 different HCAs formed from cooked meats that potentially cause cancer. A recent case-control study from the NCI found that people who consumed beef medium-well or well-done increased their risk of stomach cancer by more than three times in comparison to those who consumed rare or medium-rare beef. Other NCI studies have shown that a high intake of well-done, fried, or barbecued meats is associated with an increased risk of developing colorectal, pancreatic, and breast cancer.

Carbohydrates, Fiber, and Whole Grains

The protective effects of eating whole grains to prevent cancer are not clearly established. However, many case-controlled studies have shown an association between high intakes of whole grains and low incidence of several types of cancer. A meta-analysis of 40 case-control studies that looked at 20 different types of cancer found that those with high whole grain intake had a 34 percent lower overall cancer risk than those with low whole grain intake. While a decrease risk of gastrointestinal tract cancers is most commonly associated with whole grain intake, the lignans in whole grains (phytoestrogens) may affect hormone dependent cancers as well.

Fiber is known to provide many health benefits such as reduce the risk of heart disease and diabetes and prevent constipation. Because fiber increases stool bulk and speeds the journey of food through the colon, many hypothesize that it may help reduce the exposure to carcinogens by the colon mucosa. However, many current studies show that fiber seems to have little impact on colon cancer risk. Recently, The Nurses Health Study conducted by Harvard University failed to show a link between colon cancer and fiber intake. Researchers followed 80,000 female nurses for 16 years and found no strong association between dietary fiber and a reduced risk for colon cancer. In contrast, many case-control studies conducted prior to 1990 did find a lower incidence of colon cancer in people with high fiber intake. These discrepancies indicate that more research is needed before conclusions may be drawn, and the notion that fiber reduces the risk for colorectal cancer is not definitely established. It is important to note that the type and amount of fiber consumed vary among different studies.

Fats

While total fat intake does not seem to alter cancer risk, diets high in animal fats are positively associated with colorectal and prostate cancer. Recently, omega-3 fatty acids from fish oils have received a lot of attention for their heart health and anti-inflammatory benefits. Omega-3 fatty acids, DHA and EPA, are converted into anti-inflammatory prostaglandins, which researchers believe may reduce tumor growth. Now, research suggests that while omega-3 fatty acids may be beneficial, omega-6 fatty acids may actually be harmful and promote prostate cancer. Omega-6 fatty acids cause the production of a family of eicosanoids including prostaglandins, which affect immunity and promote inflammation. The health impact of these various fatty acids is related to the ratio of omega-6: omega-3 fatty acids consumed. In the United States, 60 years ago, people consumed a dietary ratio of omega-6 to omega-3 that was about 2:1. Today, the ratio is roughly 25:1. Over these 60 years, the incidence of prostate cancer in the United States has grown steadily. Scientists have demonstrated in cell culture that omega-6 fatty acids cause increased production of cytosolic phospholipase A2 (cPLA2), which causes the production of the enzyme Cyclooxygenase-2 (COX2). COX2 stimulates the release of prostaglandin E2 (PGE2) and promotes cell growth, a process that may ultimately lead to cancer.

Phytochemicals

Phytochemicals are compounds found in plants that have the ability to protect the plant against disease and bacterial or fugal infections. Research shows that these compounds may play an important role in preventing tumor growth in humans. Over 4000 different types of plant phytochemicals have been identified. Two main classes of phytochemicals include, carotenoids and flavonoids, as shown in Table 11-1, but there are several other families of phytochemicals including other polyphenols, sulfur compounds, and saponins.

Flavonoids are found in grapes, apples, berries, green tea, and red wine, and many other foods. The chemical structure of these polyphenols makes them ideal for absorbing free radicals, making them effective antioxidants. Free radicals are unstable molecules produced by the cell that ultimately lead to cell damage and may cause cancer. Antioxidants interact with and stabilize free radicals and thus prevent them from causing harm to cells.

Soy and Breast Cancer

Soybeans are legumes used to make tofu, soymilk, miso, tempeh, soy burgers, soy sauce, and soynut butter. Soy contains a class of phytochemicals called isoflavones. The main isoflavones in soybeans are genistein and daidzein. These compounds are similar in structure to human estrogen. Thus, isoflavones are often referred to as phytoestrogens. Researchers originally associated soy with reduced breast cancer risk after observations of diet differences in Eastern and Western cultural diets. The low

Table 11-1 Phytochemicals Found in Fruits and Vegetables

Family	Example	Food
Carotenoids	Beta-carotene	Carrots
	Lycopene	Tomatoes
	Lutein	Spinach
Flavonoids	Resveratrol	Red grapes
	Anthocyanidins	Blueberries
	Quercetins	Kale, Apples
	Isoflavones	Soybeans
Sulfur compounds	Sulphoraphane	Broccoli
	Indoles	Cabbage
	Ellagic acid	Strawberries
	Alliins (organic sulfur compounds)	Onions, garlic
	Glucosinolates	Cabbage, cauliflower

rate of endometrial and breast cancer in Asia may be due to women's dietary habits and their high consumption of soy. Based on these initial observations, several studies have examined the influence of soy on breast cancer risk. The prevailing hypothesis is that phytoestrogens compete with estradiol for the binding sites on intracellular estrogen receptors. These phytoestrogens are acting as selective estrogen receptor modulators (SERMs). For example, genistein binds to estrogen receptors with a weaker affinity, which does not produce as strong of a cellular response but blocks estrogen from reaching the receptors – therefore potentially protecting women from developing breast cancer. Several studies have shown that consumption of soy (55 grams per day or more) reduces women's risk of developing breast cancer. Studies have found that pre-menopausal women may benefit from eating soy foods since their natural estrogen levels are high. However, another large study showed no correlation between soy intake and the risk of developing breast cancer. These contrasting effects may be due to the amount of isoflavone consumed in the studies or the timing of soy consumption (e.g. ingestion during adolescence). There may be a certain threshold needed for soy consumption before the protective effects are realized.

Another key factor that may influence the effect of soy on breast cancer risk is the age at which soy is introduced into the diet. Most studies have shown strong evidence for a decrease in breast cancer occurrence in women who consumed soy before puberty and during adolescence. AICR and the American Cancer Society (ACS) stress that data on soy and breast cancer are not conclusive. Additionally, many studies showing the positive impact of soy on breast cancer have been done exclusively in Asian women. Possible genetic differences in phytoestrogen metabolism make it difficult to extrapolate these results to non-Asian women. More information is needed before any dietary recommendations can be made. One exception to this rule may be for women who have estrogen-receptor positive breast cancer or those taking anti-estrogen medications such as tamoxifen or aromatase inhibitors. According to AICR, patients taking such medication should limit or avoid soy intake until further studies are conducted.

Soy and Prostate Cancer

The role of soy phytoestrogens in prostate cancer is also controversial. While treating prostate cancer with estrogens inhibits cancer growth, estrogens have also been associated with the growth of both benign prostatic hyperplasia and prostate cancer. In a small study, Australian researchers found that men consuming a soy-enriched diet had a statistically significant drop of 12.7 percent in prostate-specific antigen (PSA) levels, compared to the control group whose PSA levels rose 40 percent. Additionally, researchers showed that by adding about 2 ounces of soy grits a day to the diets of men diagnosed with prostate cancer, they could cause quick and noticeable improvements in the subjects' PSA levels. PSA is commonly used to screen for prostate cancer and for tracking the disease once it has been diagnosed. Soy grits are soybeans that have been toasted and cracked into coarse pieces. During the late 1980s, researchers found that Japanese men in Hawaii who ate tofu at least 5 times per week had 65 percent less chance of developing prostate cancer than those who ate tofu only once a week or less. In 1998, a study involving 12,395 men showed that men who drank a serving of soy milk at least once a day had a 70 percent less chance of developing prostate cancer than those who never drank soy milk. Soy has also been found to be potentially beneficial in treating prostate cancer and slowing its progression in many animal and *in vitro* studies. Lately, more human studies point to similar results. Despite these optimistic results, another study that followed 5855 Japanese American men for over 20 years found no association between tofu intake and prostate cancer risk. It is important to note the limitations of any cohort case study in which the data is based on dietary questionnaires and recall.

Several mechanisms have been proposed for how isoflavones may impact prostate cancer. These include blocking androgen receptors, inhibiting tyrosine protein kinases and growth factor receptors, and preventing tumor angiogenesis. Still, researchers are not clear whether the benefits of soy seem to have on men's health are due to the soy protein, the isoflavones, daidzein, and genistein, or a combination. What is clear is that there are far more prostate cancers in the West compared to the East, and this may be attributable, in part, to the differences in diet and lifestyle.

Berries

Blackberries, raspberries, strawberries, blueberries, cranberries, lingonberries, and deerberries (either winter green berry or partridge berry) all have a high content of flavonoids that absorb free radicals. Berries contain a unique phytochemical compound known as ellagic acid that may have the capacity to interfere with tumor genesis. Ellagic acid is a polyphenol antioxidant found in high concentrations in raspberries, pomegranates, and strawberries. In a recent study from the Hollings Cancer Institute, researchers demonstrated that ellagic acid can stop cancer cells from dividing for 48 hours. Ellagic acid can also cause apoptosis (cell death) within 72 hours in cultures of breast, pancreas, esophageal, skin, colon, and prostate cancer cell lines. Additionally, ellagic acid prevents the oxidation of the p53 gene that may lead to cancer. It is important to note that most studies investigating the properties of ellagic acid have been conducted in cell cultures and laboratory animals. While human research with ellagic remains preliminary, there are several theories about the mechanism of action of this phytochemical. Ellagic acid may work by preventing the activation of carcinogenic substances in the body. Ellagic acid may also be a powerful inhibitor of tumor angiogenesis.

Raspberries and blueberries contain another class of polyphenol compounds called anthocyanidins, which are responsible for the blue and red colors of berries. Anthocyanidins are among the most potent antioxidants ever discovered. In isolated laboratory cancer cells, anthocyanidins stopped cells from synthesizing DNA and caused apoptosis. Anthocyanidins may also inhibit tumor angiogenesis. Other laboratory studies have shown that these phytochemicals inhibit the growth of lung, colon, and leukemia cancer cells while sparing healthy cells. This evidence puts berries at the top of the list of potential cancer-fighting foods.

Fruits and Vegetables

Vegetables Both the ACS and AICR recommend maintaining a diet rich in fruits and vegetables to reduce the risk of cancer. In particular, several cohort case studies suggest that fruits and vegetables may protect against cancers of the oropharynx, esophagus, stomach, colon, rectum, and lung. However, overall, the results of studies linking cancer prevention to fruit and vegetable consumption have been inconclusive and inconsistent. Specifically, prospective cohort studies show a weak link between cancer risk reduction and fruit and vegetable intake. Despite weak data from prospective cohort studies concerning overall vegetable intake, there is significant evidence that high intakes of cruciferous vegetables may reduce cancer risk. Cruciferous vegetables include cabbage, broccoli, Brussels sprouts, cauliflower, collard greens, kale, mustard, rutabaga, turnips, bok choy, Chinese cabbage, arugula, radishes, and several others. Such vegetables contain high concentrations of a group of sulfur compounds called glucosinolates. The breakdown of glucosinolates results in the release of indoles and isothiocyanates. This hydrolysis may be accomplished when these vegetables are chopped or chewed and come in contact with a plant enzyme called myrosinase. Indoles and isothiocynates may help prevent cancer by eliminating carcinogens, altering cell signaling pathways, or changing the metabolism and activity of certain hormones. For example, one study showed that consumption of 250 g/day broccoli and 250 g/day of Brussels sprouts caused an increase in the urinary excretion of a possible carcinogen found in well-done meat. This suggests that such high intakes of cruciferous vegetable may decrease colorectal cancer risk by helping to eliminate carcinogens found in food. Some studies have shown that cruciferous vegetables may also help prevent breast and prostate cancer, but currently the data remain inconsistent and indefinite.

Two other molecules have received attention for their potential cancer fighting properties: sulforaphane and indole-3-carbinol (I3C). Studies show that sulforaphane, an isothiocynate found in high concentrations in broccoli, has the ability to both cause excretion of toxic, cancer-causing substances from the body and cause cell death in tumor cells. Indole-3-carbinol is produced by the hydrolysis of glucosinolates but contains no sulfur atoms. Recent research has focused on I3C's ability to influence estrogen metabolism. I3C may play an important role in cancers that are dependent on estrogen such as breast, cervical, and uterine cancers. Several factors must be considered to maximize the indole and isothiocyanate content in these vegetables. Glucosinolates are extremely water soluble and boiling cruciferous vegetables in water for more than ten minutes may reduce the amount of glucosinolates by half. Steaming or stir-frying is a more effective way to maximize the amount of cancer-fighting compounds present in these vegetables. While NCI recommends consuming 5 to 9 servings of fruits and vegetables, there is currently no specific recommendation on cruciferous vegetable consumption.

Tomatoes Tomatoes have a high concentration of the carotenoid lycopene. Carotenoids are the molecules in fruits and vegetables that are responsible for their vibrant colors such as red, oranges, and yellows. Some carotenoids, such as beta-carotene, are precursors to vitamin A. Lycopene is not related to vitamin A, but it may be the carotenoid with the greatest cancer fighting potential. The association between lycopene and prostate cancer came from observations that countries where there is high tomato consumption such as Italy, Spain, and Mexico have much lower rates of prostate cancer compared to the United States or England. Several studies have shown that individuals who consume large amounts of tomato products have a reduced risk of developing prostate cancer. However, different tomato products contain variable concentrations of lycopene. For example, while tomato paste may contain 29.3 mg per 100 grams, canned tomatoes may contain only 9.7 mg per 100 grams. This variability makes it difficult to come to any definitive conclusions linking tomato products and prostate cancer prevention.

Not all carotenoids demonstrate promising anticancer effects. Beta-carotene is a carotenoid found in many foods that are orange in color, including sweet potatoes, carrots, cantaloupe, squash, apricots, pumpkin, and mangos. In 1994, a cancer prevention study known as the Alpha-Tocopherol (Vitamin E)/Beta-Carotene Cancer Prevention Study (ATBC) found that lung cancer rates of male smokers actually increased with beta-carotene supplementation. Smokers should now be warned not to take beta-carotene supplements. Thus, current research suggests that any benefit from foods containing phytonutrients cannot automatically be related to their individual constituents.

Garlic Garlic is part of a larger group of vegetables known as the Allium family, which includes onions, scallions, leeks, and chives. Allium vegetables possess a sulfur-containing compound called alliin that is converted to allicin when raw garlic is crushed, chewed, or chopped by an enzyme known as allinase. Allicin then quickly converts to a number of other compounds including diallyl sulfide (DAS), diallyl disulfide (DADS), and ajoene.

In the lab, DAS and DADS have shown promising effects on cancer prevention and progression through two main mechanisms: the ability to prevent the activation of carcinogenic substances and the potential to induce apoptosis in tumor cells. In laboratory studies, DAS inhibits cancer progression and onset in animals in which cancer was induced by carcinogenic substances. Garlic seems especially protective against cancers caused by nitrosamines, which are chemical compounds commonly found in preserved meat products such as salami, bacon, and sausage. In addition to garlic's action on carcinogenic substances, researchers believe that garlic may have the ability to directly attack and destroy tumor cells. Cancer is characterized by unregulated cell division, and organosulfur compounds such as DADS and ajoene have the ability to induce cell cycle arrest when added to cancer cells in cell culture. Additionally, DAS seems to have the greatest ability to induce apoptosis in cancer cells grown in culture. Specifically, according to AICR, DAS has actually killed leukemia cells in the laboratory, and ajoene has shown some similar effects. While more studies are needed before dietary recommendations can be made, garlic continues to hold a place in the list of foods that fight cancer.

Vitamins and Cancer Prevention

The ATBC Cancer Prevention Study found that 50 milligrams a day of alpha-tocopherol, a form of vitamin E, had no effect on lung cancer incidence. They also found that 20 milligrams of beta-carotene, a precursor of vitamin A, actually increased lung cancer incidence in smokers by 18 percent. Despite these disappointing vitamin supplementation studies, research shows that vitamin D may actually possess cancer fighting properties. "Vitamin D" refers to both vitamin D_3 (also known as cholecalciferol), which is created by skin cells called keratinocytes after exposure to UVB light, and vitamin D_2 (or ergocalciferol). Vitamin D2 comes from from a plant sterol and is slightly structurally different from vitamin D_3. Neither compound is biologically active in the body. First, these compounds must be modified by hydroxylase enzymes and converted to 25-hydroxyvitamin D ($25(OH)D$) and then 1,25-dihydroxyvitamin D ($1,25(OH)_2D$). Sunlight is the main source of vitamin D, but it is also found in foods such as salmon, tuna, mackerel, sardines, and cod liver oil. Milk is irradiated to increase its vitamin D content. Other fortified foods include cereal, orange juice, soymilk, and margarine. People who live in the northern regions of the United States and Europe do not receive as much sunlight and are more prone to vitamin D deficiencies.

In the north of the United States, the population rates of cancers of the bladder, breast, colon, ovary, and rectum are twice what they are in southern regions. Race also plays a role because the higher levels of melanin in dark skin prevent UV penetration and thus vitamin D synthesis. In fact, white skin synthesizes vitamin D six times faster than dark skin. Those with more skin pigmentation are at an increased risk of vitamin D deficiency. Recently, researchers reviewed 63 observational studies that examined the protective effects of vitamin D against various types of cancer including breast, ovarian, prostate, and colon cancers. They found that the majority of these studies did show that vitamin D protects against cancer. This review suggests that taking 1000 international units (IU) (or 25 micrograms) of vitamin D_3 per day could lower one's risk of colon cancer by 50 percent, and by 30 percent for breast and ovarian cancer.

In laboratory studies, mice were induced with cancer and then treated with a synthetic compound that mimicked $1,25(OH)_2D$. The compound reduced tumor growth in mice by about 80 percent. Researchers found that $1,25(OH)_2D$ seems to turn on certain genes that are responsible for causing cells with damaged DNA to stop growing. Thus, $1,25(OH)_2D$ may inhibit the uncontrolled growth of tumor cells and thus stop cancer. Clinical interventions will ultimately provide the best evidence to determine vitamin D's role in cancer prevention, but until those studies have been completed, an adequate dose of vitamin D certainly seems important.

Minerals

Selenium is an essential micronutrient for all people. Selenium is thought to help control cell damage that may lead to cancer because it boosts the body's antioxidant capacity. Most people do not obtain the recommended dose of 200 micrograms a day from their typical diet. Selenium has been shown in multiple studies to be an effective tool in warding off various types of cancer, including breast, esophageal, stomach, prostate, liver, and bladder cancers. Selenium may also act in other ways to stop early cancer cells in their development. Specifically, several studies have shown that when selenium is used in conjunction with vitamin C, vitamin E, and beta-carotene, it works to block free radical formation. Several promising studies have shown potential benefits of selenium in the prevention of prostate cancer. One epidemiological study suggested that men with high blood levels of selenium were about half as likely to develop advanced prostate cancer as the men with lower blood selenium. Selenium is found in nuts, cereals, meat, fish, and eggs. Vegetables such as garlic, onions, broccoli, asparagus, and tomatoes can also be good sources of selenium. While selenium may be an important mineral for preventing cancer, it may also be helpful for those suffering from cancer. Some believe that the use of selenium during chemotherapy in combination with vitamin A and vitamin E can reduce the toxicity of chemotherapy drugs.

Alcohol and Wine

Alcohol consumption is linked to an increased risk of cancer of the mouth, throat, larynx, esophagus, breast, and liver. According to ACS, alcohol users experience oral cancers six times more often than non-alcohol users. Alcohol is also the primary cause of liver cancer. By altering the liver's ability to eliminate toxins and carcinogenic substances, alcohol may also affect many other cancers in addition to liver cancer. For example, the findings from the Women's Health Study (1999 to 2004) suggest that moderate alcohol consumption increases the risk of breast cancer. The higher the alcohol consumption, the greater the risk of breast cancer. Additionally, recent studies have also shown strong correlations between high-alcohol and low-folate intake and increased cancer risk.

While alcohol may have detrimental consequences for human health, specific compounds in certain wines may actually have the potential to help fight cancer. Resveratrol, a cancer-fighting polyphenol found in nature, is produced by some plants when under attack from bacteria and fungi. This antibacterial chemical is found in the skin of grapes and therefore is a small component of red wine. Red wine is a unique alcohol. The distinctive properties of red wine are due to the long process of grape fermentation, which allows certain polyphenols to be extracted from the grape's skin and allows the wine to absorb resveratrol. Despite this fact, resveratrol remains a minor component in wine (1 to 7 mg per liter). In 1996, researchers showed that resveratrol was able to inhibit initiation, promotion, and progression of cancer. In laboratory studies, resveratrol triggered cell death in leukemic and colon cancer cells. Studies also show it slows the growth of cancer cells in the liver, stomach, and breast. Laboratory studies of isolated cell cultures have revealed several possible mechanisms of action for resveratrol. These mechanisms include modulation of the transcription factor NF-kB, inhibition of the cytochrome P450 isoenzyme CYP1A1, and expression and activity of COX enzymes.

In other laboratory studies with isolated cancer cells, resveratrol caused apoptosis specifically by inducing Fas/Fas ligand mediated apoptosis, p53, cyclins, and cdk (cyclin-dependent kinases). In addition, resveratrol has also proven to be a potent antioxidant and may possess anti-angiogenic properties. Despite resveratrol's potential anticancer benefits, laboratory studies show that it may not be sufficient to explain what is known as the French Paradox, which is the observation that there is a relatively low incidence of coronary heart disease in regions of southern France and other areas where wine consumption is high. . The French Paradox is the observation that many studies have shown that when humans ingest resveratrol, most of the compound seems to be rapidly metabolized and excreted. In 2004, a study investigating human metabolism of resveratrol found that when humans were given 25 mg doses, resveratrol was quickly metabolized and only trace amounts were found in human plasma. Studies associating red wine consumption and cancer in humans are in their preliminary stages. As has been noted, consumption of large amounts of alcoholic beverages may actually increase the risk of some cancers. Advise those who drink alcohol to do so in moderation – less than one drink per day for women and two drinks per day for men.

Food Processing and Preparation

The processing and preparation techniques used on foods can influence quality and may have protective, causative, or neutral effects on the risk of cancer. According to AICR, current evidence suggests that salt and salt-preserved foods are potential causes of stomach cancer, and that foods contaminated with aflatoxins are a cause of liver cancer. Although salt is necessary for human health, the total amount consumed is a critical factor and needs to be monitored. The US Dietary Guidelines limit sodium to less than 2300 mg per day. This goal can be achieved by avoiding salt-preserved, salted, or salty foods, limiting consumption of foods processed with added salt, and use of preservation methods that do not require salt. Limiting consumption of foods that have been improperly processed, stored, or prepared is critical in order to avoid microbial contamination and adverse outcomes.

Physical Activity Recommendations

Being physically active is a key component of a healthy lifestyle and recommended for the prevention of many chronic diseases, including cancer. Sedentary lifestyles associated with weight gain, overweight, and obesity increase the risk of certain cancers. Regular physical activity is an important component of cancer prevention. AICR recommends that all individuals incorporate moderate levels of physical activity, equivalent to brisk walking, for at least 30 minutes every day. As fitness levels improve, individuals should aim for 60 minutes or more of moderate, or 30 minutes or more of vigorous physical activity every day.

Nutrition in Cancer Treatment

Malnutrition in Cancer Patients

Malnutrition is prevalent among patients with certain types of cancer, including gastrointestinal, pancreatic, head and neck, and lung cancers. Thirty to ninety percent of patients with cancer face some degree of clinical malnutrition. At the time of diagnosis, approximately 75 percent of cancer patients are malnourished. Malnourished patients have significantly lower fat-free mass than healthy individuals. This lower fat-free mass increases the risk of morbidity and mortality. In fact, 20 to 40 percent of cancer patients die from the effects of malnutrition and its complications rather than their malignancy. Maintaining good nutritional status during cancer treatment is critical to increase the likelihood of successful completion of prescribed therapies and to improve quality of life.

Significant reductions in energy and protein intake are observed in some patients depending upon on the type and stage of cancer. Patients with stage III/IV disease may have significant reductions from their usual energy and protein intakes. Reduced nutritional intake may be a consequence of anorexia, taste changes, dysphagia, nausea, vomiting, and diarrhea and/or other disease and treatment-related factors. These symptoms can result in impairments in physical structure, function, and well-being of the cancer patient, and may contribute to the malnutrition that is already commonly observed in these patients. The nutritional status of cancer patients is also influenced by the disease stage and treatment associated sideeffects. The 10 most common symptoms among advanced cancer patients are pain, fatigue, weakness, anorexia, weight loss, lack of energy, dry mouth, constipation, dyspnea, and early satiety, each of which can significantly impact nutritional status. Managing these symptoms is therefore important to improve the cancer patient's nutritional status, treatment outcomes, and quality of life. Helping patients maintain adequate dietary intake to help promote maintenance and/or gain of body weight can reduce malnutrition, the incidence and severity of anorexia and diarrhea, and improve quality of life.

Weight Loss

Weight loss is the outcome parameter relied upon most in assessing the nutritional status of patients with cancer. Up to two-thirds of patients with advanced cancer have some degree of weight loss. A study conducted with ambulatory patients with cancer showed that 59 percent had decreased appetite, 67 percent had decreased food intake, and 54 percent were underweight. Patients diagnosed with malignant solid tumors of the colon, prostate, lung, pancreas, or gastrointestinal tract frequently experience weight loss. The frequency of weight loss ranges from 31 percent in patients with non-Hodgkin's lymphoma to 87 percent in patients with gastric cancer. Segura et al. noted that patients with the highest weight loss were those with tumors of esophagus (57 percent), stomach (50 percent), and larynx (47 percent). Significant weight loss is associated with body protein loss, increased cancer morbidity, and mortality. Weight loss is greater in patients with stage III/IV disease than in those with stage I/II disease. The weight loss observed in cancer patients may be progressive if appropriate interventions are not implemented to prevent and/or slow the rate.

Cancer Cachexia

Cancer cachexia is a complex syndrome that occurs in 50 to 80 percent of cancer patients. Features of cancer cachexia include loss of muscle mass, visceral protein, and body fat, which are all used to meet the energy demands of the body. Muscle wasting in the presence of significant weight loss is a hallmark of cachexia. Cachexia is most prevalent among patients with gastrointestinal and lung cancers. With the exception of breast cancer, patients with solid tumors are at greater risk of developing cachexia. Cancer cachexia should be suspected when an involuntary weight loss of greater than 5 percent of pre-morbid weight is observed within the past month.

Lung cancer patients, who lost 30 percent of their pre-illness body weight, experienced an 85 percent reduction in total body fat and a 75 percent reduction in skeletal muscle protein. This loss of lean tissue leads to reduced organ functional capacity and weakness, which ultimately results in immobility and death due to loss of respiratory muscle function. A weight loss of greater than 15 percent in cancer patients typically causes impaired physiological function, with death occurring in up to 30 percent of patients. Many of the changes in body composition and the severe weight loss of cancer cachexia are thought be the result of tumor-induced pathophysiological changes in normal metabolism. Many metabolic changes occur in cancer patients; for example, some patients with advanced cancer become hypermetabolic. This leads to increased energy requirements with impaired response to starvation, altered insulin sensitivity, increased protein use, and increased cytokine synthesis. The increased metabolic rate and reduced food intake contribute to an overall negative energy balance and accelerated weight loss in cancer patients. Additional features associated with cachexia include anorexia, nausea, weakness, fatigue, depression, and overall reductions in quality of life.

Substrate Metabolism

Cancer patients experience an increased rate of body protein breakdown (by 50 to 70 percent) while protein synthesis fails to keep up. These individuals are unable to conserved body protein stores and are breaking down muscle protein to provide energy for use in glucose synthesis. This results in an accelerated rate of muscle protein breakdown and reduced rate of protein synthesis, causing an elevated state of protein catabolism. Adipose tissue is also broken down to provide energy as the disease progresses; this accounts for the greatest reduction in body mass.

This increased breakdown of body fat sores can also result in elevated blood lipid levels in cachectic patients. Cancer patients may also suffer from abnormal glucose metabolism. Glucose intolerance, hyperglycemia, and delayed glucose clearance are frequently observed in cancer patients. In addition, insulin resistance has also been observed in patients with gastrointestinal cancer.

Nutrition-Related Side Effects of Cancer Treatment

Nausea and vomiting are the two most common side effects of cancer treatment, occurring in 21 to 68 percent of advanced cancer patients. Nausea and vomiting can affect the amount and types of food eaten during treatment. Uncontrolled nausea and vomiting can interfere with the patient's ability to receive cancer treatment and care for himself or herself by causing chemical changes in the body, loss of appetite, physical and mental difficulties, a torn esophagus, broken bones, and the reopening of surgical wounds. Therefore, it is very important to prevent and control nausea and vomiting in patients with cancer. Other gastrointestinal complications (constipation, diarrhea, and bowel obstruction) are common problems in cancer patients. The growth and spread of cancer as well as its treatments can contribute to these conditions.

Cancer patients may also develop treatment induced oral or intestinal mucositis, which is an inflammation of the lining of the mouth and gastrointestinal tract and is a common side-effect of cancer chemotherapy and/or radiation therapy. Severe inflammation, lesions, ulceration, and bleeding can occur in the mouth, esophagus, and intestine. Patients can experience intense pain, cramping, nausea, and gastroenteritis. The severity and nature of the mucositis varies based on the patient's treatment regimen. Among patients with mucositis, food and fluid intake may be drastically limited and nutrient absorption may be reduced. Oral mucositis is observed in 100 percent of head–neck cancer patients undergoing radiation therapy, 70 to 80 percent of hematopoietic stem cell transplant recipients, 40 percent of patients receiving primary chemotherapy, and 10 percent of patients receiving adjunctive chemotherapy. Oral mucositis related pain affects the patient's ability to eat, drink, speak, and sleep, and thus negatively influencing the patient's nutritional status, quality of life, and treatment regimen.

Gastrointestinal cancer patients who experience weight loss, impaired functional performance, and poor nutritional status do not respond well to their cancer treatment. Individuals with poor nutritional status and weight loss before they start chemotherapy or radiation therapy experience severe toxicity, poorer quality of life, and increased mortality than those who did not experience weight loss preceding chemotherapy.

The metabolic and nutritional abnormalities associated with cancer can cause severe fatigue and reduction in functional ability. Functional capacity for all types of cancer patients is substantially influenced by deficits in current intake and recent weight loss. Better quality of life is observed in well-nourished cancer patients, compared to malnourished cancer patients. At the end of radiation therapy, increased nutritional intake was associated with improvement in quality of life among high-risk cancer patients.

Table 11-2 Goals of Medical Nutrition Therapy for Cancer Patients

- Support adequate calorie and nutrient intake
- Prevent weight loss and promote weight gain
- Prevent malnutrition, anorexia, and cachexia
- Reverse malnutrition and weight loss that have already occurred
- Improve body composition
- Enhance immune function
- Maximize tolerance to cancer therapies
- Improve functional or performance status
- Reduce fatigue
- Improve the physical functioning and quality of life

Medical Nutrition Therapy for Cancer Patients

Medical nutrition therapy (MNT) can play an important role in the management of cancer patients, from the initial phases of treatment and recovery through the long-term continuum of care as shown in Table 11-2. Maintenance of nutritional status during cancer treatment is essential to increase the likelihood of successful completion of prescribed cancer therapies and to improve the patient's quality of life during and after treatments. Adequate and appropriate MNT therapy can help slow or minimize reduction in body weight, reduce incidence and severity of cachexia and anorexia, reduce cancer treatment associated side-effects, improve quality of life, reduce risk of other co-morbid diseases, and increase likelihood of survival.

Maintaining Energy and Protein Intake

Nutritional status has an important effect on a patient's quality of life, sense of well-being to fight disease, and ability to withstand the rigors of anticancer treatments. Early and sustained nutritional support is one of the most valuable adjuncts to the optimal management of cancer. Health care professionals should help patients aim to prevent weight loss, reduce muscle wasting, and avoid nutrient deficiencies. Weight management and weight gain should be considered primary goals for cancer patients. Preventing weight loss is simpler, safer, and less expensive than trying to regain lost weight. Sufficient calories and protein should be provided to meet the complete nutritional and energy needs of each patient and to minimize protein catabolism and the use of stored energy reserves. In order to support protein synthesis and minimize the magnitude of the nitrogen deficit, sufficient protein should be provided. Requirements for protein in most patients range from 1.0 to 1.5 g/kg per day. Carbohydrates should provide the primary source of energy and fat should represent 25 to 30 percent of calories to provide essential fatty acids and meet energy demands, while providing adequate protein, vitamins, minerals, and trace elements. Additionally, to address treatment induced side-effects such as constipation and diarrhea, adequate dietary fiber and fluid intake should be ensured. Since patients may frequently experience a feeling of early satiety, nutrient dense foods may be necessary.

For patients with inadequate ad libitum food intake, oral nutritional supplements may be appropriate. Use of high-protein and energy-dense oral nutritional supplements have been observed to contribute to increased energy and protein intake, improvements in nutritional status, body weight, and quality of life and reductions in incidence and severity of anorexia, diarrhea, and radiation toxicity and treatment. In addition, for patients with cancer cachexia, the omega-3 fatty acid eicosapentaenoic acid (EPA) has been observed to help reduce weight loss. Consumption of high-protein, energy-dense oral supplements with EPA (2.1 g/day) was observed to promote weight gain in cachectic pancreatic cancer patients.

Managing Gastrointestinal Side Effects

Appropriate nutrition can also play a role in controlling nausea and vomiting, thus reducing the need for drugs. There are several ways to control or relieve nausea such as consuming clear or ice-cold drinks, eating slowly, drinking beverages slowly, and eating smaller, more frequent meals. Persistent vomiting combined with diarrhea can result in dehydration. Ways to relieve vomiting include gradually drinking small amounts of clear liquids, avoiding solid food until the vomiting episode has passed, resting and temporarily discontinuing all oral medication, which can irritate the stomach and make the vomiting worse. If vomiting and diarrhea last more than 24 hours, an oral rehydration solution should be used to replace electrolytes. Consumption of adequate fluids, replacement of fluid losses with sodium and potassium-containing fluids, and consumption of clear liquids are critical to avoid dehydration associated with diarrhea. Additionally, consumption of soluble fiber can help control the frequency of diarrhea. Ensuring adequate fiber intake is crucial for patients suffering from either constipation or diarrhea.

Conclusion

Maintaining healthy lifestyle practices plays a critical role in the prevention of cancer. Appropriate food choices not only play a major role in cancer prevention but also in the treatment and management of individuals with cancer.

Chapter and Case References

American Institute for Cancer Research (AICR). Food, Nutrition, Physical Activity and the Prevention of Cancer: a Global Perspective. Second Expert Report. Available from http://www.aicr.org/site/PageServer?pagename=res_report_second.

Argilles J, Busquets S, Garcia-Martinez C, Lopez-Soriano FJ. Mediators involved in the cancer anorexia-cachexia syndrome: past, present, and future. *Nutrition*. 2005;21;977–985.

Barber MD, Fearon KC, Tisdale MJ, McMillan DC, Ross JA. Effect of a fish oil enriched nutritional supplement on metabolic mediators in patients with pancreatic cancer cachexia. *Nutr Cancer*. 2001;40:118–124.

Barrera R. Nutritional support in cancer patients. *JPEN*. 2002;26(5 Suppl):S63–S71.

Beliveau R, Gingras D. *Foods to Fight Cancer*. Dorling Kindersley: New York, 2007.

Beresford SAA, Johnson KC, Ritenbaugh C, et al. Low-fat dietary pattern and risk of colorectal cancer. The Women's Health Initiative Randomized Controlled Dietary Modification Trial. *JAMA*. 2006;295:643–654.

Berkiw SE, Barnard ND, Saxe GA. Diet and survival after prostate cancer diagnosis. *Nutr Rev*. 2007;65:391–403.

Bianchini D, Kaaks R, Vainio H. Overweight, obesity, and cancer risk. *Lancet Oncology.* 2002;3(9):565–574.

Calle EE, Rodriquex C, Walker-Thurmond K, Thun MJ. Overweight, obesity, and mortality from cancer in a prospectively studied cohort of U.S. adults. *N Engl J Med.* 2003;348:1625–1638.

Chen YQ, Berquin IM, Daniel LW, et al. Omega-3 fatty acids and cancer risk. *JAMA.* 2006;296(3):282.

Cheng C, Michaels J, Scheinfeld N. Alitretinoin: a comprehensive review. *Expert Opin Investig Drugs.* 2008;17(3):437–43.

Doyle VC. Nutrition and colorectal cancer risk: a literature review. *Gastroenterol Nurs.* 2007;30(3):178–82.

Duffy C, Perez K, Partridge A. Implications of phytoestrogen intake for breast cancer. *A Cancer J Clin.* 2007;57:260–277.

Farwell WR, Gaziano MJ, Norkus EP, Sesso HD. The relationship between total plasma carotenoids and risk factors for chronic disease among middle-aged and older men. *Br J Nutr.* 2008;100(4):883-9.

Feskanich D, Ziegler RG, Michaud DS, et al. Prospective study of fruit and vegetable consumption and risk of lung cancer among men and women. *J Natl Cancer Inst.* 2000;92:1812–1823.

Fimognari C, Lenzi M, Hrelia P. Chemoprevention of cancer by isothiocyanates and anthocyanins: mechanisms of action and structure-activity relationship. *Curr Med Chem.* 2008;15(5):440–7.

Fuchs C, Giovannucci E, Colditz G, et al. Dietary fiber and the risk of colorectal cancer and adenoma in women. *NEJM.* 1999;340:169–176.

Givannucci E, Rimm EB, Liu Y, Stampfer MJ, Willett WC. A prospective study of tomato products, lycopene, and prostate cancer risk. *J Natl Cancer Inst.* 2002;94:391–398.

Grainger EM, Schwartz SJ, Wang S, et al. A combination of tomato and soy products for men with recurring prostate cancer and rising prostate specific antigen. *Nutr Cancer.* 2008;60(2): 145– 54.

Greenwald P. Clinical trials in cancer prevention: current results and perspectives for the future. *J Nutr.* 2004;134(12 Suppl):3507S–3512S.

Holzbeierlein JM, McIntosh J, Thrasher JB. The role of soy phytoestrogens in prostate cancer. Preventive and alternative medicine. *Curr Opin Urology.* 2005;15(1):17–22.

Huang CS, Liao JW, Hu ML. Lycopene inhibits experimental metastasis of human hepatoma SK-Hep-1 cells in athymic nude mice. *J Nutr.* 2008;138(3):538–43.

Huang ZSE, Hankinson GA, Colditz, et al. Dual effects of weight and weight gain on breast cancer risk. *JAMA.* 1997;278(17):1407–11.

Kirsh VA, Peters U, Mayne ST, Subar AF, Chatterjee N, Johnson CC, Hayes RB, on behalf of the Prostate, Lung, Colorectal and Ovarian Cancer Screening Trial. Prospective study of fruit and vegetable intake and risk of prostate cancer. *J Natl Cancer Inst.* 2007;99:1200–1209.

Kushi LH, Byers T, Doyle C, Bandera EV, McCullough M, Gansler T, Andrews KS, Thun MJ, and The American Cancer Society 2006 Nutrition and Physical Activity Guidelines Advisory Committee. American Cancer Society guidelines on nutrition and physical activity for cancer prevention: reducing the risk of cancer with healthy food choices and physical activity. *CA Cancer J Clin.* 2006 56: 254–281

Lanza E, Jartman TJ, Albert PS, et al. High dry bean intake and reduced risk of advanced colorectal adenoma recurrence among participants in the Polyp Prevention Trial. *J Nutr.* 2006;136:1896–1903.

Lethaby AE, Brown J, Marjoribanks J, Kronenberg F, Roberts H, Eden J. Phytoestrogens for vasomotor menopausal symptoms. *Cochrane Database Syst Rev.* 2007;(4):CD001395.

Lin J, Zhang SM, Cook NR, et al. Dietary intakes of fruit, vegetables, and fiber, and risk of colorectal cancer in a prospective cohort of women (United States). *Cancer Causes Control.* 2005;16(3):225–233.

Linos E, Willett WC. Diet and breast cancer risk reduction. *J Natl Compr Canc Network.* 2007;5(8):711–718.

Linseisen J, Piller R, Hermann S, Chang-Claude J. Dietary phytoestrogen intake and premenopausal breast cancer risk in a German case-control study. *Intern J Cancer.* 2004;110(2): 284–290.

Liu C, Russell RM. Nutrition and gastric cancer risk: an update. *Nutr Rev.* 2008;66(5):237–49.

Liu S, Willett WC. Dietary glycemic load and atherothrombotic risk. *Current Atherosclerosis Reports.* 2002;4(6):454–461.

MacLean CH, Newberry S, Mojica WA, et al. Effects of omega-3 fatty acids on cancer risk. A systematic review. *JAMA.* 2006;295:403–415.

Mason JB, Cole BF, Baron JA, Kim YI, Smith AD. Folic acid fortification and cancer risk. *Lancet.* 2008;371(9621):1335.

McCann SE, Moysich KB, Freudenheim JL, Ambrosone CB, Shields PG. The risk of breast cancer associated with dietary lignans differs by CYP17 genotype in women. *J Nutr.* 2002;132(10):3036–3041.

Michels KB, Mohllajee AP, Roset-Bahmanyar E, Beehler GP, Moysich KB. Diet and breast cancer. A review of the prospective observational studies. *Cancer.* 2007;109(12 Suppl):2712–2749.

Millen AE, Subar AF, Graubard BI, Peters U, Hayes RB, Weissfeld JL, Yokochi LA, Ziegler RG; PLCO Cancer Screening Trial Project Team. Fruit and vegetable intake and prevalence of colorectal adenoma in a cancer screening trial. *Am J Clin Nutr.* 2007;86(6):1754–64.

Miller MF, Bellizzi KM, Sufian M, Ambs AH, Goldstein MS, Ballard-Barbash R. Dietary supplement use in individuals living with cancer and other chronic conditions: a population-based study. *J Am Diet Assoc.* 2008;108(3):483–94.

Nagini S. Cancer chemoprevention by garlic and its organosulfur compounds – panacea or promise? *Anticancer Agents Med Chem.* 2008;8(3):313–21.

National Cancer Institute. Nutrition in Cancer Care (PDQ®). Available from http://www. cancer.gov/cancertopics/pdq/supportivecare/nutrition/healthprofessional.

Neto CC. Cranberry and blueberry: evidence for protective effects against cancer and vascular diseases. *Mol Nutr Food Res.* 2007;51(6):652–64.

Ngo SN, Williams DB, Cobiac L, Head RJ. Does garlic reduce risk of colorectal cancer? A systematic review. *J Nutr.* 2007;137(10):2264–9.

Omenn GS, Goodman GE, Thornquist MD, et al. Effects of a combination of beta carotene and vitamin A on lung cancer and cardiovascular disease. *N Eng J Med* 1996;334(18):1150–1155.

Pandalai PK, Pilat MJ, Yamazaki K, et al. The effects of omega-3 and omega-6 fatty acids on in vitro prostate cancer growth. *Anticancer Research.* 1996;16(2):815–20.

Park Y, Hunter DJ, Spiegelan D, Bergkvist L, Berrino F, van den Brandt PA, Buring JE, Colditz GA, Freudenheim JL, Fuchs CS, et al. Dietary fiber intake and risk of colorectal cancer. A pooled analysis of propsective cohort studies. *JAMA.* 2005;294:2849–2857.

Parsons JK, Newman V, Mohler JL, Pierce JP, Paskett E, Marshall. The Men's Eating and Living (MEAL) Study: A cancer and leukemia group B pilot trial of dietary intervention for the treatment of prostate cancer. *J. Urology.* 2008; 72(3):633–7.

Perabo FG, Von Löw EC, Ellinger J, von Rücker A, Müller SC, Bastian PJ. Soy isoflavone genistein in prevention and treatment of prostate cancer. *Prostate Cancer Prostatic Dis.* 2008;11(1):6–12.

Pierce JP, Natarajan L, Caan BJ, et al. Influence of a diet very high in vegetables, fruit, and fiber and low in fat on prognosis following treatment for breast cancer. The Women's Healthy Eating and Living (WHEL) Randomzied Trail. *JAMA.* 2007;298:289–298.

Pittler MH, Ernst E. Clinical effectiveness of garlic (*Allium sativum*). *Mol Nutr Food Res.* 2007;51(11):1382–5.

Ravasco P, Monteiro-Grillo I, Camilo ME. Does nutrition influence quality of life in cancer patients undergoing radiotherapy? *Radiother Oncol.* 2003;67:213–220.

Ravasco P, Monteiro-Grillo I, Vidal PM, Camilo ME. Cancer: disease and nutrition are key determinant of patient quality of life. *Support Care Cancer.* 2004;12;246–252.

Ravasco P, Monteiro-Grillo I, Vidal PM, Camilo ME. Dietary counseling improves patient outcomes: a prospective, randomized, controlled trial in colorectal cancer patietnes undergoing radiotherapy. *J Clin Oncol.* 2005;23:14131–1438.

Rennert G. Prevention and early detection of colorectal cancer – new horizons. *Recent Results Cancer Res.* 2007;174:179–87.

Rieck G, Fiander A. The effect of lifestyle factors on gynecological cancer. *Best Prac Res Clin Obs Gyn.* 2006;20(2):227–251.

Rock CL. Dietary counseling is beneficial for the patient with cancer. *J Clin Oncol.* 2005;23;1348–1349.

Ross D.D, Alexander CS. Management of common symptoms in terminally ill patients: Part I. Fatigue, anorexia, cachexia, nausea and vomiting. *Am Fam Physician.* 2001;64:807–814.

Ryan-Harshman M, Aldoori W. Diet and colorectal cancer: Review of the evidence. *Can Fam Physician.* 2007;53:1913–1920.

Schatzkin A, Mouw T, Park Y, Subar AF, Kipnis V, Hollenbeck A, Leitzmann MF, Thomposin FE. Dietary fiber and whole-grain consumption in relation to colorectal cancer in the NIH-AARP Diet and Health Study. *Am J Clin Nutr.* 2007;85:1353–1360.

Schnäbele K, Briviba K, Bub A, Roser S, Pool-Zobel BL, Rechkemmer G. Effects of carrot and tomato juice consumption on faecal markers relevant to colon carcinogenesis in humans. *Br J Nutr.* 2008;99(3):606–13.

Segura A, Pardo J, Jara C, et al. An epidemiological evaluation of the prevalence of malnutrition in Spanish patients with locally advanced or metastatic cancer. *Clin Nutr.* 2005;24:801–814.

Simopoulos AP, Leaf A, Salem N, Jr. Workshop statement on the essentiality of and recommended dietary intakes for omega-6 and omega-3 fatty acids. *Am Coll Nutr.* 1999; 18(5):487–489.

Singletary KW, Jung KJ, Giusti M. Anthocyanin-rich grape extract blocks breast cell DNA damage. *J Med Food.* 2007;10(2):244–51.

Slavin JL. Mechanisms for the impact of whole grain foods on cancer risk. *Am Coll Nutr.* 2000;19(3 Suppl):300S–307S.

Stan SD, Kar S, Stoner GD, Singh SV. Bioactive food components and cancer risk reduction. *J Cell Biochem.* 2008;104(1):339–56.

Tanabe K, Utsunomiya H, Tamura M, Niikura H, Takano T, Yoshinaga K, Nagase S, Suzuki T, Ito K, Matsumoto M, Hayashi S, Yaegashi N. Expression of retinoic acid receptors in human endometrial carcinoma. *Cancer Sci.* 2008;99(2):267–71.

Thorne J, Campbell MJ. The vitamin D receptor in cancer. *Proc Nutr Soc.* 2008;67(2):115–27.

Tulio AZ Jr, Reese RN, Wyzgoski FJ, et al. Cyanidin 3-rutinoside and cyanidin 3-xylosylrutinoside as primary phenolic antioxidants in black raspberry. *J Agric Food Chem.* 2008;56(6):1880–8.

Van Gils CH, Peeters PH, Bueno-de-Mesquita HB, et al. Consumption of vegetables and fruits and risk of breast cancer. *JAMA.* 2005;293(2):183–193.

Walters DG, Young PJ, Agus C, et al. Cruciferous vegetable consumption alters the metabolism of the dietary carcinogen 2-amino-1-methyl-6-phenylimidazo[4,5-b]pyridine (PhIP) in humans. *Carcinogenesis.* 2004;25(9):1659–1669.

Wu AH, Yu MC, Tseng CC, Pike MC. Epidemiology of soy exposures and breast cancer risk. *Br J Cancer.* 2008;98(1):9–14.

Zafra-Stone S, Yasmin T, Bagchi M, Chatterjee A, Vinson JA, Bagchi D. Berry antho-cyanins as novel antioxidants in human health and disease prevention. *Mol Nutr Food Res.* 2007;51(6):675–83.

Zhang S, Lee I, Manson J, et al. Alcohol consumption and breast cancer risk in the women's health study. *Am J Epid* 2007;165(6):667–676.

Zhang Y, Tang L. Discovery and development of sulforaphane as a cancer chemopreventive phytochemical. *Acta Pharmacol Sin.* 2007;28(9):1343–54.

12 Enteral Nutrition Support

Judith Fish[1] and Douglas Seidner[2]

[1] Private Practice, Asheville, NC
[2] Vanderbilt University Medical Center, Nashville, TN

OBJECTIVES *

- Describe the indications and contraindications for enteral nutrition.
- Identify the appropriate enteral formula to meet individual patients' requirements.
- Identify the most appropriate route for tube feeding based on a patient's clinical condition.
- Determine the most appropriate administration method based on feeding route and the patient's clinical condition.
- Select appropriate monitoring tools and methods to identify, treat, and prevent complications of tube feeding.

*Source: Objectives for chapter and cases adapted from the NIH Nutrition Curriculum Guide for Training Physicians. (http://www.nhlbi.nih.gov/funding/training/naa)

Tube feeding, or enteral nutrition, is a method of providing nutrition support to patients who are unable to ingest adequate nutrients by mouth. A functional gastrointestinal (GI) tract is necessary to successfully support a patient on tube feeding. This usually means that a patient must have at least 100 cm of small bowel and the condition of the bowel must be adequate for absorption of nutrients. Short-term tube feeding is often used in acute-care settings in patients who are incapable of oral intake due to changes in mental status, poor appetite, or other therapies that prevent eating, such as mechanical ventilation. Guidelines established by the American Society of Parenteral and Enteral Nutrition (ASPEN) recommend initiating nutrition support when patients are expected to (or have) not received adequate oral intake for 7 to 14 days. However, patients who are malnourished or stressed may require earlier initiation of nutrition support. Most institutions provide nutrition screening for patients so that nutrition support can be initiated when appropriate.

Indications and Advantages of Tube Feeding

Patients with a functional GI tract can be fed with a feeding tube. The presence of adequate GI functionality may not be apparent after initial evaluation. In these situations, a cautious trial of tube feeding may be warranted and failure would

---

Medical Nutrition and Disease: A Case-Based Approach, 4th edition. Edited by Lisa Hark.
© 2009 Wiley-Blackwell Publishing, ISBN: 978-1-4051-8615-5.

be a good indication for initiating parenteral nutrition. Tube feeding should not be initiated if a patient has diffuse peritonitis, intestinal obstruction, intractable vomiting or diarrhea, paralytic ileus, or GI ischemia, or if the patient is refusing nutrition support. Advances in tube feeding have made enteral nutrition possible in conditions such as acute pancreatitis and high-output enterocutaneous fistulae.

Tube feeding offers many potential advantages over parenteral nutrition including lower rates of infectious and metabolic complications, decreased hospital length of stay, and reduced cost. Research in animals suggests that critical illness leads to a translocation of bacteria and endotoxin from the lumen of the intestine across the mucosal barrier and that this leads to activation of inflammatory pathways and subsequent multisystem organ failure. Antigen sensitized T and B cells travel from gut-associated lymphoid tissue (GALT) to mucosal tissues. Here antigen-specific IgA is produced by plasmacytes. Lack of enteral stimulation alters the GALT, resulting in disruption in intestinal and other mucosal immunity. It has been proposed that the benefits of enteral feeding are, in part, due to a preservation of gut integrity. Studies in patients with burns, head injury, and trauma have shown decreased rates of infection in those receiving enteral nutrition compared to those given parenteral nutrition. Although insufficient numbers of randomized controlled trials are available to draw definitive conclusions on the superiority in outcomes of enteral feeding compared to parenteral feeding across all disease states, tube feeding is generally thought to have the least risk for major complications with decreased cost and therefore the nutrition support therapy of choice when feasible and safe.

Selecting Tube Feeding Formulas

Tube feeding formulas can be grouped according to their composition and caloric density. There are a multitude of formulas available for enteral nutrition. Since there are a variety of companies that manufacture these products, many formulas are similar between companies. For this reason, many institutions have a formulary that offers a selection of formulas to meet most patients' needs without maintaining an excessive inventory. Modular components are also available to add to tube feeding formulas to modify calorie and protein content to better meet many patients' needs. Some formulas may not fit into one category and therefore it is best to understand the composition and advantages of each formula.

Appropriate formulas can easily be selected after defining a patient's nutrient requirements and understanding the composition of available formulas. Nutrient composition and density are important factors to consider when selecting tube-feeding formulas. Other factors that may influence formula decisions include gut function and disease state.

Properties of Tube Feeding Formulas

Tube feeding formulas come in a variety of caloric densities (0.8 to 2.0 kcal/mL). Most patients with standard fluid requirements will tolerate a 1.0 to 1.2 kcal/mL formula. Formulas with a caloric density greater than this are well suited for fluid-restricted patients. These formulas provide less water and tend to have a higher viscosity and osmolality. If patients are placed on nutrient-dense formulas to decrease infusion time or volume of tube feeding and additional water is not provided, they are likely to become dehydrated. The amount of water provided by the tube feeding can easily be calculated from the product literature. Most products contain 60 to 80 percent water. Additional water to meet fluid requirements can be administered as water flushes through the tube during the day or when applicable, intravenous fluids.

At one time it was thought that tube-feeding formulas with high osmolalities were poorly tolerated. However, tube-feeding formulas generally have osmolalities that are easily tolerated when administered correctly and therefore there is no reason to dilute a formula.

Medications with osmolalities over 2000 mOsm may contribute to diarrhea but tube feeding formulas of 700 or less mOsm (which account for the majority of tube feeding formulas) should not contribute to increased stool output.

Nutritional Content of Tube Feeding Formulas

The type and quantity of carbohydrate, protein, and fat can vary among tube feeding formulas and should be well understood so an appropriate formula can be selected for a patient in a given clinical situation.

The amount of protein contained in a tube feeding formula can range from 8 to 25 percent of total calories. Nitrogen in tube feeding formulas can be supplied as whole protein or partially hydrolyzed protein (peptides) or fully hydrolyzed protein (crystalline amino acids). The products containing hydrolyzed proteins tend to be more expensive. Hydrolyzed proteins are utilized for patients with inability to fully digest and absorb protein, such as in Crohn's disease. Formulas containing hydrolyzed proteins should be limited to use for patients who cannot tolerate standard polymeric formula or where a clear-cut advantage for a given indication has been shown (Table 12-1).

Crystalline amino acids are also found in formulas that are designed to have a specific amino acid composition. For example, products designed for hepatic encephalopathy have a very specific branch chain to aromatic amino acid ratio. These formulas should be used only for patients with advanced liver disease and hepatic encephalopathy who fail to respond to conventional therapy. Some formulas designed for patients with renal failure restrict fluids, potassium, phosphorus, and magnesium to meet the dietary restrictions of this population. These products should be used only in renal disease when dialysis is inadequate. These products are not nutritionally complete for patients without the appropriate indications and are significantly more expensive.

Individual amino acids have recently been added to some formulas with whole protein. For example, glutamine has been supplemented in formulas to promote immune function and improve bowel integrity. It is well documented that under appropriate conditions, glutamine is essential for cell proliferation, it can act as a respiratory fuel, and it can enhance the function of stimulated immune cells. Many studies have been done to measure the benefits of immune enhancing formulas. Meta-analyses document that these formulas can be beneficial in lowering infection rates, reducing infectious complications, and shortening length of stay when used

Table 12-1 Classification of Tube Feeding Formulas

Formula type	Characteristics
Polymeric	Whole protein, polysaccharide, and mixture of fat sources
Nutrient dense	Polymeric with reduced water (60 to 70%)
High nitrogen	Over 15% of calories as protein
Chemically defined	Oligo-peptides and free amino acids (elemental) in place of whole proteins, low fat, and/or higher concentration of medium chain triglycerides (MCT)
Immunomodulating	Added glutamine, arginine, RNA, or marine oils
Hepatic disease	Increased branch chain amino acids and reduced aromatic amino acids
Renal disease	Reduced protein, water, electrolytes and minerals. May contain few non-essential amino acids
Glucose intolerance	High-fat, low carbohydrate, fiber
Pulmonary disease	High-fat, low-carbohydrate, n-3 fatty acids, and antioxidants
Inflammatory bowel disease	Elemental/peptides, soluble fiber, higher concentration of MCT, n-3 fatty acids, and antioxidants

MCT = medium chain triglycerides
Source: Douglas Seidner, MD, FACG, and Judith Fish, MMSC, RD, CNSD. Used with permission.

in certain population groups. Patients that seem to benefit most from glutamine-containing formulas are those with trauma, postoperative wound infection, cancer requiring surgery, massive blood infusions, and acutely ill immunosuppressed patients. Arginine has also been supplemented in some formulas to prevent muscle wasting and promote wound healing and immune function. The benefits of arginine have been best demonstrated in surgical patients. The benefit in critically ill patients is still not clear. Again, these special products are more expensive so it is best to use them in well-defined situations.

Carbohydrate and Fat

Carbohydrate and fat are the primary calorie sources in tube feeding formulas. Most patients will tolerate a standard formula that is 40 to 50 percent carbohydrate and 25 to 35 percent fat. Formulas designed for specific disease states may have proportions of carbohydrate and fat content that fall outside this range. Carbohydrate sources come from large molecules such as glucose oligosaccharides, maltodextrin, and hydrolyzed corn starch. Smaller molecules such as mono- and disaccharides are also available. These molecules require a smaller amount of pancreatic enzymes and intestinal mucosal disaccharidases for adequate digestion. Most commercially made tube feeding formulas are lactose and gluten free. Some supplements designed for oral intake and infant formulas may contain lactose. Specialty formulas designed to improve glucose control in diabetic patients contain lower concentration of carbohydrate and are supplemented with fiber. These formulas are useful in those patients who cannot be controlled with a standard polymeric formula and an oral hypoglycemic medication or insulin. These products should not be routinely used for all diabetic patients as they tend to be higher in fat and are more expensive.

The fat component in tube feeding formulas has recently been the focus of much research. Previously, most tube feeding formulas contained one fat source, primarily omega-6-fatty acids. Typical sources included corn oil and soybean oil. Recent research has shown the importance of other fatty acids such as omega-3 and medium chain triglycerides (MCT) in maintaining immune function and maximizing absorption and metabolic efficiency. Now, most tube feeding formulas contain a mixture of fat sources such as canola oil, sunflower oil, MCT, and marine oils in addition to corn and soy oils. Many of the formulas designed for patients with malabsorption are low in fat or are supplemented with MCT to minimize symptoms of malabsorption. Formulas should contain a minimum of 4 percent of calories as long chain fatty acids to provide a sufficient quantity of essential fatty acids and fat-soluble vitamins.

Formulas designed for respiratory insufficiency contain 40 to 50 percent of total calories as fat to minimize the production of carbon dioxide through carbohydrate metabolism. These formulas are also nutrient dense for fluid restriction in patients with pulmonary edema. The use of these formulas is usually limited to patients that continue to have respiratory difficulty in spite of standard treatments. Recently, some pulmonary enteral formulas have been supplemented with n-3 fatty acids and antioxidants to down regulate the inflammatory response in patients with acute respiratory distress syndrome (ARDS).

Fiber

Some formulas contain added fiber (4 to 20 g/L). Many contain a mixture of fibers, both soluble and insoluble. Fiber's benefits include an increase in stool bulk and a source of energy for colonocytes, which may help to normalize bowel function. Certain fibers can have a "probiotic" effect by altering intestinal flora. These fibers such as fructooligosaccharides and inulin are metabolized by intestinal flora that produce short-chain fatty acids (acetate, proprionate, and butyrate) that lower the intraluminal pH, causing changes in the bacterial flora makeup. Butyrate also acts as an anti-inflammatory substrate. Fiber has also been promoted for the management of diabetics' blood sugar control. The benefits of fiber are most useful for patients requiring long-term tube feeding. Fiber does increase the viscosity of formulas and can contribute to the clogging of feeding tubes. It is best to administer fiber-containing formulas through a tube that is large enough to avoid tube clogging.

Vitamins, Minerals, and Trace Elements

Vitamins, minerals, and trace elements are all included in standard tube feeding formulas. Most formulas meet the United States Dietary Reference Intake for these nutrients in 1.0 to 1.5 liters of formula. A vitamin and mineral supplement is appropriate for patients receiving less than the necessary volume to meet the requirements. Antioxidant vitamins (vitamin C and E) have been added to formulas to treat specific diseases associated with oxidative stress such as inflammatory bowel disease and ARDS.

Selecting the Feeding Route

Several factors are considered when selecting a route for tube feeding. First, it is important to consider the potential duration of tube feeding. Patients requiring only four to six weeks of therapy are managed with a nasogastric or nasoenteric tube, which can be placed with little risk to the patient. These tubes can be easily removed when tube feeding is no longer needed. Patients who require long-term tube feeding often prefer a tube that is less visible and more comfortable. Surgical gastrostomy and jejunostomy tubes are frequently placed in patients requiring long-term tube feeding. Because these procedures are performed in the operating room, they are frequently done at the time the patient is scheduled for another surgical procedure. For patients who are not scheduled for a surgical procedure, a percutaneous endoscopically placed gastrostomy (PEG) or PEG with jejunostomy tube (PEG/J) can be placed without general anesthesia. The surgical and endoscopic methods of tube placement carry some risks, which include bleeding, wound infection, and bowel obstruction. However, these risks are minimized when an experienced physician is performing the procedure and the patient's clinical and nutritional status is not severely compromised.

A feeding tube placed with the tip of the tube in the stomach offers many advantages over a tube placed in the small bowel. Feeding into the stomach is more physiologic and allows feeding to be administered without a feeding pump. Gastric feeding tubes are common in patients who receive home tube feeding. Small bowel feeding tubes, which are ideally placed past the ligament of Treitz, are frequently used for patients with tracheal aspiration, reflux esophagitis, gastroparesis, gastric outlet obstruction, previous gastric surgery, and early postoperative feeding. Tubes have been designed to meet this need and can be placed temporarily via a nasoenteric route or long-term through the abdominal wall. Although controversial, many clinicians feel that small bowel tube feeding may decrease the risk of aspiration. Temporary small bowel feeding tubes are generally more difficult to place than nasogastric feeding tubes.

Feeding tubes can be manually advanced into the small bowel at the bedside. Several reports using these techniques have shown good success; however, this requires protocols and adequately trained staff. Radiologic and endoscopic techniques are also used for small bowel tube placement. Nasoenteric feeding tubes can also be directly placed in the operating room if a patient is undergoing abdominal surgery. Confirmation of nasogastric and nasoenteric tube position can be made using a plain film of the abdomen. Radiographic confirmation is recommended when tubes are placed or repositioned.

Administering Tube Feeding

Tube feeding schedules should be designed around the patient's clinical condition, physical activity, and the feeding access. Feeding tubes placed in the stomach allow a large volume (200 to 500 mL) of formula to be administered over 20 to 40 minutes. The small bowel cannot tolerate large volumes given over a short period of time. For this reason, small bowel tube feeding must be administered with a pump over a prolonged time period (8 to 24 hours). Most patients who are critically ill receive tube feeding continuously over 24 hours. Patients who are more mobile are good candidates for tube feeding that is cycled nocturnally. This also allows patients who are transitioning to oral intake to avoid suppressing their appetite during the day. Patients with gastric feeding tubes who are physically active may prefer to administer their tube feeding over a short period of time 3 to 5 times daily, similar to eating meals. This method, referred to as intermittent gravity feeding, offers flexibility, minimal equipment, and is popular with patients receiving home tube feeding.

In order to allow for GI adaptation to tube feeding, continuous tube feeding is generally initiated at 30 mL per hour. The feeding volume is increased in a stepwise fashion by 30 mL per hour every 6 to 8 hours to a goal rate by the second or third day, depending on tolerance. Intermittent feedings, via gastric feeding tubes, are usually initiated at 150 to 200 mL over 20 to 40 minutes. The feeding is then advanced by 50 to 100 mL with every feeding to the eventual goal volume as tolerated. Mild bloating and loose bowel movements are common when tube feeding is initiated. If the patient shows any signs of severe intolerance to the feeding, such as diarrhea, elevated gastric residuals, or vomiting, the administration should not be further advanced and may be discontinued temporarily while appropriate clinical evaluation is done.

Monitoring and Complications

Outcome measures, such as length of hospital stay, morbidity, mortality, and costs, are important to track to determine the efficacy of enteral nutrition support. Other measures are used to monitor nutrition support to optimize therapy and minimize complications. Clinical monitoring of patients receiving tube feeding should include metabolic, GI, and mechanical assessment. Feedings received should be compared to prescribed calorie and protein goals. Adjustments in prescriptions should be made with changes in clinical status and activity. If a patient is not responding to the therapy, indirect calorimetry can be used to better define energy needs. Need for nutrition support should also be routinely reevaluated. Acutely ill patients require daily to weekly monitoring of serum electrolytes, blood urea nitrogen (BUN), creatinine, and glucose. Stable outpatients may only need laboratory tests performed every month.

Because of the risk of refeeding syndrome, it is important to begin tube feeding cautiously and to monitor serum potassium, magnesium, phosphorus, and calcium closely in patients with severe undernutrition. Patients with pre-existing diabetes or significant stress may develop hyperglycemia. These patients can be managed with enteral hypoglycemic agents or insulin and frequent blood glucose monitoring. Excessive carbon dioxide production caused by overfeeding can cause difficulty in ventilatory support and weaning. Calories and carbohydrate provided from tube feeding and other sources such as intravenous fluids should be routinely monitored and adjusted to avoid the complications of overfeeding.

Assessing GI tolerance should include noting any reports of abdominal pain, nausea, vomiting, abdominal distention, or change in stool patterns. Precautions should be undertaken to prevent aspiration. This includes elevating the head of the

Table 12-2 Aspiration Precautions

- Elevate the head of the bed to at least 30 to 45 degrees.
- Monitor for aspiration contents in the lungs.
- Direct observation
- Monitor gastric residuals (greater than 200 mL warrants holding tube feeding and considering promotility agents).
- Consider use of dual lumen tubes when gastric emptying is poor or aspiration risk is high (small bowel feeding with continuous gastric decompression).
- Monitor feeding tube placement:
- Radiography
- Auscultation of insufflated air
- Observation of fluid pulled from the feeding tube
- Check pH of fluid aspirated from the tube
- Monitor and maintain adequate airway cuff pressure

Source: Douglas Seidner, MD, FACG, and Judith Fish, MMSC, RD, CNSD. Used with permission.

bed to 30 degrees or greater while the feeding is administered, monitoring for high gastric residual volumes, use of post-pyloric feeding tubes in high risk patients and adequate airway management (Table 12-2). The precise amount of gastric residual volume used to judge whether gastric feeding should be withheld is controversial. Other methods to reduce the incidence of aspiration pneumonia have included the examination of endotracheal aspirates for pH value and glucose concentration but these are now felt to lack the sensitivity or specificity to be of clinical value. The addition of blue dye number 1 to tube feeding formulas to help monitor aspiration of tube feeding should no longer be done as it is also a poor predictor of aspiration pneumonia and there are several case reports of mortality due to dye.

In order to monitor hydration, it is helpful to routinely evaluate input/output and daily weight. A rapid change in weight may suggest an alteration in hydration and should prompt further investigation.

For those patients who are transitioning to an oral diet, it is important to monitor their oral intake and adjust tube feeding volume accordingly so as to avoid suppressing their appetite or overfeeding. The most common complication of tube feeding in the hospital setting is diarrhea, which is rarely caused by the tube feeding formula. Likely causes of diarrhea are medications, *C. difficile* colitis, underlying or unrecognized GI disorders, and sometimes the rate of tube feeding delivery. Medications that may cause diarrhea include antibiotics and elixirs that contain sorbitol (Table 12-3). If a patient develops diarrhea while receiving tube feeding, it is important to evaluate all the potential causes and treat them appropriately. Administering antidiarrheals before checking stool for *C. difficile* toxin, and when appropriate, bacterial cultures, can be risky and may lead to toxic megacolon. Constipation is a more common symptom in patients receiving long-term tube feeding, patients receiving high doses of pain medications, and those who are immobile. Fiber-containing formulas and adequate water are most useful in preventing constipation in this population.

Dehydration can occur when patients do not receive adequate fluid via tube feeding, intravenous fluid, and water flushes through the tube. This can occur in patients receiving diuretic therapy and those patients with unusual losses from

Table 12-3 Examples of Medications Associated with Diarrhea

Sorbitol-containing medications
Propranolol solution
Acetaminophen elixir
Cimetidine solution
Ranitidine syrup
Bactrim suspension
Furosemide solution

Antibiotics
Ampicillin
Amoxicillin
Clindamycin
Tetracycline
Cephalosporins

Others
Potassium oral solutions
Oral phosphate supplements
Magnesium-based antacids
Promotility agents
Solubilizers such as propylene glycol and polyethylene glycol

---

Source: Douglas Seidner, MD, FACG, and Judith Fish, MMSC, RD, CNSD. Used with permission.

drains, stool output, or emesis. Routine monitoring of weight, blood pressure, heart rate, laboratory measures, and clinical status help to identify this problem before it becomes critical.

Clogged and displaced feeding tubes are frequent problems for patients receiving tube feedings. Patients may pull out nasal feeding tubes either intentionally or inadvertently. It is important to secure feeding tubes in place and avoid excess tubing that can be tangled with other objects. Percutaneously placed tubes can be displaced as well. If this occurs, a temporary tube must be placed in the ostomy immediately because the site can close quickly. Feeding tubes can become clogged when water flushes are inadequate or medications are administered in the feeding tube inappropriately. It is recommended that feeding tubes be flushed daily and at any time the feeding is stopped or a medication is administered. Medications should be in a liquid form whenever possible and the tube should be flushed with water after each separate medication administration (Table 12-4). Although there are many theories about how to unclog feeding tubes, warm water or pancreatic enzymes with sodium bicarbonate are the only two methods proven to be effective. It is best to avoid colas and cranberry juice due to their likelihood of leaving a residue that can cause further clogging.

Conclusion

Tube feeding offers a method of nutrition support to patients who are unable to consume adequate nutrition but have a functional GI tract. There are many advantages to tube feeding over parenteral nutrition and therefore it should be used

Table 12-4 Administering Medication through a Feeding Tube

- Use liquid form of medication whenever possible.
- Consult pharmacy on availability of liquid medication and if tablets are crushable.
- If crushing a medication, crush finely and disperse in warm water if clinically appropriate.
- Flush the feeding tube before and after each medication.
- Consult pharmacy on the timing of medications in relationship to the feeding to avoid drug–nutrient reactions.
- Consult pharmacy before administering drugs through a small bowel feeding tube. Some medications require the acidic stomach pH for proper action.
- Medications should not be mixed with enteral formulas.
- Do not crush enteric coated, sustained released, or timed-released tablets or capsules.
- Do not mix medications together.

Source: Douglas Seidner, MD, FACG, and Judith Fish, MMSC, RD, CNSD. Used with permission.

whenever feasible and clinically safe. There are a wide selection of formulas, tubes, and administration methods. Detailed assessment of the patient's clinical condition, nutrient requirements, and activity will direct selection of feeding route, formula, and administration method. Monitoring metabolic, mechanical, and GI tolerance to tube feeding will guide adjustments in tube feeding therapy. Following these principles, tube feeding can support patients successfully for as long as the therapy is indicated.

Case 1 **Enteral Feeding and Esophageal Cancer**

Lisa D. Unger[1] and M. Patricia Fuhrman[2]

[1] University of Pennsylvania School of Medicine, Philadelphia, PA
[2] Nutrition Services DCRX Infusion, Ballwin, MO

OBJECTIVES

- Assess the nutritional status of patients with esophageal cancer.
- Assess the nutrition-related metabolic abnormalities that can affect patients with cancer.
- Identify appropriate dietary recommendations for patients with odynophagia due to radiation therapy.
- Understand clinical and metabolic monitoring of patients receiving enteral nutrition support.
- Recognize the benefits of enteral nutrition support in a patient receiving radiation therapy to the head and neck.

CD is a 50-year-old white male inpatient at a university hospital. He has recently been diagnosed with esophageal cancer and reports a 25-pound weight loss over the past 6 months due to dysphagia (difficulty swallowing) and loss of appetite. CD is status-post esophagectomy with jejunostomy tube placement. Chemotherapy and radiation therapy are planned. During this hospitalization, a swallowing study was performed to rule out a postoperative leak and to assess whether it was safe for CD to resume eating and drinking. After he passed the swallowing test, a liquid diet was initiated, and he was eventually advanced to a regular diet.

Past Medical History

CD has no significant past medical history.

Medications

CD takes no medications.

Social/Diet History

CD lives alone. He denies intravenous drug use and drinks one beer in the evening. CD smoked two packs of cigarettes per day for 30 years (60 pack-year history). He quit 2 years ago. CD's dysphagia worsened over the past 6 weeks, and his appetite became very poor. He reports limiting his intake to juices, broth, and tea over the past month.

Medical Nutrition and Disease: A Case-Based Approach, 4th edition. Edited by Lisa Hark.
© 2009 Wiley-Blackwell Publishing, ISBN: 978-1-4051-8615-5.

Review of Systems
General: Fatigue, weight loss
Gastrointestinal: Poor appetite, dysphagia
Neurologic: No sensory loss
Musculoskeletal: No muscle or joint pain

Physical Examination
Vitals Signs
Temperature: 99.0 °F (37.2 °C)
Heart rate: 80 BPM
Respiratory rate: 14 BPM
Blood pressure: 120/80 mm Hg
Height: 5'11" (180 cm)
Current weight: 130 lb (59 kg)
Usual body weight: 155 lb (70 kg)
BMI: 18 kg/m^2
Percent weight change: 16% over 6 months $[(155–130)/155] \times 100$

Exam
General: Cachectic male in no acute distress
Head/neck: Bilateral temporal wasting
Cardiac: Regular rate and rhythm; no rubs, gallops, or murmurs
Chest: Status-post esophagectomy with wound site clean, dry, and intact
Abdomen: Soft, non-tender, non-distended; bowel sounds present; jejunostomy; tube site clean and dry
Extremities: No edema; general decrease in muscle mass
Neurologic: Alert and oriented to person, place, and time; no abnormalities noted

Laboratory Data

Patient's Values	Normal Values
Albumin: 3.1 g/dL	3.5–5.8 g/dL
Hemoglobin: 13.5 g/dL	13.5–17.5 g/dL
Hematocrit: 40%	40–52%
BUN: 13 mg/dL	10–20 mg/dL
Creatinine: 0.8 mg/dL	0.8–1.3 mg/dL
Potassium: 3.6 mmol/L	3.5–5.3 mmol/L
Sodium: 136 mmol/L	133–143 mmol/L

Go to Questions 1–2

Follow-up Description
CD was discharged from the hospital able to eat an adequate oral diet. His jejunostomy tube was not removed because in 4 weeks he would be receiving chemotherapy and radiation therapy that could adversely affect his oral intake. CD was instructed to flush his jejunostomy tube daily with 60 cc of water to keep it patent (open). Four weeks later, CD began receiving chemotherapy and radiation therapy, and

after 2 weeks of these treatments, he developed severe odynophagia (painful swallowing). As a result, his oral intake greatly diminished. Based on a 24-hour recall and usual intake over the past week, CD reported consuming $\frac{1}{2}$ cup of flavored gelatin and 6-ounces of applesauce daily, which totals about 200 calories per day with no significant amount of protein, vitamins, or minerals.

Go to Questions 3–8
Case Questions

1. What factors are helpful in diagnosing malnutrition in this patient?
2. What nutritional and nutrition-related metabolic abnormalities can affect patients with cancer?
3. What are the possible adverse effects of radiation therapy for esophageal cancer patients and how can they affect CD's nutritional status?
4. In general, what dietary recommendations alleviate odynophagia, as experienced by a patient receiving radiation therapy for esophageal cancer?
5. Since CD developed severe odynophagia secondary to radiation therapy and is eating only approximately 200 kcal/day, what alternative feeding options are available for him?
6. How should an enteral formula be selected and what issues related to fluid balance should be considered?
7. What clinical and laboratory parameters should be monitored for patients who receive tube feeding?
8. CD asks how long enteral nutrition support is planned. What factors determine when CD's jejunostomy tube can be removed?

Answers to Questions: Case 1
Part 1: Diagnosis

1. What factors are helpful in diagnosing malnutrition in this patient?

Based on CD's medical history, he has had a decreased appetite and dysphagia for the past 6 months, with worsening dysphagia over the past 6 weeks. This has limited his intake to juices, broth, and tea over the last month. His diet is inadequate in protein, calories, vitamins, and minerals, and has contributed to CD's severe weight loss resulting in a 16 percent weight change over the past 6 months. In addition, his BMI is only 18 kg/m^2, indicating that he is currently underweight. Additional evidence that supports a diagnosis of malnutrition includes his cachectic appearance and temporal wasting found on physical examination. Laboratory data shows a decreased albumin level of 3.1 g/dL. Although hypoalbuminemia is often used as a nutrition indicator in clinical practice, its lack of sensitivity and specificity for nutritional changes limit its clinical use as an indicator of nutritional status.

2. What nutritional and nutrition-related metabolic abnormalities can affect patients with cancer?

Patients with cancer and those undergoing treatment can experience symptoms that decrease oral intake, such as dysphagia, alterations in taste and smell, and obstruction of the GI tract, which can be caused by tumor growth. In addition, the release of cytokines, such as tumor necrosis factor and interleukins, can lead to decreased intake. Psychological factors, such as depression and anxiety, may also contribute to a decreased appetite.

Of note, there may be an increase in resting energy expenditure in some oncology patients. Furthermore, an alteration in carbohydrate metabolism with an impaired sensitivity to endogenous insulin and an alteration in lipid metabolism may cause patients with progressive disease to metabolize more fat (have an increased rate of lipolysis), thus depleting fat reserves. The catabolism of endogenous protein and accelerated gluconeogenesis can occur because the normal starvation adaptive mechanism of protein-sparing and reduced energy expenditure may not take place in the cancer patient.

Go to Follow-up Description on page 5
Part 2: Medical Nutrition Therapy

3. What are the possible adverse effects of radiation therapy for esophageal cancer patients and how can they affect CD's nutritional status?

Radiation therapy for esophageal cancer can cause adverse effects including odynophagia, nausea, vomiting, dysphagia, maldigestion, malabsorption, enteritis, fatigue, and anorexia. Each of these effects can significantly diminish CD's oral intake and eventually affect his nutritional status.

4. In general, what dietary recommendations alleviate odynophagia, as experienced by a patient receiving radiation therapy for esophageal cancer?

For odynophagia, the patient should avoid foods with extreme temperatures; foods that are spicy, hot, tart, or high in acid; raw fruits and vegetables; and dry, coarse, and highly salty food. It is recommended that the patient drink liquid nutritional supplements to increase their energy and nutrient intake. Suggest that the patient try soft, blended foods such as casseroles, mashed potatoes, soups, scrambled eggs, and yogurt.

5. Since CD developed severe odynophagia secondary to radiation therapy and is eating only approximately 200 kcal/day, what alternative feeding options are available for him?

Because of severe odynophagia resulting from radiation therapy, CD is not consuming adequate energy and nutrients. Therefore, he will continue to lose weight and become more malnourished if he depends nutritionally on oral intake alone. Since his radiation therapy is planned for several more weeks and he has a functional GI tract, he is a potential candidate for enteral nutrition support using his jejunostomy tube, which is a long-term feeding tube. After determining his nutrient goals, choose an enteral formula that best meets these goals. According to the American Dietetic Association Evidence Analysis Library Oncology Guideline, enteral nutrition can maintain weight by providing energy and protein for patients with stage III or IV head and neck cancer receiving intensive radiation therapy. However, enteral nutrition has not been shown to increase tolerance to therapy or survival in patients with esophageal cancer.

6. How should an enteral formula be selected and what issues related to fluid balance should be considered?

There are a variety of enteral formulas available, each of which provides different concentrations of macro- and micronutrients to meet patients' requirements. The enteral formula for CD should be selected based on his estimated energy and nutrient needs for weight gain and nutrient repletion, the function of his GI tract and its ability to digest and absorb nutrients, and his current oral intake. In most cases, a standard polymeric enteral formula is well tolerated. Patients with severe enteritis may require a monomeric (elemental) enteral formula. There is an insufficient amount of evidence to recommend enteral formulas that contain omega-3 fatty acids and other immuno-enhancing nutrients in this patient population. Gastric feedings can be provided either as continuous, intermittent, or bolus feedings. Jejunal feedings should be given continuously or cycled with a controlled volumetric rate. Patients at home should be considered for nocturnal cycled infusions.

Fluid balance is important to consider, particularly when enteral nutrition is the sole source of fluid intake. It is therefore important to monitor fluid status in all patients receiving tube feedings in order to prevent dehydration. Fluid loses from diarrhea, vomiting, ostomies, fistulas, and GI drains can increase fluid requirements. Patients may also require additional fluid if the enteral formula is enriched with fiber or high in protein. If the patient cannot or does not consume adequate fluids orally, and if the tube-feeding regimen does not supply enough water to meet patient's fluid requirements, additional fluid can be provided with water flushes via the feeding tube several times throughout the day.

7. What clinical and laboratory parameters should be monitored for patients who receive tube feeding?

It is very important to monitor patients for tube feeding tolerance, hydration, electrolytes, and nutritional status. Physical symptoms that should be monitored include incidence of nausea, vomiting, stool frequency, diarrhea, and abdominal pain. Physical examination should include assessing for abdominal distention or tenderness and evidence of edema or dehydration. Weight changes should also be noted. In addition, serum electrolytes (sodium, potassium, chloride, bicarbonate), calcium, magnesium, phosphorous, BUN, creatinine, and glucose should be monitored daily when the patient begins receiving enteral nutrition support. Parameters that can be monitored on a weekly basis include albumin, prealbumin, and transferrin.

It is important to note that in the first few days of initiating the tube feeding, malnourished patients such as CD may exhibit a refeeding syndrome in which extracellular to intracellular electrolyte shifts of potassium, phosphorous, and magnesium may occur, requiring prompt repletion. Initiating enteral nutrition at a low rate with gradual advancement based on tolerance and electrolyte levels can reduce the risk of refeeding syndrome.

Once the patient is metabolically stable, the frequency of monitoring can be decreased as appropriate. The adequacy of energy and nutrients in the tube feeding can be assessed by stabilization or increase in weight, depending on clinical goals for the patient.

8. CD asks how long enteral nutrition support is planned. What factors determine when CD's jejunostomy tube should be removed?

After his radiation therapy is completed, as CD's odynophagia decreases and his oral intake improves, the tube feedings should be decreased accordingly. Upon follow-up 2 weeks after radiation therapy was completed, CD reports less odynophagia and is able to increase his oral intake. He also followed up with a dietitian who offered suggestions and recipes for high-calorie, high-protein, soft, easy-to-swallow foods. He was therefore instructed to decrease his tube feeding regimen through the jejunostomy tube since his oral intake had greatly improved. The patient's weight should also be monitored and should increase with adequate nutritional intake.

Two weeks later, he was able to substantially increase his oral diet and began to drink two cans (480 cc) of a nutritional supplement daily for additional energy and nutrients. An 8-ounce can of this supplement (240 cc) provides about 14 grams of protein and 365 total calories along with vitamins and minerals. Since his oral intake was deemed adequate to meet his nutritional needs, his tube feeding regimen was discontinued. He was monitored for 4 weeks off tube feeding. His oral intake remained excellent and he continued to gain weight. Since no further radiation therapy was planned, the decision was made to remove the feeding tube.

Chapter and Case References

American Dietetic Association. Evidence Analysis Library. Oncology Guideline. Available from http://www.adaevidencelibrary.com.

ASPEN Board of Directors. Guidelines for the use of parenteral and enteral nutrition in adults and pediatric patients. *J Parenter Enteral Nutr.* 2002;26:1,9SA–138SA.

Braga M, Gianotti L, Vignali A, Cestari A, Bisagni P, DiCarlo V. Artificial nutrition after major abdominal surgery: impact of route of administration and composition of the diet. *Crit Care Med.* 1998;26:24–30.

Braunschweic C, Levy P, Sheean P, Wang X. Enteral versus parenteral nutrition: a meta analysis. *Am J Clin Nutr.* 2001;74:534–542.

Campbell S. An anthology of advances in enteral tube feeding formulations. *Nutr Clin Prac.* 2006:21:411–415.

Eisenberg PG. Causes of diarrhea in tube-fed patients: a comprehensive approach to diagnosis and management. *Nutr Clin Pract.* 1993;8:119–123.

Fearon KC, Voss AC, Hustead S. Definition of cancer cachexia: effect of weight loss, reduced food intake, and systemic inflammation on functional status and prognosis. *Am J Clin Nutr.* 2006;83:1345–1350.

Frankel EH, Enouw NB, Jackson KC, et al. Methods for restoring patency to occluded feeding tubes. *Nutr Clin Pract.* 1998;13:129–131.

Fuhrman MP, Charney P, Mueller CM. Hepatic proteins and nutrition assessment. *J Am Diet Assoc.* 2004;104(8):1258–1264.

Garrell DR, Razi M, Lariviere F, et al. Improved clinical status and length of care with low fat nutrition support in burn patients. *J Parenter Enteral Nutr.* 1995;19(6):482–491.

Gassull MA, Mane J, Elisabest P, Cabre E. Macronutrients and bioactive molecules: is there a specific role in the management of inflammatory bowel disease? *J Parenter Enteral Nutr.* 2005;29:S179–183.

Hasselman M, Reimund J. Lipids in the nutritional support of the critically ill patients. *Curr Opin Crit Care.* 2004;10:449–455.

Hernandez G, Velasco N, Wainstein C, et al. Gut muscosal atrophy after a short enteral fasting period in critically ill patients. *J Crit Care.* 1999;14:73–77.

Heyland DK, Drover JW, Dhaliwal R, Greenwood J. Optimizing the benefits and minimizing the risks of enteral nutrition in the critically ill: role of small bowel feeding. *J Parenter Enteral Nutr.* 2002;26:S51–55.

Kang W, Kudsk KA. Is there evidence that the gut contributes to mucosal immunity in humans? *J Parenter Enteral Nutr.* 2007;31:246–258.

Kirby DF, Delegge MH, Fleming CR. American Gastroenterological Association technical review on tube feeding for enteral nutrition. *Gastroenterol.* 1995;108(4):1282–1301.

Kudsk KA, Schloerb PR, DeLegge MH, et al. Consensus recommendations from the US summit on immune-enhancing enteral therapy. *J Parenter Enteral Nutr.* 2001;25:S61–62.

Lipman TO. Grains or veins: is enteral nutrition really better than parenteral nutrition? A look at the evidence. *J Parenter Enteral Nutr.* 1998;22:167–182.

Magnuson BL, Timothy MC, Lora AH, Bernard A. Enteral nutrition and drug administration, interactions, and complications. *Nutr Clin Prac.* 2005;20:618–624.

Matarese LE, Seidner DL, Steiger E. The role of probiotics in gastrointestinal disease. *Nutr Clin Prac.* 2003;18:507–516

McClave SA. Nutrition support in acute pancreatitis. *Gastroenterol Clin North Am.* 2007;36(1):65–74.

McCowen KC, Bistrian BR. Immunonutrition: problematic or problem solving? *Am J Clin Nutr.* 2003;77:764–770.

Metheny NA. Preventing respiratory complications of tube feedings: evidence-based practice. *Am J Crit Care.* 2006;15(4):360–369.

Newsholme P. Why is l-glutamine metabolism important to cells of the immune system in health, post injury, surgery or infection? *J Nutr.* 2001;131:S2515–S2522.

Pearce CB, Duncan HD. Enteral feeding, nasogastric, nasojejunal, percutaneous endoscopic gastrostomy, or jejunostomy: its indications and limitations. *Postgrad Med.* 2002;78:198–204.

Pontes-Arruda A, Aragao AM, Albuquerque JD. Effects of enteral feeding with eicosapentaenoic acid, gamma-linolenic acid, and antioxidants in mechanically ventilated patients with severe sepsis and septic shock. *Crit Care Med.* 2006;34:2325–2333

Robinson CA. Enteral nutrition in adult oncology. In: Elliott L, McCallum PD, editors. *The Clinical Guide to Oncology Nutrition*, 2nd ed. Chicago, IL: American Dietetic Association, 2006:138–155.

Savy G. Enteral glutamine supplementation: clinical review and practical guidelines. *Nutr Clin Pract.* 1997;12:259–262.

Schloerb P. Immune-enhancing diets: products, components, and their rationales. *J Parenter Enteral Nutr.* 2001;25:S3–7.

Senkal M, Mumme A, Eickhoff U, et al. Early postoperative analysis in surgical patients. *Crit Care Med.* 1997;25:1489–1496.

Stechmiller JK. Childress B, Porter T. Arginine immunonutrition in critically ill patients: a clinical dilemma. *Am J Crit Care.* 2004:13;17–23.

Stiegmann GV, Goff JS, Silas D, Pearlman N, Sun J, Norton L. Endoscopic versus operative gastrostomy; final results of a prospective randomized trial. *Gastrointest Endosc.* 1990;9:172–182.

Talpers SS, Pomberger DJ, Bunce SB, Pingleton SK. Nutritionally associated increased carbon dioxide production: excess total calories vs. high proportion of carbohydrate calories. *Chest.* 1992;203:551–555.

Trujillo E, Nebeling L. Changes in carbohydrate, lipid, and protein metabolism in cancer. In: Elliott L, McCallum PD, editors. *The Clinical Guide to Oncology Nutrition,* 2nd ed. American Dietetic Association, Chicago, IL. 2006:17–27.

13 Parenteral Nutrition Support

Laura Matarese[1], Robert DeChicco[2], and Ezra Steiger[3]

[1] Thomas E. Starzl Transplantation Institute, Pittsburgh, PA
[2] Cleveland Clinic, Cleveland, OH
[3] Lerner College of Medicine of Case Western Reserve University, Cleveland, OH

OBJECTIVES *

- Describe the indications and contraindications for parenteral nutrition support.
- Determine the composition of parenteral nutrition formulas and how the macronutrient, micronutrient, and fluid requirements are calculated.
- Describe appropriate methods for monitoring and management of the complications associated with parenteral nutrition support.

*Source: Objectives for chapter and cases adapted from the *NIH Nutrition Curriculum Guide for Training Physicians*. (WWW.nhlbi.nih.gov/funding/training/naa)

Parenteral nutrition (PN) supplies protein in the form of amino acids, carbohydrate as dextrose, fat, vitamins, minerals, and trace elements to patients when the gastrointestinal (GI) tract is not functional, accessible, or safe to use. It can be infused via peripheral or central veins. The exact route of administration will depend on the length of therapy, nutrition requirements, goal of nutrition therapy, availability of intravenous (IV) access, severity of illness, and fluid status.

Indications and Contraindications

Indications
Enteral nutrition is always preferable to PN if the GI tract is functional, accessible, and safe to use. Due to its expense and potential for serious complications, PN should be used only when enteral feedings are not possible in patients who require nutrition support. The following conditions may warrant the use of PN:

- Paralytic ileus
- Mesenteric ischemia
- Small bowel obstruction
- High output GI fistula

Contraindications
Parenteral nutrition is contraindicated when the GI tract is functional and safe to use, when the patient's prognosis is not consistent with aggressive nutrition support, or when the risks outweigh the benefits.

Medical Nutrition and Disease: A Case-Based Approach, 4th edition. Edited by Lisa Hark.
© 2009 Wiley-Blackwell Publishing, ISBN: 978-1-4051-8615-5.

Central Parenteral Nutrition

Central PN is indicated in patients requiring long-term therapy or a concentrated formula. The solution may be dextrose-based (2-in-1) or lipid-based (3-in-1) and is infused via a central vein. Intravenous fat emulsions (IVFE) can be admixed into the solution or administered separately. Stability of the PN formula becomes a concern with the addition of IVFE due to the presence of destabilizing cations such as magnesium and calcium. The IVFE manufacturer's guidelines should be followed to ensure stability of 3-in-1 formulas.

Lipid-based solutions are indicated in situations where restricting carbohydrate load is desirable, as in patients with persistent hyperglycemia. Reducing carbohydrate intake may also decrease the production of carbon dioxide, which may facilitate weaning from the ventilator (Chapter 9). There is no limit on osmolarity of central PN since the solution is rapidly diluted by the high flow rate of blood returning to the heart. Central PN is generally indicated when any of the following conditions are present:

- Long-term (>7 days) PN support is anticipated
- Moderately-to-severely elevated metabolic rate
- Moderate-to-severe malnutrition
- Fluid restriction
- Poor peripheral access
- Central access available

Peripheral Parenteral Nutrition

Peripheral PN is usually reserved for patients requiring short-term nutrition support who are not markedly hypermetabolic or fluid-restricted and have adequate peripheral venous access. Osmolarity should be considered in peripheral PN because infusion of a hypertonic solution through a peripheral vein may result in phlebitis. To prevent this, solutions should have less than 900 mOsm per liter. Dextrose and amino acids are limited because they increase the osmolarity of the solution. Therefore, peripheral PN is usually lipid-based because IVFE is isotonic. Peripheral PN usually cannot provide adequate calories and protein for hypermetabolic, fluid-restricted patients but can be helpful for several days until GI function returns or central access is obtained. The osmolarity of a PN solution can be estimated using the conversions shown in Table 13-1.

Table 13-1 Conversions for Estimating PN Solution Osmolarity

Amino acids: 1 g = 10 mOsm
Dextrose: 1 g = 5 mOsm
20% IVFE: 1 g = 0.71 mOsm
Calcium gluconate: 1 mEq = 1.4 mOsm
Magnesium sulfate: 1 mEq = 1 mOsm
Potassium: 1 mEq = 2 mOsm
Sodium: 1 mEq = 2 mOsm

Macronutrient Requirements

Energy

Estimation of energy expenditure is difficult in the healthy non-stressed individual but becomes even more complex during illness and injury. Yet this portion of the PN prescription is critical in order to avoid the complications associated with overfeeding and underfeeding. It is important to note that the stress response is different from starvation. The stress response is characterized by increased metabolic rate, increased glucose production, protein catabolism, hyperglycemia, increased catecholamines, increased glucocorticoids, and hyperinsulinemia. Starvation is characterized by decreased energy expenditure and decreased protein wasting which is adaptive and aimed at preserving lean body mass. Glycogen stores are depleted in 24 hours; gluconeogenesis decreases and fatty acids and ketones provide energy later in the process. Meeting or exceeding goal calories and protein during stress response will not improve nitrogen balance or decrease catabolic rate as compared to starvation.

Energy expenditure can be measured directly or indirectly by providing accurate assessments of the patient's requirements at a given point in time. However, due to the cost of the equipment required and limited availability, calculation methods to determine energy expenditure are often employed. These equations provide estimates of the patient's energy requirements. Many of these equations are cumbersome to use and most clinicians prefer a more convenient technique. The American Society for Parenteral and Enteral Nutrition recommends a range of 20 to 35 kcal per kg daily for adults. However, the nutrition prescription should be adjusted based on the patient's response to the therapy.

Harris–Benedict Equation This resting energy expenditure (REE) equation, first published in 1919, was derived from energy expenditure measurements on 239 adult men and women during resting conditions. The study population also included some obese individuals.

REE equation for males:
$$66 + [13.7 \times \text{weight (kg)}] + [5.0 \times \text{height (cm)}] - [6.8 \times \text{(age)}] = \text{kcal/day}$$

REE equation for females:
$$655 + [9.7 \times \text{weight (kg)}] + [1.85 \times \text{height (cm)}] - [4.7 \times \text{(age)}] = \text{kcal/day}$$

These equations remain among the most commonly employed predictive methods for determining energy expenditure today. However, they do not represent the height, weight, age, and racial diversity of the current population as these equations were developed nearly a century ago.

Mifflin–St. Jeor Equations These equations were derived from experiments of 247 women and 251 adult men and included both obese and non-obese individuals. Fat-free mass was found to correlate with total body weight and resting metabolic rate. The Mifflin–St. Jeor equations predict resting metabolic rate (RMR) within 10 percent of actual in most individuals.

Men: Energy expenditure $= 5 + 10$ (wt in kg) $+ 6.25$ (ht in cm) $- 5$ (age)

Women: Energy expenditure $= -161 + 10$ (wt in kg) $+ 6.25$ (ht in cm) $- 5$ (age)

Both the Harris–Benedict and the Mifflin–St. Jeor equations were derived from healthy individuals based on gender, weight, height, and age but do not represent the energy needs during critical illness. Consequently, they are often modified by various stress factors to account for sickness and injury.

In order to better assess the energy requirements of stressed patients, equations such as Swinamer and Ireton-Jones have been developed to account for the factors that often change in severe illness such as body temperature, respiratory rate, tidal volume, and minute ventilation.

Swinamer Equation

RMR (kcal/d) $=$ BSA(941) $-$ age (6.3) $+$ T(104) $+$ RR(24) $+$ V$_t$$(804)$ $- 4243$

Penn State: RMR (kcal/d) $=$ HBE (0.85) $+$ V$_t$ (33) $+$ T$_m$ (175) $- 6433$

BSA $=$ Body surface area (m^2)

T $=$ Body temperature (centigrade)

RR $=$ Respiratory rate (breaths/min)

V$_t$ $=$ Tidal volume (L)

HBE $=$ Harris–Benedict equation using actual body weight

VE $=$ Minute ventilation (L/min)

T$_m$ $=$ Maximum body temperature in previous 24 hours (centigrade).

Ireton-Jones Equation

Spontaneous Breathing:

IJEE (s) $= 629 - 11$(A) $+ 25$(W) $- 609$(O)

Ventilator-Dependent:

IJEE (v) $= 1784 - 11$(A) $+ 5$(W) $+ 244$(S) $+ 239$(T) $+ 804$(B)

where IJEE $=$ kcal/day; s $=$ spontaneously breathing; v $=$ ventilatory-dependent; A $=$ age (years); W $=$ actual body weight (kg), S $=$ sex (male $= 1$, female $= 0$); T $=$ diagnosis of trauma (present $= 1$, absent $= 0$); O $=$ obesity greater than 30 percent above IBW from 1959 Metropolitan Life Insurance Tables or BMI greater than 27 (present $= 1$, absent $= 0$).

Carbohydrate

Carbohydrate is provided as an energy substrate and is supplied as dextrose monohydrate in concentrations ranging from 5 to 70 percent. Dextrose monohydrate used in PN solutions yields 3.4 kcal per gram. A 10 percent solution yields 100 g of carbohydrate per liter of solution. The use of carbohydrate (100 g daily for a 70 kg person) ensures that protein is not catabolized for energy during conditions of normal metabolism. Higher dextrose concentrations can be used when fluid volumes need to be restricted.

Dextrose infusion should be limited to 7 mg per kg per minute in stable hospitalized patients and <4 mg per kg per minute in the critically ill. When glucose oxidation rates are exceeded, fat synthesis will occur, a process that may generate excessive CO_2. This may contribute to CO_2 retention in patients with respiratory disease. In addition, exceeding glucose oxidation rates may also contribute to hepatic steatosis or fat deposition in the liver. Patients are more likely to experience other complications with high dextrose infusions such as hyperglycemia and electrolyte shifts. Consideration should be given to the dextrose content of other intravenous fluids which may be infusing simultaneously.

Lipids

Intravenous fat emulsions (IVFE) supply lipids, which are a source of essential fatty acids (EFAs) and a concentrated source of calories. In addition to providing a source of EFAs and supply of non-protein calories, the use of IVFE may aid in blood glucose control in the hyperglycemic patient.

IVFE are available in 10 and 20 percent concentrations for infusion and 30 percent for compounding. They are composed of aqueous suspensions of soybean or safflower oil, with egg yolk phospholipid as the emulsifier. Patients who are allergic to eggs should not be given IVFE. Glycerol is added to make an isotonic solution. A 10 percent emulsion provides 1.1 kcal/mL; a 20 percent emulsion provides 2 kcal/mL; and 30 percent emulsion provides 3 kcal/mL. About 10 percent of calories per day from fat emulsions provide the 2 to 4 percent of calories from linoleic acid required to prevent EFA deficiency.

Linoleic acid has been shown to alter prostaglandin metabolism, thereby producing both proinflammatory and immunosuppressive effects, particularly at high doses and at faster infusion rates. Therefore infusion of currently available soybean or safflower oil lipid emulsions over 24-hour periods should be limited to a maximum of 1 g of lipid per kg per 24 hours. In order to avoid the deleterious effects often observed on the liver, daily infusion of lipid should be avoided in long-term PN-dependent patients. Lipid emulsions should not be given in hypertriglyceridemia-induced pancreatitis or when serum triglyceride values are greater than 400 mg per dL.

Protein (Amino Acids)

The primary function of protein in PN solutions is to maintain nitrogen balance and promote maintenance of lean body mass. Parenteral protein is provided in the form of synthetic amino acids and contains a mixture of essential and non-essential amino acids. The concentration of amino acids in these solutions ranges from 3 to 20 percent. Thus, a 10 percent solution of amino acids supplies 100 g of protein per liter. Each gram of protein supplies 4 calories. In general, 15 to 20 percent of the total energy prescription should be supplied as protein. Protein is often administered based on body weight and stress level:

Mild stress: 0.8 to 1.0 g per kg per day

Moderate stress: 1.5 g per kg per day

Severe stress: 2.0 g per kg per day

Adjustments in protein load should be made according to the patient's tolerance and clinical response, and through monitoring of serum transport proteins, nitrogen balance results, and renal and liver function.

Fluid and Electrolyte Requirements

Once the macronutrient portion of the PN prescription has been established, the day-to-day management centers on fluid and electrolytes. Daily fluid requirements can be estimated from the sum of urine output, gastrointestinal losses, and insensible water losses from the skin and respiratory tract. Weighing the patient daily is the best means of assessing net gain or loss of fluid. Rapid weight gain or loss (more than 4 pounds (1.8 kg) in 1 week) generally represents fluid changes and not tissue synthesis. Vital signs, such as blood pressure and heart rate, and physical examination changes (e.g. edema, ascites, and skin turgor) also offer evidence of fluid status. In general, young adults require 30 to 40 mL per kg per day and the elderly require 20 to 30 mL per kg per day.

Electrolytes are routinely added to the PN solutions in amounts sufficient to provide for daily needs (Table 13.2). Electrolyte requirements will vary depending on the patient's current electrolyte, renal, and fluid status, as well as the patient's underlying disease process. If the patient had been receiving maintenance IV fluids prior to starting PN, it is helpful to note the electrolyte composition of these fluids and use this as a guide to prescribe the PN formula. Patients receiving PN may have higher intracellular electrolyte requirements than patients receiving standard IV fluids.

Calcium is an extracellular cation that is essential for normal muscle contraction, nerve function, blood coagulation, and bone mineralization. The usual dose is 10 to 15 mEq per day. Sixty percent of serum calcium is bound to protein, primarily albumin. Therefore in the presence of a low serum albumin level, a low serum calcium level needs to be adjusted for hypoalbuminemia.

$$\text{Adjusted calcium level} = (4.0 - \text{serum albumin}) \times 0.8 + \text{serum calcium}$$

Table 13-2 Daily Electrolyte Requirements during Parenteral Nutrition in Adults

Electrolyte	Parenteral Equivalent of RDA	Standard Intake
Calcium	10 mEq	10–15 mEq
Phosphate	30 mMol	20–40 mMol
Magnesium	10 mE	8–20 mEq
Sodium	NA	1–2 mEq/kg + replacement
Potassium	NA	1–2 mEq/kg + replacement
Acetate	NA	As needed to maintain acid-base balance
Chloride	NA	As needed to maintain acid-base balance

Source: National Advisory Group on Standards, and Practice Guidelines for Parenteral Nutrition, ASPEN: Safe practices for parenteral nutrition formulations, *J Parenter Enteral Nutr.* 2004; 28(suppl):S38–S70.
NA: Not applicable

Table 13-3 Prevention of Calcium–Phosphorus Precipitation

Calcium mEq/L + (2 X total phosphate mM) ≤45
Calcium mEq/L × mEq phosphorus/L <200
Calcium mEq/L × potassium as phosphate mEq/L <250
Calcium mEq/L × sodium as phosphate mEq/L <225
Calcium mEq/L × phosphate mM/L <150
Calcium mM/L × potassium as phosphate mEq/L <125
Calcium mM/L × phosphate mM/L <75

Source: Laura Matarese MS, RD, LDN, FADA, CNSD, Robert DeChicco
MS, RD, CNSD, and Ezra Steiger, MD. Used with permission.

This equation provides an estimate of the adjusted calcium level in the presence of hypoalbuminema. When in doubt and when the serum albumin is less than 2.8 grams per dL, an ionized calcium level should be obtained. Along with calcium, phosphorus is the major component of bone hydroxyapatite and teeth. Phosphorus is the primary intracellular anion and functions in the metabolism of carbohydrate, fat, and protein. The usual dose is 20 to 40 mM per day. The combination of calcium and phosphorus in PN formulas has the potential of forming a precipitate. Thus, it is important to follow appropriate and safe guidelines for maximum calcium and phosphorus additives in a PN formula. Numerous equations are available to test calcium–phosphorus solubility, which are shown in Table 13.3.

Magnesium functions in enzyme reactions such as glycolysis and in all reactions involving adenosine triphosphate (ATP). Magnesium is often depleted in patients with protein calorie malnutrition and prolonged IV fluid therapy. Magnesium may also appear low in patients with hypoalbuminemia.

Corrected magnesium level = Mg + 0.005 (4.0 − serum albumin)

Patients may also have excessive losses from prolonged gastric suction, fistulas, and diarrhea. The usual dose of magnesium sulfate is 8 to 20 mEq per day. Magnesium sulfate provides 8.12 mEq per gram of magnesium.

Sodium is a major extracellular cation and functions in the maintenance of osmotic pressure and in acid–base balance. The usual dose is 1 to 2 mEq/kg per day. Requirements may be increased when there are excess losses from urine, ostomies, or fistulas or decreased in renal, cardiac, or hepatic failure.

Potassium is the major cation of intracellular fluid. The normal dose is 1 to 2 mEq per kg. Hypokalemia may result from diuretics, amphotericin B, nasogastric suction, or vomiting. Other medications such as cyclosporine and tacrolimus may cause hyperkalemia. The PN solution should provide maintenance potassium requirements. Acute deficits of potassium should be corrected outside of the PN with an IV replacement dose.

Sodium and potassium may be added to PN solutions in the form of chloride or acetate salts. Chloride is a major extracellular anion and functions in the maintenance of osmotic pressure and acid–base balance. Acetate maybe added to PN solutions when clinically appropriate since it is converted to bicarbonate in the

Table 13-4 Adult Parenteral Multivitamins: Guidelines and Products

Vitamin	NAG-AMA Guidelines	FDA Requirements	MVI-12	MVI-13
A (retinol)	3300 units (1 mg)	3300 units (1 mg)	3300 units (1 mg)	3300 units (1 mg)
D (ergocalciferol cholecalciferol)	200 units (5 mcg)	200 units (5 mcg)	200 units (5 mcg)	200 units (5 mcg)
E	10 units (10 mg)	10 units (10 mg)	10 units (10 mg)	10 units (10 mg)
B1 (thiamin)	3 mg	6 mg	3 mg	6 mg
B2 (riboflavin)	3.6 mg	3.6 mg	3.6 mg	3.6 mg
B3 (niacinamide)	40 mg	40 mg	40 mg	40 mg
B5 (dexpanthenol)	15 mg	15 mg	15 mg	15 mg
B6 (pyridoxine)	4 mg	6 mg	4 mg	6 mg
B12 (cyanocobalamin)	5 mcg	5 mcg	5 mcg	5 mcg
C	100 mg	200 mg	100 mg	200 mg
Biotin	60 mcg	60 mcg	60 mcg	60 mcg
Folic acid	400 mcg	600 mcg	400 mcg	600 mcg
K	150 mcg	0		150 mcg

Source: National Advisory Group; American Medical Association; U.S. Food and Drug Administration; MVI-12 and MVI-13, multivitamin injections.

liver and functions as a systemic alkalinizer. Bicarbonate should never be added to PN solutions since it is not compatible with other additives and may form a precipitate.

Vitamins, Minerals, and Trace Elements

Vitamins, minerals, and trace elements are essential for humans and should be added daily to the PN solution in order to prevent deficiencies. Guidelines and products for adult parenteral multivitamins are shown in Table 13.4. Since they are provided parenterally and therefore bypass the digestive and absorptive process, the amounts are lower than the Dietary Reference Intakes (DRI). Parenteral vitamins and trace elements are given as standard multiple-vitamin and trace element preparations. In the event that vitamin, mineral, or trace element deficiencies or unusual losses occur, they can sometimes be supplemented above the amount normally added to the PN solution as shown in Table 13.5.

Medications

PN solutions are complex formulations designed to deliver fluid, electrolytes, and nutrients. Most medications should not be added to the PN solution due to potential instability and incompatibility. Heparin and, when necessary, insulin can be added to the PN solution. Only regular human insulin should be added to PN solutions. Other medications, such as histamine H2 receptor antagonists and octreotide, can be added to the PN solution when needed.

Table 13-5 Daily Trace Element Requirements

Trace Element	ASPEN Recommendations*	GI Losses
Chromium	10–15 mcg	20 mcg/day
Copper	0.3–0.5 mg	500 mcg/day
Manganese	60–100 mcg	
Selenium	20–60 mcg	
Zinc	2.5–5mg[a]	Additional zinc[b]

a: Additional 2 mg/day in hypermetabolic states
b: Additional 12 mg/L of small bowel losses and 17 mcg/kg of stool or ileostomy losses
Source: A.S.P.E.N. Board of Directors and the Task Force for the revision of safe practices for parenteral nutrition. *J Parenter Enteral Nutr.* 2004; 28(suppl):S38–S70.

The PN Prescription

The base solution can be specified by the actual grams of dextrose, fat, amino acids, and calories, or it can be prescribed as final concentrations. Individual electrolytes and minerals can be specified or a selection can be made from several standard solutions. In most institutions, the PN prescription is ordered for a 24-hour period. Initiation is based on patient tolerance. The initial dextrose concentration is generally less than 200 grams per day. For patients with diabetes or stress-induced hyperglycemia, initial dextrose concentrations of 100 to 150 grams are recommended. In most patients the goal concentration can be achieved by the second day. Serum blood glucose levels should be less than 150 mg/dL and all electrolytes within normal limits before advancing the PN concentration.

Infusing Parenteral Nutrition

When using a continuous PN regimen, it is important to determine the desired volume to be delivered at the maintenance rate of infusion to fulfill the patient's caloric and protein needs over a 24-hour period. Occasionally, patients who are clinically and metabolically stable and who exhibit no complications with continuous 24-hour PN may benefit from cycled PN to increase mobility and ease of care. Cycled PN generally is infused over a 10- to 16-hour period. This provides patients with time away from the pump, which enhances their quality of life. It is also more physiologic in that it mimics normal eating patterns and may decrease the incidence of cholestasis that is associated with long-term continuous infusions of dextrose, lipids, and amino acids.

Discontinuation of PN

As gastrointestinal function returns, the patient can be transitioned to enteral nutrition by tube or oral nutrition. When oral intake approximates 500 kcal/day, decrease carbohydrate and protein in PN to equal amount consumed daily. Continue to decrease PN as oral intake improves. Discontinue PN when the patient meets 60 to 80 percent of energy goal enterally or orally. If acceptable oral intake is not achieved within a few days, tube feeding should be considered.

Monitoring and Management of Complications

Catheters

Central access for administering PN can be obtained via the subclavian or jugular veins using a temporary central venous access device (CVAD) or via the basilic or cephalic vein using a peripherally inserted central catheter (PICC). A tunneled catheter or implanted port may also be used for long-term access. The most common complications associated with the percutaneous placement of a CVAD are pneumothorax and arterial puncture. A chest X-ray should be obtained before using a new CVAD to ensure that the line was correctly placed and that no internal injuries occurred during insertion. The tip of a CVAD should be located in the distal superior vena cava adjacent to the right atrium to reduce the risk of catheter-related deep venous thrombosis.

Infectious Complications

Hospitalized patients receiving PN have many potential reasons for elevations in temperature and sepsis including intra-abdominal infections, wound infections, urinary tract infections, pneumonia, phlebitis, and drug fever. However, a sudden change in the patient's usual temperature, especially in combination with new onset shaking chills, leukocytosis, or unexplained hyperglycemia, may be an indication of catheter-related blood stream infection (CRBSI). The catheter can be the primary source of infection or seeded by a remote source. An infected catheter should be removed and re-sited. A long-term CVAD may be treated *in situ* providing the patient's symptoms improve after treatment is started. The main risk of leaving the catheter in place for patients who respond to antibiotics is a higher rate of recurrent bacteremia, especially if the infection is due to gram-negative bacilli. The prevalence of CRBSI can be reduced with proper catheter insertion technique and strict adherence to catheter care protocols.

Metabolic

Hyperglycemia is a common adverse consequence of PN and has been associated with increased morbidity and mortality in hospitalized patients. Close monitoring of blood sugars along with aggressive treatment reduces hyperglycemia and improves outcomes. Blood glucose levels should be checked frequently, usually four times daily in patients starting on PN until adequately controlled. Blood sugars in hospitalized patients should be less than 150 mg/dL.

PN-associated hyperglycemia may be treated with a combination of basal, nutritional, and correction insulin in insulin-deficient patients. Basal insulin is the amount of exogenous insulin required to maintain blood sugar levels when not eating and is usually given as long-acting insulin administered subcutaneously once or twice per day. Nutritional insulin is the amount of insulin required to cover the dextrose in the PN and is usually given in the form of regular insulin added directly to the solution. Correction insulin is the amount of insulin given to treat unexpected hyperglycemia and is usually given in the form of short-acting insulin administered subcutaneously based on a sliding scale. In some instances it may be necessary to reduce dextrose calories and replace with lipid calories to aid in blood glucose control.

Hypoglycemia may occur in patients if an excessive amount of insulin is added to the PN solution or after abrupt discontinuation of high-dextrose PN infusion. To avoid these problems, insulin should be added in increments to the PN solution and blood sugars monitored frequently until the appropriate dose is determined. To prevent rebound hypoglycemia, PN infusions should be tapered down over a period of 1-to-2 hours to allow for serum insulin adaptation.

Electrolyte imbalances may occur in severely stressed patients, both before and after PN begins. It is best to correct any existing electrolyte abnormalities before PN is initiated. Close monitoring of electrolytes, especially potassium, magnesium, and phosphorus during the first few days of PN, is important. Corrections for severe electrolyte imbalances must be made promptly with IV replacements to avoid serious complications such as seizures, arrhythmias, or even death.

Dehydration and fluid overload are potential complications when PN is the primary source of fluid. Fluid overload or edema may be seen in patients with renal failure, liver failure, congestive heart failure, and hypoalbuminemia. Excessive PN volume can significantly exacerbate fluid retention states. Under these circumstances, a concentrated PN solution may be used. Fluid status should be evaluated daily to determine if the patient is dehydrated or at risk for fluid overload. Monitor intake, output, and body weight records daily. The physical examination should note the presence of edema, rales, ascites, distended neck veins, and other signs of fluid retention.

Preventing Refeeding Syndrome

Refeeding syndrome may occur when starting PN in a patient after a period of prolonged starvation resulting in fluid retention and hyperglycemia in addition to severe imbalances of serum phosphorus, potassium, and magnesium. Once PN begins, increased cellular uptake of electrolytes may cause extremely low serum levels. This dramatic shift can lead to generalized fatigue, lethargy, muscle weakness, cardiac dysfunction, and potentially death. The risk of refeeding syndrome can be minimized by initially providing the patient a low-dextrose PN solution for the first several days while closely monitoring phosphorus, potassium, magnesium, glucose, and fluid status (Chapter 4: Case 4.2).

Case 1 Colon Cancer and Post-Operative Sepsis

José Antonio Ruy-Díaz

Anahuac University School of Medicine, Mexico City, Mexico

OBJECTIVES

- Describe the appropriate parenteral nutrition recommendations for a patient with colon cancer.
- Assess the nutritional status of a critically ill patient.
- Identify clinical and metabolic parameters used to monitor patients receiving parenteral nutrition.
- Recognize the adverse effects of undernutrition and the associated benefits of providing appropriate nutrition support.
- Recognize the benefits of parenteral nutrition in a malnourished, critically ill, surgical patient.

AJ is a 73-year-old Mexican man who presents to the Emergency Department with 72-hours of abdominal pain of increasing severity. He describes his pain as radiating through the entire abdomen. He also reports nausea and vomiting of gastric contents at least five times, during the last three days. AJ also reports liquid greenish stools on about eight occasions. He mentions that he has been losing weight for the last six months without any explanation.

Past Medical History

AJ had a stroke two years ago leaving him with weakness of his right leg. He currently takes coumadin and digoxin. He denies drug or food allergies. He had an appendectomy three years ago.

Social History

AJ is currently retired from his job as an employee for a commercial organization. He was a heavy alcohol consumer, drinking up to 1 liter of tequila daily until 10 years ago when on advice from his physician, he stopped drinking. AJ smoked 20 cigarettes every day until about 10 years ago.

Review of Systems

The review of systems was unremarkable except for nausea, abdominal pain, and unintentional weight loss.

Medical Nutrition and Disease: A Case-Based Approach, 4th edition. Edited by Lisa Hark.
© 2009 Wiley-Blackwell Publishing, ISBN: 978-1-4051-8615-5.

Physical Examination
Vital Signs
Temperature: 100 °F (38 °C)
Heart rate: 112 BPM
Respiration: 23 BPM
Blood pressure: 100/60 mm Hg
Height: 5′6″ (170 cm)
Current weight: 99 lb (45 kg)
BMI: 16 kg/m^2
Usual weight: 132 lb (60 kg) 1 year ago
Percent weight change: 25% over 6 months (132 − 99)/132

Exam
General: Thin male who appears in severe distress.
Skin: Pale, cold and dry.
HEENT: Anicteric.
Cardiac: Regular rate and rhythm, no murmurs or extra sounds.
Pulmonary: Decreased breath sounds bilaterally, with rales.
Abdomen: Marked abdominal tenderness, particularly in the hypogastrium with guarding and rebound; distended; no bowel sounds.
Extremities: No cyanosis or edema. Paresis of right leg.
Neurologic: Awake, alert, non-focal, no asterixcis.
Clinical studies: An abdominal X-ray shows severely distended loops of the small bowel in right upper quadrant and no air in the rectum. An abdominal ultrasound reveals distended loops of small intestine. No evidence of cholelithiasis (gallstones). Bile ducts and liver appear normal.

Laboratory Data

Patient's Values	Normal Values
Sodium: 139 mEq/L	133–145 mEq/L
Potassium: 5.8 mEq/L	3.5–5.3 mEq/L
Chloride: 110 mEq/L	97–107 mEq/L
CO_2: 27 mEq/L	24–32 mEq/L
BUN: 41 mEq/L	10–20 mEq/L
Creatinine: 2.5 mg/d	0.8–1.3 mg/dL
Glucose: 137 mg/dL	70–99 mg/dL
Albumin: 2.8 g/dL	3.5–5.8 g/dL
Calcium: 7.6 mg/dL	9–11 mg/dL
Adjusted calcium: 8.1 mg/dL	9–11 mg/dL
Magnesium: 1.7 mg/dL	1.8–2.9 mg/dL
Phosphorus: 2.7 mg/dL	2.5–4.6 mg/dL
Amylase: 48 U/dL	60–180 U/dL
Bilirubin: 0.57 mg/dL	0.2–1.2 mg/dL
AST: 36 U/L	0–40 U/L
ALT: 14 U/L	0–36 U/L
Hemoglobin: 7.9 g/dL	13.5–17.5 g/dL

Patient's Values	Normal Values
Hematocrit: 29%	41–53%
White blood cells: 32 tho/μL	4.0–11.0 tho/μL
Prothrombin time: 27 seconds	<15 seconds
Platelet count: 1,315,000/mm^3	150,000–450,000/mm^3

Hospital Course and Therapy

Upon admission to the hospital, a nasogastric tube was placed and his nausea and vomiting resolved. He was also placed on NPO (nothing to eat or drink) restrictions. His nasogastric tube drained 800 to 1200 mL of feculent fluid the first day. At the same time, he was rehydrated with IV fluids consisting of D$_5$1/2 normal saline. However, 24 hours after admission he continued to experience abdominal pain and his nausea and vomiting recurred when the nasogastric tube was clamped.

The surgical team decided to take AJ to the operating room to perform an exploratory laparotomy. The findings of the procedure were an occlusive tumor mass of 3.9 centimeters located at the sigmoid colon, with necrosis of the entire colon proximal to the tumor. AJ had a total colectomy, with Hartmann's procedure and an ileostomy. The histopathological examination reported a well differentiated adenocarcinoma of the colon, Dukes–Ashley B, with free surgical margins and acute necrotizing colitis proximal to obstructing neoplasm. AJ was transferred to the ICU after surgery. He required mechanical ventilation for 5 days. After correction of his volume deficit, AJ's serum creatinine dropped to 1.2 mg/dL. There was no evidence of renal failure.

Case Questions

1. List AJ's possible medical problems demonstrated by his overall clinical picture.
2. What are the possible etiologies of AJ's bowel obstruction?
3. What additional evidence from AJ's physical examination could be used to assess his nutritional status prior to initiating parenteral nutrition?
4. Why is parenteral nutrition the most appropriate form of nutritional intervention at this point in AJ's clinical course?
5. Using the Harris–Benedict equation, calculate AJ's resting energy expenditure (REE); also calculate AJ's protein requirement, and maximum carbohydrate and lipid oxidation rates. How much dextrose and lipid should be ordered in the PN?
6. What biochemical laboratory data should be used to monitor AJ while he is on PN?
7. Once AJ's abdominal sepsis and septic complications resolved and his bowel sounds showed increased activity, he was advanced to an oral diet. How should AJ's feeding begin and what recommendations are appropriate upon discharge?

Answers to Questions: Case 1

1. List AJ's possible medical problems demonstrated by his overall clinical picture.

- Bowel obstruction (mechanical?) as evidenced by distended loops of small intestine and no air in rectum on abdominal X-rays and feculent fluid obtained from the nasogastric tube.

- Mesenteric thrombosis? (Consider his past medical history of stroke.)
- Severe electrolyte imbalance demonstrated by hyperkalemia, elevated BUN and creatinine.
- Bilateral pneumonia?
- Unintentional weight loss and severe undernutrition.

2. What are the possible etiologies of AJ's bowel obstruction?

In a compilation of the overall causes of intestinal obstruction (both small and large bowel), taken from thirteen reported series comprising a total of 12,731 adult patients, hernia accounted for 40 percent of the causes of the obstruction; adhesions 29 percent, 12 percent intussusception, and cancer 10 percent. However, in elderly patients, the main cause of large intestinal obstruction is colon cancer (70 percent of the cases), followed by diverticulitis (5 percent), and volvulus (10 percent). The symptoms are often insidious, though in most cases acute obstruction is the direct reason for calling a surgical consult. Diarrhea, with the passage of blood and mucus, may result from an ulceration of the bowel. The occurrence of diarrhea may lead patients to assert that their bowel function is regular, whereas the looseness is secondary to the irritation caused by constipation as in AJ's case.

3. What additional evidence from AJ's physical examination could be used to assess his nutritional status prior to initiating parenteral nutrition?

Evidence of undernutrition includes decreased food intake, significant unintentional weight loss, decreased albumin level, and thin appearance. Serum albumin is low, which could indicate undernutrition, but could also indicate hemodilution or the presence of an inflammatory response. Undernutrition plays an important role in the rate of post-operative complications that interfere with surgical activity, impairing immune response mechanisms. Synthesis and regeneration processes are affected and the ability to fight infection is altered. The GI tract must be supported during critical illness to accomplish rapid cellular turnover rate and the metabolic and immunologic adaptation to severe stress. Disruption in the ecologic equilibrium of the GI tract often occurs during critical illness. This damaged equilibrium may cause bacterial translocation, sepsis, and the systemic inflammatory response syndrome (SIRS). Bacterial translocation occurs from the small intestine to the mesenteric lymph nodes, triggering a whole cascade of deleterious events that could lead to multi-organic dysfunction syndrome (MODS) and death.

4. Why is parenteral nutrition the most appropriate form of nutritional intervention at this point in AJ's clinical course?

AJ has malnutrition, inflammatory metabolism, abdominal sepsis, cancer, and impaired intestinal function. Therefore, PN should be initiated to prevent further undernutrition and as a method for nutrition support.

Immunonutrition could be considered as an alternative approach for this case. In a meta-analysis of 11 randomized controlled trials accounting of 1009 patients, immunonutrition proved to be effective in reducing the risk of infectious complications and length-of-stay in "critically ill" patients and in patients with GI cancer, as compared with patients receiving standard nutritional support.

5. Using the Harris–Benedict equation, calculate AJ's resting energy expenditure (REE); also calculate AJ's protein goal and maximum carbohydrate and lipid oxidation rates. How much dextrose and lipid should be ordered in the PN?

$$\text{REE} = 66 + 13.7 \text{ (weight in kg)} + 5 \text{ (height in cm)} - 6.8 \text{ (age)} =$$
$$66 + 13.7 \text{ (45)} + 5 \text{ (170 cm)} - 6.8 \text{ (73)} = 1035 \text{ kcal/day}$$

Total daily calorie needs with activity factor for in-bed patient = REE $\times$ 1.45 = 1500 kcal/day

Protein goals = Current weight X 1.3 g/kg = 45 kg X 1.45 g/kg = 65 g/day

(Protein restriction is based on patient's initial renal parameters; when renal function normalizes, protein goal can be increased to 1.5 g/kg per day.)

Maximum glucose oxidation rate is 5 to 7 mg per kg per minute in hospitalized patients but parenteral carbohydrate infusion should not exceed 4 mg per kg per minute in the critically ill. At 3.4 kcal per gram hydrated dextrose, the maximum dextrose infusion should not exceed 880 kcal/day. Maximum lipid oxidation rate is 2.5 grams per kg per day and fat has 9 kcal per gram. The caloric equivalent of this lipid load is 1000 kcal. Many nutrition support specialists advocate an upper limit of 1.0 grams lipid per kg body weight, which for AJ would be 45 g (405 kcal per day). There could be some consideration to eliminate or severely limit IV fat for the first week, in an attempt to avoid stimulating eicosanoid pathways that would promote inflammation and down-regulate cellular immunity, especially when a long chained triglycerides mixture of lipid emulsion is used. Dextrose infusion should be started in the PN (aim to keep serum glucose maintained at less than 150 mg per dL). With a goal of 1500 kcal per day, a protein calorie contribution of 280 kcal per day (70 grams amino acid $\times$ 4.0 kcal per gram), and a lipid intake of 1.0 grams per kg body weight, dextrose calorie infusion will be 660 kcal per day (3.0 mg per kg per minute). The initial infusion can be lower than goal to assess the metabolic response to the PN especially in a chronically malnourished patient who is at risk for refeeding syndrome. Insulin may be necessary to control the blood glucose. Insulin can be added directly to the PN bag based on initial use of sliding scale if requirements remain stable.

6. What biochemical laboratory data should be used to monitor AJ while he is on PN?

- Sodium, potassium, chloride, CO_2, BUN, creatinine, calcium, magnesium, phosphorus, and glucose should be measured daily. Daily electrolyte replacement in PN solution is designed to replenish any losses noted in the previous day's labs. When these laboratory data become stable and normal, frequency of checking may be able to be reduced.
- Liver function tests, albumin or prealbumin weekly; transferrin, and triglycerides every few weeks.
- A 24-hour urine collection can be made weekly for measurement of urine urea nitrogen. With this information, nitrogen balance can be calculated (nitrogen

balance = nitrogen intake − nitrogen excretion), and the protein content of the PN can be adjusted as required. To calculate nitrogen excretion the recommended formula is

- Nitrogen urinary excretion (g/dL) = Urinary nitrogen × 1.25 + 4

7. Once AJ's abdominal sepsis and septic complications were resolved and his bowel sounds showed increased activity, he was advanced to an oral diet. How should AJ's feeding begin and what recommendations are appropriate upon discharge?

Oral feedings should begin with a clear liquid diet and be gradually advanced as tolerated, eventually to regular food. PN should not be discontinued until AJ tolerates 75 percent of his requirements through the oral diet, however, PN should be weaned accordingly as oral intake increases in order to avoid overfeeding. Tube feeding should be considered if the patient cannot consume adequate nutrition by mouth but has a functional GI tract. Evaluation of the patient's nutritional progress should be included in any follow-up visits to his physician.

Chapter and Case References

A.S.P.E.N. Board of Directors and the Task Force for the revision of safe practices for parenteral nutrition. *J Parenter Enteral Nutr.* 2004;28(suppl):S38–S70.

Berenholtz SM, Pronovost PJ, Lipsett PA, et al. Eliminating catheter-related bloodstream infections in the intensive care unit. *Crit Care Med.* 2004;32:2014–2020.

Centers for Disease Control and Prevention. Guidelines for the prevention of intravascular catheter-related infections. *MMWR.* 2002;51(No. RR-10).

Clement S. Better glycemic control in the hospital: Beneficial and feasible. *CCJM.* 2007;74:111–120.

Donnelly SF, Foster SM, Bannon MP. 5 steps to prevent CVC-related infections. *Contemporary Surgery Online.* 2007.

Frankenfield DC, Roth-Yousey L, Compher C. Comparison of predictive equations for resting metabolic rate in healthy nonobese and obese individuals, a systematic review. *J Am Diet Assoc.* 2005;105:775–789.

Furnary AP, Zerr KJ, Grunkemeier GL, Starr A. Continuous intravenous insulin infusion reduces the incidence of deep sternal wound infection in diabetic patients after cardiac surgical procedures. *Ann Thorac Surg.* 1999;67:352–362.

Furnary AP, Gao G, Grunkemeier GL, et al. Continuous insulin infusion reduces mortality in patients with diabetes undergoing coronary artery bypass grafting. *J Thorac Cardiovasc Surg.* 2003;125:1007–1021.

Garber AJ, Moghissi ES, Bransome ED, et al. American College of Endocrinology position statement on inpatient diabetes and metabolic control. *Endocr Pract.* 2004;10(suppl 2):4–9.

Hanna H, Afif C, Alakech B, et al. Central venous catheter-related bacteremia due to gram-negative bacilli: significance of catheter removal in preventing relapse. *Infect Control Hosp Epidemiol.* 2004;25:646–649.

Harris JA, Benedict FG. A biometric Study of Basal Metabolism in Man. Publication No. 279. Washington, DC: Carnegie Institute; 1919.

Heys SD, Walker LG, Smith I, Eremin O. Enteral nutritional supplementation with key nutrients in patients with critical illness and cancer: a meta-analysis of randomized controlled trials; *Ann Surg.* 1999;229(4):467–77.

Issacs JW, Millikan WJ, Stackhouse J, et al. Parenteral nutrition of adults with 900-milliosmolar solution via peripheral vein. *Am J Clin Nutr.* 1977;30:552–559.

Kusminsky RE. Complications of central venous catheterization. *J Am Coll Surg.* 2007;204:681–696.

Lee S, Gura KM, Kim S, et al. Current clinical applications of omega-6 and omega-3 fatty acids. *Nutr Clin Pract.* 2006;21(4): 323–41, 417.

McMahon MM. Diabetes Mellitus. In: The A.S.P.E.N. Nutrition Support Practice Manual, 2nd ed., Merritt R (ed.). American Society for Parenteral and Enteral Nutrition, 2005;317–323.

McGee DC, Gould MK. Preventing complications of central venous catheterization. *N Engl J Med.* 2003;348;1123–1133.

Mifflin MD, St. Jeor ST, Hill LA, et al. A new predictive equation for resting energy expenditure in healthy individuals. *Am J Clin Nutr.* 1990;51:241–247.

Mirtallo JM. Overview of Parenteral Nutrition. In: The A.S.P.E.N. Nutrition Support Core Curriculum: A Case-Based Approach, Gottschlich MM (editor). American Society for Parenteral and Enteral Nutrition, 2007;264–276.

Mizock BA, DeMichele SJ: The acute respiratory distress syndrome: role of nutritional modulation of inflammation through dietary lipids. *Nutr Clin Pract.* 2004;19;563.

Pomposelli JJ, Baxter JK, Babineau TJ, et al. Early post-operative glucose control predicts nosocomial infection rate in diabetic patients. *J Parenter Enteral Nutr.* 1998;22:77–81.

Thomas MC, Mathew TH, Russ GR, Rao MM, Moran J. Early peri-operative glycemic control and allograft refection in patients with diabetes mellitus: a pilot study. *Transplantation.* 2001;72:1321–1324.

Umpierrez GE, Issacs SD, Bazaragan N, et al. Hyperglycemia: an independent marker of in-hospital mortality in patients with undiagnosed diabetes. *J Clin Endocrinol Metab.* 2002;87:978–982.

van den Berghe G, Wouters P, Weekers F, et al. Intensive insulin therapy in the critically ill patient. *N Engl J Med.* 2001;345:1359–1367.

Waitzberg DL, Torrinhas RS, Jacintho TM. New parenteral lipid emulsions for clinical use. *JPEN.* 2006;30(4):351–67

Whitman ED. Complications associated with the use of central venous access devices. *Curr Probl Surg.* 1996;33:311–378.

Appendices

Developed by Susan Zogheib and Lisa Hark

Appendix A: Food sources of vitamin A

Appendix B: Food sources of vitamin D

Appendix C: Food sources of vitamin E

Appendix D: Food sources of vitamin K

Appendix E: Food sources of vitamin C

Appendix F: Food sources of folate

Appendix G: Food sources of calcium (dairy)

Appendix H: Food sources of calcium (non-dairy)

Appendix I: Sources of high-sodium foods

Appendix J: Food sources of potassium

Appendix K: Food sources of magnesium

Appendix L: Food sources of iron

Appendix M: Food sources of omega-3 fatty acids

Appendix N: Sources of high oxalic acid-foods and beverages

Appendix O: Food sources of dietary fiber

Appendix P: Food sources of purine

*Appendices A–P used *www.nutritiondata.com*

Appendix A Food sources of vitamin A.

Food, Standard Amount	Serving Size	Vitamin A (μg RE)
Margarine	1 Tbsp	
Liver (beef, veal, goose, and turkey)	3 oz	13,000–19,000
Liver (chicken, lamb)	3 oz	6000–10,000
Various ready-to-eat cereals, with added Vitamin A	1 oz	180–376
Instant cooked cereals, fortified	1 packet	285–376
Beets	1 cup	3.4
Apricots, dried	$\frac{1}{2}$ cup	80
Broccoli, fresh, cooked	1 cup	120.2
Herring, Atlantic	3 oz	219
Cantaloupe, raw	$\frac{1}{4}$ medium melon	233
Chinese cabbage, cooked	1 cup	360
Red sweet pepper, cooked	1 cup	371
Peppers, chili	1 cup	405
Mustard greens, cooked	1 cup	442
Milk, (all types) with added vitamin A	1 cup	478
Winter squash, cooked	1 cup	535
Turnip greens, cooked from frozen	1 cup	549
Collards, cooked from frozen	1 cup	771
Kale, cooked from frozen	1 cup	885
Spinach, cooked from frozen	1 cup	943
Mixed vegetables, canned	1 cup	949
Pumpkin, canned	$\frac{1}{2}$ cup	953
Carrots, raw	1 cup	1026
Sweet potato with peel, baked	1 medium	1096
Mango, raw	1 cup	1262
Carrot juice	$\frac{3}{4}$ cup	1692
Tomatoes and vegetable juice	1 cup	3770
Fish oil, cod liver	1 Tbsp	4051

Source: www.nutritiondata.com

Appendix B Food sources of vitamin D.

Food, Standard Amount	Serving Size	Vitamin D (IU)
Herring, Atlantic	3 oz	1384
Fish oil, cod liver	1 Tbsp	1350
Fish, sardines, salmon, codfish	3 oz	649–71.4
Catfish	3 oz	425
Oysters	3 oz	268.8
Egg, yolk, raw, fresh	1 large	260
Milk (all types)	1 cup	299–97.6
Milk, whole	1 cup	100
Margarine	1 Tbsp	60
Cereals ready-to-eat	1 cup	126–88
Butter, salted	1 Tbsp	7.8
Cheddar Cheese	1.5 oz	5.1

Source: www.nutritiondata.com

Appendix C Food sources of vitamin E.

Food, Standard Amount	Serving Size	Alpha Tocopherol (mg)
Fortified ready-to-eat cereals	1 cup	33.8–13.5
Sunflower seeds, dry roasted	1 oz	7.4
Almonds	1 oz	7.3
Sunflower oil	1 Tbsp	5.6
Tomato sauce	1 cup	5.0
Safflower oil	1 Tbsp	4.6
Spinach, frozen, cooked	1 cup	3.7
Swiss chard, cooked	1 cup	3.3
Mixed nuts, dry roasted	1 oz	3.1
Turnip greens, frozen, cooked	1 cup	2.7
Pine nuts	1 oz	2.6
Peanut butter	2 Tbsp	2.5
Canola oil	1 Tbsp	2.4
Wheat germ, toasted, plain	2 Tbsp	2.3
Peanuts	1 oz	2.2
Avocado, raw	½ avocado	2.1
Carrot juice, canned	¾ cup	2.1
Corn oil and olive oil	1 Tbsp	1.9
Mustard greens, frozen, cooked	1 cup	1.7
Sardine, Atlantic, in oil, drained	3 oz	1.7
Radicchio	1 cup	0.9
Herring, Atlantic	3 oz	0.9
Margarine	1 Tbsp	0.8
Salad dressing (Italian)	1 Tbsp	0.7

Source: www.nutritiondata.com

Appendix D   Food sources of vitamin K.

Phyloquinone per Food, Standard Amount	Serving Size	serving (μg)
Kale, frozen, cooked	1 cup	1062
Collard greens, frozen, cooked	1 cup	1060
Spinach, frozen, cooked	1 cup	889
Turnip greens, frozen, cooked	1 cup	529
Mustard greens, frozen, cooked	1 cup	419
Parsley, raw	¼ cup	246
Brussels sprouts, fresh	1 cup	218
Broccoli, fresh	1 cup	110
Asparagus, fresh	1 cup	91
Okra, frozen, cooked	1 cup	88
Cabbage, fresh	1 cup	67.6
Green peas, frozen, cooked	1 cup	38.4
Cauliflower	1 cup	17.2
Celery, raw	1 medium stalk	17
Carrot, raw	1 cup	16.1
Grapes, red/green, seedless, raw	1 ½ cup	12
Plums, raw	2 medium	11
Pear, raw	1 medium	8.1
Tomato juice, bottled	8 fluid oz	5.6
Tomato, red, raw	1 medium	4.4
Avocado, raw	⅕ medium	4.3
Apricot, raw	½ cup	2.5

Source: www.nutritiondata.com

Appendix E Food sources of vitamin C.

Food, Standard Amount	Serving Size	Vitamin C (mg)
Guava, raw	½ cup	188
Peppers (all types), raw	1 cup	155
Peppers (all types) cooked	1 cup	150
Broccoli, cooked	1 cup	101.2
Strawberries, raw	1 cup	100
Brussels sprouts, cooked	1 cup	96.8
Kohlrabi, cooked	1 cup	90
Broccoli, raw	1 cup	81.2
Peas, Snowpeas, Sugar snap peas, cooked	1 cup	76.6
Kiwi fruit	1 medium	70
Orange, raw	1 medium	70
Orange juice	¾ cup	61–93
Peas, edible-podded, raw [Snowpeas, Sugar snap peas]	1 cup	58.8
Tangerines, (mandarin oranges), raw	1 cup	52.1
Green pepper, sweet, cooked	½ cup	51
Grapefruit juice	¾ cup	50–70
Vegetable juice cocktail	¾ cup	50
Cantaloupe	¼ medium	47
Papaya, raw	¼ medium	47
Tomato juice	¾ cup	33
Raspberries, raw	1 cup	32.2
Melons, honeydew, raw	1 cup	31.9
Sweet potato, cooked	1 medium	22.3

Source: www.nutritiondata.com

Appendix F Food sources of folate.

Food, Standard Amount	Serving Size	Folate (μg)
Ready-to-eat cereals	1 cup	1010
Chicken liver	3 oz	495
Beef liver	3 oz	243.6
Spinach, frozen, cooked	1 cup	230
Lentils, cooked	½ cup	180
Tomato	1 medium	75–97
Mustard and turnip greens, frozen, cooked	1 cup	170
Seaweed, kelp, raw	1 cup	144
Chickpeas, canned	½ cup	140
Okra, frozen, cooked	1 cup	134
Collard greens, frozen, cooked	1 cup	129
Asparagus, fresh, cooked	1 cup	121.2
Peas, green, boiled	1 cup	94.4
Brussels sprouts, raw	1 cup	93.6
Broccoli, fresh, cooked	1 cup	84.2
Lettuce, romaine	1 cup	63.9
Orange juice	6 oz	55.8
Cauliflower	1 cup	54.6
Potato, baked with skin	1 medium	40
Egg, boiled	1 large	24

Source: www.nutritiondata.com

Appendix G Food sources of calcium (dairy).

Food, Standard Amount	Serving Size	Calcium (mg)
Lactose-Free Calcium Fortified Milk	1 cup	500
Plain yogurt, non-fat	8 oz	452
Romano cheese	1.5 oz	452
Plain yogurt, low-fat	8 oz	415
Soy Milk, calcium fortified	1 cup	368
Fruit yogurt, low-fat	8 oz	345
Swiss cheese	1.5 oz	336
Ricotta cheese, part skim	½ cup	335
Pasteurized process Swiss cheese	1.5 oz	324
Provolone cheese	1.5 oz	321
Egg, yolk, raw, fresh	1 large	313
Mozzarella cheese, part-skim	1.5 oz	311
Cheddar cheese	1.5 oz	307
Fat-free (skim) milk	1 cup	306
Muenster cheese	1.5 oz	305
1% low-fat milk	1 cup	290
Low-fat chocolate milk (1%)	1 cup	288
2% reduced fat milk	1 cup	285
Reduced fat chocolate milk (2%)	1 cup	285
Buttermilk, low-fat	1 cup	284
Chocolate milk	1 cup	280
Whole milk	1 cup	276
Yogurt, plain, whole milk	8 oz	275
Ricotta cheese, whole milk	½ cup	255
Pasteurized process American cheese food	1.5 oz	232
Blue cheese	1.5 oz	225
Mozzarella cheese, whole milk	1.5 oz	215
Feta cheese	1.5 oz	210

Source: www.nutritiondata.com

Appendix H Food sources of calcium (non-dairy).

Food, Standard Amount	Serving Size	Calcium (mg)
Soy beverage, calcium fortified	1 cup	368
Collard greens, frozen, cooked	1 cup	357
Sardines, Atlantic, in oil, drained	3 oz	325
Tofu, firm, prepared with nigari	1/2 cup	253
Spinach, frozen, cooked	1 cup	245
Turnip greens, frozen, cooked	1 cup	197
Pink salmon, canned, with bone	3 oz	181
Okra, frozen, cooked	1 cup	176
Molasses, blackstrap	1 Tbsp	172
Beet greens, fresh, cooked	1 cup	164
Pak-choi, Chinese cabbage, cooked from fresh	1 cup	158
Soybeans, green, cooked	1/2 cup	130
Ocean perch, Atlantic, cooked	3 oz	116
White beans, canned	1/2 cup	96
Kale, frozen, cooked	1 cup	93.6
Clams, canned	3 oz	78
Nuts, almonds, oil roasted	1 oz	74.5
Rainbow trout, farmed, cooked	3 oz	73
Oatmeal, plain and flavored, instant, fortified	1 packet prepared	99–110

Source: www.nutritiondata.com

Appendix I Food sources of sodium.

Food, Standard Amount	Serving Size	Sodium (mg)
Salt (sodium chloride)	1 tsp	2325
Pickle relish, sweet	1 cup	1987
Soup, canned (all types)	1 cup	850–2500
Tomato sauce	1 cup	1284
Soy sauce made from soy (tamari)	1 Tbsp	1006
Sauerkraut, canned	1 cup	939
Chicken Pot pie, frozen entree	1 pie	841
Potato chips, regular and baked	1 bag (1 oz)	837
Pretzels, hard, plain, salted	10 twists	814
Cheese American	1.5 oz	670
Tomato juice, canned, with salt added	1 cup	654
Vegetable juice cocktail, canned	1 cup	653
Pickles, kosher dill	1 medium	569
Beef frankfurter, hot dog	1 frank	461
Olives, canned or bottled, green	1 oz	440
Scrapple, pork	2 oz	369
Gravy, canned	$\frac{1}{4}$ cup	352
Canned tuna	3 oz	320
Canned vegetables	1 cup	243
Lunch meats (turkey, ham, salami, pastrami)	3 slices	250–500
Barbeque Sauce	1 Tbsp	212
Noodles, Chinese, chow mein	1 cup	198
Cheese Pizza	1 slice	194
Beef sausage, fresh, cooked	1 oz	184
Salad dressings	1 Tbsp	147
Peanuts, oil-roasted, with salt	1 oz	121
Frozen Dinner	1 dinner	360–768

Source: www.nutritiondata.com

Appendix J Food sources of potassium.

Food, Standard Amount	Serving Size	Potassium (mg)
Beet greens, cooked	1 cup	1309
Spinach, cooked	1 cup	839
Tomato sauce	1 cup	810
Sweet potato, baked	1 medium	694
Potato, baked, flesh	1 medium	610
White beans, canned	½ cup	595
Yogurt, plain, non-fat	8 oz	579
Tomato puree	½ cup	549
Clams, canned	3 oz	534
Yogurt, plain, low-fat	8 oz	531
Prune juice	¾ cup	530
Carrot juice	¾ cup	517
Apricots, dried	½ cup	514
Blackstrap molasses	1 Tbsp.	498
Halibut, cooked	3 oz	490
Soybeans, green, cooked	½ cup	485
Tuna, yellow fin, cooked	3 oz	484
Lima beans, cooked	½ cup	484
Artichokes, (globe or French), raw	1 artichoke	474
Winter squash, cooked	1 cup	449
Soybeans, mature, cooked	½ cup	443
Rockfish, Pacific, cooked	3 oz	442
Cod, Pacific, cooked	3 oz	439
Bananas	1 medium	422
Tomato juice	¾ cup	417
Peaches, fresh	1 medium	398
Prunes, stewed	½ cup	398
Milk, non-fat	1 cup	382
Pork chop, center loin, cooked	3 oz	382
Rainbow trout, farmed, cooked	3 oz	375
Pork loin, center rib (roasts), lean, roasted	3 oz	371
Buttermilk, cultured, low-fat	1 cup	370
Cantaloupe	¼ medium	368
1%–2% milk	1 cup	366
Honeydew melon	⅛ medium	365
Lentils, cooked	½ cup	365
Plantains, cooked	½ cup slices	358
Kidney beans, cooked	½ cup	358
Orange juice	¾ cup	355
Split peas, cooked	½ cup	355
Yogurt, plain, whole milk	8 oz container	352

Source: www.nutritiondata.com

Appendix K Food sources of magnesium.

Food, Standard Amount	Serving Size	Magnesium (mg)
Beet greens, cooked	1 cup	97.9
Okra, cooked from frozen	1 cup	93.8
Halibut, cooked	3 oz	91
Quinoa, dry	¼ cup	89
Almonds	1 oz	78
Soybeans, mature, cooked	½ cup	74
Nuts, (various types)	1 oz	70–107
White beans	½ cup	67
Pollock, walleye, cooked	3 oz	62
Black beans, cooked	½ cup	60
Oat bran, raw	¼ cup	55
Soybeans, green, cooked	½ cup	54
Tuna, yellow fin, cooked	3 oz	54
Lima beans, baby, cooked from frozen	½ cup	50
Navy beans, cooked	½ cup	48
Tofu, firm, prepared with nigari	½ cup	47
Soy beverage	1 cup	47
Cowpeas, cooked	½ cup	46
Hazelnuts	1 oz	46
Great northern beans, cooked	½ cup	44
Oat bran, cooked	½ cup	44
Buckwheat groats, roasted, cooked	½ cup	43
Brown rice, cooked	½ cup	42
Haddock, cooked	3 oz	42
Spinach, frozen, cooked	1 cup	157
Pumpkin and squash seed kernels, roasted	1 oz	151
Bran ready-to-eat cereal (100%)	1 oz	103

Source: www.nutritiondata.com

Appendix L Food sources of iron.

Food, Standard Amount	Serving Size	Iron (mg)
Spinach, frozen, cooked	1 cup	6.4
Liver (various types) cooked	3 oz	5.0–9.9
Fortified instant cooked cereals (various)	1 packet	5.0–8.1
Soybeans, mature, cooked	½ cup	4.4
Pumpkin and squash seed kernels, roasted	1 oz	4.2
White beans, canned	½ cup	3.9
Blackstrap molasses	1 Tbsp	3.5
Lentils, cooked	½ cup	3.3
Fortified ready-to-eat cereals (various)	1 cup	19–28
Clams, canned, drained	3 oz	23.8
Clams, canned	3 oz	23.8
Kidney beans, cooked	½ cup	2.6
Sardines, canned in oil, drained	3 oz	2.5
Chickpeas, cooked	½ cup	2.4
Duck, meat only, roasted	3 oz	2.3
Prune juice	¾ cup	2.3
Shrimp, canned	3 oz	2.3
Cowpeas, cooked	½ cup	2.2
Ground beef, 15% fat, cooked	3 oz	2.2
Tomato puree	½ cup	2.2
Lima beans, cooked	½ cup	2.2
Soybeans, green, cooked	½ cup	2.2
Navy beans, cooked	½ cup	2.1
Refried beans	½ cup	2.1
Tomato paste	¼ cup	2.0
Oysters, eastern, wild, cooked	3 oz	10.2
Beef, lean ground, raw	3 oz	1.5
Beef, sirloin steak or filet mignon, raw	3 oz	1.2
Lamb, shoulder, arm, raw	3 oz	1.1

Source: www.nutritiondata.com

Appendix M Food sources of omega-3 fatty acids.

Food, Standard Amount	Serving Size	Omega-3 FA (g)
Flaxseed oil	1 Tbsp	6.7
Salmon, Atlantic, wild, cooked	3.0 oz	2.198
Flaxseeds	1 Tbsp	2.63
Walnuts	1 oz	2.5
Soybeans, cooked	½ cup	2.1
Canola oil	1 Tbsp	1.4
Walnut oil	1 Tbsp	1.3
Sardine	3.0 oz	1.2
Tuna, white, canned in water	3.0 oz	0.81
Wheat germ oil	1 Tbsp	0.86

Source: www.nutritiondata.com

Appendix N Food sources of oxalic acid.

Food, Standard Amount	Serving Size	Oxalic acid (mg)
Spinach, frozen	1 cup	1230
Beans in tomato sauce	1 cup	1148
Beetroot, pickled	1 cup	1135
Chard, Swish, boiled	1 cup	1129
Spinach, boiled	1 cup	420
Okra, boiled	1 cup	234
Chard, Swiss, raw	1 cup	232
Tea, Indian, 6 minute infusion	1 cup	185
Potato, sweet, boiled, mashed	1 cup	184
Peanuts, roasted	2 oz	137
Cocoa, dry powder	¼ cup	134
Berries, green goose	1 cup	132
Crackers, soybean	2 oz	118
Pecans	2 oz	111
Leeks, raw, boiled	1 cup	110
Grits, white corn, cooked	1 cup	99
Collards, raw, boiled	1 cup	95
Chocolate, plain	2 oz	66
Raspberries, black	1 cup	65
Parsley, raw	1 cup	64
Grapes, concord	1 cup	40
Squash, summer	1 cup	40
Berries, black	1 cup	26
Celery	1 cup	24
Berries, blue	1 cup	22
Wheat germ	1 Tbsp	19
Raspberries, red	1 cup	18
Eggplant, boiled	1 cup	17
Dandelion greens, raw	1 cup	14
Pepper, green	1 cup	12
Escarole, raw	1 cup	9

Source: www.nutritiondata.com

Appendix O   Food sources of dietary fiber.

Food, Standard Amount	Serving Size	Dietary Fiber (g)
Cereal, All-Bran	1 cup	25.8
Wheat bran	1 cup	24.6
Cereal, Fiber One	1 cup	23.8
White beans, great-northern, canned	1 cup	14.4
Kidney beans, red, cooked	1 cup	13.8
Navy beans, cooked	1 cup	13.0
Black beans, cooked	1 cup	12.2
Pinto beans, cooked	1 cup	11.8
Lentils, cooked	1 cup	10.4
White beans, great northern beans, cooked	1 cup	10.0
Lima beans, canned	1 cup	8.6
Chickpeas, cooked	1 cup	8.6
Peas, cooked	1 cup	8.6
Peas, green, cooked	1 cup	8.6
Okra, frozen, cooked	1 cup	8.2
Brussels sprouts, cooked	1 cup	7.6
Split peas, cooked	1 cup	6.2
Pear, fresh with skin	1 small	6.0
Cracker, Matzo	6 crackers	6.0
Bread, pumpernickel	2 slices	5.4
Spaghetti, whole-wheat, cooked	1 cup	5.4
Figs, dried	3 pieces	4.6
Carrots, cooked	1 cup	4.0
Applesauce, canned, unsweetened	1 cup	4.0
Prunes, dried, stewed	6 pieces	3.4
Raspberries, fresh	1 cup	3.3
Spinach, cooked	1 cup	3.2
Orange, fresh without skin	1 small	3.0
Carrots, canned	1 cup	3.0
Apple, fresh with skin	1 small	2.8

Source: www.nutritiondata.com

Appendix P Food sources of purine.

Food, Standard Amount	Purine (mg/100 g)
Sweetbreads	825
Anchovies	363
Brains	363
Sardines	295
Scallops	295
Liver, calf/beef	233
Mackerel	233
Kidney, beef	200
Game meats	200
Herring	200
Asparagus	50–150
Bread and cereals, whole grain	50–150
Cauliflower	50–150
Fish, fresh and saltwater	50–150
Legumes, beans/lentils/peas	50–150
Meat-beef/lamb/pork/veal	50–150
Mushrooms	50–150
Oatmeal	50–150
Peas, green	50–150
Poultry, chicken/duck/turkey	50–150
Shellfish, crab/lobster/oysters	50–150
Spinach	50–150
Wheat germ and bran	50–150

Source: www.nutritiondata.com

Review Questions

Chapter 1 Overview of Nutrition Assessment in Clinical Care

1. When reviewing a patient's medical record, where would information regarding the patient's use of vitamins, minerals, or dietary supplements be found in the chart?

a. Past medical history
b. Family history
c. Social history
d. Review of systems

2. Body mass index (BMI) may not accurately reflect body fat in which of the following individuals?

a. Underweight individuals
b. Normal weight individuals
c. Overweight individuals
d. Obese individuals

3. Why should waist circumference (WC) be measured only in patients with a BMI measurement less that 35 kg/m²?

a. WC measurement is not accurate in obese patients
b. Because it confers little additional information about risk
c. WC cutoff thresholds do not apply in obese patients
d. Tape measures are difficult to find at that length

4. Which of the following tissues are most sensitive to vitamin and mineral deficiencies and likely to appear abnormal on physical examination?

a. Skin
b. Nails
c. Mouth
d. All of the above

5. When interpreting serum albumin in hospitalized patients, levels may decrease irrespective of nutritional status in which of the following conditions?

a. Dehydration
b. Liver disease
c. Diabetes
d. Stroke

6. The energy and protein requirements of hospitalized and critically ill patients should be calculated separately. Which of the following value ranges is recommended to calculate the protein needs of post-surgical patients who are not highly catabolic?

a. 0.6–1.0 grams/kg per day
b. 1.0–1.4 grams/kg per day
c. 1.5–2.0 grams/kg per day
d. 2.0–2.5 grams/kg per day

7. Diagnosis of underweight patients includes assessment of a patient's BMI. Which of the following BMI values would indicate a risk of undernutrition in a patient who is consistently underweight?

a. $<18.5 \text{ kg/m}^2$
b. $<19.5 \text{ kg/m}^2$
c. $<20.5 \text{ kg/m}^2$
d. $<21.5 \text{ kg/m}^2$

8. The healthcare costs associated with obesity in the United States have skyrocketed due to the increased prevalence of obesity. Economists estimate that medical expenses and loss of productivity will cost US businesses approximately how much money on an annual basis in 2009?

a. $100 million/year
b. $500 million/year
c. $20 billion/year
d. $45 billion/year

9. According to the CDC, more than 30 percent of US adults are obese. Which of the following age groups had the highest prevalence of obesity compared to other age groups in 2006, even after controlling for gender, race, and ethnicity?

a. 20–29 years
b. 30–39 years
c. 40–59 years
d. 60–79 years

10. MG is a 55-year-old woman who has been overweight most of her adult life. She comes to her internist for her annual physical examination and laboratory data reveal the following results:

Blood pressure: 133/86 mm Hg   WC: 36" Triglycerides: 230 mg/dL
HDL-C: 60 mg/dL   Glucose: 98 mg/dL

Her doctor suspects she has metabolic syndrome. How many of the metabolic syndrome criteria does she meet based on these results?

a. 1
b. 2

c. 3
d. 4

11. FL is a 48-year-old obese man who questions his doctor about the side effects and benefits of bariatric surgery. Which of the following procedures has been shown to have the least amount of postoperative side effects?

a. Gastric banding
b. Gastric bypass
c. Roux-en-Y procedure
d. Whipples procedure

12. Side effects associated with Roux-en-Y bariatric surgery frequently include the GI tract. Which of the following GI side effects occurs in approximately 70 percent of patients following this type of procedure?

a. Inflammatory bowel disease
b. Irritable bowel syndrome
c. Dumping syndrome
d. Lactose intolerance

13. JT is a 39-year-old female who recently underwent gastric bypass surgery. She presents to her primary care physician 6 months postoperatively complaining of headaches, fatigue, and being cold all the time. Which of the following deficiencies is most likely associated with these symptoms in patients who have undergone gastric bypass surgery?

a. Vitamin C
b. Riboflavin
c. Zinc
d. Iron

14. PC is a 26-year-old male who attends a worksite wellness program at his place of employment. He is motivated to lose weight and attempts to follow a strict diet. After one month he has lost 20 pounds but is diagnosed with kidney stones, which have been extremely painful. Blood and urine tests reveal uricosuria and hyperuricemia. Which of the following diet programs was PC most likely adhering to?

a. Low-fat, high-fiber
b. Low-carbohydrate, high-protein
c. Low-sodium, low-protein
d. Juice detox

Chapter 2 Vitamins, Minerals, and Dietary Supplements

1. EF is a 56-year-old male who was treated for Crohn's disease with a resection of his terminal ileum. He has not taken any vitamin supplements following this procedure. He presents to his primary care physician complaining of numbness and tingling in his hands and feet. Which of the following vitamin deficiency should be suspected?

a. Vitamin C
b. Vitamin D
c. Vitamin B_{12}
d. Vitamin K

2. CF is an 18-year-old teenager who comes to his primary care physician complaining of headaches and blurred vision. He has started taking large doses of vitamins because he read on the Internet that it would improve his acne. Mega doses of which of the following vitamins could contribute to headaches and blurred vision (above the tolerable upper limit recommendation)?

a. Vitamin A
b. Vitamin B_{12}
c. Vitamin E
d. Vitamin B_6

3. NS is an 16-year-old teenage boy who has been taking the antibiotic Minocycline for acne for the past 5 years. What vitamin deficiency is NS at risk of developing?

a. Vitamin B_{12}
b. Vitamin C
c. Vitamin K
d. Vitamin A

4. GM is a 35-year-old homeless man who presents to the Emergency Department with a red, swollen tongue, soreness of the lips and mouth, dermatitis, and diarrhea. Which of the following vitamin deficiencies should be suspected in this patient?

a. Vitamin C deficiency
b. Iron deficiency
c. Niacin deficiency
d. Folate deficiency

5. Which of the following minerals functions as an antioxidant as a component of enzymes that protect cells from the damaging effects of free radicals?

a. Zinc
b. Selenium
c. Potassium
d. Chromium

6. According to the 2005 *U.S. Dietary Guidelines*, what is the recommended sodium intake for the population?

a. Less than 1500 mg/day
b. Less than 2300 mg/day
c. Less than 3200 mg/day
d. Less than 4400 mg/day

7. LF is a 22-year-old female who complains of weakness, fatigue, and feeling cold. When asked about her diet, she admits that she switched to a vegetarian diet six months ago and has been avoiding meat, chicken, and fish. Which of the following mineral deficiencies should be suspected in this patient?

a. Magnesium
b. Phosphorus
c. Iron
d. Calcium

8. DC is a 65-year-old female who complains of weakness and shortness of breath. She has been taking large doses of magnesium and aluminum containing antacids at each meal for dyspepsia. For the past two years, she has also been following a bland diet. Which of the following mineral deficiencies should be suspected in this patient?

a. Chromium
b. Phosphorus
c. Calcium
d. Selenium

9. TL is a 74-year-old female with a medical history of osteoporosis and a hip fracture two years ago. She has been taking 1000 mg/day of calcium for at least 10 years and now requests information about vitamin D. She lives in an independent living facility in Boston. How much vitamin D_3 should be prescribed to TL based on the RDA?

a. 200 IU/day
b. 300 IU/day
c. 500 IU/day
d. 800 IU/day

10. Which of the following laboratory measures is the best determinant of iron status in a normal 18-year-old female with regular menses and no chronic health problems?

a. Ferritin
b. Transferrin saturation
c. Hemoglobin
d. Total iron-binding capacity

11. VF is a 43-year-old female with a history of hypertension who is managed with a diuretic and beta-blocker. She presents to her primary care physician complaining of weakness. She is diagnosed with hypokalemia. Which of the following foods should she be advised to increase?

a. Tunafish
b. Orange juice
c. Oatmeal
d. Eggs

12. HV is a 42-year-old male who recently broke his hip after falling off his bike during a race. He is currently taking warfarin to reduce his chance of blood clotting. The function of which of the following vitamins is inhibited by warfarin therapy?

a. Vitamin E
b. Vitamin A
c. Vitamin D
d. Vitamin K

13. When taken alone, in doses ranging from 300 to 900 mg/day, St. John's Wort has been shown to be moderately effective in the treatment of which for the following conditions

a. Mild-to-moderate depressive symptoms
b. Type 2 diabetes
c. Hypertension
d. Osteoarthritis

Chapter 3 Nutrition in Pregnancy and Lactation

1. BC is a 16-year-old teenager who comes to her family doctor for the first time at 12 weeks gestation. She has gained only a few pounds since she became pregnant. Based on her pre-pregnancy BMI ($22 kg/m^2$) what is the total amount of recommended weight gain during pregnancy according to the Institute of Medicine?

a. 10–15 pounds
b. 15–20 pounds
c. 20–30 pounds
d. 25–35 pounds

2. TC is a 28-year-old woman who has just found out that she is pregnant and asks her obstetrician about caffeine intake during pregnancy. She has had two previous miscarriages. She is very concerned about recent reports describing the increased risk of miscarriage related to excess caffeine intake. According to the

March of Dimes what is the current recommendation for limiting caffeine intake during pregnancy?

a. Less then 200 mg/day
b. Less then 300 mg/day
c. Less then 400 mg/day
d. Less then 500 mg/day

3. CT is a 31-year-old pregnant woman who comes to see her obstetrician for a routine prenatal visit. She is complaining of fatigue and her hemoglobin and hematocrit results indicate that she is anemic. Pregnant women are more likely to experience anemia in which of the following trimesters?

a. 1st trimester
b. 2nd trimester
c. 3rd trimester
d. There is no difference in the prevalence of anemia during pregnancy

4. DW is a 32-year-old obese woman who is 25 weeks in gestation. She is being screened for gestational diabetes by her obstetrician since she has a family history of type 2 diabetes. Which of the following results for a 1-hour, 50 gram glucose load would be considered a positive diagnosis for gestational diabetes?

a. 100–110 mg/dL
b. 110–120 mg/dL
c. 120–130 mg/dL
d. 130–140 mg/dL

5. Breast-fed infants may feed more often than formula-fed infants because breast milk empties from an infant's stomach slightly more rapidly than formula-fed infants. On average, what is the approximate time for emptying?

a. 1 hour
b. 1.5 hours
c. 2 hours
d. 3 hours

6. Nutritional requirements for certain macronutrients and micronutrients increase significantly during pregnancy. Which of the following nutrient requirements increases the most during pregnancy?

a. Protein
b. Fat
c. Carbohydrates
d. Fiber

7. JH is a 23-year-old woman who recently delivered a healthy, full-term infant. She is breastfeeding her 2-month old and complains to her family doctor about sore nipples. Which of the following strategies could help JH prevent and treat sore nipples associated with breastfeeding?

a. Apply moisturizer to the breast after feeding.
b. Clean the breasts with a washcloth and soap after breastfeeding.
c. Apply heat to the nipple area after feeding.
d. Make sure the infant is tummy to tummy and latching on properly.

8. PR is a 29-year-old female who has been successfully breastfeeding her infant since she gave birth four weeks ago. This week she notices a red mark on her right breast and she has flu-like symptoms. She is diagnosed with mastitis and prescribed an antibiotic. Which of the following is the most appropriate recommendation for breastfeeding women with mastitis?

a. Switch to infant formula until the mastitis is resolved.
b. Discontinue breastfeeding.
c. Continue breastfeeding and nurse frequently.
d. Avoid breastfeeding with the infected breast.

9. The US Public Health Service recommends that women of childbearing age take supplements containing folic acid during which of the following time periods?

a. Before becoming pregnant and during the first trimester
b. During the second trimester of pregnancy
c. During the third trimester of pregnancy
d. Never, if they are consuming a high-folate diet

10. According to the CDC, to reduce the risk of bearing a child with a neural tube defect, what is the minimum amount of folic acid a woman of childbearing age should consume on a daily basis prior to becoming pregnant?

a. 400 μg/day
b. 600 μg/day
c. 800 μg/day
d. 1000 μg/day

11. Which of the following population groups in the United States has the highest prevalence of neural tube defects?

a. Non-Hispanic white women
b. Non-Hispanic black women
c. Asian women
d. Hispanic women

12. BR is a 24-year-old female who has recently found out that she is pregnant. She questions her obstetrician about which exercises are appropriate during pregnancy. Which of the following exercises would not be considered safe during pregnancy?

a. Rebounding on a trampoline
b. Walking
c. Yoga
d. Swimming

13. CJ is a 26-year-old woman who has been breastfeeding for the past 3 months. She questions her pediatrician about whether she is able to provide enough nutrition for her infant. What parameters should be used to determine if breastfeeding is providing adequate nutrition for an infant or child?

a. Monitoring growth and development on the growth charts
b. Measuring the amount of milk being produced by the mother
c. Tracking the frequency that the infant feeds
d. Assessing the number of bowel movements of the infant

14. CJ asks how quickly after delivery she can return to her pre-pregnancy weight while she is breastfeeding. Which of the following would be considered a safe weight loss while breastfeeding?

a. 1–2 pounds/week
b. 1–2 pounds/month
c. 6–8 pounds/month
d. Women should not lose weight during breastfeeding

Chapter 4 Infants, Children, and Adolescents

1. Body mass index (BMI) is an important growth assessment tool in children over the age of two. Which of the following is the correct way to determine height for use in calculating BMI?

a. Using the height stick on the scale
b. Without shoes using a wall-mounted stadiometer
c. By weight-for-length
d. By asking the parent

2. Head circumference measures brain growth in infants and children. Assessing head circumference is recommended for infants and children up to what age?

a. 6 months
b. 12 months
c. 2 years
d. 3 years

3. Dry, scaly dermatitis, alopecia, and easily pluckable, dull hair may be signs of which of the following deficiencies?

a. Protein deficiency
b. Essential fatty acid deficiency
c. Vitamin and mineral deficiency
d. All of the above

4. Pasteurized cow's milk is an important source of calories, protein, and calcium for children, but should not be introduced until a child is how old?

a. 6 months
b. 9 months
c. 12 months
d. 18 months

5. According to the American Academy of Pediatrics (AAP), intake of 100 percent juice should be limited in children. What is the AAP's recommendation for daily juice intake for children aged 12 months to two years of age?

a. Less than 4 ounces/day
b. Less than 6 ounces/day
c. Less than 8 ounces/day
d. Less than 12 ounces/day

6. KS is a 13-year-old boy with hypercholesterolemia and a positive family history of heart disease (his dad had a heart attack at age 50). What is the recommended initial medical nutrition therapy for children with hypercholesterolemia over the age of two years?

a. The Atkins diet
b. Therapeutic Lifestyle Changes (TLC) diet
c. The South Beach diet
d. The DASH diet

7. Children under the age of two should not follow a low-fat diet because normal fat intake is required to maintain the development of which of the following systems?

a. Central nervous system
b. Respiratory system
c. Musculoskeletal system
d. Digestive system

8. JK is a 16-year-old boy who has been diagnosed as obese according to his BMI greater than the 95th percentile. Obesity intervention for children and adolescents has been found to be most effective when:

a. The provider/program, child, and parents have a high degree of contact.
b. The provider/program, child, and parents have a low degree of contact.
c. The program is fairly unstructured.
d. The parents are not involved at all.

9. JK's parents ask if he could try a medication for weight loss. Which weight loss drug is approved for children over the age of 16?

a. There are no weight loss medications approved for children under the age of 18
b. Sibutramine
c. Orlistat
d. Both Sibutramine and Orlistat

10. TP is an 8-year-old girl who comes to see her pediatrician for a well-childcare visit. Her height is 127 cm and her weight is 25 kg. Her BMI is 15.7 kg/m^2. Which of the following weight classifications is correct for this child?

a. Underweight
b. Normal weight
c. Overweight
d. Obese

11. DR is an 18-year-old overweight teenager who is diagnosed with non-alcoholic fatty liver disease (NAFLD) by his family physician. Which of the following is the most appropriate therapy for DR at this time?

a. Immediate drug therapy
b. Immediate drug therapy combined with weight loss
c. Weight loss
d. There is no treatment for this condition

12. According to the CDC and AAP, the maximum amount of time a child should spend engaging in sedentary activities, such as watching TV and playing computer and video games, on a daily basis is:

a. 1 hour/day
b. 1.5 hours/day
c. 2 hours/day
d. 2.5 hours/day

13. CT is a 2-year-old child who presents to the hospital with wasting and apparent emaciation, yet serum albumin and protein values are normal. It is suspected, however, that protein status may be depleted. What is the most likely explanation for these normal serum values?

a. Inaccurate test procedure
b. Decreased blood volume (hemoconcentration)

c. Protein malnutrition
d. Increased blood volume

14. The "hallmark sign" of refeeding syndrome, an imbalance that may lead to cardiac, neuromuscular, hepatic, hematologic, and respiratory dysfunction, and ultimately organ failure, involves which of the following?

a. Potassium, sodium iron, biotin
b. Phosphate, magnesium, calcium, potassium
c. Magnesium, niacin, folate, zinc
d. Calcium, zinc, iron, pyridoxine

15. DF is an 18-year-old female whose parents suspect she has an eating disorder. Her symptoms include esophagitis and electrolyte abnormalities, suggesting which of the following?

a. DF is using laxatives in an effort to keep her weight down
b. DF is vomiting in an effort to keep her weight down
c. DF has amenorrhea
d. DF has been taking mega doses of vitamins.

16. DF's parents request that she be hospitalized immediately for observation and treatment. Which of the following criteria should be used to determine if DF needs to be managed in an in-patient hospital setting rather than on an out-patient basis?

a. DF is medically unstable
b. DF is psychiatrically unstable
c. DF is 25 to 30 percent below her ideal weight
d. All of the above

Chapter 5 Older Adults

1. TP is an 85-year-old female who is brought to her primary physician by her daughter and son-in-law. They explain that TP has not been feeling well and they are concerned. Which of the following pairs of assessment parameters are most consistently correlated with poor nutritional status?

a. Visual and hearing deficits
b. Alcohol use and polypharmacy
c. Poverty and social isolation
d. Involuntary weight loss and lack of appetite

2. DA is a 74-year-old man with type 2 diabetes. He is currently being treated with metformin. Which of the following vitamin deficiencies is associated with long-term metformin therapy due to reduced vitamin absorption?

a. Vitamin A
b. Vitamin D

c. Vitamin B_{12}
d. Vitamin C

3. ML is an 82-year-old female who is living in an assisted living facility. Her family questions about how to reduce her risk of falling and how much vitamin D she should have. Which of the following vitamin D_3 doses should be recommended for fracture prevention in older adults?

a. 200 IU/d
b. 300 IU/d
c. 500 IU/d
d. 800 IU/d

4. RB is a 69-year-old man who lives with his wife. They come together to the physician's office and she expresses concern about her husband's daily drinking. According to the American Geriatrics Society (AGS), risky alcoholic beverage drinking in an older adult man is defined as which of the following?

a. More than 1 drink/day or more than 4 drinks/week
b. More than 2 drinks/day or more than 5 drinks/week
c. More than 3 drinks/day or more than 7 drinks/week
d. There is no limit for alcohol consumption in older adults.

5. Which of the following groups in the United States are at increased risk of malnutrition due to inadequate funds to purchase food?

a. Female
b. Minority
c. Urban dwelling
d. All of the above

6. JN is an 88-year-old man who is living in a nursing home. He has experienced a loss of 10 percent of his body weight over the past six months. This unplanned weight loss in older adults is most likely related to which of the following?

a. Normal age-related changes
b. Underlying disease processes
c. Increased metabolic rate
d. Changes in fat-to-lean ratio

7. Malnutrition in the elderly is associated with which of the following factors?

a. Poor appetite
b. Problems with chewing and swallowing
c. Medical illness
d. All of the above

8. CJ is an 81-year-old female who lives in an assisted living facility. Her daughters visit frequently and determine that she is having a bowel movement only once or twice a week. Which of the following should be prescribed for CJ to address her constipation?

a. Increasing consumption of garlic
b. Decreasing consumption of fried foods
c. Increasing consumption of whole grains
d. Decreasing consumption of dairy foods

9. The older adult population is rapidly increasing in the United States. Minorities, which include Hispanics, African-Americans, Asian/Pacific Islanders, and Native Americans, are expected to represent approximately what percentage of the elderly population by 2030?

a. 10%
b. 15%
c. 25%
d. 35%

10. Dehydration in older adults has been linked to impaired cognition, kidney stones, and constipation. Older adults are less likely to experience signs and symptoms of dehydration because of which of the following physiological changes associated with aging?

a. Increased total body water
b. Reduce tolerance to fluid
c. Increased taste sensation
d. Decline in thirst perception

11. Oral health problems are very common in the older adults and 26 percent are endentulous. The incidence of periodontal disease is higher in older adults who have which of the following chronic conditions? (Select two answers.)

a. Arthritis
b. Cardiovascular disease
c. Diabetes
d. Cancer

12. RF is an 83-year-old female who is living in an assisted living facility. Her recent blood tests results show a low vitamin B_{12} level even though her dietary intake of vitamin B_{12} is adequate. Which of the following mechanisms most likely explains the cause of RF's low vitamin B_{12} levels?

a. Decreased ability to absorb protein-bound vitamin B_{12}
b. Increased conversion to the inactive form of vitamin B_{12}
c. Increased HCL which interferes with vitamin B_{12} absorption
d. Decreased vitamin C intake which is required for vitamin B_{12} absorption

13. HJ is a 91-year-old man living in a nursing home. His family comes to visit this week and notices that his clothes are fitting more loosely and he seems to have lost some weight. They ask the nursing staff to weigh him. He weighs 150 pounds (68 kg) and has experienced a ten-pound weight loss since their last visit one month ago. What is HJ's estimated total daily protein requirements for repletion, using his current weight?

a. 50 grams/day
b. 77 grams/day
c. 102 grams/day
d. 150 grams/day

Chapter 6 Cardiovascular Disease

1. According to the NCEP Therapeutic Lifestyle Changes (TLC) diet, what is the recommended range for total dietary fat as a percentage of the total calorie intake?

a. Less than 20% of total calories
b. 20–30% of total calories
c. 25–35% of total calories
d. 30–40% of total calories

2. Which of the following metabolic diseases can cause a secondary hyperlipidemia?

a. Diabetes mellitus
b. Obesity
c. Hypothyroidism
d. All of the above

3. Recent evidence suggests that *trans* fatty acids raise LDL-C levels when compared to unsaturated fatty acids. Which statement is true concerning *trans* fatty acids?

a. *Trans* fats are found in partially hydrogenated margarines and shortenings
b. *Trans* fats add shelf life and flavor to foods
c. *Trans* fats may reduce HDL-C levels
d. All of the above

4. TK is a 49-year-old man with hyperlipidemia. He frequently eats in fast food restaurants. Which of the following dietary factors is most likely contributing to TK's elevated LDL-C level?

a. Unsaturated fat
b. Saturated fat
c. Protein
d. Simple sugar

5. JF is a 35-year-old man with hypercholesterolemia. He requests information about vitamins that can help reduce his cholesterol. Which of the following vitamins are used to treat hypercholesterolemia when used in pharmacological doses?

a. Vitamin C
b. Folate
c. Vitamin B$_6$
d. Niacin

6. Which of the following foods contains the highest amount of omega-3 polyunsaturated fat per serving?

a. Salmon
b. Soybeans
c. Yogurt
d. Olive oil

7. BR is a 50-year-old female with hypertriglyceridemia. She requests information about the benefits of taking omega-3 fatty acids to reduce her risk of cardiovascular disease. In addition to lowering triglyceride levels, what additional cardiovascular benefits are seen with omega-3 fatty acids?

a. Decreased platelet aggregation
b. Decreased clotting time
c. Increased foam cell production
d. Increased free radical formation

8. JB is a 35-year-old female who has an LDL-C of 145 mg/dL and HDL-C of 30 mg/dL. She does not smoke but has a family history of heart disease. What is her target LDL-C level according to the National Cholesterol Education Program (NCEP) ATP III guidelines?

a. <100 mg/dL
b. <130 mg/dL
c. <160 mg/dL
d. <190 mg/dL

9. PR is a 25-year-old man who presents with a BMI of 30 and a recent diagnosis of hypertension. He has a family history of hypertension. He is 5′7″ and 210 lbs. What is the most likely etiology of this patient's hypertension?

a. Genetics
b. Gender
c. Obesity
d. Age

10. Alcohol consumption has been shown to have both positive and negative effects on the heart. Which of the following statements is correct regarding excessive alcohol consumption (>2 drinks/day for men; >1 drink/day for women)?

a. Excess alcohol increases blood pressure
b. Excess alcohol is cardioprotective
c. Excess alcohol reduces the risk of cardiomyopathy
d. Excess alcohol reduces triglyceride levels

11. AM is a 54-year-old female who is pre-hypertensive (blood pressure: 135/85 mmHg). She requests advice about how to lower her blood pressure without medication. Which of the following medical nutrition therapies would likely reduce her hypertension?

a. Reduce saturated fat intake
b. Increase low-fat-dairy foods
c. Increase fruits and vegetables intake
d. All of the above

12. SL is a 74-year-old man who has been discharged from the hospital after being diagnosed with heart failure. What is the most appropriate medical nutrition therapy for a patient with heart failure?

a. Limit sodium intake to 2000 mg/day
b. Limit total fat intake to less than 30% of total calories
c. Limit potassium intake to less than 2000 mg/day
d. Limit cholesterol intake to less than 200 mg/day

13. Soluble fiber has been shown to reduce serum LDL-C levels when consumed on a regular basis. Which of the following best explains the mechanism of how soluble fiber reduces LDL-C?

a. Increasing bile salt production
b. Binding with bile salts
c. Increasing fat excretion
d. Binding with iron

14. SR is a 59-year-old female who has recently been diagnosed with hyperlipidemia. Which of the following physical examination findings should be checked? (Select two answers.)

a. An eye examination for corneal arcus senilis
b. A mouth examination for glossitis or cheilosis
c. A skin examination for xanthelasmas or xanthomas
d. An extremity examination for edema in the limbs

15. Heart failure affects approximately 5 million adults in the United States. Which of the following medical nutrition therapies should be prescribed for patients with heart failure?

a. Control sodium and fluid retention
b. Provide adequate energy, vitamins, and minerals
c. Replete protein stores
d. All of the above

16. Which of the following risk factors for metabolic syndrome has different criteria among various ethnic groups?

a. Hypertension
b. Fasting plasma glucose levels
c. Waist circumference
d. HDL-C levels

17. Which of the following ethnic groups are at highest risk for hypertension?

a. African-Americans
b. Caucasians
c. Asian-Americans
d. Hispanics

Chapter 7 Gastrointestinal Disease

1. CB is a 24-year-old woman with unintentional weight loss of 30 pounds (13.6 kg) over the past four months despite a normal intake. CB also complains of foul-smelling stools and after several days of work-up, she is diagnosed with Crohn's disease. Which of the following is the most likely cause of her weight loss?

a. Bowel obstruction
b. Perforated colon
c. Vitamin deficiency
d. Malabsorption

2. TR is a 48-year-old man recently diagnosed with peptic ulcer disease. Medical nutrition therapy for patients with peptic ulcer disease includes which of the following?

a. Reducing alcohol
b. Reducing tobacco
c. Reducing caffeine
d. All of the above

3. Individuals who are lactose intolerant and choose to avoid products containing lactose may not meet daily calcium requirements. Which of the following is the best non-dairy source of calcium to recommend to patients who are lactose intolerant?

a. Soy milk (enriched)
b. Spinach
c. Fortified whole-wheat bread
d. Ice cream

4. SH is a 60-year-old man with chronic liver disease and ascites. He has lost a significant amount of weight and is at risk of malnutrition. Which of the following is most likely contributing to his poor dietary intake?

a. Hyperkalemia
b. Hypoglycemia
c. Dehydration
d. Early satiety

5. PV is a 35-year-old obese woman, recently diagnosed with gastroesophogeal reflux disease (GERD). She states that her symptoms mostly occur in the middle of the night. Which of the following recommendations may be most helpful in alleviating her symptoms?

a. Avoid eating at least two hours before bedtime.
b. Sleep with at least two pillows at night.
c. Drink warm milk before bed.
d. Take an over-the-counter sleeping pill.

6. According to the CDC, what level of weight loss helps to define an AIDS diagnosis?

a. Greater than 20% with diarrhea or fever for more than 30 days
b. Greater than 10% with diarrhea or fever for more than 30 days
c. Greater than 10% with diarrhea or fever for more than 60 days
d. Greater than 25% with diarrhea or fever for more than 60 days

7. MG is a 29-year-old man who is HIV positive. He complains of poor appetite, decreased food intake, and frequent diarrhea. However, after testing it is noted that his extracellular fluids are elevated. What does this indicate?

a. Non-compliance with HIV medication
b. Abnormal lipid levels
c. Malabsorption
d. The presence of an underlying infection

8. Which nutritional measure is frequently abnormal in the presence of advanced HIV?

a. Low albumin
b. Low cholesterol
c. Anemia
d. All of the above

9. HN is a 68-year-old man with severe liver disease. Recent labs show an elevated prothrombin time (PT). Why are PT levels elevated in patients with advanced/end stage liver disease?

a. Vitamin B_{12} deficiency
b. Fat malabsoprtion
c. Reduced production of clotting factors
d. Weight loss

10. AL is a 45-year-old male who presents to the emergency department after falling. AL admits to drinking at least five alcoholic drinks daily and having failed several rehab attempts. Lab data indicates an elevated mean corpuscular volume (MCV), a characteristic finding in megaloblastic anemia. Which of the following is the most likely cause of this type of anemia in alcoholic patients?

a. Vitamin B_{12} deficiency
b. Iron deficiency
c. Thiamin deficiency
d. Calcium deficiency

11. LK is a 30-year-old female with severe Crohn's disease. She recently required an intestinal resection of her ileum. Which of the following is the most likely cause of fat malabsorption in patients with Crohn's disease?

a. Decreased hepatic synthesis of bile salts
b. Poor liver function
c. Inability to reabsorb bile salts
d. Decreased fat intake

12. Which of the following nutritional recommendations are correct for a patient experiencing fat malabsorption secondary to GI surgery?

a. Eat small frequent meals
b. Increase consumption of soluble fiber
c. Maintain a lactose-free diet
d. All of the above

Chapter 8 Endocrine Disease

1. What statements summarize the expected outcomes from medical nutrition therapy for diabetes? (Select two answers.)

a. It will take about six months to observe the outcomes from nutrition therapy interventions.
b. The expected outcome from nutrition therapy interventions is a 1 to 2 percent decrease in A1C.
c. Outcomes from nutrition therapy should be evaluated between 6 weeks and 3 months after initiation.
d. Nutrition therapy interventions have an immediate effect on blood pressure.

2. Which of the following statements summarizes a first priority of nutrition therapy for patients with type 2 diabetes?

a. Weight loss is essential if type 2 diabetes is to be treated effectively.
b. Nutrition strategies are implemented to correct the dyslipidemia associated with diabetes.
c. Nutrition therapy focuses on nutrition interventions that will improve glycemia, lipid profiles, and blood pressure.
d. Sugars and white foods should be eliminated from the diet.

3. Which of the following statements is correct regarding carbohydrate intake in patents with type 2 diabetes?

a. The total amount of carbohydrate ingested is more important than the source or the type.
b. Any increase in dietary fiber will improve glycemia.
c. Implementing a low glycemic index diet will improve glucose and lipid levels.
d. Bolus insulin doses are based on the total amount of carbohydrate and protein in the planned meal.

4. Nutrition recommendations from the American Diabetes Association, AHA, and the Surgeon General agree on which of the following guidelines for healthy eating?

a. Carbohydrate in the diet should be restricted.
b. A high-protein diet is best for weight reduction.
c. Saturated and *trans* fats in the diet should be restricted.
d. Only monounsaturated fats should be used to replace saturated fats.

5. Two major studies showed a 58 percent reduction in the onset of diabetes in a population of people with pre-diabetes. What percentage weight loss was necessary to achieve this risk reduction?

a. 7%
b. 15%
c. 25%
d. 58%

6. Which of the following is a correct statement about carbohydrate counting?

a. Bolus insulin doses are based on the total amount of carbohydrate and protein in the planned meal.
b. One carbohydrate serving is based on a portion of food that contains 15 grams of carbohydrate.
c. Compared to carbohydrate, protein and fat have half the expected glucose response.
d. Basal insulin doses are adjusted to cover the carbohydrate content of meals.

7. Which of the following are appropriate guidelines for treating hypoglycemia in a patient taking insulin? (Select two answers.)

a. Treat with 15 grams of carbohydrate, wait 15 minutes; if blood glucose has not increased, treat again.
b. Retest in approximately an hour after the initial treatment to see if additional carbohydrate is needed.
c. Treat with 20 grams of a fast-acting carbohydrate.
d. Treat with a food or beverage source of carbohydrate and protein.

8. Which of the following are correct statements about alcohol? (Select two answers.)

a. Moderate amounts of alcohol always raises triglyceride levels.
b. Moderate amounts of alcohol always raises blood glucose levels.
c. Moderate amounts of alcohol with food does not affect glucose or insulin levels.
d. Moderate amounts of alcohol without food for people using insulin secretagogues can lower blood glucose levels.

9. The United Kingdom Prospective Diabetes Study has demonstrated that diabetes mellitus is a progressive disease. How has medical nutrition therapy for diabetes mellitus changed over recent years based on this concept?

a. Medical nutrition therapy is aimed at an "ideal" nutrition prescription for all patients with diabetes mellitus.
b. Medical nutrition therapy is aimed at the achievement of blood glucose and lipid goals.

c. Medical nutrition therapy is aimed at reducing the source of carbohydrate in the diet, namely, simple sugars, rather than the total daily intake.

d. All of the above.

10. What is the target range for the pre-meal plasma glucose values for non-pregnant adults with diabetes mellitus?

a. 90–130 mg/dL
b. 100–140 mg/dL
c. 150–180 mg/dL
d. 180–200 mg/dL

11. What is considered an optimal HgbA1C for patients with diabetes mellitus?

a. Less than 7%
b. Less than 8%
c. Less than 9%
d. None of the above

12. Most normal weight adult patients with type 1 diabetes require 1 unit of insulin for what range of carbohydrate intake?

a. 1–10 grams CHO
b. 5–10 grams CHO
c. 8–16 grams CHO
d. 10–20 grams CHO

13. Which of the following conditions increases a patient's likelihood of developing insulin resistance?

a. Personal history of impaired glucose tolerance
b. A first-degree relative with type 2 diabetes
c. Obesity, especially abdominal or central obesity
d. All of the above

14. According to the American Diabetes Association, fiber intake for patients with type 1 and type 2 diabetes is recommended at which of the following levels?

a. 15 g/day for women and 20 g/day for men
b. 20 g/day for women and 25 g/day for men
c. 25 g/day for women and 38 g/day for men
d. 30 g/day for women and 44 g/day for men

15. Instant oatmeal contains 30 grams of carbohydrates (CHO), which would be the equivalent of how many carbohydrate servings?

a. 1 serving CHO
b. 2 servings CHO
c. 3 servings CHO
d. 4 servings CHO

Chapter 9 Pulmonary Disease

1. Respiratory quotient (RQ) is the ratio of CO_2 produced to oxygen consumed. Excess CO_2 production and increased RQ can lead to which of the following adverse effects?

a. Heart failure
b. Difficulty weaning from the ventilator
c. Increased appetite
d. Hyponaturemia

2. CK is a 71-year-old man with COPD who has been seeing a pulmonologist for several years. He recently experienced a 10-pound weight loss since his last visit a few months ago. Which of the following would most likely contribute to weight loss in patients with COPD?

a. Increased energy expenditure due to work of breathing
b. Decreased lung capacity
c. Increased FEV_1
d. Impaired cellular resistance

3. Which of the following is a potential side effect of medications used to treat COPD that may limit dietary intake?

a. Diarrhea
b. Gastric irritation
c. Dry mouth and dysgeusia
d. All of the above

4. KL is a 35-year-old man with obstructive sleep apnea syndrome (OSAS). Medical nutrition therapy for patients with OSAS should focus on which of the following?

a. Weight reduction
b. Vitamin and mineral deficiencies
c. Protein repletion
d. Fluid retention

5. LP is a 59-year-old female who successfully undergoes a lung transplant. She is prescribed long-term prednisone treatment. Which of the following is a common complication of prednisone therapy that may require nutritional intervention?

a. Hypokalemia
b. Hyperglycemia
c. Hypoglycemia
d. Hyponatremia

6. GR is a 10-year-old girl with cystic fibrosis who is brought to her pediatrician complaining of weakness and lethargy. She presents with a recent weight loss of eight pounds. In addition to adjusting her oral enzyme supplements, which of the following dietary recommendations would be appropriate to improve TL's nutritional status?

a. Extra salt
b. Addition of vitamins and mineral supplements
c. High calorie intake
d. All of the above

7. DR is a 71-year-old female who has had COPD for 10 years. She has recently lost weight most likely due to her decreased intake and increased energy expenditure due to the work of breathing. How much of an increase in energy expenditure has been reported in patients with COPD?

a. Up to a two-fold increase
b. Up to a five-fold increase
c. Up to a ten-fold increase
d. Up to a twenty-fold increase

8. DR is hospitalized for pneumonia and requires mechanical ventilation for more than 14 days. Assuming her GI tract is functioning normally, how should she receive nutritional support to sustain her caloric requirements?

a. Enteral nutrition support via nasogastric tube
b. Parenteral nutrition via central line
c. Peripheral parenteral nutrition support
d. It is not necessary to feed patients who are on a ventilator.

9. NB is a 12-year-old girl who has been diagnosed with cystic fibrosis for the past 3 years. She has had multiple infections and is taking antibiotics. Which of the following vitamin deficiencies may result in patients taking long-term antibiotics?

a. Vitamin B_{12}
b. Vitamin K
c. Vitamin A
d. Thiamin

10. Osteopenia is common in patients with cystic fibrosis. In addition to malabsorption, which of the following factors contribute to the osteopenia seen in patients with cystic fibrosis?

a. Malabsorption
b. Vitamin D deficiency
c. Delayed puberty
d. All of the above

11. FR is a 39-year-old obese male who was recently diagnosed with obstructive sleep apnea syndrome and pre-diabetes. Which of the following is considered first-line treatment for patients with OSAS?

a. Prescription sleep medication
b. Continuous positive airway pressure (CPAP) machine
c. Sleep study on a weekly basis
d. Taking a day-time nap

12. BB, a 9-year-old girl with cystic fibrosis, is brought to her pediatrician reporting weakness and lethargy. Her mother reports increased, foul-smelling stool output, and a recent loss of 7 pounds. What is the most likely cause of the patient's weight loss?

a. Heart failure
b. Malabsorption
c. Liver disease
d. Anemia

13. Which of the following increases resting energy requirements and promotes loss of weight and lean body mass in patients with COPD?

a. Increase in cytokines
b. Decrease in levels of cell derived protein
c. Frequent, recurrent respiratory infections
d. All of the above

14. AB is a 71-year-old man with COPD. Lab data reveal an elevated hemoglobin and hematocrit. What is the most likely etiology of these laboratory abnormalities?

a. Chronic hypoxia
b. Low mean corpuscular volume
c. Arterial hypoxemia
d. Dietary changes

15. MG is a 60-year-old man with COPD and congestive heart failure. His medications include furosemide and prednisone. Which of the following metabolic complications is he at risk for developing on these medications? (Select two answers.)

a. Hypertriglyceridemia
b. Hyperglycemia
c. Hyponatremia
d. Hypokalemia

Chapter 10 Renal Disease

1. BC is a 24-year-old female with acute renal failure who is admitted to the hospital. A nutrition support service consultation is requested to determine the patient's calorie requirements. Which of the following calorie requirements should be used for individuals with acute renal failure?

a. 10–20 kcal/kg per day
b. 20–35 kcal/kg per day
c. 30–50 kcal/kg per day
d. 50–60 kcal/kg per day

2. OK is a 65-year-old man with Stage 4 chronic kidney disease. He is scheduled to go on dialysis in a few months. Medical nutrition therapy for patients prior to initiating dialysis restricts protein for which of the following reasons?

a. To slow the progression of renal disease
b. To compensate for an increase in excretion of nitrogenous waste products
c. To better control hypertension
d. All of the above

3. AE is a 45-year-old male who recently passed a kidney stone. Which of the following foods contain the highest amount of oxalate and should be limited in patients with calcium oxalate kidney stones?

a. Apples
b. Yogurt
c. Tomatoes
d. Dark green leafy vegetables

4. WG is a 45-year-old female who has recently undergone renal transplantation due to kidney failure. Side effects related to some immunosuppressive agents that would require dietary recommendations include which of the following?

a. Hyperlipidemia
b. Hypermagnesemia
c. Hypoglycemia
d. Hypokalemia

5. Restricting dietary phosphate intake for individuals with chronic kidney disease to maintain proper calcium/phosphorus balance may decrease severity of which of the following medical problems?

a. Primary hyperparathyroidism
b. Vascular and soft tissue calcifications
c. Rheumatoid arthritis
d. All of the above

6. Patients in early stages of chronic kidney disease who are taking which of the following therapies to control blood pressure may be at risk for developing hyperkalemia?

a. Dietary salt substitutes
b. Angiotensin converting enzyme inhibitors
c. Potassium sparing diuretics
d. All of the above

7. GN is a 46-year-old female receiving hemodialysis (HD). She is 5′3″ (160 cm) and weighs 110 lbs (50 kg). Her lab data are BUN: 65 mg/dL; albumin: 3.7 g/dL; creatinine: 9.2 mg/dL. Considering GN is receiving HD three times per week, how much protein should GN be consuming daily?

a. <50 grams protein/day
b. 60–65 grams protein/day
c. 75–90 grams protein/day
d. >90 grams protein/day

8. The kidney plays an essential role in the metabolism of which of the following metabolic conversions?

a. Beta carotene to vitamin A
b. Oxalic acid to ascorbic acid
c. Ferrous sulfate to ferric sulfate
d. $25(OH)D_3$ to $125(OH_2)D_3$

9. DT is a 56-year-old man with nephrotic syndrome. In addition to reducing dietary fat intake, protein intake should also be limited to 0.8–1.0 g/kg per day. Which of the following mechanisms explains why moderate protein intake is advised for patients with nephrotic syndrome?

a. To reduce the amino acid load in the glomerulus
b. To increase albumin excretion
c. To reduce nitrogen balance
d. To increase hepatic protein synthesis

10. TD is a 56-year-old man with chronic kidney disease and normocytic, normochromic anemia. Which of the following mechanisms most likely explains the associated anemia in a patient with chronic kidney disease?

a. Blood loss due to dialysis procedure
b. Vitamin B_{12} deficiency
c. Decreased erythropoietin production
d. Folate deficiency

11. When assessing the nutritional status of a patient with chronic kidney disease it is important to use the patient's dry weight for all calculations. Which of the following is the best definition of "dry weight"?

a. The weight when the patient is dehydrated
b. The weight when the patient has not drunk any fluids in 12 hours
c. The weight when the patient has taken diuretics for several days
d. The weight of the patient minus the estimated amount of fluid retention

12. NW is a 46-year-old male with stage 4 chronic kidney disease. He weighs 200 lbs (90.7 kg), an ideal body weight for him, and is not retaining fluid. A 24-hour urine collection indicated a protein loss of 2.1 grams of protein lost due to proteinuria. What are his daily protein requirements?

a. 50.3 g/day
b. 56.5 g/day
c. 72 g/day
d. 121 g/day

13. AP is a 64-year-old male with type 2 diabetes who visits his internist for his yearly physical. His serum creatine and BUN levels are significantly elevated and the physician suspects renal disease. Which of the following are likely to be tested when he returns his 24-hour urine collection?

a. The presence of red blood cells
b. Protein excretion
c. Creatinine excretion
d. All of the above

Chapter 11 Cancer Prevention and Treatment

1. According to research on the link between obesity and cancer risk, which of the following women have the highest risk of developing breast cancer?

a. Pre-menopausal woman with a BMI of 30 kg/m^2
b. Pre-menopausal woman with a BMI of 22 kg/m^2
c. Post-menopausal woman with a BMI of 30 kg/m^2
d. Post-menopausal woman with a BMI of 40 kg/m^2

2. According to the National Cancer Institute, what is the strongest and most consistent predictor of breast cancer risk?

a. Amount of physical activity
b. Weight gain during adulthood
c. High intake of saturated fat
d. Irregular menstruation

3. Weight gain in which area of the body poses the highest risk for colon cancer?

a. Hips
b. Buttocks
c. Abdomen
d. Thighs

4. According to the American Institute for Cancer Research, dietary recommendations to reduce the risk of colorectal cancer include which of the following statements about red meat intake?

a. A maximum of 15 ounces of cooked red meat per week with limited processed meat consumption.
b. A maximum of 18 ounces of cooked red meat per week with no processed meat consumption.
c. Avoidance of all processed meats.
d. Avoid both cooked red meat and processed meats as much as possible.

5. Flavonoids are a class of phytochemicals that act as an antioxidant and absorb free radicals, thus potentially protecting against certain types of cancer. Flavonoids are found in high concentrations in which of the following foods?

a. Grapes and wine
b. Berries
c. Green tea
d. All of the above

6. CR is a 51-year-old female who questions her gynecologist about the pros and cons of eating more foods with soy. Consumption of foods made with soy *may* be protective against which type of cancer?

a. Breast
b. Colon
c. Stomach
d. All of the above

7. Selenium is an antioxidant that has shown promising anti-cancer properties, yet most people do not meet their requirements established by the RDA (55 µg/day). Which of the following foods is a good source of selenium?

a. Yogurt
b. Brazil Nuts
c. Blueberries
d. All of the above

8. TF is an 84-year-old man who was admitted to the hospital with dehydration and pneumonia. At what point should cancer cachexia be suspected?

a. Immediately upon diagnosis.
b. If he had experienced an unintentional weight loss greater than 5% of his weight over the previous month.
c. If he had experienced an unintentional weight loss greater than 10% of his weight over the previous year.
d. Only if nausea and fatigue are present.

9. EC is an 86-year-old man who is receiving daily radiation treatment for colon cancer. Which of the following side effects of radiation treatment is mostly likely to affect a patient's nutritional status?

a. Alopecia
b. Radiation pneumonitis
c. Nausea and vomiting
d. Oral mucositis

10. NT is a 59-year-old female who is receiving weekly chemotherapy following surgery for breast cancer. Which of the following nutrition recommendations can help control her complaints of nausea after treatment? (Select two answers.)

a. Consuming clear or ice-cold drinks
b. Eating smaller, more frequent meals
c. Eating larger meals in the middle of the day
d. Adequate fiber intake

11. Excessive alcohol consumption has been linked as the primary cause of liver cancer. Alcohol users also experience which of the following types of cancers six times more often than non-alcohol users?

a. Brain cancer
b. Colon cancer
c. Pancreatic cancer
d. Oral cancer

12. RT is a 45-year-old man with a family history of cancer. He recently quit smoking and is eating more healthy foods. He asks his physician what additional preventive steps he can take to reduce his risk of cancer. Which of the following lifestyle changes should be recommended to RT to help reduce his risk of developing cancer?

a. Eat only organic foods
b. Begin a regular physical activity program for 30 minutes every day
c. Eliminate all dairy foods
d. Take 1000 mg of vitamin C daily

Chapter 12 Enteral Nutrition Support

1. In which of the following conditions is the provision of tube feeding a useful therapy?

a. Two days after coronary bypass surgery in a well-nourished patient
b. Following surgery for ischemic bowel with 50 cm of remaining small bowel
c. Seven days after a stroke in a patient with aspiration when swallowing
d. Crohn's disease with a small bowel obstruction

2. When is a surgically placed feeding tube, such as a jejunostomy, indicated in a patient requiring long-term tube feeding?

a. Never
b. When tube feeding is expected for greater than 20 days
c. When a nasogastric feeding tube is displaced
d. When other abdominal surgery is scheduled

3. When a patient is ambulatory and eating small amounts of food, what is the best method for administering supplemental tube feeding?

a. Nocturnal cycle
b. Twenty-four hour continuous
c. Gravity feeding every 4 hours
d. One bolus feeding daily

4. What test is indicated when a patient receiving tube feeding and antibiotics develops diarrhea?

a. Bacteria culture of formula
b. Small bowel biopsy for celiac disease
c. Stool for *Clostridia difficile* toxin
d. Stool culture for ova and parasites

5. What is a proposed benefit of pre-biotics in enteral formulas?

a. Assists in treating sepsis
b. Improves wound healing
c. Improves nutrient absorption
d. Normalizes intestinal flora

6. Which of the following antioxidants are added to some enteral formulas?

a. Vitamin C and vitamin E
b. Vitamin B_{12} and vitamin D
c. Copper and manganese
d. Calcium and magnesium

7. What is the preferred feeding tube placement in an ICU patient with a large hiatal hernia and documented gastroesophageal reflux?

a. Nasogastric
b. Nasoenteric
c. Percutaneous endoscopic gastrostomy
d. Surgical gastrostomy with fundoplication

8. Lack of enteral stimulation may contribute to

a. Gut atrophy and higher infection risk
b. Hypoglycemia and higher infection risk
c. Suppressed thyroid function and muscle wasting
d. Vitamin K deficiency and bleeding

9. What formula density is appropriate for a patient with normal fluid requirements?

a. 0.5–0.8 kcal/mL
b. 0.8–1.0 kcal/mL
c. 1.0–1.2 kcal/mL
d. 1.5–2.0 kcal/mL

10. Formulas supplemented with glutamine are designed to accomplish which of the following?

a. Assist in controlling blood sugar
b. Decrease inflammation
c. Normalization of BUN and creatinine
d. Boost immune function

11. Which of the following is recommended for home infusion of an enteral formula via a jejunostomy?

a. Cycled over 12 hours at night
b. Continuous over 24 hours
c. Bolus feedings over 20 minutes, 6 times/day
d. Intermittent feedings over 30 minutes, 6 times/day

12. Which of the following does *not* increase fluid requirements in patients receiving tube feeding?

a. Fiber-enriched formulas
b. Fistula output
c. Nausea
d. Diarrhea

13. TB is a 59-year-old man who is undergoing radiation therapy for thoracic tumor. He has odynophasia and needs a nutrition consultation for a special diet. Medical nutrition therapy for a patient with odynophasia includes which of the following recommendations?

a. Low-fat foods
b. Raw fruits and vegetables
c. Spicy foods
d. Soft, blended foods

Chapter 13 Parenteral Nutrition Support

1. Parenteral nutrition is utilized in patients in which of the following situations? (Select two answers.)

a. Diminished motor capacity makes eating difficult
b. GI tract is not functional, accessible, or safe to use
c. When the patient has dementia
d. Enteral nutrition is not possible

2. Central parenteral nutrition is indicated in which of the following situations?

a. Long-term parenteral nutrition support (longer than 7 days) is anticipated
b. There is poor peripheral access
c. The patient has a moderately-to-severely elevated metabolic rate
d. All of the above

3. When using peripheral parenteral nutrition solutions, what is the maximum allowable concentration to prevent vascular damage?

a. 700 mOsm per liter
b. 900 mOsm per liter
c. 1000 mOsm per liter
d. This is not a concern with parenteral nutrition

4. According to the American Society for Parenteral and Enteral Nutrition, which of the following ranges is most commonly recommended when determining energy needs for parenteral nutrition?

a. 10 to 15 kcal/kg daily for adults
b. 20 to 35 kcal/kg daily for adults
c. 30 to 45 kcal/kg daily for adults
d. 45 to 60 kcal/kg daily for adults

5. Which of the following ranges is recommended for protein needs for parenteral nutrition in severely stressed patients?

a. 0.8–1.0 g/kg per day
b. 1.0–1.5 g/kg per day

c. 1.5–2.0 g/kg per day
d. >2.0 g/kg per day

6. In order to counter the potential side effects of linoleic acid on prostaglandin metabolism in patients receiving parenteral nutrition, the infusion of soybean or safflower oil lipid emulsions should be limited to which of the following amounts?

a. <1 g of lipid per kg per 24 hours
b. <1 g of lipid per kg per 12 hours
c. <2 g of lipid per kg per 24 hours
d. <2 g of lipid per kg per 12 hours

7. Patients receiving parenteral nutrition may experience complications that include a sudden change in their body temperature, new onset shaking chills, leukocytosis, or unexplained hyperglycemia. Which of the following is most likely to cause these complications?

a. Intra-abdominal infection
b. Urinary tract infection
c. Catheter-related blood stream infection
d. Pneumonia

8. Potential complications of parenteral nutrition that should be monitored include which of the following?

a. Hyperlipidemia
b. Electrolyte imbalances
c. Dehydration and fluid overload
d. All of the above

9. Which of the following is the most common cause of large intestinal obstruction in an adult patient?

a. Colon cancer
b. Diverticulitis
c. Volvulus
d. Hernia

10. Which of the following is the most common cause of large intestinal obstruction in an elderly patient?

a. Colon cancer
b. Diverticulitis
c. Volvulus
d. Hernia

11. Which of the following explains why low serum calcium levels need to be adjusted in patients who also exhibit hypoalbuminemia?

a. Calcium absorption decreases
b. Calcium is chelated to phosphorous
c. Calcium interferes with protein absorption
d. Calcium is bound to serum albumin

12. When a patient transitions from parenteral nutrition to oral feeding, at what point should the parenteral nutrition be discontinued?

a. As soon as the patient is able to tolerate any oral feeding
b. When the patient tolerates 50 percent of daily nutrition requirements through the oral diet
c. When the patient tolerates 75 percent of daily nutrition requirements through the oral diet
d. When the patient tolerates 100 percent of daily nutrition requirements through the oral diet

Review Answers

Chapter 1 Overview of Nutrition in Clinical Care

1. a
2. a
3. b
4. d
5. b
6. c
7. a
8. d
9. c
10. c
11. a
12. c
13. d
14. b

Chapter 2 Vitamins, Minerals, and Dietary Supplements

1. c
2. a
3. c
4. c
5. b
6. b
7. c
8. b
9. d
10. a
11. b
12. d
13. a

Chapter 3 Pregnancy and Lactation

1. d
2. a
3. c
4. d
5. b
6. a
7. d
8. c
9. a
10. a
11. d
12. a
13. a
14. b

Chapter 4 Infants, Children, and Adolescents

1. b
2. c
3. d
4. c
5. a
6. b
7. a
8. a
9. b
10. b
11. c
12. c
13. b
14. b
15. b
16. d

Chapter 5 Older Adults

1. d
2. c
3. d
4. c
5. d
6. b
7. d
8. c
9. c
10. d
11. b,c
12. a
13. c

Chapter 6 Cardiovascular Disease

1. c
2. d
3. d
4. b
5. d
6. a
7. a
8. b
9. c
10. a
11. d
12. a
13. b
14. a,c
15. d
16. c
17. a

Chapter 7 Gastrointestinal Disease

1. d
2. d
3. a
4. d
5. a
6. b
7. d
8. d
9. c
10. a
11. c
12. d

Chapter 8 Endocrine Disease

1. b,c
2. c
3. a
4. c
5. a
6. b
7. a,b
8. c,d
9. b
10. a
11. a
12. c
13. d
14. c
15. b

Chapter 9 Pulmonary Disease

1. b
2. a
3. d
4. a
5. b
6. d
7. c
8. a
9. b
10. d
11. b
12. b
13. d
14. a
15. b,d

Chapter 10 Renal Disease

1. b
2. a
3. d
4. a
5. b
6. d
7. b
8. d
9. a
10. c
11. d
12. b
13. d

Chapter 11 Cancer Prevention and Treatment

1. d
2. b
3. c
4. b
5. d
6. a
7. b
8. b
9. c
10. a,b
11. d
12. b

Chapter 12 Enteral Nutrition Support

1. c
2. d
3. a
4. c
5. d
6. a
7. b
8. a
9. c
10. d
11. a
12. c
13. d

Chapter 13 Parenteral Nutrition Support

1. b,d
2. d
3. b
4. b
5. c
6. a
7. c
8. d
9. d
10. a
11. d
12. c

Index